KU-091-840

Paediatric Emergencies

Paediatric Emergencies

Second Edition

Edited by **J. A. Black,** MD, FRCP
Late Consultant Paediatrician, The Children's Hospital, Sheffield
and Jessop Hospital for Women, Sheffield, UK

Butterworths

London Boston Durban Singapore Sydney Toronto Wellington

First published 1979
Second edition 1987

British Library Cataloguing in Publication Data

Paediatric Emergencies – 2nd ed.
1. Pediatric emergencies
I. Black, John, *1918–*
618.92′0025 RJ370

ISBN 0-407-00280-4

Library of Congress Cataloging-in-Publication Data

Paediatric Emergencies

Includes bibliographies and index.
1. Pediatric emergencies I. Black, J. A.
(John Angus) [DNLM: 1. Emergencies—in infancy & childhood.
WS 200 P124]
RJ370.P33 1986 618.92′0025 86-13625
ISBN 0-407-00280-4

Photoset by Butterworths Litho Preparation Department
Printed and bound in England by Anchor-Brendon Ltd., Tiptree, Essex

Contents

Part III: Emergencies Involving the Face and Neck

Part IV: Intensive Treatment and Emergency Anaesthesia

Part V: Respiratory Tract Emergencies

Part VI: Cardiac Emergencies

Part VII: Neurological Emergencies

Contributors

David J. Atherton, MA, MB, FRCP
Consultant Dermatologist, The Hospital for Sick Children, Great Ormond Street, London

N. D. Barnes, MA, MB, FRCP
Consultant Paediatrician, Addenbrooke's Hospital, Cambridge

J. D. Baum, MA, MSc, MD, FRCP, DCH
Professor of Child Health, Department of Child Health, Royal Hospital for Sick Children, University of Bristol

Dion R. Bell, MB, ChB, FRCP, MFCM, DTM&H
Reader in Tropical Medicine and Honorary Consultant Physician, Liverpool School of Tropical Medicine

J. A. Black, MD, FRCP
Late Consultant Paediatrician, The Children's Hospital, Sheffield and Jessop Hospital for Women, Sheffield

Andrew W. Boon, BSc, MD, MRCP, DCH
Consultant Paediatrician, Royal Berkshire Hospital, Reading

J. T. Buffin, FRCS, DLO
Consultant ENT Surgeon, Department of Communication, The Children's Hospital, Sheffield

Christine E. Candy, BA, SRN, RSCN, RNT, Dip N
Formerly Nurse Tutor, Paediatrics, Charles West School of Nursing, The Hospital for Sick Children, Great Ormond Street, London

David C. A. Candy, MSc, MB BS, MRCP, MO
Wellcome Senior Lecturer in Paediatrics and Child Health, University of Birmingham

Judith M. Chessells, MD, FRCP
Consultant Clinical Haematologist, The Hospital for Sick Children, Great Ormond Street, London

A. F. Conchie, MB, ChB, DCH, DA
Consultant Paediatrician, Doncaster Royal Infirmary, Doncaster

Roger Cudmore, FRCS, DCH
Consultant Paediatric Surgeon, Alder Hey Children's Hospital, Liverpool

D. M. Danks, MD, FRACP
Professor of Paediatric Research and Director of Murdoch Institute for Research into Birth Defects, Melbourne

J. A. S. Dickson, MB, ChB, FRCS (Ed and Lond)
Consultant Paediatric Surgeon, The Children's Hospital, Sheffield

R. C. W. Dinsdale, VRD, BChD, FDS, RCS (Eng)
Consultant Oral Surgeon, The Charles Clifford Dental Hospital, Sheffield

J. C. Fallis, BA, MD, FRCS
Director of Emergency Medical Services, The Hospital for Sick Children, Toronto

Susan Fisher-Hoch, MD, MSc, MRCPath
Special Pathogens Branch, Virology Division, Centers for Disease Control, Atlanta, Georgia, USA

Martyn Gay,
Consultant Child Psychiatrist, Bristol Royal Hospital for Sick Children, Bristol

D. N. Grant, MB, ChB, FRCS
Consultant Neurological Surgeon, The National Hospital for Nervous Diseases, London and The Hospital for Sick Children, Great Ormond Street, London

S. A. Greene,
Wellcome Lecturer in Clinical Paediatrics and Metabolic Medicine, University Department of Paediatrics, United Medical and Dental Schools of Guy's and St Thomas's Hospitals, London

G. B. Haycock, MB, BChir, FRCP, DCH
Consultant Paediatric Nephrologist, Guy's Hospital, London

J. A. Henry, MB, FRCP
Consultant Physician, National Poisons Unit, Guy's Hospital, London

B. Heyworth, MB, FRCP, FRACP, FRACMA, DCH, DRCOG, DTM&H
Professor of Child Health, National University of Malaysia, Kuala Lumpur, Malaysia

Anna Jarvis, MB BS, FRCP(C), FAAP
Supervising Paediatrician, Emergency Department, The Hospital for Sick Children, Toronto; Associate Professor of Paediatrics, University of Toronto

Gregor W. Lawrence, MD, FRACP
Senior Research Fellow, Queensland Institute of Medical Research, Brisbane

Michael Levin, MB BCh, MRCP
Consultant and Senior Lecturer in Paediatric Infectious Diseases, The Hospital for Sick Children and Institute of Child Health, London

David A. Lloyd, MChir (Cantab), FRCS(Eng), FCS(SA)
Paediatric Surgeon, The Children's Hospital of Pittsburgh; Associate Professor, University of Pittsburgh School of Medicine, Pittsburgh

Elizabeth Lund, MB BCh, BAO
Medical Officer of The Newborn Nursery, Edendale Hospital, Pietermaritzburg, South Africa

Ian A. McKinlay, MB ChB, FRCP, BSc, DCH
Consultant Paediatric Neurologist, Booth Hall Children's Hospital, Manchester

P. J. Milla, MSc, MB, BS, FRCP
Senior Lecturer in Child Health; Honorary Consultant in Paediatric Gastroenterology, Institute of Child Health, London

Colin G. Miller, MB, BS, FRCP, DCH
Consultant Paediatrician, The Warrington General Hospital, Warrington, Cheshire

R. W. S. Miller, FRCP(Ed), LRCP(Ed), LRFP&S (Glas)
Consultant Plastic Surgeon, The Children's Hospital, Sheffield

R. D. G. Milner, MD, ScD, FRCP
Professor of Paediatrics, University of Sheffield, Honorary Consultant Paediatrician, The Children's Hospital and the Jessop Hospital for Women, Sheffield

R. A. Minns, PhD, MB, BS
Consultant Paediatric Neurologist, Royal Hospital for Sick Children, Edinburgh

M. E. Imogen Morgan, MB, ChB, MRCP, DCH
Lecturer in Child Health, Alder Hay Children's Hospital, Liverpool

Alex P. Mowat, MB, FRCP, DObst, RCOG, DCH
Consultant Paediatrician, King's College Hospital, London

John Pearn, MA, MD, MB BS, BSc, FRACP, FRCP(UK), PhD(Lond), DCH
Head of Department of Child Health, Royal Children's Hospital, Brisbane; Consultant Paediatrician, Royal Children's Hospital, Brisbane

M. J. Noronha, FRCP(Lond & Ed), MRCP
Consultant Paediatric Neurologist, Royal Manchester Children's Hospital and Booth Hall Children's Hospital, Manchester

A. M. K. Rickwood, FRCS
Consultant Paediatric Urologist, Alder Hey Children's Hospital, Liverpool

Carol S. Rubidge MB ChB, MMed(Paed), DCM, RCP & S(Eng)
Late Senior Specialist/Senior lecturer, Department of Paediatrics and Child Health, Faculty of Medicine, University of Natal, Durban, South Africa

Martin O. Savage, MA, MD, FRCP
Consultant Paediatric Endocrinologist, St Bartholomew's Hospital, London; Consultant Paediatrician, Queen Elizabeth Hospital for Children, London

Ian Shellshear, MB BS, FRACP(Paediatric)
Consultant Paediatrician, Townsville General Hospital, Townsville, Australia

D. H. Smith, FRCP
Senior Lecturer in Tropical Medicine and Honorary Consultant Physician, Liverpool School of Tropical Medicine, Liverpool

Marian D. Smith, MB, ChB, MRCP(Ed)
Late Paediatrician, Patan Hospital, Kathmandu, Nepal; Senior Registrar in Paediatrics, The Children's Hospital, Sheffield

N. J. Spencer, MRCS, MRCP, DCH
Consultant Paediatrician, Northern General Hospital, Sheffield

Lewis Spitz, MB, ChB, PhD, FRCS
Nuffield Professor of Paediatric Surgery, Institute of Child Health, University of London and Honorary Consultant Surgeon, Hospital for Sick Children, Great Ormond Street, London

J. Paget Stanfield, MD, FRCPS(G), FRCP, DCH
Head, Department of Community Health, African Medical and Research Foundation, Nairobi, Kenya

David Taylor, FRCS, FRCP
Consultant Ophthalmic Surgeon, The Hospital for Sick Children, Great Ormond Street, London

F. G. Thorpe, MB, ChB, FRCPsych, DPM
Consultant in Children's Psychiatry, The Children's Hospital, Northern General Hospital, School Health Psychiatry Clinics and Shirle Hill Children's Unit, Sheffield

Richard S. Trompeter, MB, MRCP
Senior Lecturer in Paediatrics and Consultant Paediatric Nephrologist, The Royal Free Hospital and Medical School, London

Alan Usher, OBE, MB BS, FRCPath, DMJ (Clin et Path)
Professor of Forensic Pathology, University of Sheffield

John C. Vance, MB BS, FRACP
Senior Lecturer in Child Health, Department of Child Health, University of Queensland, Mater Children's Hospital, South Brisbane and Consultant Paediatrician, Mater Children's Hospital, South Brisbane

J. A. Walker-Smith, MD (Sydney) BS, FRACP, FRCP (E&L)
Professor of Paediatric Gastroenterology, Queen Elizabeth Hospital for Children, London

M. P. Ward, CBE, MA, MD, FRCS
Consultant Surgeon, St Andrew's Hospital, London; Lecturer in Surgery, London Hospital Medical College

J. O. Warner, MD, MRCP, DCH
Consultant Paediatric Chest Physician, Brompton Hospital, London

A. G. Wesley, MD, FRCP, DCH
Senior Specialist/Senior lecturer, Respiratory Unit, King Edward VIII Hospital and Department of Paediatrics and Child Health, University of Natal, South Africa

M. F. Whitfield, MD(Ed), MRCP, DCH, D(Obst)RCOG, FRCP(C)
Assistant Professor, Department of Paediatrics, University of British Columbia; Neonatologist and Director, Neonatal Follow-Up Programme, British Colmbia Children's Hospital, Vancouver

James L. Wilkinson, MB, ChB, FRCP
Consultant Paediatric Cardiologist, Royal Liverpool Children's Hospital; Lecturer in Child Health, University of Liverpool

A. Murray Wilson, MB, ChB, FFARCS, DRCOG, C Av Med
Consultant Anaesthetist, The Children's Hospital and Plastic Surgery Unit, Sheffield

Wong Hock Boon, MB BS, FRCP(Ed), FRACP, FRCP(Glas), DCH, PJG, PPA
Professor and Head, Department of Paediatrics, National University of Singapore; Director, School of Postgraduate Medical Studies, National University of Singapore

E. R. Wozniak, BSc, MB BS, MRCP, DCH
Consultant Paediatrician, Saint Mary's Hospital, Portsmouth

Preface to the second edition

In this second edition, much new material has been added, and there are many new contributors. Continuing the policy of including diseases of the tropics and subtropics, new chapters have been added, on abdominal ascariasis (Chapter 42), enteritis necroticans (Pigbel) (Chapter 44), and the viral haemorrhagic fevers (Chapter 67). There are also new chapters on raised intracranial pressure (Chapter 26), brain death (Chapter 27), acute liver failure (Chapter 47), and abuse of solvents and other volatile substances (Chapter 57). The chapter on practical procedures (Chapter 93) has been expanded to include oral rehydration at village level, nasogastric feeding and intraperitoneal fluid in dehydration.

I am grateful to all the contributors, who have taken so much trouble over writing or revising their chapters. I am specially indebted to Butterworths, for much helpful advice during the preparation of this book. My wife has, once again, provided support and encouragement throughout. My thanks are also due to Mrs Sandra Parfitt for her skill and care in typing many of the contributions.

J.A.B.

Preface to the first edition

An emergency can be defined as an acute illness in which lack of prompt and appropriate treatment may result in death, disability, or delayed recovery. In Europe and North America, of all children admitted to hospital, 60 per cent are emergencies; in Africa and Asia this proportion is much higher.

Acute disease in children develops more rapidly than in adults, but with correct treatment the child has a greater capacity for quick and complete recovery. Emergency treatment in the child must therefore be of a very high standard, and it is unfortunate that in most hospital services treatment of the emergency admission is in the hands of relatively junior staff, and the more experienced the clinician becomes, the less acute disease does he see. Normally, the Consultant or Specialist becomes directly involved in emergency treatment only when something goes wrong. It is for this reason that the management of the acutely ill child is seldom subjected to the same critical analysis as is that of the less acutely ill patient, and the traditions of emergency treatment are maintained at a sub-Consultant level, often with inadequate facilities. Thus the standard of emergency care in general paediatric departments tends to lag behind that of the more specialized units. In this book we have attempted to make available to the general paediatrician the practice of the best specialist units. With its emphasis on recognition of the emergency, we hope that this book will also be useful to those who are the first to see the acutely ill child, the family doctors, and the casualty officers. We have, where appropriate, attempted to describe the management of the emergency in sufficient detail to be of use both to medical and to nursing staff.

We have included a section on diseases of the subtropics and tropics for a number of reasons, the most important being that rapid intercontinental travel makes it essential that the paediatrician should be able to recognize conditions which are not indigenous to his own country. Also, in many parts of the world, sick children are cared for by doctors without special training in paediatrics, and it seemed essential to combine in one volume the paediatric aspects of the more important diseases of the tropics and subtropics, and the management of those emergencies such as asthma, convulsions, etc. which the non-paediatrician would have to treat. A third consideration was that, with a few notable exceptions, textbooks of tropical medicine give inadequate attention to the treatment of the sick child, and, conversely, the general paediatric textbooks deal perfunctorily with tropical disease.

I would like to thank Dr John Apley for his invaluable support and advice in putting together this book, and to express my gratitude to my family, and particularly to my wife, for their tolerance of the piles of papers which threatened for a time to become a permanent feature of our home.

I would also like to thank Miss Joan Beynon for her help with correspondence, and Miss Eve Turner, Mrs Joyce Andrews, and Mrs Sandra Parfitt for their care and patience with the typing.

I am also indebted to all the numerous contributors for their help and for their hard work.

J.A.B.

Part I

Trauma, Accident and Travel

Chapter 1

Management of acute cardiorespiratory collapse or arrest

Anna Jarvis

Figure 1.1 provides an easily memorized sequence for the management of acute cardiorespiratory failure.

Prominence has been given to this figure by placing it at the beginning of the book to emphasize that without the re-establishment of cardiorespiratory function in the desperately ill child, specific treatment related to the primary disease is ineffective.

This scheme supplies a framework of treatment which is common to any of the acute conditions associated with cardiorespiratory collapse which are described in the later chapters.

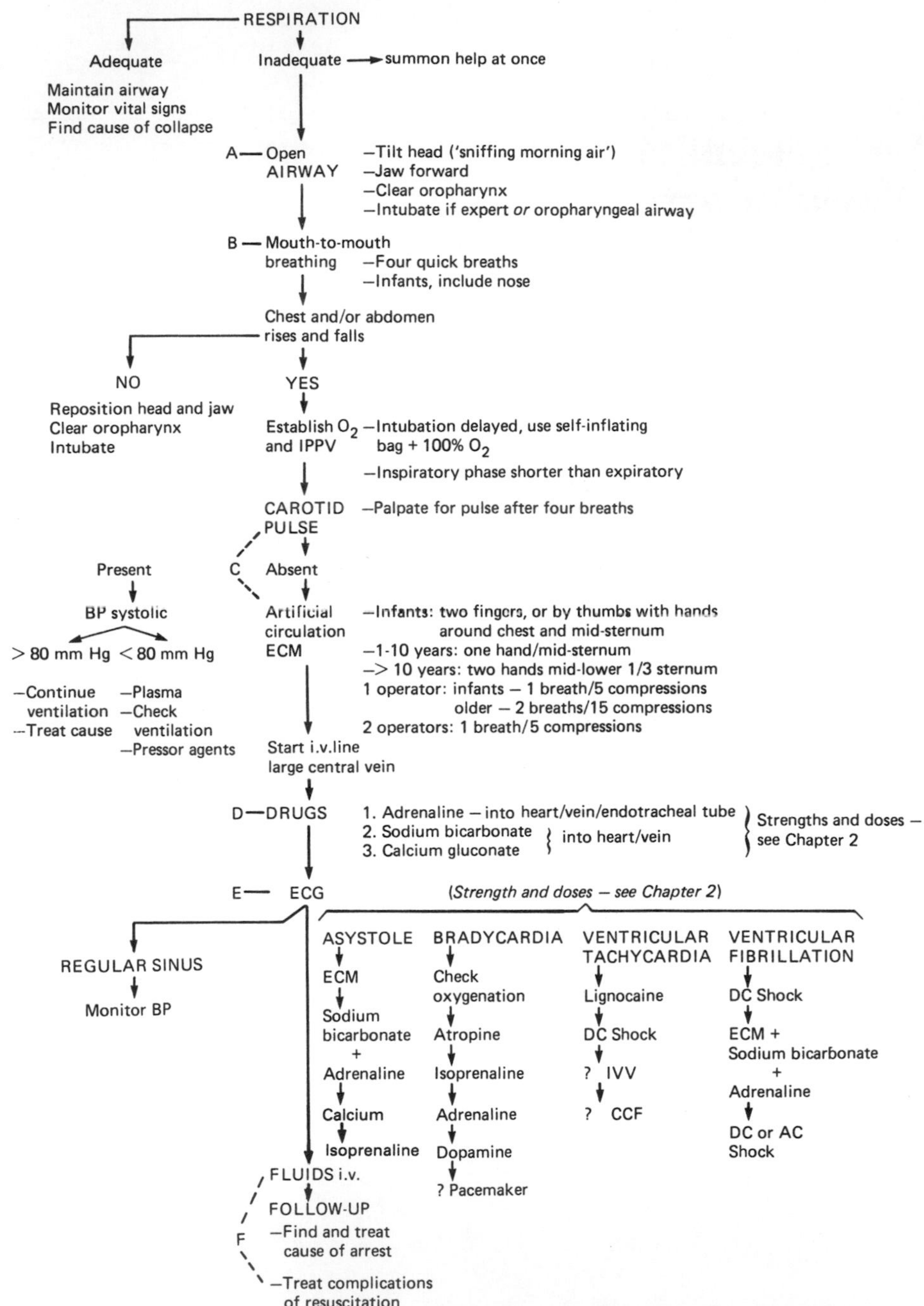

Figure 1.1 Management of acute respiratory collapse or arrest. IPPV, intermittent positive pressure ventilation; ECM, external cardiac massage or compression; IVV, intravascular volume. *Notes:*

1. When satisfactory respiration and circulation have been established, children in whom normal consciousness does *not* return, or in whom neurological damage is thought to have occurred, should be treated *immediately*, for cerebral oedema, with IV mannitol, hyperventilation and other measures as necessary. Prompt treatment in this way will prevent additional damage due to cerebral oedema (*see* Chapter 26).
2. Resuscitation of the newborn – *see* Chapter 71.
3. Drugs in resuscitation – *see* Chapter 2.
4. Use of sympathomimetics in shock – *see* Chapter 2, *Tables 2.1, 2.2* and *2.3,* and Chapter 10, pages 105–109.

Chapter 2

Drugs in resuscitation, cardiorespiratory collapse or arrest

A. M. Wilson

The tables of doses of drugs for cardiorespiratory emergencies in this chapter (*Tables 2.1–2.3*) are presented in a form that is easy to use. In an emergency often the only thing known about the patient is his age. The doses recommended are therefore based on age and the average weight of children at these ages. The dose given should be adjusted from this value for children obviously not of average weight, or for clinical states such as hypovolaemia.

Each drug is presented according to whether it is considered as first-line, immediate treatment in a cardiorespiratory arrest, or to be used subsequently, 'second line' or 'third line'. Within these sections the drugs are listed in alphabetical order. There follows the presentation of the drug as found in the *British National Formulary*, and instructions for dilution where appropriate. Where possible the dilution has been chosen so that the volume of the dose is equal to or directly related to the age, e.g. adrenaline. The range of doses is shown vertically below the age/weight row at the top. To the right are listed the pages on which further details of the administration of the drugs are to be found. These tables can form the basis for wall charts in resuscitation rooms and operating theatres. The presentation and method of dilution should be altered to suit the quantities and volumes found in ampoules supplied locally.

In all prescriptions a strong plea is made for a standardization in description of mg or μg (micrograms) per ml or per ℓ. This should replace such descriptions as % (per cent); ‰ (per mille or thousand); and ratios such as 1:1000. In children's work many drugs must be diluted and errors have occurred in the manipulation of percentages and ratios. The use of mass of drug per unit volume reduces errors in doses and facilitates the rapid calculation of such values as the volume in which the maximum dose is contained.

Drugs by infusion

Always check for compatibility before diluting drugs for infusion. This is especially important as often these drugs are used in large quantities and are expensive. For example, dopamine is incompatible with bicarbonate solutions. Drugs should be made up so that the final dilution is known in mg (or μg)/ml, and the infusion controlled as a volume per hour. To use the hour as a base is logical, as most intravenous pumps and syringe drivers are scaled in hours. Fluid balance of small children is usually adjusted by the hour. However, in an emergency, minute by minute alterations may be more appropriate, e.g. with dopamine. Several

Table 2.1 First-line treatment

	Age (years) *Average weight* (kg)	*0–½* *3.5–7*	*1* *10*	*2* *12*	*3* *15*	*4* *17*	*5* *18*	*6* *20*	*7* *22*	*8* *28*	*9* *27*	*10* *30*	*See also pages*
Drugs	*Route*												
Adrenaline*	IV or intracardiac			USE IN ASYSTOLE. Give volumes below Presentation: Ampoules 0.5 and 1.0 ml. 1 mg/ml, (1:1000), (0.1%) Dilute 0.5 ml into 10 ml saline to make 1:20 000									4, 108
		1–2 ml	1–2 ml	2 ml	3 ml	4 ml	5 ml	6 ml	7 ml	8 ml	9 ml	10 ml	
Calcium gluconate	IV or intracardiac			USE IN ASYSTOLE OR RESPIRATORY ARREST Ampoules: 5 and 10 ml 10% (0.23 mmol Ca/1 ml). Give over at least one minute									279
		0.5 ml	1 ml	2 ml	3 ml	4 ml	5 ml	6 ml	7 ml	8 ml	9 ml	10 ml	
Epinephrine – *see* adrenaline													
Sodium bicarbonate	Intravenous			USE IN ASYSTOLE OR RESPIRATORY ARREST Ampoules: 10 ml and 30 ml. Bags: 100 ml and 200 ml 8.4% (1 mmol/ml); or 7.5% (0.9 mmol/ml) Difference in dosage between these strengths is negligible. Give amount in columns times minutes of arrest. If not known, assume 3 min. If using 5% solution, multiply volumes by 1.7									4, 278
		5 ml	10 ml	10 ml	15 ml	15 ml	20 ml	20 ml	20 ml	25 ml	25 ml	30 ml	
Doxapram	Intravenous			RESPIRATORY DEPRESSION. Post-anaesthesia, poisoning Ampoules: 100 mg in 5 ml									
		5 mg	10 mg	12 mg	15 mg	15 mg	20 mg	20 mg	20 mg	25 mg	25 mg	30 mg	
Naloxone	IV or IM			OPIATE OVERDOSE Ampoules: 400 μg in 1 ml (adult strength) Dilute 1 ml into 10 ml. Give doses below in two or three divided doses, observe response.									69
		2 ml	2.5 ml	3 ml	4 ml	4 ml	4.5 ml	5 ml	5 ml	5.5 ml	6 ml	6 ml	
Nikethamide	Intravenous			USE ONLY IN RESPIRATORY ARREST WHEN NO ONE CAN INTUBATE Ampoules: 2 ml of 25% solution Dilute 2 ml to 10 ml. Give volumes below									
		0.2–0.5 ml	1 ml	2 ml	3 ml	4 ml	5 ml	6 ml	7 ml	8 ml	9 ml	10 ml	
Intubation	External diameter			Always select a low size to start. *Never* force in.									22, Appe-ndix 21
		3 mm	3.5 mm	4 mm	4.5 mm	4.5 mm	5 mm	5.5 mm	5.5 mm	5.5 mm	6 mm	6.5 mm	

* For use in shock, *see* Chapter 10 and Table 10.5.

Table 2.2 Second-line treatment

Drugs	Route	*0–½*	*1*	*2*	*3*	*4*	*5*	*6*	*7*	*8*	*9*	*10*	*See also pages*
	Age (years) / *Average weight (kg)*	*3.5–7*	*10*	*12*	*15*	*17*	*18*	*20*	*22*	*28*	*27*	*30*	
Atropine	Intravenous			USE IN BRADYCARDIA. Give dose as below Ampoules 0.4, 0.5, or 6.0 mg. Check first!									
		0.1 mg	0.2 mg	0.3 mg	0.3 mg	0.3 mg	0.3 mg	0.4 mg	0.4 mg	0.4 mg	0.5 mg	0.5 mg	
Dobutamine*	Intravenous			LOW-OUTPUT STATE Vials: 250 mg Dilute as for dopamine Normal dose range 2.5–10 μg/kg/min									106–107
Dopamine*	Intravenous infusion			CARDIAC INSUFFICIENCY. Ensure adequate blood volume Ampoules: 200 mg in 5 ml, and 800 mg in 5 ml Take three times child's weight in mg of dopamine, dilute into 50 ml. In a minidrip (60 drops per ml), 1 drop per minute = 1 μg/kg/min Normal rate = 5–25 μg/kg/min									106–107
Isoprenaline* Isoproterenol (Isoprel Suscardia)	Intravenous bolus			USE IN ASYSTOLE OR PERSISTENT BRADYCARDIA Ampoules: 200 μg in 1 ml, and 2 mg in 2 ml Dilute 100 μg into 10 ml. Give dose over 1 min. Repeat until effective									106
		0.5 ml	1 ml (10 μg)	2 ml	3 ml	4 ml	5 ml (50 μg)	6 ml	7 ml	8 ml	9 ml	10 ml (100 μg)	
	Intravenous infusion			LOW-OUTPUT STATE Dilute 1 mg into 100 ml of 5% dextrose (10 μg/ml) Use microdrop (60 drops per ml) infusion set (0.016 μg/drop) Normal range 0.5–12 microdrops/kg/min (0.008–0.19 μg/kg/min) Titrate rate of infusion against clinical response									
Lignocaine (xylocaine, lidocaine)	Intravenous			MULTIPLE VENTRICULAR EXTRASYSTOLES Ampoules and vials: 5 mg/ml (0.5%), 10 mg/ml (1%), 20 mg/ml (2%) Make a 1 mg per ml solution. CHECK *NO* ADRENALINE!! Give dose below at 1–2 mg per min									272
		3–7 mg	10 mg	10 mg	15 mg	15 mg	20 mg	20 mg	20 mg	25 mg	25 mg	30 mg	
Propranolol	Intravenous			SUPRAVENTRICULAR TACHYCARDIA Ampoules: 1 mg in 1 ml Dilute 2 mg into 10 ml of saline Inject slowly under ECG control									270
		0.5 ml	2 ml	3 ml	3.5 ml	4 ml	4.5 ml	5 ml	5.5 ml	6 ml	7 ml	7.5 ml	
Defibrillation				d.c. for fibrillation or synchronized shock									270; 272
Initial shock	Joules	5	10	20	30	40	50	60	70	80	90	100	
				a.c. for fibrillation only									
Initial shock	Volts	12	5	50	75	100	125	150	175	200	225	250	

* For use in shock, *see* Chapter 10 and Table 10.5.

Table 2.3 Third-line treatment

	Age (years) / *Average weight* (kg)	*0–½* / *3.5–7*	*1* / *10*	*2* / *12*	*3* / *15*	*4* / *17*	*5* / *18*	*6* / *20*	*7* / *22*	*8* / *28*	*9* / *27*	*10* / *30*	*See also pages*
Drugs	*Route*												
Aminophylline	Intravenous			USE IN STATUS ASTHMATICUS OR ANAPHYLAXIS WITH BRONCHIAL SPASM Ampoules: 250 mg in 10 ml (1 ml = 25 mg) Give dose *slowly* over 30 min.									234
		(0.3 mg/kg) 0.5 ml	1 ml	2 ml	3 ml	4 ml	5 ml	6 ml	7 ml	8 ml	9 ml	10 ml	
Aramine – *see* Metaraminol													
Dexamethasone	Intravenous			PREVENTION AND TREATMENT OF CEREBRAL OEDEMA Vials: 4 mg per 1 ml.									296
		2 mg	2 mg	2 mg	4 mg	4 mg	4 mg	4 mg	4 mg	4 mg	4 mg	4 mg	
Diazepam (Valium)	IV or IM			POST-HYPOXIC FITS, BUT BEWARE OF OVERDOSE AND RESPIRATORY DEPRESSION Ampoules: 10 mg in 2 ml Should not be diluted. Diazemuls less damaging to veins. Double dose intramuscular or orally									308
		0.5mg	0.5 mg	1 mg	1.5 mg	2 mg	2.5 mg	3 mg	3.5 mg	4 mg	4.5 mg	5 mg	
Frusemide	Intravenous			PULMONARY OEDEMA OR RENAL SHUTDOWN Ampoules: 20 mg in 2 ml									267, 434
		5 mg	10 mg	10 mg	15 mg	15 mg	20 mg	20 mg	20 mg	25 mg	25 mg	30 mg	
Hydrocortisone hemisuccinate	Intravenous			ANAPHYLAXIS OR ADRENAL FAILURE Vials: 100 mg and 500 mg Repeat after one hour if clinical response is not obained									114, 472
		25 mg	25 mg	25 mg	50 mg	50 mg	50 mg	100 mg	100 mg	100 mg	100 mg	100 mg	

Mannitol	Intravenous			CEREBRAL OEDEMA. Only if good renal function Bags: 500 ml of 20% Warm not over 60°C (140°F) if crystals present, cool before giving.									296
		5 mg	10 mg	10 mg	15 mg	15 mg	20 mg	20 mg	20 mg	25 mg	25 mg	30 mg	
Metaraminol (Aramine)	Intravenous			ACUTE HYPOTENSION. Ensure adequate blood volume Ampoules: 10 mg in 1 ml Dilute 10 mg into 20 ml.									
		0.25 ml	0.5 ml	0.5 ml	0.5 ml	0.5 ml	0.5 ml	0.5 ml	1 ml	1 ml	1 ml	1 ml	
Methoxamine	Intravenous			ACUTE HYPOTENSION. Ensure adequate blood volume Ampoules: 20 mg in 1 ml Dilute 20 mg into 20 ml									
		0.25 ml	0.5 ml	0.5 ml	0.5 ml	0.5 ml	0.5 ml	0.5 ml	1 ml	1 ml	1 ml	1 ml	
Paraldehyde	IV or IM			POST-HYPOXIC FITS, STATUS EPILEPTICUS Ampoules: 2, 5 and 10 ml Use glass syringe or new types of disposable syringe									309
		0.25 ml	0.5 ml	1 ml	1.5 ml	2 ml	2.5 ml	3 ml	3.5 ml	4 ml	4.5 ml	5 ml	
Plasma protein fraction	IV			LOW-OUTPUT STATE Give between 10 ml and 20 ml/kg									*Table 10.4*, p. 100
Valium – *see* diazepam													
Vasoxine – *see* methoxamine													

computer programs have been written for the calculations which relate initial drug mass, diluting volume, rate of infusion and the weight of patient. Thus the relationship between rate of infusion (ml/hour) and the dose of the active drug (mg/kg/hour) is made clear. These programs simplify the calculations but require an available computer. The Janssen Infusion Calculator, a pocket-sized circular slide rule, is readily portable and may be used rapidly in all situations.

Chapter 3

Multiple injuries

J. C. Fallis

Initial assessment

Nowhere is the accuracy of initial assessment more critical than in the management of the child with multiple injuries. The initial assessment establishes a therapeutic route which is only as correct as the assessment was accurate. Failure to recognize those injuries which may rapidly become life threatening is an important cause of morbidity and mortality. Hence the physician who cares for those with multiple injuries must remain *serious-disease conscious*. It matters little if the fracture of the clavicle or the metatarsal is not immediately detected. *But the child with a head injury which alone would not be lethal may die if a slowly expanding pneumothorax associated with it is overlooked.*

History

If a fraction of the effort expended in obtaining a history for a complicated medical illness were directed towards discovering, after major trauma, the details of the accident and the mechanism of injury, fewer important but initially obscure injuries would be missed. When an individual has landed on head or shoulder one must be alert to the possibility of an injured cervical spine. The head injury inadvertently inflicted by a golf club will rarely be associated with other major injuries. However, the child with a comparable head injury sustained when he was run over by a tractor is likely to have other visceral injuries which pose a more serious threat to life than does the head injury.

Inspection, the basis of examination

The critically ill, seriously shocked or semi-comatose child is usually too sick to make examination difficult through his unwillingness to co-operate. However, others, particularly the younger or frightened children, or those who are just ill-behaved, cry while being examined or merely at the expectation of being examined. When a child will not co-operate it is necessary to obtain as much information as possible before causing any further discomfort. This is largely achieved by standing back and looking. Cardiorespiratory function can be evaluated, at least in general terms, by inspection alone, and the early manifestations of traumatic shock in the paediatric patient are all visible.

Adult hands are large and can hide much that is useful if they are applied too soon to the small child's body.

The first moments

The most important moments during the management of a multiple injury casualty are the first few after arrival in hospital. During this brief interval all injuries causing major physiological derangement must be detected and their effects countered. Although it is difficult to ignore the grossly displaced femoral fracture,

Table 3.1 Resuscitation room equipment

A.	Shock stretcher, adult size, with radiolucent litter-top. Anaesthetic machine. Oxygen, suction outlets. ECG monitor (with printout); defibrillator. X-ray viewing-box.	
B.	Tongue depressor Electric torches Stethoscopes Sphygmomanometers	Auroscope Ophthalmoscope Reflex hammers
C.	Laryngoscope with 8, 10 and 12 cm blades (Welch–Allyn nos 1, 2, 3). Bronchoscopes, 3.5, 4, 5 mm sizes. Oropharyngeal airways, nos 00, 0, 1, 2, 3. Endotracheal tubes, 3.0 mm to 9.0 mm sizes. Stylets. Nasogastric tubes, sizes 8 to 14 FG. Tracheostomy tray with trcheostomy tubes (Hollinger type) of sizes 0, 1, 2, 3, 4 and 5. Lengths vary, 33 mm (size 0), to 60 mm (size 5).	
D.	Caps, masks, surgical gowns. Surgical gloves, gloves for rectal examinations.	
E.	Sterile water, saline for irrigating wounds. Detergent, aqueous antiseptic. Syringes, needles, of all sizes. Bandages, dressings, sterile towels, dressing trays. Laceration suture trays, variety of sutures. Minor surgical instruments. Venous cut-down trays. Chest tube trays. Chest tubes 12, 16, 20, 14 FG, Stylets. Underwater bottle system or Heimlich valve.	
F.	Venous cannulae, nos 16, 18, 20, 22. CVP line (radio-opaque catheter with stylet). Venous pressure manometer. Splints for restraining arms with infusions. Blood pump. Venous infusion lines, adult and infant (micro) drop sizes. Blood-warmer for IV line. Blood filter (maximum pore size 40 μm).	
G.	Lumbar puncture trays. Urethral catheter trays. Catheters 8, 10, 12, 14 FG Straight and Foley.	
H.	Optional items: overhead X-ray unit, electronic blood pressure recorder, Doppler equipment, refrigerator (blood, drugs)	

the degloving injury of the foot and the badly lacerated face, none of these will result in death. *The physician must single mindedly focus on a sequence of priority items critical to survival.* He must complete a mental check-list of vital functions before attending to items which are more obvious but have less influence on survival.

During these critical few minutes diagnosis merges with therapy. For example, respiration noted to be inadequate must be corrected while circulation is being evaluated. Priority assessment and resuscitation proceed simultaneously.

Critical assessment: the priority sequence

1. Airway

(a) Evidence of obstruction

Much is revealed about airway patency before palpation and auscultation. The gurgle or rattle of a partly obstructed airway is readily noted. Vigorous inspiratory effort serving only to suck in the abdomen, followed by abdominal protrusion as expiration is attempted, indicates complete obstruction.

(b) Relief of obstruction

Any degree of airway obstruction can be tolerated only briefly and must be corrected quickly while assessment is being completed. Extension of the head on the neck is often sufficient as this moves the mandible and tongue forward. Mechanical aspiration of saliva, vomitus, or other liquid may be necessary and the physician may even have to remove solid foreign bodies from mouth or pharynx.

(c) Position of the unconscious patient

A comatose subject should be maintained in the semi-prone position unless an endotracheal tube has been inserted. Although contraindicated in the presence of a cervical spine fracture and certain other injuries the semi-prone position *permits ready drainage of oral secretions and vomitus, helps to keep the jaw and tongue forward, and can provide a safe airway indefinitely while comatose subjects are being transported.*

(d) Artificial airway

If a satisfactory airway has been obtained by simple measures it is often best to delay the insertion of an artificial airway, particularly if someone skilled at intubation is expected within minutes. Too few remember that an adequate airway, even one that will permit artificial ventilation, can usually be maintained by proper head-positioning alone. However, tracheal intubation is indicated if there is coma from a head injury, or if artificial respiration will be needed for a prolonged period.

Although airway obstruction by a tongue which has fallen backwards can, theoretically, be dealt with by the insertion of an oropharyngeal airway, most anaesthetists prefer the security of endotracheal intubation if artificial airway maintenance at any level is required. Oropharyngeal airways increase airway resistance; endotracheal tubes generally reduce it and offer the advantage of isolating the airway from the oesophagus.

Tracheal intubation for more than a few days was formerly an indication for tracheostomy. More recently, nasotracheal intubation has been maintained for many days with few complications and has replaced tracheostomy in the majority of patients needing prolonged intubation. Emergency tracheostomy is now reserved for those situations in which facial or laryngeal trauma precludes the passage of a tube.

(e) Gastric decompression

In patients who are apt to vomit gastric decompression should be maintained by means of nasogastric tube. This applies particularly to children, in whom acute gastric dilatation is a very common complication of trauma to chest or abdomen. Any child with injuries which are multiple, involve chest or abdomen, or have produced peritoneal irritation to any degree, should have a nasogastric tube passed. In children who have impaired consciousness passage of the gastric tube should be preceded by tracheal intubation. A nasogastric tube should never be clamped even for brief periods. Continuous suction is preferable, but intermittent irrigation and aspiration by syringe may suffice.

(f) Airway obstruction in head injury is dangerous

When a head injury is present even minor degrees of hypoxia or hypercapnia (hypercarbia) due to partial airway obstruction can cause such an increase in cerebral oedema that the patient may die who would otherwise have survived. For this reason airway maintenance and adequate ventilation is of critical importance in craniocerebral trauma. Airway obstruction is the leading cause of the respiratory failure seen from time to time following head injuries.

(g) Diagnosis of airway obstruction in the apnoeic patient

When the apnoea is due to total obstruction this will be evident when positive-pressure insufflation is first attempted.

(h) Oxygen

Following major trauma oxygen therapy is indicated, particularly in the presence of a head injury.

2. Breathing

(a) Evaluation of respiratory function

When the airway is open and oxygen is being given, adequacy of ventilation must be assessed. Looking and listening provide the initial evaluation, although arterial blood–gas analysis should be obtained as soon as possible in order to assess gas exchange properly. Before the blood–gas analysis becomes available ventilatory assistance is indicated unless the physician is absolutely confident that ventilation is adequate. This is of particular importance when there is a head injury.

(b) Pneumothorax

After thoracic trauma grunting respirations usually signify pleural irritation and almost always indicate the presence of a pneumothorax or haemopneumothorax.

Immediate auscultation revealing decreased breath sounds on one side reinforces the diagnosis, and the equipment needed for the closed insertion of a chest tube (thoracostomy) should be requested at once. The few moments needed for the preparation of the tray permit the initial assessment of the patient to be completed. With the child supine, the physician should quickly infiltrate the second or third interspace in the midclavicular line with local anaesthetic, taking care to avoid breast tissue and the internal mammary vessels. Local anaesthesia should be used even if the child is comatose so that the intrapleural air can be sucked back through the anaesthetic liquid remaining in the syringe. The bubbling produced is confirmation of the diagnosis.

When a tension pneumothorax has produced a critical emergency, the tube may be immediately inserted in the same place. However, in most instances an axillary site is now preferred, between the mid- and anterior lines at nipple level. The tube should be connected to an underwater seal or a one-way egress valve (Heimlich valve). Evacuation of the pneumothorax is usually very rapid and almost immediately results in correction of the respiratory distress, cessation of the grunting, and restoration of air entry throughout. Suction applied to the tube will rarely be needed to empty the pleural space. *When a combination of several injuries includes a pneumothorax, and particularly when there has been cerebral trauma, there is no justification for waiting for radiographic confirmation of pneumothorax before treating it.* The first chest X-ray taken should be to show that the tube is properly located and that the lung has expanded satisfactorily.

(c) Ventilatory assistance

Ventilatory assistance may be needed for any one of several reasons. Central depression of ventilation may result from direct brainstem or medullary damage or from the effects of increased intracranial pressure due to an intracranial clot or cerebral oedema. Advanced cerebral hypoxia from asphyxia or from hypovolaemic shock will also ultimately cause respiratory arrest as the patient reaches a terminal state.

Also, positive-pressure assisted ventilation (IPPV) is the treatment of choice for the paradoxical movement of a flail chest. This condition is not frequently seen in children, in whom the chest wall is quite pliable and not prone to multiple fractures.

3. Circulation

(a) Evidence of shock

Instant evaluation of circulation is reached by inspection. *Abnormal pallor and sweating in one who is prostrate after an accident are, for practical purposes, diagnostic of hypovolaemic shock* (*see also* Chapter 10). This is particularly valid in children who usually show the pallor of shock long before tachycardia or hypotension are observed.

In children inadequate cerebral circulation secondary to hypovolaemia causes a characteristic type of behaviour. The confusion of a child fighting to pull the oxygen mask from his face or complaining bitterly of a bruised ankle when he has several other serious injuries should not be interpreted as plain cussedness. These are signs of cerebral hypoxia and signal the need for prompt action.

(b) Blood for grouping and cross-matching, Hb and haematocrit (PCV)

As this assessment is proceeding blood must be rapidly obtained for grouping and cross-matching, and determination of haemoglobin and haematocrit levels, although, if the haemorrhage is very recent, these may still be normal and serve only as a baseline.

(c) Intravenous lines

A large-bore venous cannula must be inserted in an arm vein, one in each arm if there is a risk of major blood loss. The venous cannulae now available are designed for easy percutaneous introduction, and a cut-down is rarely needed.

Jugular cannulation, perhaps with a J-wire guide, is useful in expert hands but should only be considered if there is present one skilled in the technique. A central venous line is desirable in due course although cardiac decompensation as a result of overloading is unlikely in the child and time should not be spent early on in establishing a central line at the expense of a good peripheral line.

(d) Effects of cold-stored blood (see page 22)

If a large transfusion volume is anticipated a blood-warming apparatus should be included in the infusion apparatus. The small blood volume of the child cools rapidly when mixed with cold bank blood and this has frequently resulted in cardiac arrhythmia and even arrest. A micropore filter (40 μm) should also be included in the line. It may reduce the incidence of subsequent pulmonary complications (shock lung).

(e) Monitoring with ECG

The leads from an ECG monitor with defibrillator should be attached to the patient as the venous infusions are being established.

(f) Acid–base state

When the arterial blood–gas analysis becomes available the degree of metabolic acidosis due to inadequate tissue perfusion can be estimated. In very major trauma, arterial cannulation may be desirable. This facilitates repeated sampling of arterial blood and provides a mechanism for continuous arterial pressure monitoring. In most instances the establishment of an arterial line is deferred until the child reaches the intensive care unit.

(g) External cardiac massage (see Chapter 1 and page 277)

Finally, external cardiac compression to assist a heart which has suddenly failed because of advanced hypovolaemic shock must be combined with rapid blood-volume expansion, ventilatory assistance, and control of bleeding.

4. Increased intracranial pressure (*see also* Chapter 25)

There remains one more true emergency, increased intracranial pressure. Although acute extradural and subdural haematomata are not often part of the multi-injury complex, immediate operative treatment is required when they do occur. For this reason they must never go undetected.

(a) Extradural and acute subdural haematoma (see also Chapter 25)

History is the single most important feature in the diagnosis. The classic story is that of brief depression of consciousness after the accident, followed by gradual improvement perhaps even to a normal state of alertness, followed by rapidly progressive deterioration of consciousness. Increased intracranial pressure must always be kept in mind as the course of events is not always that described above. A child may sustain seemingly minor head trauma, be only momentarily stunned, and then some hours later may develop the progressive drowsiness of an extradural haematoma. Similarly, when a subject is rendered deeply comatose in an accident, failure to improve can be at least partly due to an enlarging surface clot.

Gradual dilatation of one pupil and a decreasing responsiveness to light usually indicate an expanding clot over the ipsilateral hemisphere. This is a very important sign and, more consistently than any other, indicates the side of the haematoma. However, it heralds advanced compression and is quickly followed by hypertension, bradycardia, and then respiratory depression due to brainstem ischaemia. Both pupils soon become fixed and dilated. Therefore accurate recording is important so that treatment which has been started after both pupils have become dilated can be directed towards the correct side without delay.

Papilloedema is a sign of increased intracranial pressure. However, with acutely raised tension, papilloedema seldom has time to develop. *In most instances of acutely enlarging intracranial clot the fundi are normal.*

5. Exceptions to the sequence of priority

There are two exceptions to the above sequence of priorities which take precedence over all else.

(a) An open chest wound must be closed

However, one must also remember the possibility of an underlying lung laceration. Sealing a chest wound will prevent the escape from the pleural space of air leaking from lung. Hence one must watch for the development of a tension pneumothorax in any patient whose chest wound has been sealed.

(b) Major external haemorrhage must be controlled at once

Usually this will have been accomplished by the first-aider, ambulance attendant, or receiving nurse. If not, the physician must take the necessary action immediately.

When the priority items of airway, breathing, circulation and increased intracranial pressure have been assessed and managed appropriately, and resuscitation is proceeding, the physician can relax to some degree and complete his examination in a less hurried manner.

Completing the assessment

When the initial high-priority assessment has been completed, resuscitation is proceeding, and vital functions are stable, examination must be completed in detail. All parts of the body must be surveyed and all minor injuries itemized. Particular attention should be paid to abdomen and chest.

(a) Haemorrhage into the abdomen

Haemorrhage into the abdomen is the commonest cause of hypovolaemic shock in children. Although intraperitoneal bleeding is more common, extraperitoneal haemorrhage may be massive and is more difficult to assess. Acute gastric ileus is an almost constant manifestation of major trauma in children and gastric decompression by a nasogastric tube is usually necessary for satisfactory evaluation of the abdomen. For this reason it should be a routine measure.

(b) Sequence of examination

To ensure that no injuries are missed, it is useful to itemize them under four body zones – head, chest, abdomen, and extremities. However, two specific injury sites, *the cervical spine and the diaphragm*, are frequently neglected until some time has elapsed. As a result injuries to these structures may be diagnosed too late, with tragic results. Neither the neck nor the diaphragm is automatically included in any of the four body sections listed above. Each lies between two of the zones and is often remembered only as an afterthought. Hence the physician must look specifically for a fractured cervical spine and a ruptured diaphragm and he must do so early in order to avoid the complications which can occur if either is missed.

Investigations

(a) Blood and urine

Immediate tests necessary for the seriously injured child include blood grouping and cross-matching, haemoglobin and haematocrit determination, blood acid–base and gas analysis, and urinalysis.

(b) X-ray

Radiographic examination follows – it must never replace, physical examination. X-rays of skull, cervical spine, chest, abdomen, and any extremities suspected to be injured can usually be obtained in the resuscitation room. *Cervical spine films, particularly the lateral, should be obtained in any child whose consciousness is impaired by a head injury; these must be reviewed before the manipulations needed to obtain skull X-rays are carried out.* Intravenous pyelography and catheter cystography are essential in the evaluation of the urinary tract. Other contrast studies (barium examinations, angiography, etc.) are occasionally required in the traumatized patient to identify specific lesions (e.g. renal artery tear). More sophisticated radiographic techniques are rarely useful with the possible exception of computerized tomography (CT scan), which has proved its worth in detecting small intracranial clots before they would have been otherwise identified. The 'CT scanner' is playing an increasing role in emergency diagnosis in spite of the practical problems encountered when using it for a patient with multiple injuries and all the accompanying dressings, splints, tubes, and wires.

Ultrasound studies are rapidly invading what has hitherto been radiographic domain and have replaced some of the X-rays now considered standard procedures.

One must remember that sophisticated tests usually serve only to confirm clinical suspicions. Only rarely will an accident victim's survival be determined by, or initial handling depend on, the immediate availability of such studies, no matter how specialized or sophisticated. An occasional exception is the CT scan of the skull, with its ability to differentiate rapidly between diffuse oedema and a surgically treatable clot.

(c) Arterial blood–gas analysis

Arterial blood–gas studies are important in the assessment of cardiorespiratory function after trauma and are usually obtained by needle aspiration of an available artery (radial, temporal, femoral) (*see* page 727). More sophisticated techniques call for the insertion of an arterial line which facilitates monitoring of the arterial pressure and repeated sampling.

(d) Confirmation of intraperitoneal bleeding (see also Chapter 93, page 741)

Peritoneal aspiration or lavage has gained great popularity in adult emergency medicine as a rapid method of determining the presence of an operable lesion within the abdomen. Nevertheless, increasing awareness of the spleen's importance in the child's defence against infection has led to a policy of treating suspected splenic injuries expectantly unless, as time passes, the surgeon's hand is forced by persisting blood loss. This has resulted in many fewer splenectomies than were formerly carried out. Some attempts are also being made to repair lacerated spleens. This policy of non-intervention not only results in fewer asplenic children but also removes much of the practical value of peritoneal lavage as a tool to detect the indications for laparotomy.

Peritoneal lavage remains highly valuable in the child who is unconscious from a head injury and shows signs of hypovolaemia.

(e) Scanning and intracranial pressure monitoring

Although rarely useful in an emergency, intracranial pressure monitors are being used in some specialized centres for continuous monitoring of pressure changes within the skull (*see* page 294).

Nuclear scanning has now been applied to many solid organs, particularly liver, spleen, brain, lungs, and kidneys. Liver and spleen scans are especially useful in the acute state, and later when evidence of previous injury may be manifest.

The variety and complexity of investigative techniques available are endless. However, the simplest are of greatest value immediately after major trauma. One must guard against becoming too dependent on tests and neglecting careful, repeated clinical assessment of the patient.

Hypovolaemic shock in children (*see also* Chapter 10)

Causes

In children severe shock is rarely due to injury of the limbs. The femoral shaft fracture which, in the 25 year old, can cause enough bleeding into the thigh to produce the picture of shock, will rarely do so in the 8 or 10 year old. A child may have no evident systemic signs even in the presence of bilateral femoral fractures. When signs of blood loss do appear in such a child, one must first look elsewhere for the cause, particularly towards the abdomen. *The child who has a severe cerebral concussion and a fractured femur, who develops the picture of haemorrhagic shock, probably has a ruptured spleen.* Finally, in children as in adults, head injuries do not cause shock unless they are so serious that death is imminent.

Diagnosis

Compensatory vascular responses are so effective in the young child that a quarter or more of the circulating blood volume can be lost with little change in pulse rate or blood pressure. Progressive and very striking pallor and a cool damp skin are the chief signs of hypovolaemic shock. Before the stage of hypotension and tachycardia, *a child who becomes increasingly pale and sweaty after trauma can, in most instances, be assumed to have lost at least a quarter of his estimated blood volume.*

An unusual and striking behaviour pattern is also noted as a result of the cerebral hypoxia of shock. A child in shock will fight the oxygen mask and is likely to complain constantly of some trivial bruise or scrape, while ignoring two or three major injuries.

As blood loss continues, tachycardia, hypotension, impaired consciousness, and a declining urinary output will all occur. Nevertheless, the diagnosis of traumatic shock can be made before this stage if the history of trauma, the characteristic pallor and typical behaviour, are noted and their significance recognized.

Treatment

General aspects

Although the chief element in the management of traumatic shock is replacement of lost blood volume, other measures are important and easily neglected in the excitement of the moment.

External bleeding can usually be controlled by the application of simple pressure dressings. Operative management of internal haemorrhage is sometimes required before venous infusion can catch up with blood loss.

Oxygen administration and the other elements of respiratory support have been previously discussed but are part and parcel of the total management of hypovolaemic shock.

Small children cool rapidly when exposed and tolerate poorly this accidental cooling. Hence there must be efforts to minimize heat loss.

Splinting of fractures – Although this is not one of the immediate high-priority items it should be attended to when practicable. Persistent movement at a fracture site continues to cause pain, tissue damage, and increases blood loss.

Gentleness in handling is important and the injured child should not be jostled or moved more than is necessary. When resuscitation is complete and vital signs have been stabilized it is often beneficial to keep the patient a further half hour or so in the casualty department. During this period intravenous intake progresses and continued observation detects any delayed problems yet to be handled. In institutions where immediate transfer to intensive care or trauma-observation unit is the practice this transfer must be done as gently as possible.

During the initial management the body weight must be obtained by asking patient or parents, by weighting him if this is possible, by consulting a weight-for-age chart (*see* page 759), or by guessing. This figure should be recorded and prominently displayed as it forms the basis for all infusion volumes and drug dosages to be administered subsequently.

Pneumatic anti-shock trousers of a variety of sizes are increasingly available. These are of particular value for bleeding from fractures or open wounds of the legs, and haemorrhage into pelvis and lower abdomen. When a patient arrives in the department in anti-shock trousers which have been applied outside, their deflation and removal must be carried out gradually and only after clinical hypovolaemia has been corrected, ready venous access has been established, experienced trauma surgeons are present, and preparations are completed for immediate surgery. In most instances the pneumatic device should not be removed until the patient is on the operating table. This applies particularly to children, in whom the cause of severe traumatic shock is most likely to be haemorrhage from a major rupture of liver or spleen. In such cases definitive therapy is open operation.

Blood-volume expansion (see also pages 99–104)

TRANSFUSION

The single most important factor in survival is blood volume expansion, large enough and soon enough. The choice of the ideal fluid for initial expansion remains an unsolved and controversial issue. In most centres a crystalloid such as lactate Ringer's solution or isotonic saline is used as the initial fluid until blood is available. Others will switch to a colloid solution such as plasma, plasma protein fraction, serum albumin or dextran. At The Hospital for Sick Children, Toronto, it is usual to infuse lactate Ringer's solution while the blood grouping and cross-matching are carried out. A quick cross-matching can be finished in a little more than half an hour. If blood is needed sooner than this, group-specific but uncrossmatched blood can be obtained very quickly and in the rare critical situation group O Rhesus negative universal donor blood is given.

The ability of the child's vascular tree to compensate so effectively for quite large volume losses while maintaining an acceptable pulse rate and blood pressure has been emphasized. One must equate visible pallor after trauma in the younger child (i.e. under 10 or 11 years or older if physically small) with a blood loss of at least one-quarter the normal blood volume. *The normal blood volume should be estimated as approximately 75–85 ml/kg. One-quarter of this blood volume should be calculated and written down prominently*. This serves as an infusion unit and will be used throughout the resuscitation.

If the pallor of shock is noted, this unit of one quarter blood volume should be infused rapidly as a bolus. One should then slow the infusion down to maintenance rate and take stock. If a degree of clinical shock persists a second such bolus is needed. If the clinical situation seems to have been corrected it is wise to slow the infusion to maintenance rates. Should subsequent deterioration occur the physician may more confidently infer that bleeding is continuing. If, on the other hand, the infusion is kept running briskly continued bleeding will be partially replaced, signs of shock will be delayed, and the need for surgical intervention may be obscured, with resulting delay.

Table 3.2 Infusion fluids

Isotonic saline (0.9% NaCl)*		
Lactate Ringer's solution*		
0.45% NaCl in 2.5% glucose*		
10% Glucose*		
Plasma (pooled or protein fraction)*		
Mannitol†	50 ml vial of 25%	keep warm to prevent crystallization
	500 ml bag of 20%	
	1000 ml bag of 10%	

* See Appendix 8.
† See Chapter 2, *Table 2.2* and page 296.

SITES OF IV INFUSION

Although the long saphenous veins are customary sites for infusions in children they are not recommended when there has been trauma to the trunk. *A deep liver laceration or a tear of the inferior vena cava or one of its major tributaries can provide a route by which fluid infused into an ankle vein merely increases the volume already extravasated into the abdomen*. For this reason there must be a large bore cannula in at least one arm vein. On the other hand, one must not delay the resuscitation of a shocked child while repeated attempts are made to find an arm vein. A long saphenous cut-down (*see* page 732) is still a dependable and rapid route for infusion and must occasionally be used.

EFFECTS OF COLD BLOOD

A complication of massive transfusion seen occasionally in paediatric practice is cardiac arrythmia or arrest due to cold bank blood. The small blood volume of the child cools quickly even with small infusions if they are taken directly from the blood bank refrigerator. For this reason a blood-warmer should be installed in the infusion apparatus when large intravenous volumes are required. The simplest consists of a coil included in the venous line and placed in a water bath at 40°C (104°F).

AUTOTRANSFUSION

Rare instances occur in which rapid reinfusion of an accident victim's own blood (autotransfusion) is life saving. Ingenious autotransfusion units are available for the purpose of reinfusing large amounts of blood which have accumulated within either abdomen or chest. However, the time required to prepare the apparatus and to obtain it from storage once the decision to use it has been reached detracts from its practical value. Nevertheless, even without such equipment, direct reinjection by syringe into a large venous cannula of blood collected in a sterile basin as it drained from a chest tube is feasible. In such cases an appropriate filter may be

Table 3.3 Resuscitation drugs*

Adrenaline	1:1000 in 1 ml ampoule or 30 ml vial
Aminophylline	250 mg in 10 ml ampoule
Atropine	0.3 mg in 1 ml ampoule
Calcium chloride	(10%) 1 g in 10 ml ampoule
Calcium gluconate	(10%) in 10 ml ampoule
Dopamine	200 mg in 5 ml ampoule
Chlorpheniramine	10 mg in 1 ml ampoule
Dexamethasone	8 mg in 2 ml vial
Diazepam†	10 mg in 2 ml ampoule
Diazoxide	300 mg in 20 ml ampoule
Digoxin	0.05 or 0.25 mg in 1 ml ampoule
Frusemide (Furosemide)	20 mg in 2 ml ampoule
Glucose	(50%) in 50 ml ampoule
Hydralazine	20 mg in 1 ml ampoule
Hydrocortisone sodium	100 mg, 250 mg, or 500 mg in 2 ml vial
Isoprenaline	0.2 mg in 1 ml ampoule
Lignocaine	500 mg in 5 ml vial (other strengths also commonly used; see *Table 2.2* and page 272)
Methoxamine	20 mg in 1 ml ampoule
Morphine†	10 mg in 1 ml ampoule
Pethidine†	50 mg in 1 ml ampoule
Sodium bicarbonate	(7.5%) 44.6 mmol in 50 ml ampoule or (8.4%) containing 1 mmol of $NaHCO_3$ per 1 ml of solution
Sterile water	10 ml ampoule
Thiopentone sodium	1 g bottle
Vitamin K (phytomenadione)	5 mg in 1 ml ampoule

* For dosages *see* Chapter 2 *Tables 2.1–2.3*, or Appendix 11.
† Kept locked up for security reasons.

introduced into the venous line to remove the larger cell aggregates. In most instances autotransfusion will be a temporary measure designed to support circulation until surgical intervention can take place, and blood bank resources can be mobilized.

Acid–base changes (see also pages 117–121)

As tissue damage, blood loss and shock develop, progressive metabolic acidosis can result from the accumulation of acid metabolites. Most subjects in established hypovolaemic shock have a demonstrable metabolic acidosis. For this reason arterial sampling should be carried out as soon as possible. Indeed, it has been previously thought that administration of buffer should begin as soon as the infusions have been established for patients in hypovolaemic shock. Current trends are more towards permitting spontaneous correction of the acidosis as circulation improves, unless arterial blood studies indicate that the acidosis is excessive and jeopardizes cardiac function (pH under 7.1). It is apparent that the body's potential for buffering acidosis is very great. In addition, the alkalosis which can be the outcome of a resuscitation in which large amounts of bicarbonate have been administered is neither well tolerated nor easily corrected. It now appears that the single most important element in one's approach to the acidosis of shock is early and aggressive volume replacement.

Continuing care

As time passes serial haemoglobin and haematocrit values help in judging the amount of haemodilution that has occurred and may indicate the need for further transfusion.

Urine output per catheter must be measured from the outset in any child with multiple and serious injuries. This provides an excellent continuing indication of fluid balance (*see* Appendix 7).

Trauma team: organization and duties

Smaller hospitals may have only two or three physicians in the building at any time and their ability to handle effectively the initial resuscitation of a seriously injured casualty will be greatly increased by prearranged protocols and routines. Larger institutions may have organized trauma teams on duty at all times. In a university hospital where there is particular interest in trauma there may be full-time 'trauma fellows' who receive victims of trauma and carry out resuscitation and much of the definitive care.

The leader of the trauma team is usually a general surgeon. However, his specialty is less important than his ability to co-ordinate and to generate co-operation among the various specialists and his willingness to accept the ultimate responsibility.

In sophisticated trauma units each member of the team has a well-planned series of duties to be carried out, permitting resuscitation to proceed with a minimum of

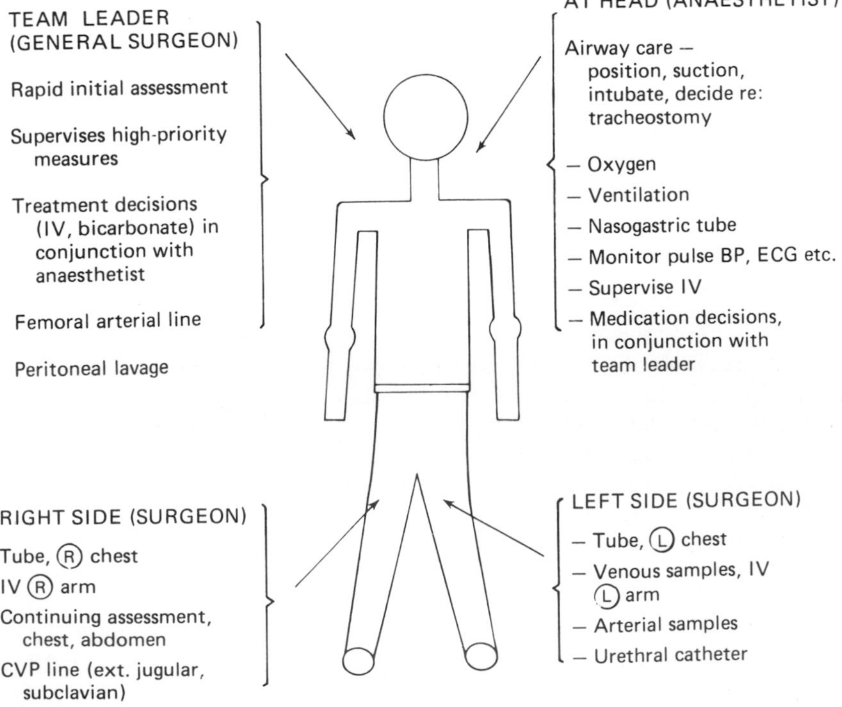

Figure 3.1 Trauma team – duty assignments

discussion and delay. The leader gives any orders necessary, supervises documentation, indicates further equipment or tests needed and makes descisions relating to further therapy.

Figure 3.1 shows one example of the various ways in which duties may be assigned to members of a trauma team.

Continuing evaluation

With the exception of those with serious head trauma, the majority of accident victims who die do so because of haemorrhage into abdomen or chest. Because of this, continuing assessment of trauma victims after resuscitation and for the ensuing few days consists largely of repeated examination of chest and abdomen.

Psychological trauma

Major and multiple injuries, unexpected hospitalization and surgery all have long-lasting emotional effects. Fractures unite, incisions heal, wound scars improve in time. However, the psychological scarring is deep seated and persists for many years. Gentleness and kindness shown by the nursing and medical staff from the moment of arrival are most effective in minimizing the psychological hurt. Painful procedures should be carried out only if really necessary. On the other hand, it is not kindness to omit a test or procedure that is important, because of the discomfort associated with it.

The psychological effects of trauma are now recognized and in many centres psychiatrists and psychologists are increasingly involved. It is hoped that this policy will become more widely accepted in the future.

Parents

The parents of the injured child are too often forgotten. Parents should be kept completely informed from the beginning. Although one is loath to cause undue concern, it is wrong to give them a falsely optimistic prognosis. It is better to expect the worst than to be given falsely high hopes initially and then have them destroyed.

One must listen to and act upon concerns expressed by parents about their child. On occasion a parent will, through an increased sensitivity, recognize a change in colour, breathing, or facial expression, which heralds an impending complication, a change which might otherwise have gone unnoticed.

Although parents will need to be excluded from particularly complicated procedures, it is reassuring both for parents and child to permit them to be together as much as possible. Most parents have the strength to enable them to remain calm and supportive while with their child and they appreciate the opportunity to observe the repeated and meticulous examinations which are so often needed. Nothing is more reassuring for parents than to see their child's condition improving before their eyes as a result of careful assessment and appropriate therapy.

Chapter 4

Burns: immediate management*

R. W. S. Miller

A burn may be caused by any of the following, the severity depending upon the duration of contact and the area of skin affected.

1. *Dry heat:*
   (a) Flash: a brief contact with a source of intense heat such as an explosion or burning petrol.
   (b) Flame: as in burning clothing.
   (c) Direct contact with a hot object.
   (d) Friction.
2. *Wet heat:*
   (a) Scald.
   (b) Steam.
3. *Chemical* – A chemical reaction generates heat. Beware of the ingestion of corrosives, strong acids or alkalis (*see also* Acute Poisoning, page 173; ENT Emergencies, page 198)
4. *Electrical:*
   (a) Arcing, which is an electric flash burn with contact completing the electric circuit. High local resistance produces localized deep burns.
   (b) Local heat, as from contact with the firebar of an electric fire.
   (c) Tetanic spasm of nerves and muscles due to the passage of current which prevents removal of the body from the electric source whilst local heat produces the burn.
5. *Ionizing* – Most forms of burn injury are obvious within seconds. Ionizing agents produce their effects in hours or days, depending upon the dosage. Long-term effects may be manifested after years.
6. *Burns combined with other injuries.*

Recognition

In extensive burns the picture is one of 'shock' becoming progressively more severe. The pulse is thready and rapid, the skin cold and clammy with little evidence of capillary filling. The breathing is at first rapid and shallow, but later

* (*See also* Chapter 5)

becomes gasping. The urine flow is inadequate for the effective clearance of waste products. Initially the patient may be alert and apprehensive, but as 'shock' progresses he becomes disturbed, noisy, disoriented and restless, complaining of thirst and cold.

Management

1. *Clear airway* – Make certain that there is a clear airway. If in any doubt call for immediate anaesthetic assistance and advice. Prepare for endotracheal intubation or tracheostomy as soon as possible.

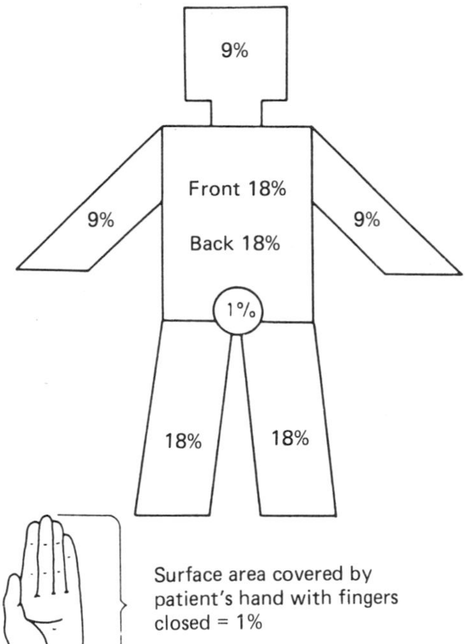

Figure 4.1 The 'Rule of Nines' assessment of burned area. For smaller areas a good guide is that the area covered by the patient's hand and fingers is 1 per cent of the body surface (Reproduced from Muir and Barclay (1974). By kind permission of authors and publishers.)

2. *Size of burned area* – Estimate the size of the burned area using Wallace's 'Rule of Nines' (*Figure 4.1*) as a rough guide, remembering that the palmar surface of the patient's hand is approximately 1 per cent of his total skin area. Compare the patient's hand with your own and roughly pat over the burned area to get an idea of the total extent. If the area is greater than 10 per cent in a child (excluding erythema) an intravenous infusion is necessary. Remember that there are variations in the area of skin of the head and lower limbs depending upon the age of the child; the 'Rule of Nines' over-estimates the area of the trunk and a more careful assessment should be done when resuscitation has started using Lund and Browder's chart (*Figure 4.2*).

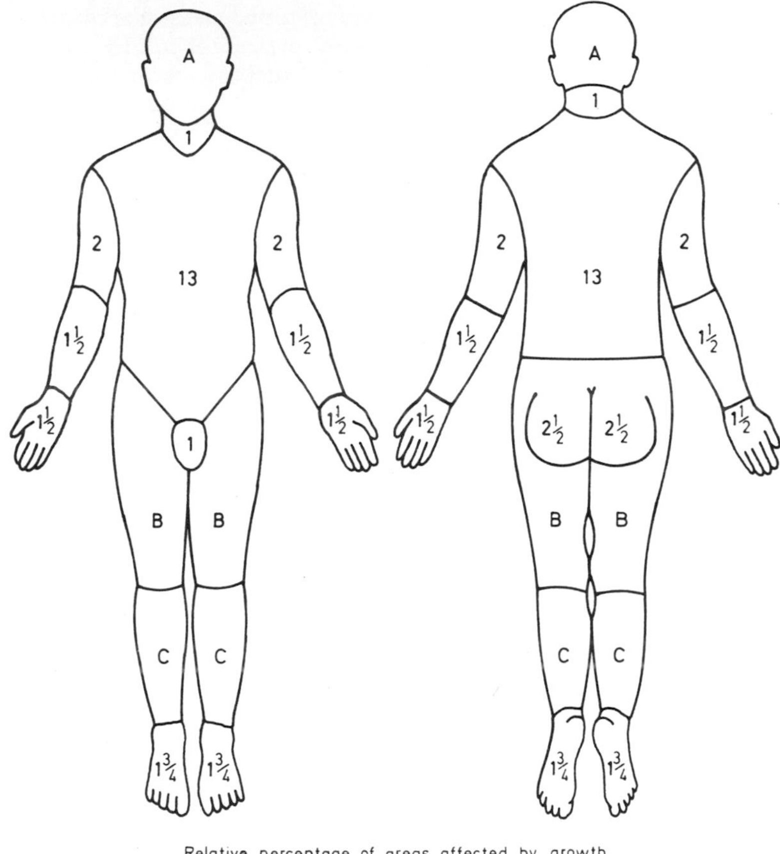

Relative percentage of areas affected by growth

Age in years	0	1	5	10	15	Adult
A - ½ of head	9½	8½	6½	5½	4½	3½
B - ½ of one thigh	2¾	3¼	4	4¼	4½	4¾
C - ½ of one leg	2½	2½	2¾	3	3¼	3½

Figure 4.2 Chart for the accurate examination of the area of burn. This can be used after resuscitation has been started (Reproduced from Lund and Browder (1944). By kind permission of Surgery, Gynecology and Obstetrics)

3. *Shock* – If the area of burn is greater than 10 per cent (excluding erythema) treat for shock:
   (a) Set up a reliable intravenous drip using the largest possible size cannula in an arm vein, securing it firmly. Use a vein beneath burned skin rather than one beneath unburned skin: no analgesics will be needed for a cut-down through burn eschar.
   (b) Withdraw a sample of blood and discard it. Then withdraw a further sample for:
      (i) Haematocrit.
      (ii) Full blood count, including platelets.
      (iii) Group and cross-matching.
      (iv) Plasma urea and electrolytes.
   (c) Put up a bottle of plasma or plasma protein fraction (PPF).

(d) Obtain a history of the accident and ascertain *the time when the accident occurred. The plan for fluid replacement is based on the time of the accident and not on the time of arrival in hospital.*

(e) Calculate the expected plasma requirement for each of five periods: 4 hours (*from the time of the accident*), 4 hours, 4 hours, 6 hours, 6 hours and 12 hours, using the formula devised by Muir and Barclay (1974):

$$\frac{\text{Total \% area burned (excluding erythema)}}{2} \times \text{weight of patient (in kg)}$$

$$= \text{ml per period}$$

Give the plasma at a rate that will ensure that the whole of the first 4-hourly quota is given in the time remaining. If more than 4 hours have elapsed since burning give the total volume in the next period. *See* page 31 for further consideration of fluid replacement.

(f) When the haematocrit is known calculate the volume of plasma deficit from the circulation, assuming that no red cell loss has occurred, by using the formula:

$$\text{Blood volume}^{*} - \frac{\text{Blood volume} \times \text{normal haematocrit}}{\text{observed haematocrit}}$$

$$= \text{deficit in ml.}$$ (**See Table 4.1.*)

Give the deficit as soon as possible in addition to the planned volumes, in each 4-hour period. If the burn is greater than 10 per cent of the total skin area there will be red cell destruction requiring blood. Blood should be ordered; the volume necessary being 1 per cent of the normal blood volume for every 1 per cent of whole skin loss burn.

(g) In addition to intravenous therapy water should be given by mouth for metabolic purposes. This should be given as 5 per cent glucose or 0.18 per cent NaCl in 4 per cent glucose. The exact amount of water necessary will depend upon the type of local treatment; exposure of the burn wound causes considerable evaporative water loss. Water should be given at the rate of 2–3 ml/kg body weight/hour initially; increasing the volume as the rate of the intravenous infusion decreases.

(h) If analgesia is required, and it rarely is once fluid is entering the circulation, give very small doses of morphine 0.1–0.2 mg/kg body weight well diluted intravenously. It will not be absorbed intramuscularly.

(i) If the burn is greater than 25 per cent insert a self-retaining catheter and lead it to a drainage bag via a burette so that the volume of urinary output can be measured hourly. (*See Table 4.1* and Appendix 7 *Table A7.2* for acceptable minimal hourly urine volumes.)

(j) Attend to the burn wound:
   (i) Assess the depth of involvement using a sterile needle. If sensation is present there will be partial skin loss only; if insensitive there is probably whole skin loss.
   (ii) Apply dressings to all burned areas except the face and perineum using an antibacterial cream or tulle, covered with gauze, Gamgee padding, and a crêpe bandage. If the hands are burned they should be smeared with an antibacterial cream and placed in a clean plastic bag taped at the wrist and elevated.

Table 4.1 Table of expected values

Age (years)	*Weight* (kg)		*Height* (cm)		*Haematocrit*		*Haemoglobin* (%)		*Blood volume* (ml)		*Metabolic water requirement 1st 24 h* (ml/h)	*Minimum hourly urine volume 1st 24 h* (ml)
	M	*F*	*M*	*F*	*M*	*F*	*M*	*F*	*M*	*F*		
Birth	3.5		50		60		145		260		30	10
6/12	7		65		36		80		520		30	11
1	10		75		38		85		750		30	12
2	12.5		87		38		85		940		30	13
3	15		95		38		85		1120		35	14
4	17		103		39		88		1270		35	15
5	19		110		39		88		1420		40	16
6	22		116		40		90		1650		45	17
7	24		124		40		90		1800		50	18
8	26		130		40		90		1950		55	20
9	30		135		40		90		2250		55	22
10	32		140		40		90		2400		60	24
11	35		145		41	40	93	90	2620		65	26
12	40		150		42	40	96	90	3000		70	29
13	45		156		43	40	98	90	3370		75	32
14	50		160		44	40	100	90	3750		80	35
15	54	52	168	161	44	40	100	90	4050	3800	85	35
16	58	53	172	162	44	40	100	90	4350	4000	90	35
17	62	54	174	163	44	40	100	90	4650	4050	95	35
18	64	55	175	163	44	40	100	90	4800	4120	95	35
Adult	70	60	175	163	44	40	100	90	5000	4500	100	35

From Muir and Barclay (1974). Reproduced by kind permission of authors and publishers.

(k) Prescribe antibiotics to prevent tetanus and staphylococcal infection. It is usual to use intramuscular benzylpenicillin, or cloxacillin if there are resistant organisms, for a limited period only.

(l) At the end of an hour reassess the patient's general condition. Estimate the fluid requirement for the next hour of the existing period and write it down on the fluid chart. Consider whether metabolic water requircments are best given orally or as additions to the intravenous regimen.

(m) Write down all that has been done, recording details of haematocrit values and volumes of fluid given together with relevant clinical findings.

4. *Hospitalization* – If the burns affect certain special sites (*see* below) it is essential that the patient should be admitted to hospital; otherwise burns of less than 7 per cent can be sent home after dressings have been applied.

Small burns and scalds

Small burns or scalds are often very painful, and there may be a considerable degree of anti-diuresis (ADH production). If electrolyte-free or electrolyte-low solutions (e.g. tea, water, fruit juice or squashes) are given by mouth in uncontrolled amounts there is a danger of fits from water intoxication and cerebral oedema (*see* Chapter 5, page 37; Chapter 26). It is just as important when giving *oral* fluids, as it is when giving IV fluids, to plan the amounts to be given, particularly over the first 48 hours, and to stick to it. For oral use a solution containing sodium chloride 5 g/ℓ and sodium bicarbonate 4 g/ℓ (Na 133 mmol/ℓ, Cl 85 mmol/ℓ, HCO_3 48 mmol/ℓ) is recommended. Acceptance is better if it is given chilled or flavoured with orange or other fruit juice. Normally the volume given per 24 hours should not exceed the child's normal requirements for age (*see* Appendix 3), but if borderline shock is present the volume can be increased to 1½ times the normal intake. For recognition and management of fits and cerebral oedema in burns, *see* page 37.

Special sites

The eye

If there is any suspicion that the eye or the eyelid has been burned, the advice of an ophthalmic surgeon should be sought urgently. As a first-aid measure instil 0.9 per cent NaCl and 1 per cent atropine eyedrops. It is essential to keep the eye moist.

The face and neck

If the burns of the neck are deep a tracheostomy is essential and should be done as soon as possible. When examining the patient it is necessary to look for evidence of burns of the tongue, singeing of the nasal hairs or soot in the airway, redness of the throat, or hoarseness. Obtain the advice of an ENT surgeon as to the best way to perform the tracheostomy. If the burn is not deep the child should be nursed on his back with his neck extended on a bolster.

The hands

The hands should be elevated. The nearest plastic surgery unit should be asked for advice about the future management.

Perineum

A burn of the perineum requires catheterization with a self-retaining catheter and sealed drainage.

Smoke inhalation (*see also* page 34)

Any person who has been in a smoke-filled room even if they have no evidence of burns on the face or elsewhere should be admitted for close observation for a period of not less than 24 hours.

Quarter-hourly examination of chest, breathing and intercostal action should be made for at least 6 hours. A watch should be made for the onset of hoarseness. Should there be intercostal indrawing or worsening of the hoarseness endotracheal intubation and tracheal toilet are urgent.

Other measures

1. If there are deep circumferential burns of the chest the burn eschar should be divided in the anterior axillary line on each side to improve breathing. No anaesthetic agent will be required. Similarly, deep circumferential burns of the limbs should be divided to prevent distal ischaemic necrosis.
2. The management of the burned child should be discussed with the parents, bringing them into the 'treatment team'. The treatment must be explained and the future outlook discussed. Parents may feel guilty about what has happened. This is manifested by questions about scarring, vision, speech, walking, etc. It is important to see both parents at the same time and to stress the importance of not looking for a scapegoat or finding someone to blame. The child needs their help during a long and painful illness as much as that of the medical and nursing staff. He must not be allowed to lose his trust in his parents. In some cases this talk will help to prevent the break-up of a family unit.
3. If the child's face is burned, it should be explained to the family that the swelling will cause an alarming appearance for a day or two, but that the swelling will go down. This should also be explained to the child if old enough to understand.
4. If there is a special unit for the treatment of burns in the area, the transfer of the child by ambulance should be arranged, but only after an intravenous infusion has been set up and been seen to be running well. A badly burned patient will travel well under these circumstances within six hours of the time of injury.

   A letter with the patient should include:

   (a) Type of accident and when it occurred.
   (b) Time when the infusion was set up, and type of fluids being given.
   (c) Volume of fluid given in ml.
   (d) Haematocrit value on admission and any other results since.

(e) The blood group, electrolyte and blood count results.
(f) Urinary output since admission.
(g) Dressings used, if any.
(h) Name and address of the nearest relatives and their telephone number.

References

LUND, C. C. and BROWDER, N. C. (1944) The estimation of areas of burns. *Surgery, Gynecology and Obstetrics,* **79,** 352–358

MUIR, I. F. K. and BARCLAY, T. L. (1974) *Burns and Their Treatment,* 2nd edn., p. 33. London: Lloyd-Luke

Chapter 5

Medical emergencies associated with burns and scalds

Roger Cudmore

Non-accidental injury (NAI) (*see also* Chapter 58)

It is important to remember that burns and scalds may be part of NAI. Suspicion should be raised if the story of how the injury occurred does not conform to the expected area of skin damage, particularly if the feet are involved in young children, who do not normally injure this area. There may be signs of other injury such as bruising or fractures, whilst the child may be withdrawn, fearful and quiet; crying is the normal reaction to a burn or scald. Cigarette burns leave clear rounded, reddened areas which can be overlooked.

After the initial assessment and resuscitation of the burned or scalded child, medical complications can occur at any time, so that their early recognition and treatment improves recovery and survival. Complications to be expected are those involving the respiratory, neurological, gastrointestinal, and renal systems, as well as septicaemia.

Respiratory complications

Any child rescued from a fire in a confined space, even though the area of skin damage may not be extensive, or one who has been scalded and possibly exposed to steam, is in danger of developing respiratory problems and needs admission with careful observation.

Carbon monoxide (CO) poisoning (*see also* Chapter 8, page 71)

Recognition

1. Confusion or unconsciousness when admitted, provided that other causes have been excluded (*see* page 36).
2. Cherry-red skin and lips. This may be obvious but is sometimes obscured by soot or burned skin. Look particularly at the back for this coloration. In pigmented skin, mucosal examination is essential.

Management

Take a specimen of blood for carboxyhaemoglobin (HbCO) by placing 2 ml blood in a heparinized tube. While awaiting the results give 100% humidified oxygen.

Intubation may be necessary and should be done early rather than wait for the blood results. A carboxyhaemoglobin level of less than 20% is unimportant. Greater than 60% is invariably fatal.

Inhalation of toxic gases

Apart from carbon monoxide, many toxic fumes are given off by burning materials. Smoke, produced before the flashpoint occurs and fire breaks out, contains poisonous substances including hydrocyanic acid.

Recognition

The history as related above should suggest the possiblity of damage from these gases which produce a loose cough and sooty sputum. Subsequently stridor, wheeziness and subcostal recession occur, but the onset may be slow with up to 24–48 hours for full respiratory distress to develop.

Management

1. Admission to an observation ward.
2. Chest X-ray. There are usually no changes on the early chest X-ray but this allows a baseline to be obtained.
3. Broad-spectrum antibiotic therapy should be started to prevent secondary infection.
4. Cautious physiotherapy should be started, for with a loose productive cough the child may produce large quantities of sputum, and even a cast of the trachea and bronchus.
5. Early intubation and bronchial lavage with the patient paralysed and ventilated may be the best treatment because of the copious secretions and oedema produced with these toxic fumes. In any case, because of carbon monoxide poisoning, the patient may already be intubated.
6. For the mild case of inhalation, corticosteroids have little part to play. Clear evidence of their usefulness in major pulmonary injury is difficult to justify. However, it is probably wise to give them at the same time as intubation and ventilation.
7. Careful intravenous fluid infusion to avoid overload.
8. Regular blood gas estimations.

Steam inhalation

The scalded child may have inhaled steam from hot liquid or swallowed some, causing damage to the upper airway.

Recognition

Careful inspection of the pharynx may indicate damage and if suspected think of early endotracheal intubation. If in humidified oxygen the child appears to be developing respiratory distress intubate early, because oedema of the larynx makes subsequent intubation almost impossible.

Pneumonia

Recognition

Lung parenchyma infections are likely to develop during the first weeks in very severe burns and particularly in those on ventilation. Rarely, empyema may occur.

Management

Frequent cultures of the sputum and upper airways will help in selecting a suitable antibiotic. Pneumothorax from a fall during burning should always be kept in mind but will be seen on an early chest X-ray.

Lung oedema

This is unlikely provided one of the standard methods of fluid replacement is used and adequate urine flow maintained. The efficacy of the fluid therapy can be easily checked by a haematocrit done at regular intervals of time. A low haematocrit (<30) indicates overload of fluid.

Recognition

The picture is one of acute pulmonary distress with a loose cough and tachypnoea, and sometimes cyanosis.

Moist sounds are heard throughout the lungs and a chest X-ray shows increased vascular markings.

Management

The intravenous fluid should be reduced in quantity and a diuresis induced by frusemide intravenously (1 mg/kg) or mannitol 10% (1 g/kg).

Neurological complications

Confusion

Recognition

1. In the initial stages after a burn or scald, confusion is likely to be due to hypoxia, from hypotension, or respiratory insufficiency. It should be borne in mind that the patient may have an associated head injury from falling while asphyxiated.
2. Confusion may also be present because of a drug, particularly morphine, having been given intramuscularly in the initial resuscitation phase.
3. Post-epileptic confusion.
4. Confusion developing after the initial resuscitation phase is over is usually due to hypoxia, often from splinting of the chest wall from burning of the skin.
5. Frequently it is a premonitory sign of septicaemia (*see* below).
6. An early sign of cerebral oedema (*see* below).

Fits

In children fits following burn injury used to be common but are now rare, due to adequate resuscitation. Fits occurring in the first 48 hours are usually due to cerebral oedema from water intoxication because of the production of ADH as a physiological response to injury and the excess of fluid that may be given by using electrolyte-free or hypotonic solutions. If plasma is given for resuscitation together with half-strength Hartmann's solution (Compound Sodium Lactate Injection; *see* Appendix 8) in 5% glucose (equal parts) hypotonicity is unlikely to occur. (*See also* page 31 for oral fluids in small burns.)

Recognition

A fit often occurs in a child with only a small area (<10%) of skin damage (*see also* Chapter 4, page 31). A base line plasma sodium level is not always available but at the time of the fit it is often under 130 mmol/ℓ and the urine shows a high osmolality.

Management

It is important to ascertain whether the child has had fits previously, particularly febrile ones, or if he is having treatment for fits. In the absence of this positive history then the fit is either due to hypotonicity or is the first febrile convulsion exhibited by the child.

1. A lumbar puncture should NOT be done since the cerebral oedema may cause coning (*see also* Chapters 26 and 93).
2. Diazepam should be given intravenously to control the fit but avoid its use with chlorpromazine.
3. Skin and rectal 'core' temperature should be recorded. Shivering and vasoconstriction may cause a low skin temperature with central hyperpyrexia. The skin is mottled and there is peripheral shutdown. Chlorpromazine may be given (10–25 mg) intravenously and slowly, but it should be remembered that the drug also lowers the blood pressure and careful monitoring is required. Extra plasma may be needed if the blood pressure falls.
4. If the sodium level is low it should be corrected with isotonic sodium chloride solution (0.9%).

Other causes of fits which must be considered

1. A febrile convulsion in a child with a previous history of similar episodes.
2. Hypertensive encephalopathy: this is a recognized complication of burns, especially in children: it appears to be related to inadequate fluid replacement.
3. Fits in a known epileptic. The burn itself may have been caused by a fit. Anticonvulsant treatment may have been stopped after admission for the burn, or hyponatraemia may have lowered the threshold for fits, even with anticonvulsant treatment.
4. Local damage to the brain in deep burns of the scalp, especially electrical.
5. Meningitis.
6. Toxic absorption of locally applied drugs. This possibility should always be considered when any new topical application is used.
7. Hypoglycaemia and hypocalcaemia are rare causes of fits in burns and scalds.

Renal complications

Haemoglobinuria

In an extensive deep burn where there is massive tissue destruction and bleeding into the tissues, haemoglobinuria is frequently seen in the first 24–48 hours after the injury.

Management

Diuresis should be induced by mannitol in a dose of 1 g/kg in 10% solution or with frusemide. Blood transfusion will be necessary to replace the rapid fall in haemoglobin as adequate oxygen transport is essential.

Renal failure

With adequate fluid replacement a urine flow of 1–2 ml/kg/hour should be maintained. If there is any difficulty in urine collection catheterization is vital (fluid replacement formulae are only a guide to treatment) and the intravenous rate will need to be adjusted with boluses of plasma to obtain this output. Oliguria can be improved with judicious injections of frusemide but if, despite adequate fluid flows and frusemide, oliguria and then anuria progress (as may happen in an extensive burn), peritoneal or even haemodialysis may be required. (*See* Chapter 48.)

Gastrointestinal complications

Children with a severe thermal injury develop an ileus and therefore oral fluids should be withheld in any large amount for the first 24–48 hours. With adequate resuscitation gastrointestinal haemorrhage or perforation is now rare.

Recognition

The patient may vomit blood or may collapse with all the symptoms of sudden haemorrhage. A silent perforation may occur, in which case the patient may become distended and abdominal X-ray will indicate the presence of free air.

Management

Blood transfusion should be started and gastroscopy will usually indicate the site of bleeding. Should the haemorrhage appear not to be decreasing despite adequate transfusion then operation is required to undersew the ulcer. Perforation will need laparotomy and possibly suture of the perforation with vagotomy and drainage.

Septicaemia

Septicaemia should always be borne in mind in a child who seems to be managing well and then becomes ill. In initial stages a burn is sterile so infection is unlikely to set in much before the third or fourth day. Frequently in a burned or scalded child there is a swinging pyrexia from the 4th to the 10th day which is due to toxins from sloughs that are separating, but blood cultures rarely show any true infection.

Recognition

Septicaemia should be suspected in the following circumstances:

1. Sudden collapse or deterioration or change in behaviour of the child.
2. A sudden rise or fall in temperature.
3. The onset of delirium.
4. The onset of oliguria.
5. The development of an ileus.

Often the child will become quiet, listless and pale.

Management

Blood cultures should be taken and a drip set up if one is not already in progress. Plasma should be given at a suitable rate appropriate for the child's weight and intravenous antibiotics such as an aminoglycoside and a broad-spectrum penicillin started immediately while awaiting the results of the blood cultures and wound swabs.

Circulatory changes

These may occur in children who have been electrocuted particularly those from transformers, overhead power lines or railway lines, in which a limb is damaged. The current flows down the vessels of the limb and although the circulation of the limb may be initially normal, peripheral gangrene sets in later.

Recognition

The limb may change colour intermittently before the periphery becomes red, blue, and then black.

Management

The changes are inevitable and infusion of heparin, low-molecular weight dextran or streptokinase have little effect, and inevitably amputation at some suitable level is indicated.

Further reading

CASON, J. A. (1981) *Treatment of Burns*. London: Chapman & Hall.

O'NEILL, J. A. (1975) Evaluation and treatment of the burned child. *Pediatric Clinics of North America,* **22,** 407–414

RAINE, P. A. and AZMY, A. (1983) A review of thermal injuries in young children. *Journal of Pediatric Surgery,* **18,** 21–26

SETTLE, J. A. D. (1974) *Burns: The First 48 Hours*. Romford, Essex: Smith & Nephew Pharmaceuticals

VIVORI, E. and CUDMORE, R. E. (1977) Managment of airway complications of burns in childhood. *British Medical Journal,* **ii,** 1462–1464

Chapter 6

Drowning and near-drowning

John Pearn

Introduction

The majority of paediatric immersion accidents are preventable and morbidity among survivors is low. A serious immersion accident is one in which consciousness is lost in the water; and the outcome may be death, delayed death due to near-drowning (Frates, 1981), survival with physical sequelae (Oakes *et al.*, 1982), survival with intellectual deficit alone, or complete recovery. Survival rates vary with age and sex, and with the temperature and osmolality (salt versus fresh) of the water involved. For young children in fresh water, survival rates approach 50 per cent. In the case of salt water at temperatures not below 15°C (59°F), survival rates approach 70 per cent. The history of the immersion incident has to be taken simultaneously with the continuation of life support in the emergency room. The interpretation of the survivor's clinical state in the hours or days after rescue depends on a knowledge of the factors surrounding the near-drowning. Children drown in a variety of sites and situations, one of which may involve non-accidental injury. Epileptic children are at increased risk from drowning (Sonnen, 1981), but the number of epileptic children who actually drown is small.

Pathophysiology

Most young children drown in chlorinated fresh-water pools, in the sea, or in bathtubs with variable concentrations of soap, but the chemical effects of chlorine or soap are not of practical clinical consequence. Oceanic sea water contains 34.5 g/kg of dissolved salts, of which 2.9 per cent is sodium chloride. Fresh water contains variable amounts of organic material, dissolved salts, and free and nascent gases. Both types contain pathogenic organisms. From the point of view of the near-drowning episode itself, the osmolality of the water is unimportant.

There are several ways in which subjects die while in the water. Brain death is the end-result, but the first link in the chain may be cerebral hypoxia, carbon dioxide narcosis, laryngeal spasm, vagal cardiac inhibition, or ventricular fibrillation. With both salt and fresh water, entry of water into the bronchial tree results within minutes in a transudation into pulmonary vein blood such that the blood looks almost water clear for a short time. At the modal age for paediatric drownings (the 2-year-old child) the diving reflex still operates to some degree. The submerged child manifests bradycardia and blood shunting from the cutaneous and visceral beds to the cerebral and coronary circulations, and blood pressure starts to rise immediately (Elsner, Gooden and Robinson, 1971). The submerged child holds his breath until the breaking point is reached. At water temperatures between 15 and 20°C (59–68°F), the immersion time necessary to cause death is believed to be between 3 and 10 minutes, but longer immersion times (5–20 minutes) are still compatible with survival. Very long immersion times (up to 40 minutes) are compatible with both survival and normal neurological function in children immersed in very cold water (0–15°C) (Conn, Edmonds and Barker, 1979).

The breaking point, when a breath must be taken, is determined by both the hypercarbic and hypoxic drives, acting synergistically, and occurs at $PaCO_2$ levels below 55 mm Hg (7 kPa) if there is associated hypoxia, and above 90 mm Hg (12 kPa) if the $PaCO_2$ exceeds 45 mm Hg (6 kPa). Gasping occurs under water, and glottal spasm may follow. The sequence of pathophysiological events in the lungs after fluid inhalation is as follows:

1. Increased peripheral airway resistance.
2. Variable degrees of laryngeal spasm.
3. Reflex pulmonary vessel vasoconstriction, leading to pulmonary hypertension.
4. Decreased lung compliance.
5. Ventilation–perfusion ratios fall.
6. Fluid shifts occur across the alveolar membrane.
7. Surfactant loss occurs (salt water), or properties alter (fresh water).
8. Foam and froth production.
9. Anatomical changes in alveolar epithelial cells.

The sequence of events in the progression from initial immersion to final brain death is as follows:

1. Voluntary apnoea.
2. Diving reflex (with shunting of blood from the cutaneous and splanchnic beds) to a variable degree.
3. Arterial hypoxaemia.
4. Tachycardia and hypertension.
5. Tissue hypoxia.
6. Tissue acidosis.
7. Inhalation with aspiration of water, or glottic spasm; leading to secondary apnoea; consciousness lost at variable places in the sequence. Decreased lung compliance.
8. Involuntary respiratory movements, continuing under water until respiratory arrest occurs.
9. Bradycardia.
10. Arrhythmias.
11. Hypotension, and loss of cerebral and coronary perfusion.
12. Cardiac arrest.
13. Brain death.

Dry drowning is NOT due to water aspiration, but results from laryngeal spasm or mechanical blockage by mucus and froth. The frequency of dry drowning is variously estimated to be from 10 to 20 per cent (Modell, 1978). A small amount of water enters the larynx or trachea, and reflex laryngeal spasm occurs, followed by an outpouring of thick mucus and development of foam and froth. When the spasm relaxes pre-terminally, further water may be prevented from entering the lungs by the foam–froth–mucus plug.

In older children, the dangerous practice of hyperventilation before underwater endurance games or dives causes the hypercarbic drive to breathe to be lost, and unconsciousness may occur (from cerebral hypoxia) before the hypoxic breakpoint is reached. Under these circumstances underwater gasping will occur with the patient unconscious. In all children who are drowning, besides gasping, large quantities of water may be swallowed even before consciousness is lost, and vomiting is likely with aspiration of gastric contents.

First aid

First aid of the apparently drowned is standard, whether at the rescue site, or in the casualty department while intubation, monitors, defibrillators and related hardware are being co-ordinated. The airway must be cleared, initial breaths given, the carotid pulse checked and (if absent) combined external cardiac compression (ECC) and expired air resuscitation (EAR) given. Even in children who are truly dead when extracted from the water, correctly administered cardiopulmonary resuscitation (CPR) should cause some lessening of pupillary dilatation, and the body should become pink to some degree. Technically poor CPR, or CPR not commenced within 10 minutes after rescue, are unfavourable prognostic factors. EAR may be difficult because of the reduced compliance of the water-containing mechanically altered lungs. The pressure used to inflate the lungs of the near-drowned subject (in both salt and in fresh water) has to be greater than that used in victims who are apnoeic from causes other than immersion. There is a danger of over-inflation during EAR, and interstitial emphysema and air embolism can be produced.

Approximately 80 per cent of victims who survive make their first respiratory gasp within 5 minutes of rescue and many do so within the first minute. It is very important that an unconscious but breathing near-drowned child be managed (both at the site of rescue, during transport, and in the emergency room or casualty department) in the coma position, as regurgitation of large amounts of water from the stomach is common.

Of all children who are pulled unconscious from the water and who do survive, less than 5 per cent will be brain damaged. Thus all children extracted from the water must be given the benefit of skilled resuscitation despite the apparent hopelessness of the situation, or of the real fears about possible prognosis. For fresh-water drowning in warm water, there is little point in continuing after 45 minutes and certainly not after 1 hour, in the absence of vital signs. It is of course essential to determine that confusing circumstances, cold water, medications, etc. are not clouding the clinical situation. If technically good resuscitation is applied, the hypothermic brain can withstand hypoxia up to 1 hour in extreme cases. For this reason there is no need to be concerned, while giving first aid, about body temperature unless this is below 28°C (82°F), until adequate ventilation in the casualty department or emergency room can be re-established. If a child regains consciousness quickly after extraction from the water, death may still occur from secondary drowning (Pearn, 1980). Thus it is essential that all near-drowned children be admitted to hospital for observation, at least for 24 hours.

Clinical history

In the emergency room or casualty department, while the child is being assessed (and life support instituted and maintained where necessary), it is important that as full a history as possible be obtained. Key factors are as follows:

1. Documented time of accident, or estimate.
2. Type of water (salt, fresh), and degree of contamination.
3. Approximate temperature of water, or estimate.
4. An estimate of the duration of the immersion, or an estimate of the bracket of time during which the child is believed to have been immersed.
5. Details of rescue.
6. Documentation of resuscitation attempts, time lapse before CPR was attempted after extraction from the water, the presence of vomiting during resuscitation.
7. Time to the first spontaneous gasp after apnoea.
8. Details of transport to hospital and maintenance of CPR (or otherwise) during transport.
9. Specific features surrounding the immersion incident itself.
10. Details of other illnesses, e.g. epilepsy, asthma.

The possibility of associated injuries should also be considered. Although they are not common, it is essential that if the near-drowning accident was precipitated by a closed head injury (e.g. by a fall, or by dumping in surf) that the medical team be aware of this. The possibility of dislocated cervical spine from diving accidents falls into this category.

Clinical examination

The near-drowned child may present to the doctor as (1) fully conscious; (2) conscious but with a blunted sensorium; (3) unconscious but breathing; or (4) comatose requiring respiratory and/or cardiac support. Special attention must be paid to examining and recording the state of respiratory, cardiovascular and neurological systems, body temperature, and to the elucidation and documentation of pulse, blood pressure and ECG, as soon as the child reaches the doctor's surgery or casualty department. This is essential, as evidence of hypoxic myocardial damage may be important when decisions about the use of barbiturates are being made.

Clinical examination for the presence of inhaled stomach contents, and for pneumothorax are important; air crepitation subcutaneously may reveal the presence of pneumomediastinum. In the central nervous system, various post-immersion syndromes may be encountered: spasms, epileptic seizures, opisthotonic stiffening, and the progressive neurological deterioration (which may lead rapidly to coma) which is secondary to pulmonary surfactant inactivation or loss. It is important to grade the level of consciousness accurately (1) to use this as a baseline in those patients where deterioration occurs; and (2) as an essential guide for triage classification which may determine the intensity of treatment. If the child is conscious but cold (and it is common for near-drowned children to be admitted with temperatures of 35°C (95°F)), it is important to realize that a blunted sensorium or unusual behaviour may be due to hypothermia rather than being the result of hypoxia. Interpretation of clinical signs is difficult if hypothermia is present (Eggink and Bruining, 1977). A proportion of near-drowned children have an elevated body temperature within three hours after rescue. Some are agitated, screaming, disoriented, depersonalized, or occasionally combative.

Tests and investigations

Chest X-rays

An urgent chest X-ray is required in all cases, however well the patient may appear at the time of admission. In the unconscious child, serial chest X-rays may be needed every 4–6 hours, or more frequently if positive end-expiratory ventilation (PEEP) is being used. Surgical emphysema may have occurred following tracheostomy, and children who have received CPR may also have a pneumothorax. Radiological changes of pulmonary oedema are seen in some 85 per cent of all cases, including (1) no findings; (2) perihilar pulmonary oedema; (3) generalized pulmonary oedema; (4) pulmonary oedema with localized floccular condensates, or any of these patterns with signs of pneumonia, aspiration, or pneumothorax superimposed. There is no difference in the radiological appearances after drowning in salt or fresh water; the heart is usually normal. Irrespective of the degree of hypoxic brain damage, radiological clearing of the lungs usually occurs within 3–5 days.

Blood gases

Assessment of the arterial PaO_2, $PaCO_2$, pH, and base excess are necessary both for (1) initial evaluation and as a guide to therapy; and (2) the establishment of baseline levels against which clinical improvement (or deterioration) can be judged. Arterial hypoxaemia is an early and sensitive indicator of lung damage; a low PaO_2 may persist even after post-aspiration intra-pulmonary shunts can no longer be demonstrated. Acidosis, rather than hypercarbia, is the critical factor which produces death. Respiratory arrest is complete when pHa levels fall to 6.5. The Siggard–Andersen nomogram can be used. The pH of the near-drowned victim varies, with an average of 7.25, and an average base deficit of 10 mmol/ℓ. Twenty per cent of all cases have an initial pH of 7.0 or less (Fandel and Bancalari, 1976). Acidosis and hypoxia are additive in the production of circulatory collapse at PaO_2 levels below 25 mm Hg (3 kPa), and at pHa levels below 6.80. When acidosis occurs there is an initial transient respiratory component, followed by a metabolic acidosis. Although there are many exceptions, a pHa of under 7.0 is a bad prognostic sign (Kruus *et al.*, 1979). In the absence of lung complications, the acidosis should be correctable and stable within six hours.

Throat and tracheal swabs

Throat and tracheal swabs should be taken on admission and daily thereafter in all but those cases who are improving rapidly. The coliform content of most swimming pools is high, and bacterial, fungal, or protozoan infections may follow near-drowning in both salt-water and fresh-water cases.

Respiratory function tests (RFT)

Respiratory function tests should be undertaken as early as is practicable in children over the age of six years. Baseline RFTs, established before the child is discharged from hospital, are a valuable method of serial documentation of convalescence, which may take many weeks to return to normal.

Blood

Baseline haemoglobin, white cell count, and electrolyte levels should be estimated although changes are rare. Blood cultures should be taken if there is any suspicion of pneumonia, and if there is any significant neurological deterioration after the first 24 hours. Serum osmolality should be measured in all cases, and checked serially if frusemide and fluid deprivation are being used to prevent raised intracranial pressure. If appropriate, plasma levels of anticonvulsants should also be measured, as should blood alcohol in children over the age of 12 years.

Electrocardiogram

An admission ECG is required in all cases, and continual ECG monitoring in all comatose patients, and in all those who are deteriorating. In the acute situation, an ECG is required to distinguish asystole from other hypoxic arrhythmias, and also to detect a hypothermic heart beating in sinus bradycardia with low output. Many arrhythmias will resolve spontaneously as the child is rewarmed.

Central nervous system

If a child remains comatose for more than six hours or so, both EEG and ICP monitoring should be initiated. Brain damage may be due not only to the primary anoxic insult, but also to reduced cerebral perfusion secondary to raised ICP. If raised ICP does develop, it is not likely to be an acute phenomenon in the first 12–24 hours after rescue. CT scanning should also be undertaken in comatose patients not responding within the first few hours after admission; uncommon cases of subarachnoid haemorrhage may also be detected, and such scanning will be required to interpret cerebral atrophy in those cases going on to a permanent vegetative existence.

Skeletal X-rays

Child abuse is a likely cause in 10 per cent of bathtub drownings. Therefore, in all but the most straightforward cases of bathtub drownings, a radiological skeletal survey should be arranged. Skull and cervical injuries may also be precipitating factors in the near-drowning episode. For this reason, especially in older children, if there is any doubt at all about what happened at the time of the drowning accident, it is desirable to X-ray the cervical spine.

Management

Admission and nursing care

Because of the potential of 'secondary drowning', all survivors should be admitted to hospital, and if the child is conscious the parent should also be admitted. In the unconscious child, tracheal toilet and suctioning must be careful and gentle, because of the tendency to increase intracranial pressure suddenly. If the child is recovering spontaneously but is hypothermic at admission and is conscious, it is best to let warming occur spontaneously. If the child remains comatose within several hours after extraction from the water, controlled hypothermia may be induced as part of a neurological-salvage plan, and under these circumstances temperature may be maintained in the region of 30–32°C (86–89.5°F).

Fluid managment

In the survivor who is conscious, no special care is required. If ICP is being monitored, and pressure is raised, this should be treated by a combination of barbiturates, hypothermia and fluid restriction (*see* page 295). If the child is being ventilated with a guarded airway, nutrition can be started early, by an intragastric tube.

Drugs

If the child is comatose on admission, and in asystole, intravenous or intracardiac adrenaline may be required: intra-tracheal instillation of 1 in 1000 adrenaline tartrate seems to be as effective. Acidosis must be corrected by intravenous bicarbonate, used empirically at first, and subsequently on a planned dosage basis if the pH falls below 7.2. Dopamine may be used but is less effective in severe acidotic states. Dexamethasone can be used after the first two hours if intracranial pressure is raised (*see also* Chapter 26), in an empirical dose of 2–4 mg eight hourly for up to two days. Prophylactic antibiotics should be used both in fresh-water and in salt-water cases. Necrotizing pneumonitis from inhaled impurities such as mud, sand, and sewage is a potentially fatal complication and under these circumstances early and vigorous antibiotic therapy should be commenced.

Ventilation

All dyspnoeic survivors, and all survivors in whom respiratory function is decreasing, should be nursed in an oxygen tent. PaO_2 of less than 60 mm Hg (8.0 kPa) breathing air, or less than 80 mm Hg (10.6 kPa) breathing oxygen, is an indication for mechanical ventilation. An arterial CO_2 tension above 56 mm Hg (7.5 kPa) is also an indication. Tidal volumes of 12–15 ml/kg are usually appropriate. Ventilator mode should be CPAP/PEEP (continuous positive airway pressure; or in the case of the intubated child with a closed circuit, positive and expiratory pressure). Although all near-drowned comatose children should be intubated and PEEP used, older children who will tolerate a mask will benefit from CPAP rather than the simple breathing of atmospheric air. PEEP is usually started at 2.5 cm H_2O, the effect on pulse and blood pressure noted and the level titrated individually up to a maximum of 10 mm Hg (0.67–1.33 kPa). PEEP is required for periods ranging between 12 and 60 hours, one day being an average. $PaCO_2$ should probably not be reduced below normal levels, as post-anoxic cerebral perfusion may be reduced. When the arterial blood gases are stable, and there are no further progressive changes in the chest X-ray, an attempt should be made to wean the patient off PEEP.

Barbiturate rescue (*see also* Chapter 26)

The use of barbiturates in the post-hypoxic phase has become well established (Smith, 1977; Hagerdal *et al.*, 1978). Recent studies on near-drowned children have used phenobarbitone in a total dose of 50 mg/kg/day on the first day, and 25 mg/kg/day for days 2–4 inclusive. It should be used only in patients who are still comatose within 2 hours or more after extraction from the water. In desperate cases (that is in those still comatose in the intensive care unit several hours after rescue, and certainly in those with fixed dilated pupils) nothing is lost by attempting barbiturate rescue, induced hypothermia and artificial ventilation.

Complications in the post-rescue period

In survivors of near-drowning in buckets, chemical disposal trenches and pits, and sewage ponds and dams, chemical necrosis of the trachea and larynx may occur, with necrotizing pneumonitis. Such cases must be treated by débridement with humidity control, steroid cover, and high dosage antibiotic cover.

Gastrointestinal bleeding occurs in up to one-third of all near-drowned children who require mechanical ventilation (Fandel and Bancalari, 1976) and prophylactic cimetidine should be used. 'Secondary drowning' (Pearn, 1980) can occur within several hours after rescue. Symptoms include developing tachypnoea, a burning retrosternal pain, rasping hoarse cough, expectoration of increasing amounts of frothy pink sputum, increasing cyanosis, respiratory failure and coma. High inspired oxygen concentrations, CPAP, or intubation with PEEP is the treatment.

When to stop therapy

In the absence of cardiac activity (on ECG monitoring) and with fixed and dilated pupils, if there is no history of hypothermia or epilepsy or alcohol ingestion, it is wise to stop resuscitation attempts after 1 hour from the time of extraction from the water.

In children with adequate cardiac perfusion, with modern therapy using barbiturate rescue with or without hypothermia, the decision to stop treatment is not appropriate in the first 3 or 4 days after rescue, as it may take this time for even a neurologically salvageable child to surface after iatrogenic coma. If the decision is made to stop therapy, it is essential that this be documented using the established criteria (*see* Chapter 27).

Prognosis

In over 90 per cent of cases, a child who is going to survive recovers rapidly without physical or intellectual sequelae. A small percentage recover without physical sequelae, but with minimal evidence of neurological impairment. In the case of near-drowned children, intellectual improvement can continue for several months after a successful rescue. Physical survival may occur, but with spastic quadriplegia and a vegetative existence. Of all children who are pulled from the water apparently dead, the incidence of this outcome is not greater than 3 per cent. Of children who are still comatose with fixed dilated pupils when they reach the intensive care unit of a referral hospital, the incidence of gross spastic quadriplegia and gross mental retardation is higher, and occurs in about 10–40 per cent of survivors.

Conclusion

The doctor involved in managing the convalescence of a near-drowned child is in a unique position to promote vigorous preventive action both in the family involved, and in the community more generally. Drowning ranks second after motor vehicle accidents as a cause of violent child death in most Western communities. Children who have survived a near-drowning episode have no greater fear of the water than before the accident, and without positive preventative action, some 6 per cent of these children will find themselves again in a life-threatening situation in the water within three years after the initial accident. Doctors caring for near-drowned children in the emergency situation are those best placed to promote, with vigour, the preventative steps of education, better safety design, and legislation which will reduce such accidents in the future.

References

CONN, A. W., EDMONDS, J. F. and BARKER, G. A. (1979) Cerebral resuscitation in near-drowning. *Pediatric Clinics of North America,* **26,** 691–701

EGGINK, W. F. and BRUINING, H. A. (1977) Respiratory distress syndrome caused by near- or secondary drowning and treatment by positive end-expiratory pressure ventilation. *Netherlands Journal of Medicine,* **20,** 162–167

ELSNER, R., GOODEN, B. A. and ROBINSON, S. M. (1971) Arterial blood gas changes and the diving response in man. *Australian Journal of Experimental Biology and Medical Science,* **49,** 435–444

FANDEL, I. F. and BANCALARI, E. (1976) Near-drowning in children: clinical aspects. *Pediatrics,* **58,** 573–579

FRATES, R. C. (1981) Analysis of predictive factors in the assessment of warm-water near-drowning in children. *American Journal of Diseases of Children,* **135,** 1006–1008

HAGERDAL, M., WELSH, F. A., KEYKHAH, M., PEREZ, E. and HARP, J. R. (1978) The protective effects of a combination of hypothermia and barbiturates in cerebral hypoxia in the rat. *Anesthesiology,* **49(3),** 165–169

KRUUS, S., BERGSTRÖM, L., SUUTARINEN, T. and HYVÖNEN, R. (1979) The prognosis of near-drowned children. *Acta Paediatrica Scandinavica,* **68,** 315–322

MODELL, J. H. (1978) Biology of drowning. *Annual Review of Medicine,* **29,** 1–8

OAKES, D. D., SHERCK, J. P., MALONEY, J. R. and CHARTERS, A. C. (1982) Prognosis and management of victims of near-drowning. *Journal of Trauma,* **22,** 544–549

PEARN, J. H. (1980) Secondary drowning involving children. *British Medical Journal,* **ii,** 1103–1105

SMITH, A. L. (1977) Barbiturate protection in cerebral hypoxia. *Anesthesiology,* **47,** 285–293

SONNEN, A. E. (1981) Epilepsy and swimming. *Monographs in Neurological Sciences,* **5,** 265–270

Further reading

BROOKS, J. G. (1981) The child who nearly drowns. *American Journal of Diseases of Children,* **135,** 998–999

CONN, A. W., MONTES, J. E., BARKER, G. A. and EDMONDS, J. F. (1980) Cerebral salvage in near-drowning following neurological classification by triage. *Canadian Anaesthetists' Society Journal,* **27,** 201–209

JENKINSON, S. G. and GEORGE, R. B. (1980) Serial pulmonary function studies in survivors of near drowning. *Chest (Chicago),* **77,** 777–780

MODELL, J. H. (1971) Definitions and descriptions. In *The Pathophysiology and Treatment of Drowning and Near Drowning,* pp. 9–12. Springfield, Il.: Charles C. Thomas

MODELL, J. H. and CONN, A. W. (1980) Current neurological considerations in near-drowning. *Canadian Anaesthetists' Society Journal,* **27,** 197–198

MODELL, J. H., GRAVES, S. A. and KUCK, E. J. (1980) Near-drowning: correlation of level of consciousness and survival. *Canadian Anaesthetists' Society Journal,* **27,** 211–215

ORLOWSKI, J. P. (1979) Prognostic factors in pediatric cases of drowning and near-drowning. *Journal of American College of Emergency Physicians,* **8,** 176–179

PEARN, J. H., DeBUSE, P., MOHAY, H. and GOLDEN, M. (1979) Sequential intellectual recovery after near-drowning. *Medical Journal of Australia,* **i,** 463–464

PETERSON, B. (1977) Morbidity of childhood near-drowning. *Pediatrics,* **59,** 364–370

POZOS, R. S. and WITTMER, L. E. (eds.) (1983) *The Nature and Treatment of Hypothermia.* London: Croom Helm

von HAERINGEN, J. R., BLOKZIJL, E. J., van DYL, W., KLEINE, J. W., PESET, R. and SLUITER, H. J. (1974) Treatment of the respiratory distress syndrome following nondirect pulmonary trauma with positive end-expiratory pressure with special emphasis on near-drowning. *Chest,* **66,** 305–345

YOUNG, R. S. K., ZALNERAITIS, E. L. and DOOLING, E. C. (1980) Neurological outcome in cold water drowning. *Journal of the American Medical Association,* **244,** 1233–1235

Chapter 7

Cold injury

M. P. Ward

Environmental cold injury may be conveniently classified into:

1. *General* – Accidental hypothermia or 'exposure'. This occurs in either wet and cold or dry and cold conditions. By definition, hypothermia occurs when the central core temperature falls below 35°C (95°F).
2. *Local:*
   (a) Immersion injury: when the tissues are at 0°–15°C (32°–59°F) for long periods.
   (b) Frostbite: when the tissues are at 0°C (32°F) – that is in dry and cold conditions. More than one type of cold injury may occur at the same time in an individual (Ward, 1975).

Environmental hypothermia

With the increasing popularity of all forms of outdoor pursuits, especially mountain-walking and sailing, as a substitute for field games, the number of children and adolescents exposed to the risks of cold injury has greatly increased in the last few years.

About 40 per cent of victims of mountain accidents in the British Isles are under 21 years of age and a number suffer from hypothermia, apart from other injuries.

As a normal part of the 'character-building' process children are exhorted to exhaust themselves physically while playing games under controlled, though often atrocious conditions. In the natural environment such exhortation can lead to hypothermia and death, and should be avoided.

Children and adolescents at risk are those who run away from home and sleep out, and youths on mountain expeditions who are inadequately prepared, or overtaken by very bad weather.

Factors important in the development of hypothermia

Fatigue

1. A recent illness may result in the unduly rapid onset of fatigue.
2. Inadequate food intake.
3. Changes in weather. The increased physical exertion necessary to walk into a gale-force wind may result in exhaustion and hypothermia.

4. Fear engendered by unfamiliar surroundings and changing weather conditions can precipitate exhaustion.
5. Adolescents may be unable to regulate energy output and have little in reserve. (In field games under controlled conditions these tendencies present no problem; in the mountains they can be disastrous.)
6. Rough, uneven ground, and deep soft snow also cause undue fatigue.

Clothing

Insulation depends on the trapped, still air in the clothes. External wind removes the warmed microclimate of the body and the heat loss increases rapidly.

As water is a good conductor of heat, water, either from outside as rain or inside as sweat, will also cool the microclimate.

Internal garments (i.e. shirt, sweater, vest) should be kept dry and protected from the wind. A water-repellant, moisture-permeable, wind-proof anorak should be used.

Eiderdown loses insulation when wet. Artificial 'down' though a less effective insulator when dry has comparatively better insulating qualities when wet.

Clothing should be put on and taken off as necessary to maintain an equable body temperature and prevent sweating. Wind-proof and water-proof clothing should be put on before the inner clothing has become wet. Boots should fit well, to prevent blisters. Mitts should be used for the hands.

Socks and stockings should have a high wool content.

Heat loss from the head may be considerable and some form of 'Balaclava' should be worn.

Environmental factors

It is not always appreciated that the environmental temperature falls by 1.5°C (3°F) for every 300 m (1000 ft) of ascent. Also a combination of wind and low temperature has an extreme chilling effect.

Recognition

The individual often starts stumbling, and there is muscular incoordination and finally rigidity. Changes in mental outlook occur, with instability and non-cooperation, apathy and confusion. Convulsions may occur followed by unconsciousness. Death has been reported within 2–3 hours of the onset of symptoms. However, 'dead' patients who are cold to the touch and apparently moribund, without respiration or pulse, have been known to recover.

Management

The commonsense precautions already outlined together with a balanced, sensible general outlook are necessary.

In the field

It is better not to try to exercise the patient 'to come out' of hypothermia. He should be sheltered from the wind, while wet clothes are removed and replaced by dry ones. External heat is applied by huddling together. Hot fluids (+ glucose) should be given if possible. The patient must be insulated from the ground as well as the wind and placed in a bag of impermeable material to prevent further heat loss.

Heat loss from the lungs occurs in a hypothermic patient despite perfect insulation. Provision of heated humidified air to breathe abolishes this loss and provides a method of central rewarming. If oxygen is breathed through soda lime, the interaction of exhaled CO_2 and soda lime provides both heat and moisture for the patient. Portable equipment is available for first aid treatment in the field (Lloyd and Frankland, 1974).

In the hospital or the 'Centre'

Central-core temperature should be measured with a low-temperature thermometer in the rectum.

Though the patient may appear dead, i.e. cold, pulseless and without respiration, recovery may still occur. The depressed respiration relates to low oxygen needs.

Hot bath treatment (rapid rewarming) (Davies, 1975; Jackson, 1975)

The unconscious patient is immersed fully clothed in a bath at 45°C (113°F) (as hot as the hand can stand). The temperature of the water should be monitored. The risks of rapid rewarming are:

1. An 'after-drop' or fall in central-core temperature. Because of surface vasodilatation deep-core blood is further cooled as it enters the chilled superficial tissues.
2. Surface vasodilatation may exaggerate hypotension.
3. Exhaustion may result in loss of thermoregulation. Hot bath treatment in these cases may be contraindicated. Once the patient has a regular heart beat and respiration, he is removed from the bath and placed flat under blankets in an air temperature of 36°–40°C (97°–104°F). An awkward movement or a poor carrying technique may further depress respiration.

Ideally all hypothermic patients should be air-lifted by helicopter to an Intensive Treatment Unit. Here facilities are available to monitor ECG, arterial pressure, plasma electrolytes, pH, PCO_2, PO_2, etc. The use of warmed IV fluids should be considered. Central warming through the airway should also be considered using an oxygen–helium mixture; alternatively a heart–lung machine could be used.

The airway must be kept clear but insertion of endotracheal tubes can cause reflex bradycardia and precipitate ventricular fibrillation, as can oesophageal thermistor probes.

Immersion injury

The mainstays of treatment are rest, analgesics, and general rewarming. If frostbite is a possiblity rapid rewarming must be undertaken. Surgery should be postponed for several weeks.

Frostbite (Ward, 1974)

This occurs in dry and cold conditions, i.e. at or below 0°C (32°F), when the tissues freeze. It is common on exposed parts such as the nose, ears, and cheeks, especially when there is a wind which lowers the effective skin temperature. Temperature variations may be considerable and individuals should dress for the temperature with which the part is likely to be in contact (e.g. while the ambient temperature may be many degrees above freezing, the feet in powder snow can be many degrees below freezing).

Clothes and boots should fit well so as to prevent any constriction of the blood supply. Insulation must be adequate for the prevailing conditions.

Pathophysiology

These are two main processes:

1. Ice crystals form and enlarge in the extracellular fluid. The intracellular osmotic pressure rises, and enzyme mechanisms are disturbed, with resulting cell death.
2. A vascular reaction occurs under the frozen tissue, with damage to the blood vessel walls. Plasma leaks into the tissues, forming blisters. The remaining intravascular blood becomes more viscous (sludging). Thus end-arteries may get blocked, with resulting tissue necrosis.

Recognition

Frostnip

This produces reversible changes. The skin blanches and becomes numb with sudden cessation of cold and discomfort.

Superficial frostbite

Damage to the tissues occurs. The adjacent skin and subcutaneous tissue are involved but the part though white and frozen is soft and pliable when pressed. Blisters may form within 24–28 hours depending on the site of the injury. Then blister fluid is absorbed leaving a black carapace which is insensitive. In certain sites carapace formation may occur without blistering. There is associated oedema and within weeks a line of demarcation forms. Throbbing and aching may persist for weeks. If the contour of the blackened carapace corresponds to the original area then loss of tissue is unlikely.

Unlike that of arteriosclerosis, the dry gangrene of frostbite is normally superficial, being only a few millimetres thick.

Deep frostbite

This involves the deeper structure, bone, muscle, and tendons. The affected part is cold, feels 'solid' and unyielding, and is a mottled blue or grey. It may remain swollen for months, and blistering is not inevitable although it can take weeks to develop. Initially the part is painless, but abnormal sensation may be present.

As tendons are more resistant to cold injury than skin, the patient will be able to move fingers and toes despite their gangrenous appearance. Thus even the most severely frostbitten patient can walk or move his fingers clumsily. Permanent loss of tissue is almost inevitable and this may be estimated from the loss of contour of the affected part.

Even with a diagnosis of deep frostbite a limb may return to normal over some months and amputation should never be carried out until a considerable period, say 6–9 months, has elapsed.

Management

Frostnip

This is the only form of frostbite that should be treated on the spot. Each person should watch for signs on the exposed portions of companions. As soon as whitening of the skin occurs, a place sheltered from the wind should be found, and the affected part warmed. Once normal colour and consistency is obtained, normal working is resumed.

Frostbite

The affected part should NOT be rubbed with snow or the normal hand. It neither melts the ice crystals, nor increases the blood supply, but only breaks the skin and increases the chances of infection. All other forms of violent therapy are open to the same objections.

Rapid warming seems the most effective treatment. It has the advantage that it can be done in primitive conditions, once a tent or similar shelter has been reached, so shortening the time that the blood vessels remain frozen.

Once active rewarming has been started it seems doubtful if any other form of treatment is beneficial.

The extent of the tissue loss may be determined by radioactive technetium. Accurate results are obtainable only some time after initial exposure.

METHOD

A container with water at 43°–44°C (111°F) should be used (measured by thermometer) as water that is too hot will damage the tissues. If a thermometer is not available the temperature should be assessed with the normal, unfrostbitten finger. It should not be too hot for comfort. If no container is available hot water poured over a towel or cloth wrapped around the part may be used. Warming should last for 20 minutes at a time. The temperature of the water should not fall below 42°C (108°F).

If rewarming by fluid is impossible, the part should be placed against a warm armpit or abdomen. It should never be placed by an open fire as it is partially anaesthetized and can be burnt without pain.

After rewarming, the part should be cleaned, and dirt removed gradually and gently. Blisters should be left as they form a covering.

Soft, dry, absorbent dressings between the fingers and toes will prevent further damage. So long as the affected part is warm and does not get rubbed it may be kept exposed. Later, active exercises will be necessary to prevent joint stiffness.

Surgical intervention must be minimal; the blackened carapace will gradually separate without interference and efforts to hasten this separation are usually ill advised and are likely to lead to infection and loss of tissue.

Rapid rewarming is the mainstay of treatment. Low molecular weight dextran and immediate sympathectomy using intra-arterial reserpine have been used (Bowman, *et al.*, 1980).

Young patients are emotionally labile and must be mentally prepared for the possibility of amputation.

Closure of amputation stumps by skin flaps is preferable to the use of grafts.

Evacuation

Once the treatment of frostbite has started, the part should be protected from any mechanical injury, such as walking. Treatment should only be started at a camp from which evacuation by helicopter, car, porter, or animal is possible.

Damage to frostbitten tissue before treatment can obviously occur, as in walking off a mountain. Yet in the mountain environment it may be quicker and safer for the frostbitten patient to reach a convenient place for evacuation by his own efforts before starting treatment.

Late effects

The skin may be scarred and hypersensitive, and the nails atrophied or deformed. Joint contractures may occur, and causalgia and hyperhidrosis have been reported.

In children, the epiphysis may be damaged, leading to deformity in adult life. The distal phalanges and joints are most commonly involved. Later, surgery may be necessary to correct deformities (Bigelow and Ritchie, 1963).

Erosive lesions in the joints with secondary arthritic changes have been reported (Welch, *et al.*, 1974; Carrera, *et al.*, 1981).

Hypothermia and frostbite

If these occur together the treatment of hypothermia should have priority as it is potentially lethal.

References

BIGELOW, D. R., BONIFACE, S. T. and RITCHIE, G. W. (1963) The effect of frostbite in childhood. *Journal of Bone and Joint Surgery,* **45B,** 122–131

BOWMAN, D. L., MORRISON, S., LUCAS, C. E. and LEDGERWOOD, A. H. (1980) Early sympathetic blockade for frostbite. Is it of value? *Journal of Trauma,* **20,** 744–749

CARRERA, G. F., KOZIN, F., FLAHERTY, L. and McCARTY, O. J. (1981) Radiographic changes in the hands following childhood frostbite injury. *Skeletal Radiology,* **6,** 33–37

DAVIES, L. W. (1975) The deep domestic bath treatment for advanced cases of hypothermia. In Clarke, C., Ward, M. P., William, E. S. (eds.). *Mountain Medicine and Physiology.* Alpine Club.

JACKSON, J. A. (1975) Personal communication.

LLOYD, E. L. and FRANKLAND, J. C. (1974) Accidental hypothermia: central rewarming in the field. *British Medical Journal,* **iv,** 717

WARD, M. P. (1974) Frostbite. *British Medical Journal,* **i,** 67–70

WARD, M. P. (1975) *Mountain Medicine. A Clinical Study of Cold and High Altitude*. St. Albans: Crosby, Lockwood, Staples

WELCH, G. S., GORMLY, P. J. and LAMB, D. W. (1974) Frostbite of the hands. *The Hand,* **6,** 33–39

Further reading

LLOYD, E. L. (1986) *Hypothermia and Cold Stress*. London: Croom Helm.

POZUS, R. S. and WITTMER, L. E. (eds.) (1983) *The Nature and Treatment of Hypothermia.* London: Croom Helm.

Chapter 8

Acute poisoning

J. A. Henry

Introduction

Poisoning in childhood is a common and important emergency. The majority of cases consist of accidental ingestion, with minimal toxicity, because the substance is non-toxic or the amount taken was small. However, serious poisoning also occurs, and prompt action to determine the likely severity and provide the appropriate treatment is necessary in all cases. A false sense of security, due to a succession of cases which present no problems, must be avoided.

The causes of poisoning in childhood are numerous (*Table 8.1*). While most cases are due to accidental ingestion in children between 1 and 4 years of age, non-accidental poisoning must be considered, and self-poisoning and drug or solvent abuse enter into the diagnosis above the age of 10. The main causes of fatal accidental poisoning are given in *Table 8.2*, and poisoning from these agents obviously deserves special attention.

Table 8.1 Aetiology of poisoning in childhood

Age (years)	*Accidental*	*Non-accidental*	*Breast milk*	*Iatrogenic*	*Deliberate self-harm*	*Substance abuse*
0–6/12		○	●	●		
6/12–4	●	●		○		
4–10		○				○
10–14					●	●

●, Common; ○, rare.

Recognition of poisoning

Diagnosis (*Figure 8.1*)

The ingested material can usually be identifed by a careful history. The drugs available in the home, any bottles or containers involved, and the place where the ingestion took place often help in identifying the poison. In plant or mushroom ingestion, a portion of the plant or a complete mushroom should be obtained if possible. Any vomit or urine should be saved.

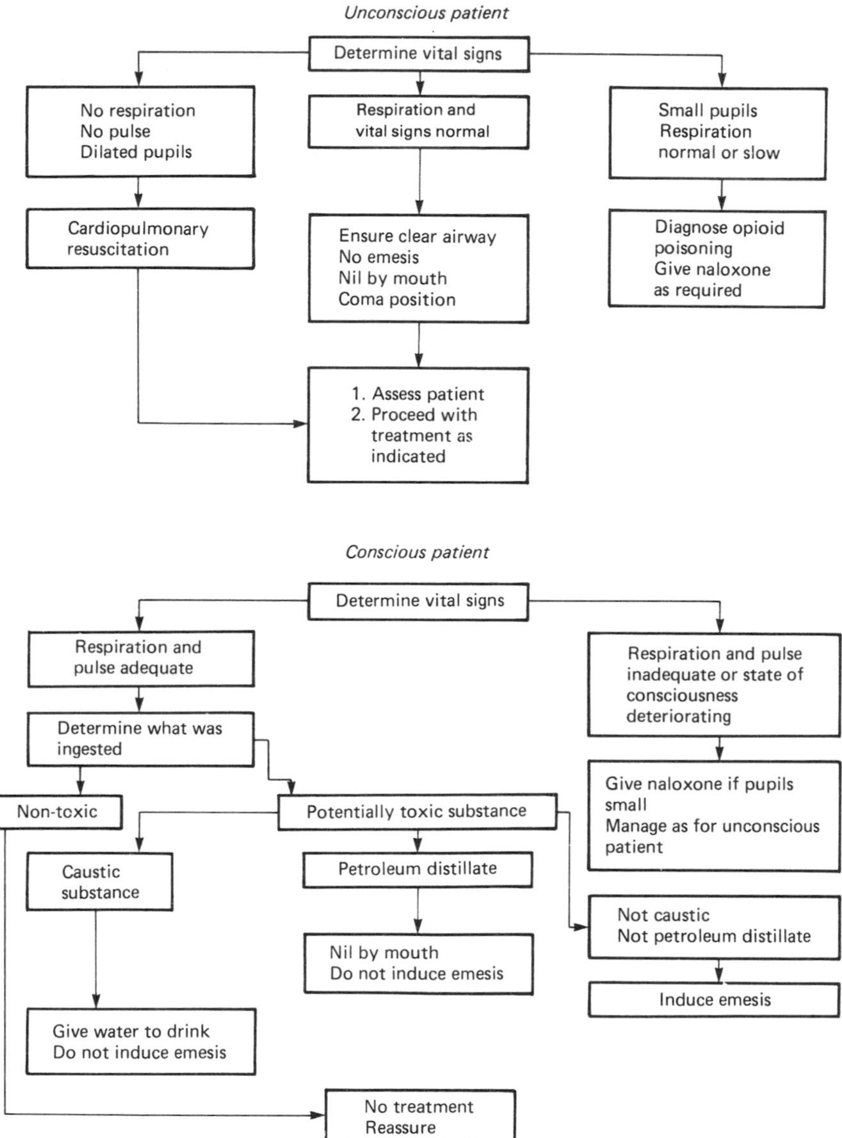

Figure 8.1 Action in suspected acute poisoning

The initial history should include what was taken and how much. With tablets, a count of those missing will provide an estimate. Where the substance taken is a liquid, a swallow for a 3 year old can be taken as approximately 4–5 ml. Frequently a child is found with part of the liquid spilt over itself or over the floor, so that the amount remaining is often a poor guide. *However, the physician should always accept the largest estimate of the amount ingested in determining the course of action.*

Table 8.2 Causes of death from accidental poisoning in children, 1974–80*

Cause		*No. of deaths*
Medicinal products		
Central nervous system drugs:		45
Tricyclic antidepressants	26	
Barbiturates	5	
Diphenoxylate	6	
Methadone	2	
Orphenadrine (Disipal)	2	
Others	4	
Analgesics:		10
Salicylates	8	
Others	2	
Other drugs		14
Quinine/chloroquine	5	
Potassium preparations	3	
Iron	2	
Others	4	
Household products		
Household products:		10
Cresol (Wright's vaporizing fluid)	2	
Acid, alkali, disinfectant	3	
Alcohol	1	
Others	4	
Other causes		
Lead poisoning		6
Carbon monoxide		5
Medical mishaps:		8
Digoxin	5	
Chloramphenicol	2	
Morphine	1	

* From Craft A. W. (1983). Circumstances surrounding deaths from accidental poisoning 1974–80. *Archives of Disease in Childhood*, **58**, 544–546.

Where the child is symptomatic, physical examination may reveal the evidence for poisoning by a particular agent, and the possibility of poisoning should always be considered in the differential diagnosis of an acute illness, especially when there are unexpected or suspicious physical signs. Many drugs and poisons produce characteristic signs of toxicity: some of the more common clinical features associated with poisoning are given in *Table 8.3*.

The lips and mouth should be inspected for burns or discoloration, and the vomitus should be inspected. There may be a smell on the breath. The general condition should be assessed, with particular attention to the level of consciousness, incoordination, tremor, or unusual behaviour, and evidence of hallucinations. Inspection of the pupils, body temperature, heart rate, and blood

Table 8.3 Symptoms and clinical and metabolic changes occurring in poisoning
(This list is not exhaustive but includes some of the major agents involved)

Vomiting	Caused by many drugs, plants and corrosive chemicals. The fact of vomiting helps to confirm suspected ingestion.
Haematemesis	Corrosives, iron, theophylline
Stuporose appearance	Sedative and hypnotic drugs, tranquillizers, opioids, antidepressants, anticonvulsants, alcohols, salicylates, solvent abuse, severe iron poisoning
Convulsions	Tricyclic antidepressants, quinine, antihistamines, theophylline, camphorated oils, lead (*see* Chapter 39)
Oculogyric spasms	Phenothiazines
Involuntary movements	Metoclopramide (Maxolon)
Hallucinations, agitation	Atropine, tricyclic antidepressants, antihistamines, amphetamines, psilocybe mushrooms ('magic mushrooms')
Pupils: dilated	Hypoxia. Hypothermia. Atropine, tricyclic antidepressants, glutethimide, antihistamines
Pupils: constricted	Opioids (including 'Lomotil'), organophosphorus compounds (insecticides)
Metabolic acidosis	Salicylates, ethanol, iron, tricyclic antidepressants, methanol, ethylene glycol, carbon monoxide
Hypoglycaemia	Insulin, oral hypoglycaemics, ethanol, ackee, salicylates
Renal failure	Salicylates, paraquat (especially Gramoxone and Dextrone X), mercury
Hepatic failure	Paracetamol, *Amanita phalloides* ('Death cap'), carbon tetrachloride

pressure are important; vomiting, diarrhoea, convulsions and coma are common in acute poisoning.

The comatose child

Drowsiness and coma should be classified by the simple system which is widely used:

Grade I – Drowsy but responsive to verbal commands.
Grade II – Responsive to mild painful stimulation.
Grade III – Minimal response to maximal painful stimulation.
Grade IV – No response to maximum painful stimulation.

Unlike adults, *children may become apnoeic even though still responsive to painful stimuli*, and a drowsy child should be admitted and kept under close observation until fully recovered. Investigations to exclude traumatic, metabolic, and infective causes of coma should not be postponed.

Non-toxic ingestions

Many cases of suspected poisoning are in fact non-toxic ingestions (and sometimes non-ingestions). It is important, once an initial history and assessment of the patient's condition have been made, to consider the maximum likely danger to the patient from this particular ingestion. If the child is asymptomatic, a simple plan of action should be followed:

1. Ascertain substance and amount taken.
2. Confirm that the ingestion is non-toxic (via literature or Poisons Information Service).
3. If non-toxic reassure parents and discharge patient.

Poisons Information Services can be of great help in determining the potential toxicity and symptoms of drugs, household agents and plants. The telephone numbers of the Poisons Information Services in the British Isles and Eire are given at the end of this chapter. Many agents are of such low toxicity as to be regarded as non-toxic, and a list of the more common substances is given in *Table 8.4*. Some of the plants may cause minor gastrointestinal irritation, which requires no treatment. Oral contraceptives can cause withdrawal bleeding in girls over 4 years of age, but hospital admission is not required. Detergents can also cause gastrointestinal irritation and possibly vomiting. In such cases reassurance of the parents and an explanation of any symptoms to be expected are all that is required.

Table 8.4 Agents of negligible acute toxicity and non-toxic agents

Non-toxic substances	*Non-toxic drugs*
Ball pen ink (less than 1 pen)	Ampicillin and other oral penicillins
Bath oil and foam	Simple antacids
Candles	Calamine lotion
Chalk	Homeopathic preparations
Cleansing cream	Laxatives
Crayons	Oral contraceptives
Dental disclosing tablets (for revealing plaque)	Prednisolone
Deodorants	Vitamins B, C, multivitamins (without iron)
Detergents	
Fish bowl additives	
Glues (water-based)	
Hair dyes and sprays	*Plants*
Hand lotion	
Ink	African violet
Lipstick	Antirrhinum
Lubricant oil	Begonia
Make-up	Berberis
Marking pens	Cacti
Matches	Coleus
Modelling clay	Cotoneaster
Oils for skin and hair	Cyclamen
Pencils	Dandelion
Putty; silly putty	Fuchsia
Shampoo	Grass
Shaving cream	Hawthorn
Silica gel (desiccant)	Mahonia (Oregon grape)
Suntan preparations	Orchids
Sweetening agents	Roses
Teething rings	Rowan
Thermometers (mercury)	*Skimmia japonica*
Toothpaste	Swiss cheese plant
Water colours	Violets

X-rays and laboratory investigations

A plain X-ray of the chest is particularly important if aspiration of vomit is suspected, and should be performed in every child who has ingested petroleum distillates. A plain X-ray of the abdomen may reveal the presence of tablets (this is particularly useful in the case of iron tablets and chloral; some phenothiazine tablets are also radio-opaque). It should be remembered that substances such as glass, mercury, paper clips, lead, and batteries are radio-opaque. Some solvents are also radio-opaque, and therefore ingestion of chemicals such as 1,1,1-trichlorethane (the solvent for typewriter correcting fluid) and carbon tetrachloride will show up like a blob of contrast medium in the stomach on X-ray of the abdomen.

Where a child is symptomatic or serious poisoning is suspected, haematological and biochemical investigations should be obtained. A metabolic acidosis is common. Some of the more important changes in laboratory tests are listed in *Table 8.3*.

Toxicology investigations

Toxicological analysis should not be requested merely to confirm poisoning, unless decisions about the child's management will need to be made on the basis of the result. Most pathology laboratories can perform assays of salicylate, paracetamol, iron, and barbiturates. Other toxicological investigations may have to be referred to a specialized laboratory. Do not hesitate to contact the doctor or biochemist of a toxicology laboratory if it is thought that they may be of help. Assays may be particularly helpful where theophylline, ethanol, methanol, ethylene glycol, solvents and metals are involved.

It is important to save samples of blood, urine and vomit on admission in case toxicological analyses are required later. These should be kept in a refrigerator at 4°C (40°F) until the episode is over and then disposed of if not required. Samples which may be required for solvent analysis or for paraquat should be taken into *plastic bottles*. Whole blood samples in an EDTA tube are necessary for carboxyhaemoglobin, mercury, and lead analysis. Consult the laboratory for details of sampling, storage and transport.

Aetiology (*see Table 8.1*)

Accidental

The commonest cause of poisoning in children aged under four years is accidental or more accurately inadvertent, where an unsupervised child is discovered ingesting something or presents subsequently with symptoms. Occasionally an older child aged 3 or 4 gives tablets or other agents to a younger child in imitation of adult behaviour. *Accidental poisoning is rare in children over 4.*

Non-accidental

Administration of poisonous agents occasionally forms part of the pattern of non-accidental injury. Other signs of non-accidental injury may be present, but poisoning may be the only manifestation, and is usually strongly denied on challenge. Common modes of presentation are repeated episodes of drowsiness, floppiness, or apnoea. Vomiting, hallucinations, or convulsions can also occur, depending on the substance given. The agents involved may be any medication prescribed to the parents (usually opioids, benzodiazepines, antidepressants, or insulin), or other substances available in the home, particularly salt. The child usually recovers in hospital but further episodes can follow visits by a parent (usually the mother). Repeated admissions with unexplained symptoms are suggestive of non-accidental poisoning (*see* Chapter 57). The earliest possible samples of blood, urine, or vomit should be collected and saved for biochemical analysis in order to confirm the diagnosis.

Iatrogenic

Both doctors and parents may be unaware of the proper dose of medicaments for children. Aspirin is the main offender, and fatal 'therapeutic' salicylate administration still occurs. Diphenoxylate is an opioid antidiarrhoeal agent which can cause severe respiratory depression. Opioid-containing cough-suppressant preparations given by the parents can also cause coma and respiratory depression. Errors can and do occur in calculating paediatric dosages. Therapeutic monitoring is essential when drugs such as theophylline, digoxin, anticonvulsants and chloramphenicol are prescribed to neonates.

Breast milk

Depending upon their physiochemical structure, drugs are excreted in breast milk in varying concentrations (*see* Appendix 15) and can cause toxicity in breast-fed children.

Deliberate self-harm

Self-poisoning can occur as part of a depressive illness in children as young as the age of 10, and parasuicidal behaviour is common in 'teenage' children (*see* Chapter 55). The acute management is similar to adult poisoning and these will not be considered further.

Addiction and abuse

Solvent abuse can occur in children of 8 years upwards (*see* Chapter 56). Abuse of heroin, cocaine, amphetamines and other drugs can occur in children as young as 10 years of age when promoted by a 'pusher'.

Resuscitation

The child who is severely ill, shocked, comatose or apnoeic needs all the usual resuscitative measures, irrespective of the cause (*see* Chapter 10). Further and more specific treatments can be given when the threat to life has been dealt with and the diagnosis is established.

Removal of the poison

Emesis

Removal of ingested poison by provoking vomiting with a finger is an acceptable procedure outside hospital but is less efficient than an emetic. Ipecacuanha, the safest and most widely used emetic, has superseded other emetic drugs. Other methods are not recommended and saline emesis can cause fatal hypernatraemia. In some countries, ipecacuanha is given to mothers to keep at home in case of accidental ingestion, when it is given after obtaining advice, over the telephone, from a poisons control centre. Once the child arrives in hospital, emesis should be induced if a toxic amount of the substance has been ingested within the last 4 hours. This should be done even if the child has reportedly vomited or been made to vomit at home. The method is to give 'syrup' of ipecacuanha (Paediatric Ipecacuanha Emetic Mixture, BP; this is equivalent in strength to Ipecacuanha Syrup, USP, and to the Adelaide Children's Hospital Formula (British National Formulary No. 11 1986)) with water or milk (do not give coloured liquids, as the colour of the vomitus may be a clue to the agent ingested or its amount). Dosages are given in *Table 8.5*. The principal contraindications to the use of emesis are:

1. Ingestion of corrosive substances, acids and alkalis.
2. Ingestion of petroleum distillates.
3. Increasing drowsiness, coma or convulsions.

Table 8.5 Use of ipecacuanha in small children (6 months to 4 years). In older children the method is similar but the dose is 30 ml syrup.

Indications

1. Conscious child
2. Suspected toxic dose of poison ingested less than 4 hours previously (longer for aspirin and tricyclic antidepressants).

Method

1. Give 15 ml ipecacuanha syrup
2. Give 200 ml water
3. Wait 15–20 minutes
4. If no vomiting give 15 ml ipecacuanha syrup
5. Wait 20 minutes
6. If no vomiting has occurred and emptying the stomach is considered essential, gastric lavage should be carried out.

Gastric lavage

Gastric lavage is rarely used in childhood poisoning, as emesis with ipecacuanha is easily performed and is efficient. However, lavage is indicated if the patient is comatose as a result of an agent ingested within the last 4 hours. Endotracheal intubation should be performed *first* to prevent aspiration of stomach contents; this is particularly important when toxic amounts of hydrocarbon have been taken. Sedation with intravenous diazepam may be necessary. A wide-gauge tube should be used, especially if the ingestion involves tablets or other particulate material.

After first aspirating all that can be removed, 50 ml amounts of water are passed into the stomach under gravity and allowed to siphon out, applying gentle suction if the tube blocks.

Activated charcoal

This is plant or petroleum residue charcoal with a large surface area and potent adsorbant capacity. Given orally, it will bind ingested poisons and prevent their absorption: it will also remove substances already absorbed, shortening their half-life and the course and severity of the poisoning. It can be given after an emetic has produced its effect, but *can bind ipecacuanha or other orally administered agents such as methionine*. Parents should be warned that the child's stools will be black. A list of substances adsorbed by charcoal is given in *Table 8.6*. Activated charcoal should be given where toxicity is anticipated and where its administration does not interfere with other courses of action. The preparations available are Medicoal (Lundbeck) in 5 g sachets as an effervescent suspension and Carbomix (Penn) in 50 g bottles. It can be given by mouth as a drink or by nasogastric tube, and can be left in the stomach at the end of lavage.

Table 8.6 Some poisons adsorbed by activated charcoal

Barbiturates	Paraquat
Dextropropoxyphene	Phenothiazines
Digoxin	Salicylates
Ethanol (ethyl alcohol)	Theophylline
Glutethimide	Trichlorethanol
Meprobamate	Tricyclic antidepressants
Methadone	Many plant toxins

As a rough guide 10 g of charcoal can be expected to bind approximately 1 g of the toxic substance, and charcoal is therefore more effective in treating poisons which are toxic in small amounts rather than those where the toxic dose is measured in grams. Doses of 5–10 g of activated charcoal should be given two hourly where indicated, usually in consultation with a poisons information service. Children over 10 should be given adult doses (50 g).

Cathartics

Where emesis or lavage are contraindicated, and also when a sustained-release or enteric-coated preparation has been ingested, the use of cathartics may be indicated. Magnesium hydroxide 10 ml should produce a purge and empty the gut within 2 hours. The dose can be given orally or left in the stomach following gastric lavage. Activated charcoal can be used as a marker and the dose repeated if necessary. This procedure can be used for poisoning with paraquat, quinine, tricyclic antidepressants and any slow-release preparation likely to cause toxicity, and when large amounts of hydrocarbons (*see below*) have been taken.

Other treatments

Drugs and antidotes should be used for the treatment of poisoning and its complications as described in the following section on specific poisons. Rarely, in life-threatening poisoning with certain agents, a specific method of drug removal may be indicated such as forced diuresis, haemoperfusion, peritoneal dialysis, haemodialysis or exchange transfusion, but these should only be carried out in consultation with a poisons information centre. These cases should be fully documented, as the literature is sparse, and a well-described case can be of great help to others. The National Poisons Information Service is grateful for all case summaries and data provided.

Specific poisons

Some of the more common poisons require special care in diagnosis or management, and are dealt with here in detail. They are listed below, together with some toxic emergencies which are covered elsewhere in this book. The possible range of poisoning problems is very great and readers are referred to texts on clinical toxicology and poisons information services for problems not dealt with here.

Drugs

Anticholinergic agents
Cardiac and respiratory drugs
Iron
Opioids
Paracetamol
Salicylates
Sedatives and hypnotics
Tricyclic antidepressants

Chemical poisoning

Alcohols and antifreezes
Battery ingestion
Carbon monoxide
Dry cleaning solvents
Essential oils
Household cleaning agents
Hydrocarbons
Paraquat

Plants

Plants, mushrooms and berries.

Poisoning problems elsewhere in the book

Acute lead poisoning (*see* Chapter 38)
Ackee poisoning (Acute Toxic Hypoglycaemia, Vomiting Sickness of Jamaica; *see* Chapter 70).
Venomous bites and stings (*see* Chapter 61).
Maternal drug dependence (*see* Chapter 92).
Solvent abuse (*see* Chapter 56).

Salicylates

Salicylates are considerably more toxic in children than in adults, and salicylate-containing preparations should never be given to children under 12 months because of the danger of iatrogenic poisoning due to accumulation, apart from the more remote risk of precipitating Reye's syndrome. Salicylates are found in aspirin (acetyl salicylic acid), oil of wintergreen, liniments, and some teething preparations though the latter rarely cause poisoning as the amount of salicylate is small.

Clinical features

Salicylates cause irritability, tremor, nausea, vomiting, and dehydration. Children old enough to speak will complain of tinnitus and deafness. Hyperpyrexia, convulsions, cerebral oedema, and renal failure may occur. Young children may become comatose, though older children usually retain consciousness, but may be confused. Salicylates can also cause an acute hepatitis and may also cause Reye's syndrome (*see* Chapter 47). Metabolic acidosis, ketosis, hypoglycaemia and hyperglycaemia may all occur. Diabetic ketoacidosis must be considered in the differential diagnosis, since the child may have acidotic (Kussmaul) breathing due to a metabolic acidosis, glycosuria, hyperglycaemia, and a positive test for ketones in the urine due to the presence of acetone.

Management

1. The child should be admitted if ingestion of over 100 mg/kg has occurred in a single overdose, or if toxicity due to therapeutic use is suspected.
2. A rapid screening check can be made by testing the urine with Phenistix or 10% ferric chloride solution. A brownish-red colour six or more hours after ingestion indicates probable salicylate toxicity, and the child should be admitted.
3. The plasma salicylate level should be measured on presentation, and again after six hours, in case it is rising. A level of 20 mg/100 mℓ in a young child receiving frequent doses of the drug therapeutically can be severely toxic. After a single overdose, levels of 30 mg/100 mℓ should be considered toxic in a child under four.
4. Emesis should be performed up to 12 hours after a single overdose or after the last therapeutic dose.
5. A Dextrostix test should be carried out in case of suspected hypo- or hyperglycaemia, and blood should be sent for biochemistry (electrolytes and glucose). INSULIN SHOULD NEVER BE GIVEN FOR HYPERGLYCAEMIA BECAUSE SEVERE HYPOGLYCAEMIA MAY DEVELOP WHICH MAY BE FATAL OR CAUSE PERMANENT BRAIN DAMAGE.
6. The child should be rehydrated with intravenous fluids and any metabolic acidosis or hypoglycaemia corrected.
7. If there are severe metabolic changes, accompanied by a salicylate level of over 30 mg/100 ml (following regular therapy for 24–48 hours or more) or over 50 mg/100 ml (after a single overdose), haemodialysis should be performed as soon as possible.

Paracetamol

Paracetamol toxicity in children is rare, possibly because the amounts ingested are relatively low, or because children are more resistant to hepatotoxicity. Liquid formulations (e.g. Calpol) are frequently taken in accidental overdoses, but the amount of paracetamol ingested is generally too small to present any risk.

Clinical features

The patient may be symptomless for the first 24 hours after ingestion, or may have nausea, vomiting, or sweating. By 24–36 hours after ingestion there may be hepatic tenderness and jaundice may be apparent. A prolonged prothrombin time is an early sign of hepatic damage, and the serum transaminases rise to a peak about 3 or 4 days after ingestion, returning to normal within a week in those who recover. Renal tubular necrosis can also occur, as shown by the development of polyuria in the absence of fluid overload or diuretics; the composition of the urine tends to approximate to that of the plasma (*see* Chapter 48, page 428).

Management

1. Emesis should be used for the patient presenting within 4 hours.
2. If a large amount has been ingested and the patient presents within 12 hours, treatment with antidotes should be started at once, without waiting for blood paracetamol levels. Methionine can be given by mouth (adult dose: 1.0 g initially, followed by 1.0 g every four hours depending on the plasma paracetamol concentration) if a patient is not comatose or vomiting; acetylcysteine should be given intravenously (initially 150 mg/kg in 200 ml 5% glucose infusion over 15 minutes, followed by 50 mg/kg in 250 ml of 5% glucose infusion over four hours and 100 mg/kg in 250 or 500 ml of 5% glucose infusion over 16 hours) if methionine is contraindicated.
3. An emergency plasma paracetamol value should be taken 4 hours after ingestion, and the antidote treatment can be stopped if the paracetamol level turns out to be below that requiring treatment.
4. Hepatic or renal failure should be treated as any case of hepatic failure (*see* Chapter 47) or acute tubular necrosis (*see* Chapter 48).

Iron

This drug is highly toxic to children, and the severity of iron poisoning should not be underestimated. Slow-release formulations are less toxic.

Clinical features

Vomiting is an early symptom and severe diarrhoea may also occur. Gastric erosions may cause haematemesis, and shock due to fluid and blood loss may develop within 6 hours of ingestion. Metabolic acidosis and convulsions may occur. The child can make an apparent recovery between 12 and 24 hours, but hepatic and renal failure are later sequelae appearing 24 hours or more after ingestion, accompanied by metabolic acidosis, hypoglycaemia and hypotension. Perforation of the bowel can occur early and intestinal stricture is not uncommon as a late complication after 2–6 weeks.

Management

1. Iron is radio-opaque, and an early abdominal X-ray may confirm ingestion and show the position of iron tablets in the gut.
2. If there are only minimal symptoms by 6 hours after ingestion of a non-slow-release formulation the patient can be sent home and late sequelae should not be anticipated.
3. Emesis should be performed unless the patient is severely shocked, when resuscitation takes precedence. Once resuscitation has been carried out, gastric aspiration and lavage should be performed in the intubated child. Oral

administration of a solution of desferrioxamine is sometimes recommended, and catharsis with magnesium hydroxide solution will help to propel tablets forward and out of the gut. This is especially useful for slow-release preparations.

4. Serum iron levels and iron binding capacity should be measured where possible. A serum iron value above 0.5 mg/100 ml is usually toxic, and a serum iron level considerably greater than serum iron binding capacity indicates serious toxicity.
5. If the plasma iron is in the toxic range and the child is symptomatic, 1 g desferrioxamine in 5 ml water should be injected intramuscularly and an IV drip set up so that desferrioxamine may be given by continuous infusion at a rate of 15 mg/kg/hour.
6. Adequate urine flow should be ensured otherwise the ferrioxamine chelate is not excreted and may cause toxicity. Haemodialysis or peritoneal dialysis are therefore required if the patient is developing renal failure.
7. Ferrioxamine chelate gives the urine a red or *vin rosé* colour, and this may be used to confirm poisoning and the need for continued treatment.

Tricyclic antidepressants

This group of drugs is the major cause of fatal childhood poisoning. Any case of ingestion should be treated seriously.

Clinical features

Hallucinations and excitability may give way to deepening coma. Muscle tone is increased and convulsions are common. Dilated pupils and tachycardia are due to the anticholinergic effects. Cardiac toxicity is shown by widened QRS complexes, arrhythmias and severe hypotension. Respiratory depression requiring ventilation is common in severe cases. The coma may last for days with full recovery.

Management

1. Any case of ingestion of over 75 mg should be admitted.
2. Emesis for a conscious child and gastric lavage for an unconscious child should be carried out up to 12 hours after ingestion of over 75 mg, and magnesium hydroxide can be left in the stomach. Activated charcoal should be given.
3. Plasma electrolytes and arterial blood gases should be measured and the electrocardiogram monitored.
4. Metabolic acidosis should be corrected.
5. Practolol should be used for arrhythmias (0.5 mg IV repeated as necessary), and if a cardiac arrest occurs, external cardiac massage should be carried out, as recovery can occur after long periods of massage.
6. Physostigmine salicylate can be used as an antidote to severe cardiac toxicity or cerebral toxicity with convulsions. The dose is 0.04–0.06 mg/kg by slow IV injection (over 3 minutes), repeated every 10 minutes to a total dose of 2 mg.
7. If there is respiratory depression with hypoxia, assisted ventilation should be commenced.

Anticholinergic agents

Phenothiazines, tricyclic antidepressants, atropine, the nightshade group of plants, delphiniums, travel sickness pills (e.g. hyoscine), some gastrointestinal sedatives and antispasmodics, stramonium, procyclidine (Arpicolin, Kemadrin), and orphenadrine (Disipal) can all cause the characteristic pattern of anticholinergic poisoning.

Clinical features

The patient is usually agitated, incoordinated, and hallucinating. The skin is warm, flushed, and dry, the pupils widely dilated, and there is a tachycardia and hypertension. In some cases there may be hyperpyrexia, convulsions, coma, and cardiovascular collapse. Symptoms may be sustained for 24–36 hours or more and may settle quite abruptly.

Management

1. Empty the stomach if the patient presents within 6 hours.
2. Most cases will resolve with conservative management. Diazepam is of little use.
3. Use sedation and external cooling if the core temperature is over 38°C (100.4°F).
4. If symptoms are judged to be life threatening, physostigmine salicylate should be given intravenously in a dose of 0.04–0.06 mg/kg by slow intravenous, subcutaneous, or intramuscular injection. This can be repeated every 10 min to a total dose of 2 mg.

Opioids

The opioids still cause deaths in children from accidental ingestion. One of the main offenders is diphenoxylate (Lomotil), but all opioids, including methadone, pentazocine, dextropropoxyphene (in Distalgesic, Cosalgesic), codeine, dihydrocodeine, and some proprietary cough mixtures can cause severe opioid toxicity.

Clinical features

Drowsiness or coma, pinpoint pupils, and slowed or irregular respiration are the cardinal features of opioid overdose. Hypotension, convulsions, vomiting and pulmonary oedema may also occur. The pupils may dilate due to anoxia or hypothermia, but may not dilate because of the atropine in Lomotil. Respiration may be rapid if a combined opioid/salicylate preparation has been taken. Symptoms may not develop for several hours after ingestion of diphenoxylate.

Management

1. Naloxone is the antidote of choice and should be given intravenously in doses of 0.2 mg as required.
2. If naloxone is not available, or if the patient is cyanosed or convulsing, assisted ventilation should be started immediately.
3. If the poisoning is severe, the patient should be intubated and gastric lavage performed.
4. An infusion of naloxone may need to be set up, particularly with long-acting agents such as methadone and diphenoxylate. The dose should be titrated against the patient's state.

Sedatives and hypnotics

Sedative and hypnotic drugs can cause excitability and occasionally hallucinations, but more often drowsiness. Larger doses cause central nervous depression, flaccidity and coma. Aspiration of vomit should be guarded against. Apnoeic spells may occur, and ventilatory support may be needed.

There are few other signs or complications. The pupils may be dilated in glutethimide poisoning and constricted in trichlorethanol poisoning. *Repeated episodes strongly suggest a highly disorganized household or non-accidental poisoning.*

Management

1. Resuscitate if apnoea occurs.
2. Mildly drowsy children can be observed while placed semi-prone to protect the airway.
3. If coma is deepening or the child is already deeply comatose, gastric lavage should be performed after first passing an endotracheal tube.
4. The endotracheal tube should be left in place and mechanical ventilation performed if respiratory depression is suspected or present.
5. In the comatose child when the possibility of accidental ingestion is denied and other diagnoses have been excluded, a toxicology laboratory should be consulted.

Cardiac and respiratory drugs

Drugs prescribed for the cardiac and respiratory illnesses of parent or grandparents may be ingested accidentally. The advice of a poisons information service should be sought for the toxic dose and likely symptoms. Three of the more common drugs are briefly mentioned here.

Beta-blocking drugs

Members of this group of drugs, particularly propranolol and oxprenolol, can cause bradycardia, hypotension, serious myocardial depression and coma.

MANAGEMENT

1. Give atropine for bradycardia, and induce emesis. Perform lavage if drowsy or comatose.
2. Glucagon (1 mg IV, repeated as required) is the agent of first choice in severe cases.
3. Alternatively, isoprenaline can be given by intravenous infusion titrating the dose against the patient's blood pressure.

Digoxin

This drug is frequently taken in accidental overdoses, but severe problems are fortunately rare, and small children usually tolerate plasma digoxin levels of 10 μg/ℓ without symptoms or electrocardiographic disturbances.

MANAGEMENT

1. Induce emesis and give activated charcoal.
2. Obtain a plasma digoxin level, and obtain a repeat level at least 12 hours after ingestion.
3. Monitor the electrocardiogram for evidence of heart block or rhythm changes.
4. Monitor plasma potassium levels. Hyperkalaemia is a complication of serious overdoses. The urgent treatment is as for hyperkalaemia (*see* page 130).
5. If there is clinical, biochemical, or electrocardiographic evidence of severe poisoning, consult a poisons information service about the use of anti-arrhythmic agents such as amiodarone and Fab antibodies for digoxin (digoxin-specific antibody fragments).

Quinidine/Quinine

Both quinidine and quinine can cause nausea and vomiting, blindness (with fixed dilated pupils and inability to follow movements), convulsions, cardiac arrhythmias, and cardiovascular collapse. The outcome may be fatal.

MANAGEMENT

1. Empty the stomach.
2. Give activated charcoal.
3. Symptoms of blindness resolve within 72 hours. Treatment is unnecessary.
4. Give diazepam for convulsions.
5. Give practolol (0.5 mg IV) for arrhythmias.
6. Prolonged cardiopulmonary resuscitation should be used if profound hypotension or cardiac arrest do not respond to conventional management.

Theophylline

Symptoms include vomiting, haematemesis, abdominal pain, irritability and hyperventilation. A sinus tachycardia is usual, and there may be hypotension, cardiac arrhythmias (usually supraventricular tachycardia), convulsions, hypokalaemia and hyperglycaemia. Coma is not common.

MANAGEMENT

1. Induce emesis, and give a purgative if the preparation is a delayed-release one.
2. Obtain a theophylline level. Over 3 mg/100 ml is a toxic plasma level in an acute overdose in children.
3. Hypokalaemia may be treated with a potassium infusion, but propranolol can reverse both the haemodynamic and metabolic changes. An infusion of 2.0 mg can be given intravenously over one hour, and may be repeated as necessary.
4. Convulsions should be treated with intravenous diazepam.
5. If there are serious symptoms (such as convulsions or cardiac arrhythmias), charcoal haemoperfusion should be considered.

Carbon monoxide (*see also* Chapter 5)

This colourless, odourless gas is produced in varying amounts when combustion of fuel occurs in the presence of oxygen. Accidental poisoning can arise whenever the products of combustion are inhaled in excess. Common sources are faulty or unflued heating apparatus, whether solid fuel, gas or paraffin; accidental poisoning occurs mainly during cold weather. Car exhaust fumes can also cause severe poisoning. Carbon monoxide combines with haemoglobin, with an affinity 240 times greater than that of oxygen, to form carboxyhaemoglobin. Transport of oxygen to the tissues is blocked, and symptoms are those of hypoxia.

Clinical features

Headache, lethargy, nausea and vomiting unaccompanied by diarrhoea, behavioural disturbances, hallucinations, convulsions, hyperventilation and tachycardia are all symptoms of moderately severe poisoning. A whole family can be affected by an illness which appears like food poisoning, and there is a wide range of other illnesses, from viral infection to an acute psychiatric disturbance, which carbon monoxide poisoning can mimic. A faulty car exhaust or a badly fitting hatchback or boot door may make the children ill in the back of a car, while the adults suffer no symptoms. The patient usually maintains a 'good colour', though the well-known pink colour of skin and mucosae may not be apparent either because of shock or when the patient has been removed from a smoke-filled house. Serious poisoning may be associated with focal neurological disurbances due to cerebral oedema or secondary to hypoxic cerebral damage. Severe poisoning can lead to cardiovascular collapse and respiratory failure, and exposure to high concentrations causes death within minutes.

Diagnosis

The circumstances and the clinical features of the poisoning should lead to the diagnosis, but a high degree of suspicion is necessary. Cellular hypoxia may lead to a metabolic acidosis, but arterial oxygen tensions are usually normal. Blood should be taken as soon as possible for carboxyhaemoglobin estimation; the normal level is about 1 per cent. Over 10 per cent carboxyhaemoglobin is diagnostic of exposure; lower levels can be produced by haemoglobin breakdown in severe haemolytic anaemia, or by smoking. Levels over 30–40 per cent indicate serious poisoning, and a carboxyhaemoglobin value of over 50–60 per cent is usually fatal. By the time the patient reaches hospital, diagnosis on the basis of the level of carboxyhaemoglobin in the blood may be difficult, even though the patient is obviously suffering from the effects of cerebral hypoxia, with or without cerebral oedema; this is because the half-life of elimination of carbon monoxide when breathing air is 250 minutes, but if he has been given 100% oxygen the half-life is reduced to 50 minutes (Meredith and Vale, 1984), so that quite low levels of carboxyhaemoglobin may be present after a short time, even when severe exposure has occurred.

Management

1. The victim should be removed from exposure.
2. Resuscitation is needed if respiratory effort is impaired.

3. Blood should be taken for carboxyhaemoglobin estimation, and 100% oxygen should be given by face mask if the patient is breathing satisfactorily or by assisted ventilation if respiration appears laboured or if resuscitation was necessary.
4. Cerebral oedema should be treated by intravenous mannitol, with intermittent positive pressure ventilation (IPPV) if necessary. Steroids are of little use. For management of cerebral oedema *see* Chapter 26 (page 295).
5. Consult a poisons information service about the use of hyperbaric oxygen.
6. Continue giving 100% oxygen for 48 hours, sedating the patient if necessary, and restrict physical activity for 2 weeks after severe exposure.

Alcohols and antifreeze

Ethyl alcohol (ethanol)

Apart from alcoholic drinks, ethyl alcohol is found in perfumes, eau-de-Cologne, and aftershave. Any case of ingestion should be taken seriously. Ethyl alcohol is a potent central nervous depressant, and after initial excitability can cause apnoea and deep coma. Hypoglycaemia is common and convulsions can occur.

Management

1. Use gastric lavage if over 0.5 ml/kg have been ingested.
2. Measure blood alcohol, blood glucose, and arterial blood gases if there is any suspicion of respiratory depression.
3. Treatment is essentially supportive and symptomatic. Intubate and ventilate if there is any evidence of respiratory depression or apnoea.
4. Although a bolus of intravenous glucose is useful initially, hypoglycaemia should be treated by an infusion of glucose, as rebound hypoglycaemia can occur.
5. Haemodialysis or peritoneal dialysis should be considered if the blood alcohol concentration is over 400 mg/100ml.

Methanol (methyl alcohol) and ethylene glycol

Both methanol and ethylene glycol are constituents of automobile antifreezes. Model aircraft fuel also contains methanol, as do screenwashes, and some varnishes and thinners. In a child, 10 mℓ of pure methanol can be fatal, causing profound metabolic acidosis. Ethylene glycol tends to cause initial intoxication followed later by acute renal failure. Methylated spirit and surgical spirit poisoning should be treated as for ethyl alcohol.

Accidental ingestion of these substances is quite common but serious poisoning is rare. The main principles of treatment are to correct acidosis, delay the metabolism of methanol or ethylene glycol to toxic metabolites by giving ethyl alcohol, and to hasten elimination.

MANAGEMENT

1. Use emesis or lavage to empty the stomach.
2. Measure arterial blood gases and electrolytes and urea. Correct acidosis with intravenous sodium bicarbonate.

3. Consult a Poisons Unit for the regimen of ethyl alcohol administration and the measurement of levels.
4. Ensure adequate fluid input and output.
5. Where serious toxicity is confirmed, haemodialysis or peritoneal dialysis are indicated.

Household cleaning agents

Detergent-based materials are in general not toxic though they may cause vomiting since they are mildly irritant. Nappy sterilizers, and denture cleaners are irritant alkaline chemicals, though some denture cleaners are acidic. Some toilet blocks contain bleaching agents, though most contain *p*-dichlorbenzene which is not corrosive and should be treated by emesis. Ingestion of a mouthful of bleach or a denture cleaning tablet may cause burns in the mouth, throat, oesophagus and stomach. The severity of corrosion is related mainly to the concentration of the agent and the duration of contact; the amount ingested is less important. Fortunately, it is very rare for children to come to serious harm after the reported ingestion of any of these materials.

Clinical features

There may be severe pain in the mouth, retrosternal area, and abdomen. Signs of burning may not appear for up to 48 hours, and the absence of burns in the mouth does not exclude damage to the pharynx, oesophagus, or stomach. Other clinical signs include vomiting, cardiovascular collapse, or coma. Perforation of the oesophagus or stomach may lead to mediastinitis or peritonitis, and pulmonary aspiration may also complicate the picture. An oesophageal stricture may develop within 2–6 weeks.

On-the-spot treatment of corrosive ingestion

Speed is important. Water or milk should be given by mouth; and the face and hands, if contaminated, should be washed with copious amounts of water. There is no point in neutralizing acids or alkalis.

Management in hospital

1. Liquid (as above) should be given at once.
2. Emesis and gastric lavage are contraindicated, as they may produce further damage. However, if the substance taken is poisonous as well as corrosive (e.g. paraquat), emesis is indicated.
3. Opioid analgesics should be used as required for pain, and plasma and saline should be given for shock. Small amounts of liquid or ice cream may be given orally, if tolerated.
4. Where there is an experienced endoscopist, endoscopy should be performed early to assess the extent of damage.
5. If perforation has occurred, urgent surgical intervention is essential. Hours of time should not be wasted in attempting to improve metabolic or cardiovascular state.

Hydrocarbons

These are found in the home as white spirit, petroleum jelly, polishes, waxes, window cleaners, turpentine substitute, paraffin, and petrol. The ingestion of petroleum distillates and hydrocarbon oils and waxes causes two main problems: if aspirated during ingestion or subsequent vomiting, they can cause pneumonitis, and if absorbed via the lungs or the gut they can cause central nervous system depression. Other effects (such as on the liver or bone marrow) are uncommon, and are not part of the emergency.

Clinical features

1. Hydrocarbon ingestion can cause irritation of mucous membranes, with coughing, choking, nausea, vomiting and diarrhoea.
2. Hydrocarbons destroy pulmonary surfactant. Aspiration of even very small amounts of paraffin or petrol can cause acute pulmonary damage similar to shock lung, developing 12–24 hours after exposure. Mineral oils and waxes cause low-grade chronic inflammation. Clinical signs include cough, a rapid respiratory rate, cyanosis, and crackles (rales). Radiological signs consist of dense patchy shadowing, usually in the lower lobes.
3. If sufficient is absorbed, central nervous system involvement can lead to restlessness, drowsiness, confusion and coma.

Treatment

1. The patient should be admitted for at least 24 hours after ingestion.
2. A chest X-ray should be performed on admission.
3. Emesis is contraindicated because of the risk of aspiration.
4. If a large amount (over 10 mℓ/kg) has been recently ingested or the patient is losing consciousness, the patient should be intubated in order to prevent aspiration of gastric contents, and gastric lavage should be performed.
5. Oxygen, humidity and bronchodilators should be used as required if aspiration is suspected or if lung damage has occurred. Recovery will take place within 1–2 weeks but may take longer with waxes and polishes. There is no specific treatment: high-dose steroids will not help.
6. If other organs are involved, management is symptomatic and supportive.

Essential oils

Like petroleum distillates, essential or volatile oils such as oil of turpentine, camphorated oil, and oil of eucalyptus, which are found in many rubs and creams, are a serious aspiration hazard when ingested. A mouthful or less of some volatile oils may cause serious systemic toxicity with convulsions, coma, and renal failure. If more than a mouthful has been swallowed, and the child is showing symptoms, gastric lavage is justified, provided the airway is protected. Other features of management are as for hydrocarbons.

Dry-cleaning solvents

Dry-cleaning agents are usually chlorinated solvents such as trichlorethylene or trichloroethane. Carbon tetrachloride is now rarely used. Chlorinated solvents are in general highly toxic, causing serious hepatic damage.

Management

1. Chlorinated solvents are radio-opaque, and significant amounts recently ingested should appear on an abdominal X-ray.
2. This type of solvent is not an aspiration risk, and so emesis can be induced safely, after first ascertaining the ingredients, since some formulations also contain petroleum distillates.
3. Acetylcysteine should be used as an antidote (*see* page 67), as in paracetamol poisoning, since the mechanism of hepatic toxicity, at least in the case of carbon tetrachloride, appears to be similar.

Paraquat

This weedkiller can cause severe burns of the skin, mouth, and gastrointestinal tract, hepatic dysfunction and renal failure; severe pulmonary damage can occur days after the initial poisoning. Poisoning in children is rare, and a poisons information service should always be consulted. The liquid concentrates (5%, 10% or 20% paraquat) are very toxic and the powder formulations are less toxic, especially when made up with water. All modern formulations of paraquat contain an emetic, and vomiting is to be expected if it has been ingested. Gramoxone (20% paraquat), Dextrone X as supplied to farmers, is extremely toxic; the granular preparations available to gardeners (2.5%) are less of a hazard.

Management

1. Remove clothing and wash off any cutaneous contamination with copious soap and water.
2. If emesis has not occurred, give syrup of ipecacuanha.
3. Obtain samples of urine and blood and save any vomitus. *All samples should be stored in plastic containers.*
4. Urine, blood and clear gastric aspirate can be subjected to the alkali dithionite test (*see* Appendix 18). A deep blue colour in urine indicates that it contains paraquat and that poisoning is significant. If plasma or serum give a positive result with the dithionite test, a fatal outcome is virtually certain.
5. If the urine test gives a positive result, a plasma sample should be analysed in a centre which carries out the assay. The result can be compared with the graph of time against plasma paraquat concentrations by Proudfoot *et al.* (1979). It should be clear that this graph refers to adults, and fatal levels in children may be very different. Not enough is known to say whether they are higher or lower than in adults.
6. Once vomiting has subsided, activated charcoal should be given in the maximum tolerated dose, together with a purgative. Ensure adequate hydration and a good urine output. Any other measures should only be carried out in consultation with a poisons information service.

Battery ingestion

Many batteries for electrical appliances such as hearing aids, watches and cameras are small enough to be ingested. There are three major problems: mechanical obstruction (usually in the oesophagus), opening of the battery and release of its contents causing corrosion of the gut (usually in the oesophagus), and release of the contents with possible systemic toxicity from the constituents of the battery.

Management

1. Batteries are radio-opaque. Confirm ingestion by X-ray.
2. Identify the type and make of battery used. A poisons information service can help. There are four main types of battery:
   (a) Mercury (one battery contains a lethal amount of mercury for a small child).
   (b) Manganese–alkali (corrosive if the battery opens when lodged but not otherwise toxic).
   (c) Nickel–cadmium (the cadmium is toxic).
   (d) Silver (non-toxic).
3. Determine the position of the battery:
   (a) If stuck in the oesophagus, endoscopic, balloon catheter or magnetic removal should be carried out as soon as possible.
   (b) If in the stomach, there is risk of corrosion of the battery case by gastric acid. Give cimetidine or ranitidine and observe radiologically (*see* below).
   (c) If the battery has passed through the stomach without radiological evidence of being corroded give purgatives and wait for it to be passed.
4. The progress of the battery should be followed up by repeated X-ray examinations. A battery with toxic contents (mercury or nickel–cadmium) should be removed by gastrotomy if it has not passed through within 36 hours, but a non-toxic battery can be left for longer. The battery's semi-liquid contents are radio-opaque and disintegration or opening of a battery can easily be diagnosed.
5. If a toxic battery has already opened, a toxicology unit should be contacted for advice on measurement of blood levels and treatment with antidotes.

Plants, mushrooms and berries

Accidental ingestion

Young children often ingest plants and berries, but this seldom gives rise to serious problems. Generally a mild gastrointestinal disturbance is the most that will occur, and symptomatic and supportive treatment is all that is required. It is important to identify the plant material in case it is one capable of causing significant or serious toxicity. The more commonly encountered toxic plants and the toxic amounts in each case are listed in *Table 8.7.* For these poisonings emesis is always recommended if the child presents within 4 hours. Subsequent treatment will then be generally supportive. If there is doubt about the ingestion, identification or the toxicity of plant material, emesis is a sensible precautionary measure, as the vomitus can be inspected and kept for identification if necessary.

Psilocybe semilanceata ('magic mushrooms')

Older children are unlikely to ingest plants accidentally, but may indulge in hallucinogenic mushrooms such as psilocybe ('magic mushrooms'). These will give rise to symptoms similar to LSD intoxication: hallucinations, aggression, nausea, dilated pupils and tachycardia, which usually resolve completely within 6 hours. Treatment should be symptomatic, suggestive and supportive, keeping the patient as quiet as possible, and offering reassurance. Gastric lavage or emesis are best avoided since either could be very distressing if the patient is hallucinating. Sedation with diazepam or chlorpromazine may occasionally be necessary.

Table 8.7 Plant ingestions for which emesis is indicated (this is NOT an exhaustive list of poisonous plants for which emesis is suggested, but includes the more common ones)

Plant	*Amount ingested*
Deadly nightshade: all parts	Any amount
Other species containing atropine-like compounds, e.g. *Datura stramonium* (thorn-apple)	Any amount
Woody nightshade: all parts	Any amount
Christmas/Jerusalem cherry: leaves or unripe berries	Any amount
Yew-leaves and seeds (the red fleshy part is not toxic)	Any amount
Snowberry	More than 3 berries
Holly berries	More than 5 berries
Foxglove: all parts	Any amount
Privet: leaves and berries	More than 1 berry
Bryony	Any amount
Daffodil bulbs	Any amount
Amanita phalloides (Death cap)	Any amount
Gyromitra esculenta (species of toadstool growing in sandy soil in conifer areas; poisonous if eaten raw)	Any amount
Laburnum: all parts	Any amount
Cuckoo pint or lords and ladies (*Arum maculatum*)	More than 1 berry
Cherry laurel	Any amount
Daphne (laureola and mezereum): all parts	Any amount
Mistletoe	More than 10 berries

Poison Information Services in the UK and Eire

Centre	*Hospital*	*Telephone*
Belfast	Royal Victoria Hospital	0232 240503
Cardiff	Cardiff Royal Infirmary	0222 569200
Dublin	Jervis Street Hospital	Dublin 745588
Edinburgh	Edinburgh Royal Infirmary	031 229 2477
London	Guy's Hospital	01 635 9191
		01 407 7600
Poisons information also available from other centres		
Birmingham	Dudley Road Hospital	021 554 3801
Leeds	Leeds General Infirmary	0532 432799
Newcastle	Royal Victoria Infirmary	0632 325131

References

BRITISH NATIONAL FORMULARY No. 12 (1986). p. 35. London: British Medical Association and The Pharmaceutical Society of Great Britain

MEREDITH, T. and VALE, A. (1984) Antidotes. *Medicine International*, Vol. 2, No. 9 (Sept. 1984), pp. 363–367

PROUDFOOT, A. T., STEWART, M. S., LEVITT, T. and WIDDOP, B. (1979) Paraquat poisoning. *Lancet*, **ii**, 330–332

Further reading

BREISBACH, R. H. (1986) *Handbook of Poisoning,* 12th Edn. Los Altos, Ca: Lange Medical Publications. (Small but useful reference handbook.)

CHEMIST AND DRUGGIST DIRECTORY (1985) London: Contract Pharmaceutical Services. (Tablet identification guide.)

COOPER, M. R. and JOHNSON, W. (1984) *Poisonous Plants in Britain and Their Effect on Animals and Man.* London: Ministry of Agriculture, Fisheries and Food, Her Majesty's Stationery Office

DEPARTMENT OF HEALTH AND SOCIAL SECURITY (1983) *Pesticide Poisoning – Notes for the Guidance of Medical Practitioners.* London: Her Majesty's Stationery Office

DIRECTORY OF GARDEN CHEMICALS, 7th edn. (1982) London: British Agrochemicals Association.

GOSSELIN, G. E., HODGE, H. C. and SMITH, B. P. (1984) *Clinical Toxicology of Commercial Products,* 5th edn. Baltimore, Md: Williams and Wilkins

HADDAD, L. M. and WINCHESTER, J. F. (eds.) (1983) *Clinical Management of Poisoning and Drug Overdose.* Philadelphia: Saunders. (A more comprehensive text on poisoning.)

HENRY, J. A. and VOLANS, G. N. (1984) ABC of Poisoning. London: BMA Publications. (Basic textbook.)

MEDICAL INDEX OF MEDICAL SPECIALITIES (MIMS) COLOUR INDEX. (1986) London: Medical Publications. (Tablet identification guide.)

POISONING. Medicine International; Vol. 2, No. 9 (Sept. 1984)

PROUDFOOT, A. (1982) *Diagnosis and Management of Acute Poisoning.* Oxford: Blackwell Scientific Publications. (Useful textbook.)

TABLIDENT. Princes Risborough, Bucks, England: Edwin Burgess. (Tablet identification system.)

VALE, J. A. and MEREDITH, T. J. (1981) *Poisoning – Diagnosis and Treatment.* London: Update Books. (Useful textbook.)

WADE, A. and REYNOLDS, J. E. F. (eds.) (1982) *Martindale. The Extra Pharmacopoeia,* 28th edn. London: Pharmaceutical Press. (General reference work on drugs and antidotes.)

Chapter 9

Travel

A. F. Conchie

Motion or travel sickness

This can occur when travelling by land, sea or air. The young child is the usual sufferer, but infants can also be affected.

Recognition

The major symptom is self-evident. Before vomiting the child sweats and appears pale. Older children may complain of nausea and upper abdominal pain.

Management

Travel sickness develops into an emergency when repeated vomiting leads to dehydration. Oral fluids are often retained better after a vomit. Plain water, boiled and cooled for the infant, should be given. Prevention is more effective than treating established travel sickness. Avoidance of a large meal before a journey, adequate fresh-air ventilation, games to occupy the attention, and on car trips, frequent stops may help. Drugs are effective. Hyoscine hydrobromide 0.15–0.3 mg or cyclizine 25 mg should be taken 30–60 minutes before starting the journey (*see Table 9.1* for list of commonly used preparations).

Table 9.1 Preparations used to prevent motion sickness

Approved name	*Proprietary name*
Cyclizine hydrochloride	Valoid (Calmic) Marzine (Wellcome)
Dimenhydrinate	Dramamine (Searle)
Hyoscine hydrobromide	Joy-Rides (Stafford-Miller) Quick Kwells (Nicholas)
Meclozine hydrochloride	Ancoloxin (Duncan Flockhart)
Promethazine theoclate	Avomine (May & Baker)
Promethazine hydrochloride	Phenergan (May & Baker)
Chlorpheniramine	Piriton (Allen & Hanburys)

Drug reactions

Hyoscine is available in proprietary travel sickness preparations. Accidental overdose can lead to tachycardia, flushed and dry skin, dilated pupils and an acute confusional state with hallucinations. Mild symptoms can be treated expectantly but the acutely disturbed child requires hospital care.

Metoclopramide (Maxolon) is also an anti-emetic. In normal dosage in children it can cause severe and painful dystonic spasms involving the head and neck and should be avoided for the prevention of travel sickness.

Traveller's diarrhoea

This is a common problem, especially in countries where the hygiene is poor.

Recognition

The diarrhoea may be accompanied or preceded by vomiting. The majority of episodes settle in 1–3 days. With those travelling in or who have been to the Middle or Far East, bacillary or amoebic dysentery, giardiasis, cholera and typhoid fever must be considered.

Management

The younger the child, the greater is the possibility of dehydration. If there is no vomiting, hydration can be maintained by giving water orally. This should be boiled and cooled for the infant, and also for the older child if the water supply is at all suspect. Vomiting usually settles within 24 hours, but small amounts of oral fluids may be given and retained while the child has this symptom.

In non-specific traveller's diarrhoea drugs are ineffective and therefore unnecessary. In particular clioquinol (Entero-Vioform) is contraindicated and there is no evidence that this drug or antibiotics are effective prophylactically in this condition.

Sleep disturbances

Many children have a sleep ritual. This often includes cuddling a particular blanket or toy. If this is not taken on a journey or is mislaid the child may have difficulty in getting to sleep. In addition travelling often causes a disturbance in the daily routine of a child so that he is not able to follow his usual pattern of sleeping.

Recognition

The child with a sleep disturbance is usually fractious and may shown signs of anxiety as well as having difficulty in falling to sleep.

Management

Parents should be advised to take any object associated with the child's sleep ritual with them when they go on a journey. If this is not done or the comfort object is mislaid it is worth trying to find a substitute. Effort should be made to make the child's routine as much as possible like that established at home. The problem is usually a temporary one but chloral mixture (500 mg × 5 ml) in a dosage 30–50 mg/kg 30 minutes before bedtime for a few nights will help resolve the difficulty of getting to sleep. Dichloralphenazone (Welldorm) (225 mg/5 ml) 30–50 mg/kg or Triclofos Elixir (500 mg/5 ml) 30–50 mg/kg are equally effective and are less likely to cause gastrointestinal upsets than chloral.

Emotional disturbances

Travelling may involve the child in having to contend with marked changes in his emotional as well as his physical environment. He may have to cope with unusual foods, hotels in which the geography is unfamiliar and communication problems because of language difficulties. At the same time his parents may have similar anxieties and be preoccupied with their own problems associated with the journey.

Recognition

The child may respond by displaying signs of anxiety with frequent and often prolonged outbursts of crying. He may become aggressive and rebellious or withdrawn and uncommunicative.

Management

Much can be done to avoid emotional problems if the parents have been advised of this possibility. The child, as far as possible, should be involved in planning and recognizing the difficulties, including emotional ones, that may arise during the course of the journey.

If the child's behaviour has become disturbed a full explanation of the cause should be given to the parents. They should be reassured that with understanding and sympathetic handling the problem is usually a temporary one. Associated sleep disturbances can be helped with chloral or dichloralphenazone as suggested above.

Car travel

Heat exhaustion and heat stroke (*see also* pages 545 and 547)

These are likely to occur when a child, particularly an infant, is left in a closed car on a hot day. The higher the temperature and the greater the humidity, the greater is the probability of symptoms. The mildest form is heat exhaustion. Electrolytes and water are lost through sweating. The child is not in a situation to replace the water loss and so there is a tendency to develop hypertonic dehydration (*see* page 126).

Recognition

The child appears flushed and irritable.

Management

Removal from the car, placing in a cool shaded area, and giving water by mouth overcomes the problem.

In heatwaves the more severe condition of heat stroke may occur. (For the symptoms, signs and management *see* page 547.) It should be noted that drugs of the hyoscine group given for the prevention of travel sickness may increase the risk of causing heat stroke by reducing sweating.

Carbon monoxide poisoning (*see also* pages 34 and 71)

Leaking and inefficient exhaust systems can cause carbon monoxide to seep into the travelling compartment of cars, and the problem is exaggerated if the ventilation system is poor and the windows are kept closed.

Recognition

The severity of the symptoms depends upon the duration of exposure. The initial symptom is headache of which the older child may complain. Irritability and mental confusion may be followed by drowsiness and vomiting.

Management

Once the condition is recognized the car should be stopped, the engine turned off and the occupants taken into the open air.

Aircraft travel

Food poisoning

With the catering techniques employed for aircraft travellers there is a possibility of food poisoning occurring during flight. The commonest agent responsible is staphylococcal enterotoxin.

Recognition

Symptoms appear 1–3 hours after eating the contaminated food. Vomiting and abdominal pain are more prominent features than diarrhoea.

Management

The illness usually settles within a few hours. A careful watch should be kept for signs of dehydration and arrangements should be considered for the most severely affected to be given parenteral saline at the next airfield (*see also* page 404).

Aural pain

Aural pain is frequently experienced on the descent of an aircraft despite pressurization of the passenger compartment. It is due to sudden changes in the pressure relationships between the middle ear and the auditory meatus. The problem is more pronounced and more likely to occur if the Eustachian canal is obstructed due to an upper respiratory infection.

Recognition

The infant may scream on the descent of the aircraft. The older child may clutch his ears and complain of aural discomfort.

Management

Attempts should be made to restore the balance of pressure on either side of the tympanic membrane. The child should be urged to swallow repeatedly to achieve this or even to perform Valsalva's manoeuvre by forcibly expiring into the nostrils which have been occluded between finger and thumb. With an infant the problem can be resolved by offering a feed. All the measures can be employed prophylactically when the aircraft begins to descend. Ephedrine nasal drops or similar preparations can be used prophylactically and will also relieve the pain and deafness.

Sea travel

As in closed motor cars, the temperature and humidity in some cabins can be high and lead to heat exhaustion and even heat stroke (*see* page 547).

Part II

Shock, Acidosis and Electrolyte Disorders

Chapter 10

Shock

D. M. Levin

Introduction

Shock is a pathological state of impaired cardiovascular function, resulting in inadequate tissue and organ perfusion. Diminished supply of oxygen and nutrients to the tissues leads to local hypoxia, anaerobic metabolism and impaired cellular function. If perfusion is not restored, cell death occurs, with organ failure and release of proteolytic enzymes and toxic metabolites into the circulation. These toxic products further impair cardiovascular function, perfusion worsens, and ultimately death occurs (Ledingham, 1976a).

The management of shock requires a clear understanding of normal cardiovascular physiology and its derangement in the shocked state. Early recognition and prompt treatment are essential if the process is to be reversed.

Physiology; determinants of tissue oxygenation

Oxygenation and nutrition of the tissues depend on adequacy of: (1) oxygenation; (2) oxygen carrying capacity; (3) cardiac output; and (4) distribution of cardiac output within the body. Severe derangement of any of these variables will result in shock. Relevant aspects of cardiovascular physiology and blood-flow distribution are discussed below.

Cardiac output

The cardiac output is the volume of blood ejected from the heart in a given time, and is therefore the product of: (1) heart rate and (2) stroke volume (*Figure 10.1*) (Guyton, Jones and Coleman, 1973).

Heart rate

Heart rate is determined by vagal (cholinergic) activity, slowing the heart, and by sympathetic (adrenergic) activity increasing heart rate. If stroke volume remains constant, cardiac output will increase linearly with increasing heart rate up to 160–180 beats per minute. At higher rates, inadequate ventricular filling time

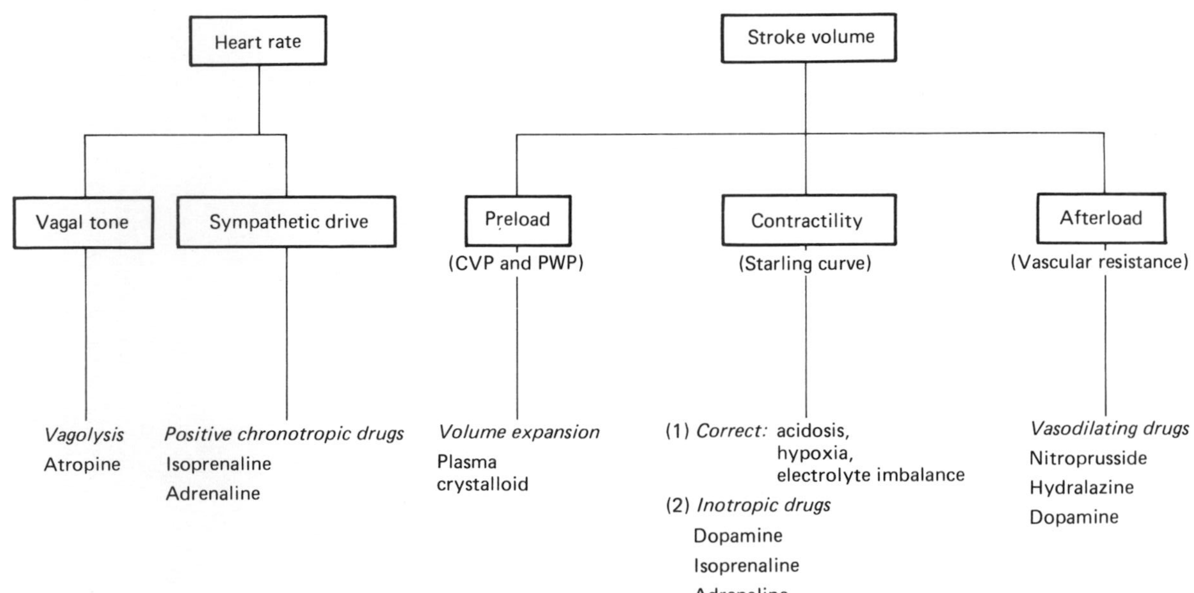

Figure 10.1 Determinants of cardiac output (Modified from Crone (1980).)

results in a fall in stroke volume. An increase in heart rate is the earliest compensatory response in shock. Administration of vagolytic or positive chronotropic drugs may improve cardiac output by increasing heart rate. (Chronotropic drugs alter the heart rate; positive chronotropic drugs *increase* the heart rate.)

Stroke volume

Stroke volume is dependent upon (1) preload; (2) myocardial contractility; and (3) afterload (Perkin and Levin, 1982a, b).

Preload

Preload is defined as the myocardial end-diastolic fibre length, and is measured clinically in terms of the filling pressures of the left and right ventricles. As the intraventricular pressures are seldom measured directly, preload is usually estimated by measurement of the pressures in the great vessels or the atria (central venous pressure, CVP). In most situations both ventricles function in concert, and thus an adequate preload of the right ventricle (CVP) also reflects adequacy of left ventricular filling. Occasionally, the two ventricles may fail independently as in pulmonary hypertension, pulmonary embolus, or severe sepsis. In these situations the CVP will not reliably reflect left ventricular filling, and a more direct measurement of left ventricular preload is required. The pulmonary wedge pressure (PWP) provides a more accurate indication of the left atrial pressure. It is obtained by floating a balloon catheter from the right ventricle into a distal pulmonary artery and measuring the pressure when the artery is occluded by inflating the balloon. This pressure closely approximates the left atrial pressure. Although the use of PWP requires considerable expertise, it is useful in management of severe shock, and is being used with increasing frequency in children (Todres *et al.*, 1979).

The major determinant of preload is the venous return to the heart which depends on the blood volume, and the capacitance of the vasculature. The post-capillary venules function as a blood storage system, the capacity of which can be altered by changes in vascular tone and sympathetic activity. Normally a considerable proportion of the total blood volume is stored in the venous beds. Rapid compensation for blood loss can be achieved by contraction of these vessels in response to increased sympathetic activity. Conversely, a loss of vascular tone, as may occur in sepsis or anaphylaxis, may result in a considerable increase in the capacity of the vasculature, and therefore a fall in venous return.

The relationship between ventricular preload and stroke volume is shown in *Figure 10.2* and is known as Starling's law of the heart (Crone, 1980). Stroke volume and cardiac output rise progressively with increasing preload (CVP or PWP) until ventricular filling is optimal: this occurs at CVP pressures between 8 and 15 mm Hg(11–21 cm H_2O) or PWP pressures between 12 and 18 mm Hg (16–24.5 cm H_2O). A further increase in filling pressures results in a decline of cardiac output due to overdistension of the ventricles.

Myocardial contractility

Myocardial contractility depends on the inherent properties of the myocardial fibres. It is decreased by hypoxia, acidosis, electrolyte imbalance, anaemia, and

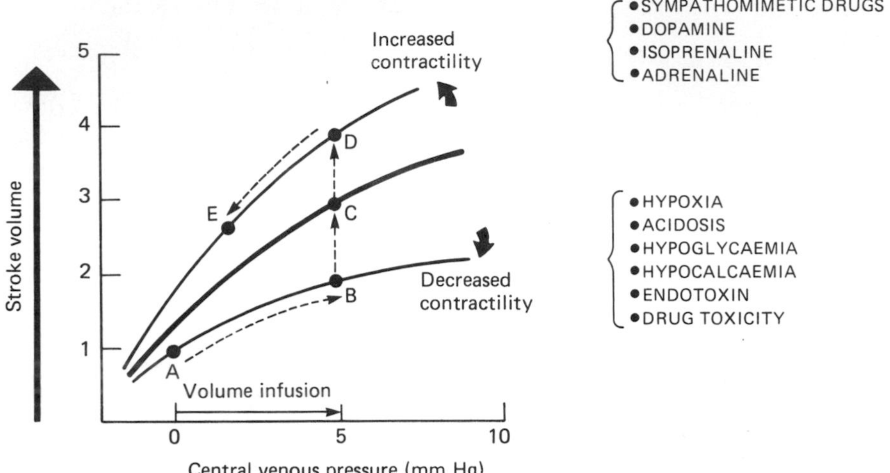

Figure 10.2 Relationship between preload (CVP) and stroke volume (Starling's law). Volume infusion increases CVP and consequently stroke volume (points A–B). Correction of acidosis, hypoxia and electrolyte imbalance improves contractility and stroke volume (points B–C). Inotropic drugs shift the myocardial function curve upwards (points C–D). Afterload reduction with vasodilating drugs produces a more favourable position on the myocardial function curve (D–E) (Modified from Crone (1980).)

disease such as myocarditis or cardiomyopathy. Decreased contractility shifts the Starling curve downwards (*Figure 10.2*). Contractility and stroke volume can be improved by correcting acidosis, hypoxia, and anaemia, and can be increased further by positive inotropic drugs (*Figure 10.2*) (Taylor, 1982).

Afterload

Afterload is defined as the ventricular wall tension during systole and depends on the resistance to blood flow from the ventricle. Arterial wall compliance and vascular resistance are its major determinants (Milnor, 1975). Afterload increases when systemic and pulmonary vascular resistance are increased by α-adrenergic activity, angiotensin II, and vasoconstrictor substances such as thromboxane A_2. It is reduced by β-adrenergic activity, α-blocking drugs and vasodilators. A rise in afterload increases both the work of the ventricle and the myocardial oxygen consumption. Stroke volume falls if the ventricle is unable to eject blood in the face of high resistance. Afterload reduction can lead to considerable improvement in cardiac output together with reduced myocardial oxygen consumption.

Distribution of cardiac output

Blood flow to the tissues is regulated by changes in tone of the pre-capillary arterioles and post-capillary venules. Even if cardiac output is normal, local abnormalities in vascular tone may produce inadequate perfusion. Excessive vasoconstriction, mediated by locally produced or circulating vasoactive substances may reduce perfusion. Conversely, vasodilation may result in pooling of blood in the tissues, and in arteriovenous shunting, which allows blood flow to bypass the tissues.

Pathophysiology

Impaired cardiac output and abnormal blood-flow distribution are common to all forms of shock. Regardless of the initiating event, the body will respond to the reduction in cardiac output by a series of homeostatic vasoconstrictor responses, which attempt to maintain cerebral and coronary perfusion at the expense of less vital tissues (*Figure 10.3*) (Hackel, Ratcliff and Mikat, 1974). If the initiating insult is maintained, the compensatory vasoconstriction leads to a progressive reduction in organ perfusion. Anoxia in the underperfused tissues results in impaired cellular metabolism and ultimately in cell death. Proteolytic enzymes and other toxins are released from damaged cells. They increase vascular permeability, activate the clotting and kinin pathways and diminish vascular tone. Increased capillary permeability leads to further losses of colloid from the vascular space. Platelets are aggregated by endothelial damage and tissue thromboplastins, resulting in the formation of microthrombi in the capillaries of the lungs, kidneys and other organs. Late shock is characterized by generalized hypoperfusion, increasing acidosis and disseminated intravascular coagulation (DIC). Respiratory, renal and hepatic failure cause further metabolic derangement. Cardiac function is impaired by hypoxia and acidosis, as well as the reduced cardiac filling and elevated peripheral resistance. Ultimately the compensatory mechanisms are overwhelmed, coronary and cerebral perfusion fall, and irreversible cardiac and cerebral damage occur (Ledingham, 1976a).

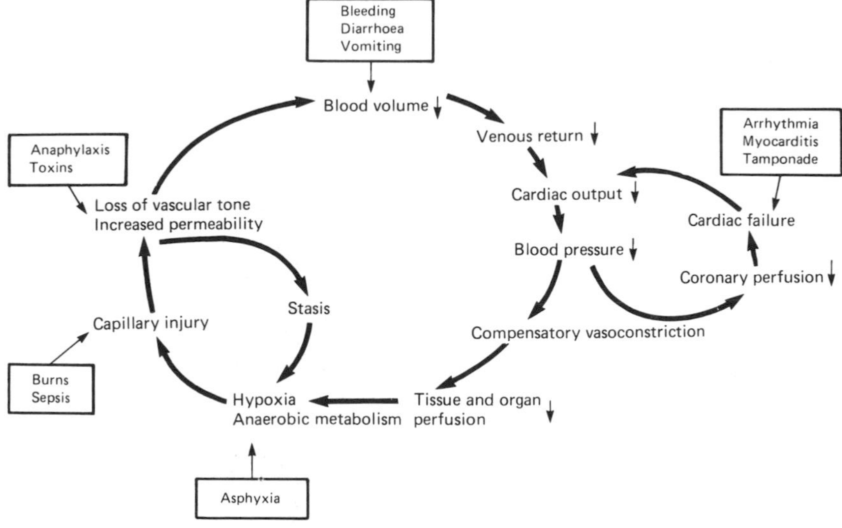

Figure 10.3 Cyclic mechanisms in shock (Modified from Hackel *et al.* (1974) and Ledingham (1976a).)

Aetiology

Shock can be initiated by four main groups of disorders (*Figure 10.4*):

1. Fluid, blood, or electrolyte loss (which may be either external or internal).
2. Cardiac failure.
3. Loss of vascular tone.
4. Combinations of all the above three groups (Perkin and Levin, 1982a, b).

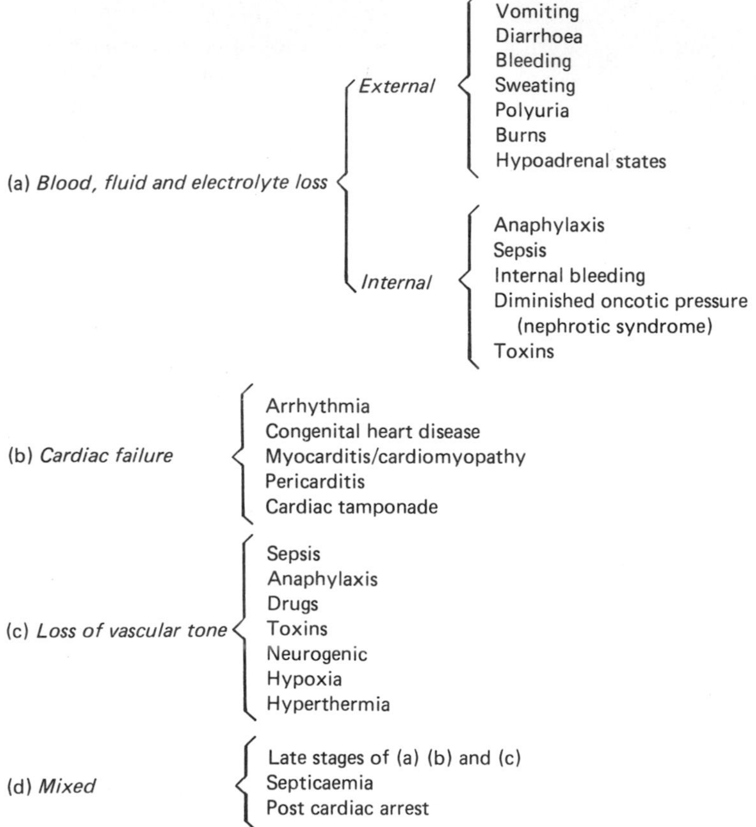

Figure 10.4 Shock: pathophysiological and aetiological classification

Fluid, blood or electrolyte loss

External losses

Gastrointestinal disorders – The commonest initiating event is loss of fluid and electrolytes due to vomiting and diarrhoea. The composition of the fluid depends upon whether gastric, pancreatic, small- or large-bowel secretions are lost. Infective diarrhoeas, pyloric stenosis, and intestinal obstruction are the major causes.

Renal disorders – Excess urinary loss of water and electrolytes occurs in chronic renal failure, obstructive uropathy, diabetes insipidus, diabetes mellitus and tubular disorders such as Bartter's syndrome and Fanconi's syndrome. Salt and water loss from the kidney may also be due to adrenal insufficiency. The underlying disease determines whether water, or electrolyte loss predominates and thus whether the dehydration is hypotonic, isotonic, or hypertonic.

Skin disorders – Significant fluid and electrolyte loss may occur from the skin in normal individuals in hot climates. Skin losses are increased in diseases such as eczema, psoriasis, fever, and cystic fibrosis. Burns are a major cause of colloid and fluid loss.

Trauma – Trauma is the commonest cause of bleeding. Loss of as little as 20 ml/kg of blood can induce shock, and loss of 50 ml/kg is usually fatal (Morse, 1983). The possibility of a coagulation or platelet disorder should be considered if severe bleeding occurs following minor trauma.

Fistulae, ileostomy and drains – Fluid losses from fistulae, drains, ileostomies and nephrostomies are easily overlooked and can account for large deficits.

Internal losses

Into the extravascular tissues – Loss of fluid or colloid from the vascular compartment into the extravascular tissues may be due either to increased permeability or to diminished oncotic pressure. Increased vascular permeability occurs in sepsis, anaphylaxis, hypoxia and burns. It is also seen in conditions such as dengue shock (*see* page 589), hyperthermia and the toxic shock syndrome. (Oncotic pressure is the effect of macromolecules in retaining fluid within the intravascular compartment. Osmotic effect refers to the effect of small molecules which freely traverse the vascular wall.)

Into the body cavities – Local accumulation of fluid in the body cavities occurs in pancreatits, peritonitis, volvulus and intussusception, or in pleural inflammations or malignancy.

Diminished intravascular oncotic pressure – Hypovolaemia due to diminished colloid oncotic pressure occurs in the nephrotic syndrome, chronic malabsorption, burns and malnutrition.

Internal bleeding – Internal bleeding into organs or tissues usually follows trauma. Subcapsular haematoma of the liver, splenic or hepatic rupture, and adrenal haemorrhage may cause sudden shock in the absence of visible bleeding. Intraventricular haemorrhage and necrotizing enterocolitis are common sites of volume loss in the asphyxiated newborn.

Cardiac failure

Shock occurs in all states of diminished cardiac output. Moreover, impaired myocardial function follows the metabolic derangements and decreased coronary perfusion in severe shock (*see Figure 10.3*).

Common causes of cardiogenic shock are:

1. Arrhythmia.
2. Structural cardiac abnormalities.
3. Myocarditis.
4. Cardiomyopathy.
5. Pericardial disease.

Cardiac tamponade should always be considered, as it is readily treated (Fulton and Grodin, 1983) (*see* page 275).

Loss of vascular tone

Loss of the normal vascular tone results in an increase in the capacity of the vascular bed and diminished venous return to the heart. This occurs in: (1) anaphylaxis, (2) neurogenic shock, and (3) poisoning with barbiturates and vasodilating drugs.

Loss of vascular tone may also lead to opening of pre-capillary arteriovenous shunts, allowing blood to bypass the tissues. This is responsible for the 'warm' phase of septic shock, where arteriovenous shunting results in impaired tissue perfusion despite a high cardiac output.

Mixed

The late stages of all forms of shock are characterized by a combination of fluid loss through damaged capillaries, loss of vascular tone in some areas (despite vasoconstriction of others) and cardiac decompensation.

Recognition

History

Early recognition of shock is imperative if major organ damage is to be avoided. Shock should be anticipated in situations such as burns, trauma or diarrhoea (*Figure 10.4*).

1. The duration, severity and previous treatment of the initiating illness should be established.
2. The parents' description of changes in the child's appearance, level of consciousness, and urine output will give an indication of the rate of progression.
3. Septic shock should be suspected in children with a history of immune deficiency, immunosuppression, or recent surgery.

Early shock

Clinical features (*see also* Chapter 3)

The early clinical features reflect the compensatory vasoconstrictor responses which maintain vital organ perfusion at the expense of peripheral perfusion. *A low blood pressure is not a feature of early shock, and arterial blood pressure may be maintained by vasoconstriction, even in severely shocked patients*. Some children even become hypertensive in response to volume loss. Reduction of blood pressure may only occur when the compensatory vasoconstriction is overwhelmed, and is often a preterminal event.

1. In early shock the child is restless and anxious (*Table 10.1*).
2. Blood pressure is normal, but tachycardia and tachypnoea are present.
3. Peripheral perfusion is poor, with a gradient above 4°C (8°F) between the central (rectal) temperature and peripheral (great toe) temperature.
4. Capillary filling is sluggish. It is best assessed by pressure over the skin or nail beds and observation of the time for the capillaries to fill.
5. Oliguria (*see* page 427) is present unless the kidney is unable to respond to volume depletion (as in chronic renal failure or diabetes insipidus).
6. There may be signs of the initiating illness such as dehydration (following fluid loss) or pallor if blood loss or cardiac failure has occurred.

Table 10.1 Recognition of shock – clinical features

Early shock	*Late shock*
BP normal	BP ↓
Tachycardia	Increasing tachycardia
Tachypnoea	Respiratory distress
Poor perfusion	Perfusion ↓ ↓
Slow capillary filling	Worsening capillary filling
Central temperature normal or ↑	Central temperature ↑ or ↓
Peripheral temperature ↓	Cyanosis
Restlessness	Coma
Anxiety	Extreme pallor
Pallor	Anuria
Oliguria	

Laboratory findings

1. Haemoconcentration, with elevation of haemoglobin and packed cell volume, is common if shock follows fluid loss.
2. However, anaemia may also be present if bleeding or haemolysis has occurred.
3. Plasma sodium concentration is normal if fluid loss has been isotonic, but may be increased or diminished depending upon the relative loss of water and electrolytes.
4. Impaired renal perfusion results in a progressive rise in plasma urea concentration, associated with the production of a highly concentrated urine. Urine urea and electrolytes are helpful in determining the cause of oliguria (*Table 10.2*).

Table 10.2 Urine electrolytes and osmolality in the assessment of oliguria

Urine Na (mmol/ℓ)	*Urine osmolality* (mosm/kg)	*Urine/plasma urea ratio*	*Diagnosis*	*Treatment*
<10	>600	>10	Pre-renal	Volume expansion; diuretics, dopamine
10–20	300–400	4–10	Incipient acute renal failure	Cautious volume expansion, dopamine, diuretics
>20	<300	1–4	Established renal failure	Dialysis, fluid restriction
>20	>600	>10	Inappropriate ADH secretion	Fluid restriction

Late shock

Clinical features

1. The clinical features in late shock reflect severely diminished perfusion of all tissues and organs.
2. Peripheral perfusion is extremely poor with an increasing difference (often >10°C or 18°F) between central and peripheral temperature.
3. Capillary filling is slow and areas of bluish discoloration, due to stagnation of blood in dilated capillaries, are superimposed upon areas of extreme pallor.
4. There is increasing tachycardia, hypotension, and eventually signs of cardiac failure.
5. The respiratory rate rises as shock and acidosis worsen. Cyanosis develops, despite increasing concentrations of inspired oxygen. Later, as the child becomes exhausted, breathing becomes laboured, and respiratory arrest occurs unless assisted ventilation is started.
6. Restlessness and confusion are followed by drowsiness, coma, and occasionally by convulsions. Once coma is present, cerebral damage and death are imminent unless cerebral perfusion is rapidly restored.
7. Severe shock is invariably accompanied by oliguria or anuria. Initially this is pre-renal in origin, but later acute tubular necrosis results in renal failure which cannot be reversed simply by improving perfusion (*Table 10.2*). Fluid overload occurs if fluid replacement is not adjusted to allow for the anuria.
8. Abdominal distension and ileus are common, and watery or bloody diarrhoea are often preterminal events.

Laboratory findings

1. Haemoglobin and platelet count fall in late shock.
2. Prolongation of prothrombin time, partial thromboplastin time and thrombin time, with elevated fibrin degradation products indicate disseminated intravascular coagulation.
3. Cellular ischaemia impairs the sodium–potassium pump. Plasma sodium level falls, and potassium level rises. Hyperkalaemia is aggravated by acidosis.
4. Plasma urea and creatinine concentrations rise progressively as renal function declines.
5. Derangement of blood glucose, calcium, phosphate and magnesium concentrations are common.
6. Ischaemia of the liver and pancreas results in elevation of plasma transaminases, ammonia and pancreatic enzyme activities.
7. Blood gases show a progressively falling po_2, rising pco_2, and metabolic acidosis.
8. Chest X-ray may show the appearance of pulmonary oedema and shock lung.
9. The ECG indicates both electrolyte imbalance, and the ischaemia caused by impaired coronary perfusion.
10. Arrhythmia is a common terminal event.

Management (*Figure 10.5*)

General principles

The shocked child presents a complex array of clinical and metabolic derangements. It may be difficult to decide which of those to treat first. THOSE

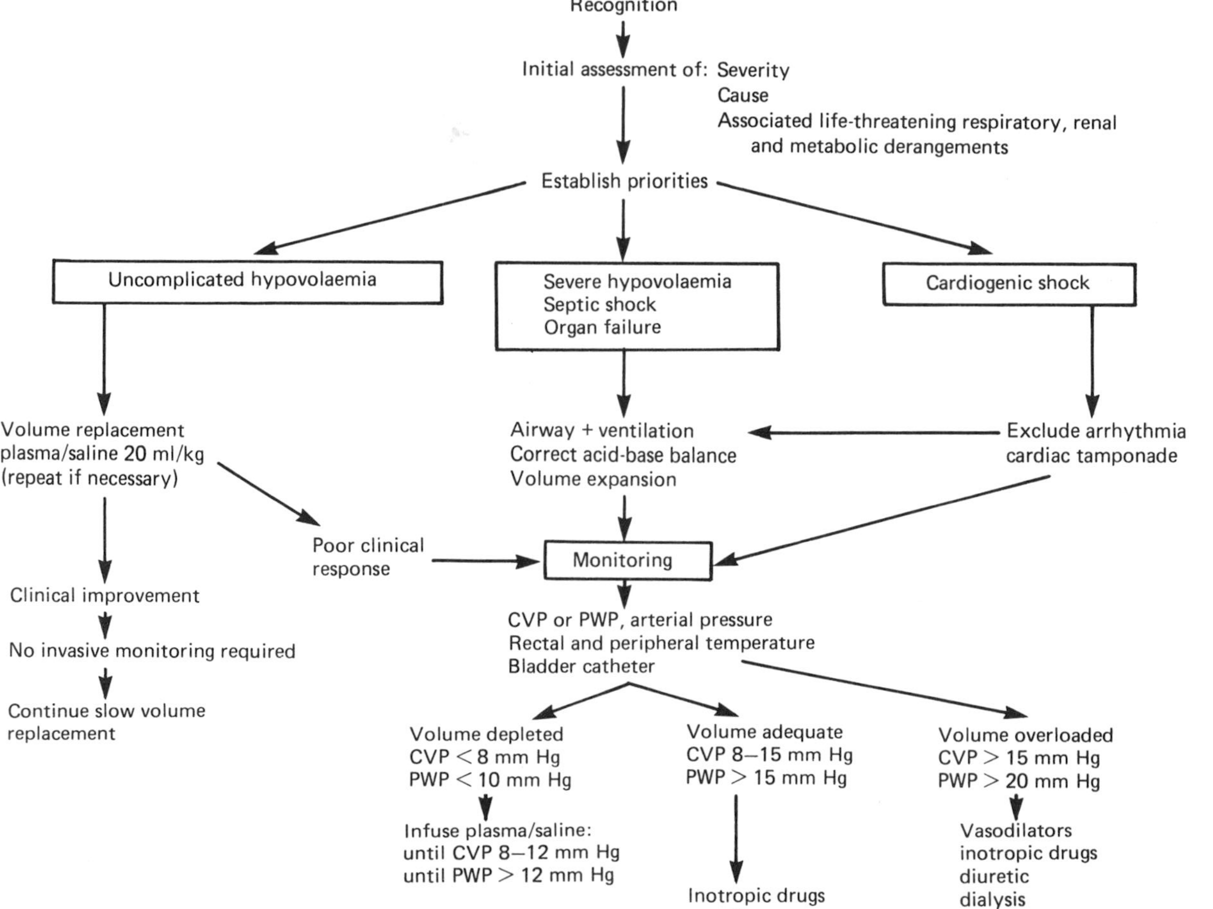

Figure 10.5 An approach to diagnosis and treatment of the shocked child

CONDITIONS WHICH IMMEDIATELY THREATEN LIFE MUST BE IDENTIFIED AT THE OUTSET (*see also* Chapter 3). This is done by a brief but thorough initial clinical assessment, at which time blood is taken for blood count and cross-matching, plasma urea and electrolyte concentrations, blood glucose concentration, and blood cultures. *Once this assessment is completed, a clear order of priorities must be established. Maintenance of the airway and effective ventilation are always the primary objectives* (Orlowski, 1983).

The aims of treatment are:

1. To improve oxygenation, oxygen-carrying capacity, cardiac output and blood-flow distribution.
2. To treat the cause of the shock. If the cause is not immediately apparent, additional investigations such as X-rays, ECG, cultures, and metabolic studies should be undertaken while treatment is initiated. Treatment cannot be delayed while awaiting results.
3. To support vital organ function while awaiting recovery.

Vascular access

Vascular access for fluid and drug administration, as well as for monitoring, is an essential early step in the management of shock. It may be difficult to secure even a peripheral venous line. In severe shock any available route may be used. Percutaneous cannulation of internal or external jugular, femoral or subclavian veins can be rapidly performed by those familiar with the techniques. However, there is a high risk of complications (pneumothorax, carotid artery puncture and haematoma) when these routes are attempted by the inexperienced, and surgical cut-down on to the saphenous vein is a safer alternative. The umbilical vein is the easiest route in the collapsed neonate. Rapid volume expansion with plasma 10–20 ml/kg or 0.9% NaCl will often improve perfusion sufficiently to enable a more secure line to be inserted.

Monitoring

1. In most cases of early shock due to hypovolaemia, invasive monitoring is unnecessary. Careful clinical assessment of central and peripheral temperature and capillary filling, pulse rate and volume, blood pressure, skin turgor, urine output, and level of consciousness are generally adequate.
2. However, the managment of severe shock with multiple organ failure requires regular monitoring of right ventricular preload using the CVP.
3. In cases of cardiogenic shock, shock lung, or septicaemia the CVP may not accurately reflect left ventricular filling, and pulmonary wedge pressure measurement (*see* page 89) is necessary.
4. Management of severe shock is facilitated by continuous monitoring of intra-arterial pressure through a radial artery catheter, and measurement of core and peripheral temperature via rectal and big toe temperature probes.
5. Urine output should be estimated at least every hour with an indwelling catheter (Hilberman and Osborn, 1976).
6. Interpretation of information derived from pressure and temperature monitoring is discussed below and outlined in *Figure 10.5* and *Table 10.3*.

Table 10.3 Use of blood pressure, CVP and central/peripheral temperature gradient to guide treatment in shock

BP	*CVP*	*Central/peripheral temperature gradient >5°C (>9°F)*	*Diagnosis*	*Management*
↓	↓	↑	Volume depleted	Plasma/saline infusion
↓	↑	↑	Cardiogenic shock	Inotropic support, consider vasodilators
N or ↑	N or ↑	↑	Vasoconstricted	Vasodilators
N or ↑	↑	N	Overloaded	Diuretics, dialysis, fluid restriction

N, normal.

7. Laboratory monitoring in all cases should include blood count, haemoglobin, packed cell volume, platelet count, urea and electrolytes, blood glucose, calcium, and urine electrolytes. In severe shock, blood gases, clotting studies and fibrin degradation products, liver function tests, and calcium, phosphate and magnesium levels are also necessary. Chest X-ray and ECG should always be performed.

Correction of reduced preload (*volume replacement*)

Choice of fluid

The choice of fluid for initial resuscitation in shock depends on the nature of the fluid lost (blood, plasma, water, or electrolytes). However, the following factors must also be considered:

1. *The need to restore oxygen-carrying capacity* – Blood loss or haemolysis occurs in many forms of shock. Restoration of oxgyen-carrying capacity with whole blood or packed red cells is necessary if the packed cell volume falls below 35 per cent, or if there is continuing blood loss. Tissue perfusion is maximal at a haematocrit between 35 and 45 per cent, but higher levels may be desirable if hypoxia due to pulmonary insufficiency is also present. Unless anaemia itself is life threatening (haemoglobin <5 g/100 ml) plasma or crystalloid should be used for volume expansion while awaiting cross-matched blood. *However, in an emergency, group O Rh negative blood can be given*. The infusion of cold stored blood may precipitate arrhythmia in shocked, acidotic, and hyperkalaemic patients, and blood should be as fresh as possible and warmed before use.
2. *Colloid oncotic pressure* – Plasma proteins, and in particular albumin, are responsible for the colloid oncotic forces retaining fluid within the intravascular space. Loss of colloid is common in shock and further dilution of plasma proteins may occur if crystalloids are used for resuscitation. When the colloid oncotic pressure falls below the capillary hydrostatic pressure, water is lost to the extravascular space, resulting in tissue or pulmonary oedema. Colloids, such

Table 10.4 Fluids available for resuscitation

Fluid	*Oncotic effect*	*Osmolality*	*Sodium content* (mmol/ℓ)	*Indications – advantages*	*Disadvantages*
Plasma protein fraction (PPF) (5% albumin)	Iso-oncotic (albumin)	Isosmolar (300 mosm/kg)	140–160	Preferred fluid for initial volume expansion. Immediately available, no cross-match required. Replaces colloid	More expensive than crystalloid. May aggravate hypernatraemia
Fresh frozen plasma (FFP)	Iso-oncotic (albumin)	Isosmolar	138–148	Replacement of clotting factors, colloid and volume	Requires blood grouping, and thawing. Hepatitis risk
20% albumin (salt poor albumin), in 5% glucose or 0.9% NaCl	Hyperoncotic	Isosmolar	140–150 if in 0.9% NaCl. ≯17 if in 5% glucose	Replacement of colloid. Mobilization of oedema fluid in hypoalbuminaemic states	Expensive. Hyperoncotic; should not be used for initial resuscitation unless diluted 1:4 with crystalloid
Dextran 40 or 70 in 0.9% NaCl (synthetic plasma substitute)	Hyperoncotic (Dextran)	Isosmolar	140–150	Volume expansion, initial colloid replacement. Beneficial effect on viscosity. Mild anticoagulant effect	May increase bleeding. Anaphylactic reactions. Interferes with cross-matching
Hydroxyethyl starch in 0.9% (synthetic colloid substitute)	Iso-oncotic (hydroxyethyl starch)	Isosmolar	140–150	Cheap plasma substitute	Anaphylactic reactions
Whole blood	Iso-oncotic	Isosmolar	138–148	Replacement of oxygen carrying capacity; volume and colloid	Requires cross-matching. Hepatitis risk. Stored blood aggravates electrolyte and metabolic derangement

Packed red blood cells	Iso-oncotic (albumin)	Isosmolar	138–148	Replacement of oxygen-carrying capacity	Requires cross-matching. Hepatitis risk. Stored red cells aggravate electrolyte derangement
Normal saline (0.9% NaCl)	Nil	Isosmolar	138–148	Suitable for initial resuscitation. Readily available, cheap	Freely distributed in extracellular fluids. Dilution of plasma proteins → oedema. Larger volumes required than when plasma is used
Ringer's lactate* balanced salt solution with lactate (28 mmol/ℓ) and potassium (4 mmol/ℓ)†	Nil	Isosmolar	130	Suitable for initial resuscitation. Readily available, cheap	Freely distributed in extracellular fluids. Dilution of plasma proteins. Dangerous in lactic acidosis and hyperkalaemia
2.5% glucose 0.45% sodium chloride	Nil	Isosmolar	77	Replacement of fluid and electrolytes after initial resuscitation	Not suitable for initial resuscitation (inadequate sodium)
4% glucose 0.18% sodium chloride	Nil	Isosmolar	30	Maintenance fluid. Suitable for replacement of physiological losses	Not suitable for initial resuscitation (inadequate sodium)
5% glucose	Nil	Isosmolar	Nil	Use only to replace water losses in excess of electrolyte loss	Not suitable for initial resuscitation. May cause hyponatraemia

* See Appendix 8 for complete electrolyte composition and for other solutions for IV use.
† Almost identical with Hartmann's solution (Ca, 2 mmol/ℓ; Na, 131 mmol/ℓ; K, 5 mmol/ℓ; Cl, 111 mmol/ℓ; lactate, 29 mmol/ℓ; Appendix 8).

as plasma, should therefore be given during initial resuscitation, with the aim of maintaining oncotic pressure and plasma albumin at near normal levels. Possible exceptions are burns or sepsis associated with severe capillary leakage. In these situations plasma proteins are continually lost across damaged capillaries and accumulate in the extravascular compartment where they exert an oncotic effect, drawing fluid out of the vascular space. In these patients volume expansion with crystalloid may be preferable but some still favour the use of colloid (Shoemaker and Hauser, 1979; Harms *et al.*, 1981).

3. *The presence of coagulation disorders* – Coagulation abnormalities occur in a high proportion of patients with severe shock. This is aggravated by replacement of losses by fluids deficient in clotting factors. In the presence of severe DIC or bleeding, fresh frozen plasma infusion is necessary to replace clotting factors.
4. *Electrolyte value derangements* (*see above*) – Patients in shock may be hypernatraemic sodium level over 150 mmol/ℓ), isonatraemic (sodium 135–150 mmol/ℓ) or hyponatraemic (sodium < 130 mmol/ℓ), depending upon the relative quantities of water or electrolytes lost. Sudden shifts in intracellular fluid and electrolytes may result in cerebral oedema if deficits are corrected too rapidly. Solutions which are both isotonic and isonatraemic (and preferably containing colloid, e.g. albumin is a synthetic plasma substitute), should always be used for initial cardiovascular stabilization in preference to isotonic but hyponatraemic solution such as 0.18% NaCℓ in 4% glucose, to minimize fluid shifts. Once perfusion has improved and cardiac output stabilized, the water deficit in hypernatraemic states can be gradually corrected over 24–48 hours using mildly hyponatraemic solutions (sodium chloride 0.45% in 2.5% glucose, sodium chloride 0.18% in 4% glucose). If hyponatraemia is not due to fluid overload, it can be corrected by infusing normal saline or plasma protein fraction (Weil and Henning, 1979).
5. *Properties of the fluids available*. A wide variety of fluids (*see* Appendix 8) are available (*Table 10.4*). *Rapid correction of the volume deficit is more important than the type of fluid used.* Volume replacement should never be delayed while awaiting blood or a fluid which has theoretical advantages over others which are immediately available.
   (a) *In severe shock*, solutions containing colloids are preferable because they retain fluid in the intravascular space, resulting in greater volume expansion than is achieved with crystalloid solutions. Blood should be taken for cross-matching before dextran is infused, as dextran may interfere with the cross-matching process.
   (b) *Isotonic crystalloids* such as normal saline (sodium chloride 0.9%), Ringer's lactate or Hartmann's solution are readily available, cheap and generally adequate for initial resuscitation. Since they are freely distributed between the intravascular and the extravascular spaces, two or three times more crystalloid than colloid is required for equivalent volume expansion. Oedema and rapid shifts of cerebral and intracellular volumes are therefore more likely with crystalloid (Shoemaker and Hauser, 1979).
   (c) *Hyponatraemic solutions* such as sodium chloride 0.45% in 2.5% glucose, or 0.18% sodium chloride in 4% glucose should be avoided for initial resuscitation, as they may cause cerebral oedema. However, once the circulation has been stabilized they are suitable for slow correction of residual water and electrolyte deficits, and for maintenance requirements.

Quantity of fluid

1. The correction of hypovolaemia is the single most important therapeutic measure in the treatment of shock. Even in cardiac failure, the failing myocardium may require a higher than normal filling pressure to achieve optimal cardiac output, and a trial of volume expansion with careful monitoring is justified unless pulmonary oedema or cardiomyopathy is present. The aim of volume replacement therapy is to adjust the preload on the left and right ventricles in order to achieve maximum cardiac output (Perkin and Levin, 1982a, b). In severe shock (such as that due to septicaemia) where fluid is continually lost across damaged capillaries, and loss of vascular tone increases the capacitance of the vasculature, several times the estimated total blood volume may be required to raise the CVP to optimal levels.
2. Volume replacement should begin as soon as vascular access has been established (*see Figure 10.5*).
3. Shock due to simple volume depletion from diarrhoea, vomiting or blood loss will respond rapidly to the infusion of plasma 10–20 ml/kg or normal saline (sodium chloride 0.9%) over 10–20 minutes. The response can be judged by improvement of pulse pressure, capillary filling, increased peripheral temperature and urine output, and improved level of consciousness. If a satisfactory response is obtained, a further 20 ml/kg may be given rapidly. If the child continues to improve invasive monitoring is unnecessary and fluid replacement can be continued at a slower rate over the next 24 hours, aiming to replace the estimated deficit, plus continuing losses and maintenance requirements.
4. A failure to respond to initial volume expansion may indicate severe volume depletion or continuing losses, necessitating additional volume replacement. However, *it may also be due to cardiac failure or the development of pulmonary oedema*. The clinical distinction between these two possibilities may be extremely difficult, and monitoring of CVP or PWP becomes essential to guide further volume replacement and drug therapy (*see Figure 10.5*). A clinical re-assessment and a search for sites of continuing blood or fluid loss, as well as a chest X-ray are also necessary at this stage. With careful monitoring, volume expansion should be continued until CVP or PWP reach levels at which ventricular preload is adequate. Cardiac output is generally optimal at a CVP between 8 and 15 mm Hg (11 and 20 cm H_2O) and a PWP between 15 and 20 mm Hg (20 and 27 cm H_2O). More information is obtained from serial measurements of CVP following fluid challenge than from a single reading.
5. With CVP monitoring, a third fluid challenge should be performed as follows (Levin, 1979; Perkin and Levin, 1982a, b):
   (a) If CVP is under 5 mm Hg or PWP under 8 mm Hg infuse 10 ml/kg over 10 minutes.
   (b) If CVP is under 10 mm Hg or PWP under 12 mm Hg infuse 5 ml/kg over 10 minutes.
   (c) If CVP is over 10 mm Hg or PWP over 12 mm Hg infuse 3 ml/kg over 10 minutes.

   Following each fluid challenge, the CVP or PWP are repeated. If the CVP returns to within 2 mm Hg, or the PWP to within 3 mm Hg, of the pre-infusion pressure within 10 minutes of completing the infusion, then further fluid is infused. Fluid administration is continued until either the haemodynamic signs of shock are corrected, or until the CVP and PWP exceed their initial values by 2 mm Hg and 3 mm Hg, respectively.

6. Once the optimal preload has been achieved, fluids should be given to cover maintenance requirements, losses from stool, urine or secretions, and to replace any remaining volume deficit.

Myocardial contractility improvement

Once volume deficits have been corrected, further improvement in cardiac output and tissue perfusion is obtainable by improving myocardial contractility. This can be achieved by:

1. Correction of acidosis, hypoxia, anaemia and electrolyte imbalance.
2. Administration of specific positive inotropic agents.
3. Reduction of afterload (*see Figure 10.2*).

(Inotropic drugs influence and modify the contractility of the heart muscle. A positive isotropic drug strengthens and improves its contractility.)

***Correction of acidosis and electrolyte imbalance (see also* Chapter 11)**

1. Metabolic acidosis is due to poor tissue perfusion. Mild degrees of metabolic acidosis are adequately compensated by hyperventilation, but in severe shock the pH falls. Reduction of pH below 7.2 is associated with impaired myocardial function, arrhythmia, and poor cardiovascular responses to sympathomimetic drugs. Mild reductions in pH will respond to improvement of perfusion following volume replacement. Severe acidosis (pH < 7.2) should be corrected by the infusion of sodium bicarbonate (Hazard and Griffin, 1980). *Respiratory acidosis* (PCO_2 *above* 50 mm Hg (7 kPa)) *must always be treated by ventilation before administering bicarbonate*. Sodium bicarbonate is metabolized to CO_2 and water; PCO_2 will rise following bicarbonate administration if ventilation cannot be increased, causing a worsening of respiratory acidosis.
2. Bicarbonate should be given initially as an infusion of 1–2 mmol/kg over 10 minutes. Subsequent correction of acidosis should be guided by frequent determination of blood gases. The formula – mmol of bicarbonate required = wt (kg) × base deficit × 0.3 – is a useful guide. Half the required volume is infused slowly either in repeated small boluses or as an infusion over 2–3 hours, to partially correct the acidosis to pH levels above 7.25. The remainder can be given over the next 12 hours (*see also* Chapter 11, page 119).
3. Rapid correction of the base deficit may cause hypernatraemia and an increase in osmolality. This is particularly hazardous in premature infants in whom it may precipitate intraventricular haemorrhage. Bicarbonate should be infused slowly and the 8.4% solution diluted with an equal volume of 5% glucose to give a 4.2% solution. If severe acidosis and persistent shock necessitate very large quantities of bicarbonate, peritoneal dialysis with a bicarbonate-containing fluid may be preferable, to minimize hypernatraemia.

Rapid correction of acidosis may result in a failure of respiratory drive, and therefore a rise in PCO_2. This may cause a worsening of cerebrospinal fluid acidosis, as HCO_3 enters the cerebrospinal fluid less readily than CO_2. Respiration must be carefully watched during HCO_3 therapy, and elective ventilation instituted early if the CO_2 rises.

CALCIUM

Shock is commonly associated with hypocalcaemia which further decreases myocardial contractility and increases the risk of convulsions and arrhythmia.

Hypocalcaemia should be corrected by slow infusion of $CaCl_2$ 10%, 0.1–0.2 ml/kg (10–20 mg/kg). Calcium gluconate may be used as an alternative, but it is less rapidly effective and larger volumes are required (calcium gluconate 10%, 0.5–1 ml/kg). Additional doses are given as required. Calcium should be given slowly, over 5–10 minutes, to avoid bradycardia. It cannot be given into a line used for bicarbonate infusion as precipitation may occur, and a central line should be used if one is available.

MAGNESIUM

Hypomagnesaemia may coexist with hypocalcaemia in shock. It is treated by injection of 24% magnesium sulphate 0.2 mEq/kg (0.1 mmol/kg) intramuscularly. The same dose can be given as a slow intravenous infusion over 6 hours. For further consideration of hypomagnesaemia, *see* Chapter 11 page 138.

PHOSPHATE

Hypophosphataemia may be associated with impaired cellular function, poor cardiac contractility and neuromuscular dysfunction. It is treated by infusion of dipotassium hydrogen phosphate 5–10 mg/kg over 4–6 hours. Disodium hydrogen phosphate should be used if hyperkalaemia is present.

GLUCOSE

Hypoglycaemia is often present in shocked patients on admission, and is treated by infusion of glucose. Conversely, sympathetic overactivity in shock may cause hyperglycaemia and relative insulin deficiency. If hyperglycaemia is severe small boluses of insulin 0.05 u/kg/hr should be given intravenously. *Repeated assessment of blood glucose using Dextrostix is essential.*

Inotropic drugs

GENERAL COMMENTS

Positive inotropic drugs improve myocardial contactility, and therefore produce an increased stroke volume for a given ventricular preload (*see Figure 10.2*). They are indicated if poor perfusion persists *after* volume correction, or if there is evidence of cardiac failure (*see Figure 10.5* and *Table 10.3*). *Arrhythmia and cardiac tamponade must always be excluded before embarking upon inotropic therapy, as these require specific treatment.* Inotropic agents should only be used in conjunction with vigorous treatment of metabolic factors which depress contractility, such as hypoxia, anaemia, acidosis, and electrolyte imbalance.

Inotropic agents of use in shock are natural or synthetic sympathomimetic agents, which act primarily on α and β-adrenergic and dopaminergic receptors in the cardiovascular system. Stimulation of α-adrenergic receptors is associated with cutaneous, splanchnic, and renal vasoconstriction, and elevation of peripheral vascular resistance. β_1 receptor activation increases heart rate, and contractility, but also increases cardiac work and oxygen consumption. β_2 receptors mediate peripheral and skeletal muscle vasodilatation and bronchodilation, and therefore reduce peripheral vascular resistance. Dopaminergic (δ) receptors mediate splanchnic and renal vasodilation (Antonaccio, 1977).

CHOICE OF INOTROPIC DRUG

Sympathomimetic agents differ in their relative effects on α, β, or δ receptors. Pure α-adrenergic drugs cause exclusively vasconconstriction, whereas a pure β stimulant causes predominantly vasodilatation and increased contractility. Often the predominant effect alters at different dosage. The choice of agent, and the dosage, must therefore include a careful consideration of the beneficial effects, as well as the possible adverse effects (Antonaccio, 1977; Storstein and Taylor, 1982). Although improved myocardial contractility is the major desired effect, the more powerful inotropic drugs (such as adrenaline or high-dose dopamine) also have significant effects on α receptors. Consequently the improved contractility may be associated with a rise in peripheral vascular resistance, and an increase in afterload, myocardial work, and oxygen consumption, which may all be detrimental to a failing heart. Furthermore, as shock is generally associated with considerable catecholamine release and intense vasoconstriction, the addition of an α-stimulating inotropic agent may further reduce peripheral and organ perfusion.

Table 10.5 Inotropic and vasodilating drugs of use in shock

Drug	*Dose*	*Action*	*Comments*
Dopamine*	Low (1–6 μg/kg/min)	δ and β stimulation (vasodilator)	Improves renal, mesenteric and peripheral perfusion, and reduces afterload.
	Moderate (6–12 μg/kg/min)	β stimulation	Improves cardiac contractility and perfusion.
	High (12–30 μg/kg/min)	α and β stimulation	Stimulates cardiac contractility but with increasing vasoconstruction at higher doses
Dobutamine*	1–2.5, up to 10 μg/kg/min	Selective β_1 stimulation	Improves myocardial contractility with minimal vasoconstriction
Isoprenaline*	0.02–0.5 μg/kg/min	β stimulation	Increases myocardial contractility and heart rate. Peripheral vasodilation. May increase cardiac work
Adrenaline†	0.02–0.5 μg/kg/min	α and β stimulation	Strong inotrope. Increases contractility. Increasing vasoconstriction at high doses. Used in anaphylactic shock and cardiogenic shock with hypotension. May be combined with nitroprusside
Sodium nitroprusside	0.5–8 μg/kg/min	Arterial and venous vasodilator	Reduces afterload and improves perfusion. May cause hypotension at high dose
Hydralazine	0.1–0.5 mg/kg IV bolus 3–6 hourly	Arterial vasodilation	Reduces afterload and improves perfusion. May cause hypotension and tachycardia
Prostacyclin	5–20 ng/kg/min	Vasodilator antiplatelet action	Improves perfusion and reduces afterload. Expensive and not yet widely used

* *See also* Chapter 2, *Table 2.2* for additional infusion solutions and drip rates.
† *See also* Chapter 2, *Table 2.1* for additional information.

Although blood pressure may be increased by vasoconstriction, *this does not necessarily indicate increased flow to the tissues*, and in fact perfusion may worsen. Some of these adverse vasoconstrictor effects may be avoided by choice of agents with predominantly β effects, or by the use of a combination of inotropic agent and a vasodilator.

The positive inotropic and vasodilator drugs should be given as continuous infusions. No other drugs should be given through the same line since interruption of the infusion or flushing of the line may cause sudden changes in blood pressure, or arrhythmia. The powerful inotropic drugs may cause major haemodynamic changes and should only be given with close monitoring of CVP, blood pressure and perfusion.

SPECIFIC POSITIVE INOTROPIC DRUGS (*Table 10.5*)

Dopamine

Dopamine is the naturally occurring precursor of adrenaline which has dopaminergic, α-adrenergic, and β-receptor stimulating activities. Its cardiovascular effects are dose related: at low doses (1–6 μg/kg/min) the primary effect is vasodilatation which increases renal, mesenteric, coronary and cerebral blood flow, with minimal increase in heart rate. Peripheral vascular resistance may fall, and therefore cardiac output increases owing to the decrease in afterload. At higher doses (6–30 μg/kg/min) there is increasing β receptor stimulation, causing increased myocardial contractility, and heart rate. However, there is also increasing α-stimulation with vasoconstriction and increased peripheral resistance. The rise in peripheral resistance may increase myocardial oxygen consumption.

Dopamine can be used at different doses to obtain a variety of effects on the circulation (Table 10.5). Dopamine can also be used in high doses (12–30 μg/kg/min) in combination with a vasodilator (such as nitroprusside) to obtain its inotropic effect, but to minimize the unwanted α effects of vasoconstriction.

Dopamine has few toxic effects in low doses. In moderate dosage (6–12 μg/kg/min) and at higher doses (12–30 μg/kg/min) tachycardia and arrhythmia may occur, with unwanted vasoconstriction. Dopamine is given by either central or peripheral infusion. An easy formula for calculation of dosage is:

$$6 \times \text{weight in kg} = \text{mg dopamine}$$

This dose is diluted to 100 ml in 5% glucose. The rate of infusion in ml/hr equals the dosage in μg/kg/min, e.g. 4 ml/hr = 4 μg/kg/min.

More concentrated solutions can be used if volume restriction is necessary.

Dobutamine

Dobutamine is a synthetic catecholamine which increases myocardial contractility by direct action on β-adrenergic receptors, and has minimal α effects. Unlike isoprenaline dobutamine only occasionally causes tachycardia, and unlike noradrenaline it produces little vasoconstriction at usual therapeutic doses. Dobutamine does not dilate renal and mesenteric vessels, but renal and mesenteric flow may improve as a consequence of improved cardiac output.

Side-effects include hypertension, arrhythmia, nausea, vomiting and headache.

Positive inotropic effects occur at doses as low as 0.5 μg/kg/min. The usual effective range is 1.0–2.5 μg/kg/min but the dose may be increased up to 10 μg/kg/min if necessary. Dobutamine has no advantages over dopamine, which in general is the preferred drug.

Isoprenaline

Isoprenaline is a synthetic sympathomimetic drug with almost pure β-receptor stimulating effect. It increases heart rate, myocardial contractility, and oxygen consumption. The peripheral β effect causes vasodilatation, bronchodilatation, and a reduction in vascular resistance, which may diminish venous return to the heart. The increased contractility usually compensates for the vasodilatation, so blood pressure does not fall. However, increased muscle blood flow may divert blood from more vital areas.

The starting dose should be 0.02 μg/kg/min. The dose may be increased to 0.5 μg/kg/min. Tachycardia, arrhythmia and increased myocardial oxygen consumption are the main unwanted effects.

Adrenaline

Adrenaline has both α- and β-receptor stimulating effects. In low dosage its inotropic action increases cardiac output while peripheral vascular resistance falls slightly. α-stimulation is greater with increasing dose. At high doses intense vasoconstriction may severely reduce tissue perfusion, despite considerable elevation of blood pressure. Adrenaline is primarily indicated for treatment of anaphylactic shock, where its vasoconstrictor effects are necessary to restore blood pressure to levels adequate to sustain coronary perfusion. In most other situations, the vasoconstrictor effects are undesirable, and can be diminished by combination of adrenaline with a vasodilator.

The starting dose for continuous infusion is 0.02 μg/kg/min. This can be increased to 0.2–0.5 μg/kg/min. Doses exceeding 0.5 μg/kg/min are associated with poor peripheral perfusion.

Unwanted effects are tachycardia, arrhythmia, peripheral vasoconstriction, and hyperglycaemia. *Adrenaline must be given into a central line because the intense vasoconstriction it induces may cause peripheral gangrene.*

Digitalis

The cardiac glycosides have in the past been used to increase myocardial contractility in shock. However, they are less effective than the other agents discussed above, and their long serum half-life and numerous toxic effects are major drawbacks. Digitalis should NOT be used, as other less toxic and rapidly acting agents are available.

Afterload reduction: vasodilatation

GENERAL COMMENTS

Vasodilator drugs cause smooth-muscle relaxation in the arterial and venous circulation. They reduce the resistance to blood flow from the heart and therefore increase cardiac output with decreased myocardial oxygen requirements. Vasodilatation may improve tissue perfusion, and reduce elevated left and right ventricular pressures in severe heart failure (Cohn and Franciosa, 1977).

The indications for vasodilator therapy are:

1. Persistent vasoconstriction and poor perfusion in the presence of adequate circulating volume.
2. Severe cardiac failure with elevated CVP or PWP.

3. Hypertension and/or cardiac failure.
4. Reduction of unwanted vasoconstriction in combination with inotropic drugs (*see Figure 10.5* and *Table 10.3*).

Vasodilatation is dangerous in the presence of hypovolaemia. It should not be attempted if severe hypotension is present, but may be used cautiously in the presence of mild hypotension. Close monitoring of arterial pressure, CVP or PWP, and central and peripheral temperature is essential.

VASODILATOR DRUGS (*Table 10.5*)

Dopamine
In doses of 1–6 μg/kg/min dopamine functions mainly as a vasodilator through its β and δ-receptor stimulating activity. Renal, splanchnic, and peripheral vasodilatation occur with a mild increase in cardiac output. These effects are often beneficial in improving perfusion in shock.

Sodium nitroprusside
Nitroprusside is a potent rapidly acting vasodilator, with effects on both the arterial and venous circulations. Its activity is very short lived, and it must therefore be given as a constant infusion. The dose range is between 0.5 and 8.0 μg/kg/min. The infusion must be commenced at the lower dose and increased slowly until the desired improvement in perfusion is obtained. If hypotension occurs, the infusion rate should be reduced, any volume depletion treated, and inotropic support considered. Nitroprusside is unstable in solution, and must be protected from light. The end-product of metabolism is thiocyanate, which is toxic in high doses. Blood levels of thiocyanate should be monitored in patients receiving high doses for prolonged periods (more than 3 days) and the drug stopped if levels exceed 10 mg/100 ml or blood cyanide levels exceed 0.34 mg/100 ml.

Hydralazine
Hydralazine is a vasodilator acting directly on arterial smooth muscle. It has a duration of action of 2–6 hours. Intravenous doses of 0.1–0.5 mg/kg every 3–6 hours may be used. It is less easily controlled than nitroprusside as the effect is more prolonged. Pronounced tachycardia and hypotension may occur.

Prostacyclin
Prostacyclin is a recently developed naturally produced prostaglandin (epoprostenol) with both vasodilating and anti-platelet actions. It has shown promising effects in doses of 5–20 ng/kg/min given as a constant infusion. Side-effects include hypotension, bleeding (owing to its antiplatelet action) and bradycardia at high doses.

Chlorpromazine
The α-blocking action of this major tranquillizer has been used to reduce afterload and vasoconstriction. However, the drug is unpredictable in its action, and severe hypotension may occur. It should NOT be used, as more easily controlled agents are available.

Phentolamine
Phentolamine is a direct-acting α-receptor blocking drug. Dosages of 1–20 μg/kg/min are infused. Duration of action is 20–40 minutes. It has no advantages over nitroprusside.

Treatment of organ failure

Ventilation

Respiratory failure is invariably present in severe shock, and is a common cause of death (Sykes, 1976). It is caused by damage to the pulmonary vasculature and declining level of consciousness, which impairs ventilatory drive and the ability to maintain an airway. In early shock patients usually hyperventilate, and have a normal PO_2, low PCO_2, and normal chest X-ray. However, as shock worsens, increasing interstitial oedema results in a fall of lung compliance. Obstruction of lung capillaries by platelet–fibrin microthrombi causes increasing ventilation–perfusion imbalance. There is a progressive fall in PO_2, increase in oxygen requirements and ultimately a rise in PCO_2. Pulmonary oedema, shock lung, and respiratory arrest rapidly supervene.

Control of the airway and positive pressure ventilation allows resuscitation to continue without fear of sudden arrest, and also allows sedation and paralysis, which decrease oxygen requirements.

Elective ventilation should be undertaken in all severely shocked patients if the level of consciousness declines and there is no response to simple volume expansion. Any reduction of PO_2 below 60 mm Hg (8 kPa) or a rising PCO_2 should immediately be treated with oxygen and ventilation.

Shock lung

Shock lung is a syndrome of severe respiratory failure with markedly decreased lung compliance, poor oxygenation despite high concentrations of inspired oxygen, and X-ray appearances of diffuse interstitial oedema. Pathologically, there is damage to the alveolar epithelium and capillary endothelium, causing increased permeability to proteins. Fluid accumulates in the interstitial spaces and alveoli. Leukocyte, platelet and fibrin aggregates occlude the capillaries, and pulmonary vasoconstriction occurs due to hypoxia and the release of vasoactive mediators of inflammation (Bone, 1980).

Management

The management of shock lung is difficult, and consists primarily of ventilatory support. High concentrations of oxygen, and high-pressure ventilation are often required for long periods. Positive and end-expiratory pressures help to prevent intra-alveolar fluid accumulation. Vigorous chest physiotherapy and tracheal toilet are essential, and any infection must be treated with antibiotics.

Fluid accumulation in the extravascular pulmonary spaces can be minimized by maintaining a normal colloid oncotic pressure and by reducing hydrostatic pressure in the pulmonary capillaries. Pulmonary wedge pressure measurement is useful; PWP should be kept as low as possible without impairing left ventricular function. Water restriction, diuretics, and dialysis may help to reduce extravascular pulmonary fluid, and improve lung compliance (Shoemaker and Hauser, 1979).

Renal support

Impaired renal perfusion and oliguria occur early in shock. Initially the kidney responds by maximal sodium and water retention. If renal hypoperfusion persists, acute renal failure occurs, indicated by a declining urine/plasma urea ratio and rising urine sodium level (*see Table 10.2*). In early shock, volume expansion and inotropic support will improve urine flow. Dopamine, in doses of 1–6 μg/kg/min, is useful in improving renal blood flow. Frusemide (1–5 mg/kg IV) and mannitol (1 g/kg IV) increase urine flow and lessen the risk of acute tubular necrosis. However, once renal failure is established, peritoneal dialysis should be started. Dialysis is urgently indicated if urine flow is less than 0.5 ml/kg/hr, potassium rises above 6 mmol/ℓ, or if acidosis or fluid overload supervene (*see* page 434).

Inappropriate antidiuretic hormone secretion (ADH)

Inappropriate ADH secretion commonly occurs in shocked patients, with both cerebral and pulmonary involvement. It is manifested by oliguria, declining plasma sodium concentration and fluid overload. It can be distinguished from pre-renal oliguria by urine electrolyte findings (*see Table 10.2*) and by clinical and CVP evidence of fluid overload. It is treated by fluid restriction to less than maintenance requirements plus urine output (*see* page 126).

Central nervous system

Deterioration of cerebral function, manifested by restlessness, confusion and coma, is common in shock. It may be the result of the initiating insult (such as encephalitis, or Reye's syndrome) or of cerebral hypoperfusion. Elective intubation and ventilation must be performed early in comatose patients. Electrolyte imbalance, hypoglycaemia, and hypocalcaemia should be corrected and convulsions controlled. Cerebral oedema should be treated by controlled ventilation to maintain CO_2 between 25 and 30 mm Hg, mannitol infusion (0.5–1 g/kg 6 hourly), fluid restriction and barbiturates. In severe cases intracranial pressure monitoring is necessary (*see* Chapter 26, page 295 for detailed managment of cerebral oedema).

Nutrition

Severely shocked patients are in a highly catabolic state and may visibly waste away within a few days of intensive care. Endogenous protein and energy stores are rapidly consumed, and there is poor wound healing, increased risk of infection and poor recovery from organ failure. Nutritional support should be started after initial resuscitation in all severely shocked patients likely to require prolonged intensive care. High concentrations of glucose (10–15% solutions) with at least 1 g/kg of protein (given as an amino acid solution) are necessary (*see Appendix 5*). Insulin 0.05 units/kg/hr intravenously may be required if hyperglycaemia develops. Vitamins and trace metals must be provided in patients requiring prolonged intravenous nutrition. Enteral feeding by nasojejunal or nasogastric tube is preferable as soon as gastric motility returns.

Disseminated intravascular coagulation (DIC) (*see also* Chapter 54)

DIC is invariably present in severe shock, and is associated with many of the initiating illnesses such as septicaemia, burns, and major trauma. It is treated by correction of the shock and replacement of clotting factors with fresh frozen plasma. Treatment with heparin is controversial, and it should be used only if DIC cannot be controlled by clotting factor replacement, as it may be associated with severe haemorrhage. Heparin in doses of 25 units/kg/hr is usually adequate. Exchange transfusion with fresh blood may be effective in treating DIC, and is relatively easy in children, whose small blood volume may be readily exchanged.

Pain relief

Many of the initiating events such as severe injury or burns may cause pain. The sympathetic response to pain increases vasoconstriction and tachycardia. Morphine (0.1 mg/kg IV) or pethidine (0.5 mg/kg IV) are suitable analgesics, but may depress respiration. Elective ventilation, however, should enable adequate analgesia to be given. Analgesia should always be given when the patient is paralysed for ventilation.

Treatment of the primary disease

Treatment of the primary disease should be undertaken simultaneously with resuscitation. When the diagnosis is not obvious, appropriate investigations must be undertaken to establish the aetiology (*see Figure 10.4*). Infection should always be suspected as a precipitating factor. After appropriate cultures have been taken, treatment with broad-spectrum antibiotics should be commenced without delay. A combination of a penicillin (100 mg/kg/day) and gentamicin (7 mg/kg/day) is suitable for initial therapy.

Septic shock

The general principles of cardiovascular and organ support outlined previously are applicable to septic shock. However, its pathophysiology and presenting features may differ from most other forms of shock, and even with intensive support the mortality remains high (Ledingham, 1976b).

Septic shock occurs either as a primary illness, (such as Gram-negative septicaema in the newborn), or as a complication of immune deficiency, immunosuppressive therapy, surgery or trauma.

Recognition

Patients with septicaemia present either with hypotension and poor peripheral perfusion typical of other forms of shock, or as 'warm shock' with elevated central temperature, warm extremities, bounding pulses, normal capillary refilling and a normal systolic blood pressure. In the latter instance the only signs of shock are tachypnoea, tachycardia, oliguria, restlessness and confusion. Laboratory features indicate hypoxaemia and metabolic acidosis with compensatory respiratory alkalosis. Mild coagulation disturbance and thrombocytopenia are common.

As septic shock worsens, features of the 'warm' phase are replaced by those typical of other forms of severe shock. Respiratory and renal failure are common, with deepening coma.

The initial warm phase of septic shock is due to arteriovenous shunting in the precapillary vessels. Thus, despite a high cardiac output and a hyperdynamic circulation, organ perfusion is impaired. As perfusion worsens, there is organ failure, with loss of vascular tone, capillary damage and activation of clotting. In the late stages, cardiac output falls and the physiology then resembles other forms of shock.

Management

Treatment is aimed at careful volume replacement guided by CVP monitoring, PWP monitoring, or both. Pulmonary oedema may develop at normal or low levels of PWP, and elective ventilation should be started early if PO_2 cannot be maintained above 60 mm Hg (8 kPa). Ventilation allows fluid replacement to proceed with less risk of sudden pulmonary oedema. Once volume has been corrected, perfusion should be improved, using low-dose dopamine or isoprenaline and vasodilation with nitroprusside. Acidosis and electrolyte imbalance must be treated early, with dialysis if necessary. DIC is treated with fresh frozen plasma and blood and heparinization may be considered (25 units/kg/hr). Broad-spectrum antibiotics should be started with a combination of a cephalosporin or penicillin and an aminoglycoside. Where adrenal haemorrhage is suspected (as in meningococcal septicaemia) replacement hydrocortisone should be given (*see* page 472).

Anaphylactic shock

The basic principles of shock management apply to anaphylactic shock, but specific features of its management are discussed here.

Anaphylactic shock may occur following:

1. Drugs (especially antibiotics) given orally or intravenously.
2. Radiological contrast media.
3. Desensitization.
4. Injection of blood or blood products.
5. Food allergies.
6. Insect stings.

Recognition

The earliest symptoms are swelling of tissues, sweating, restlessness, itching, nausea, vomiting, diarrhoea, coughing or wheezing. Hypotension, circulatory failure and cardiac arrest may occur suddenly, often associated with bronchial spasm or laryngeal oedema.

Management

During early symptoms

1. The offending drug should be stopped immediately.
2. Adrenaline (1 in 1000 = 0.1% = 1.0 mg in 1 ml) should be given subcutaneously in a dose of 0.01 mg (0.01 ml)/kg. The maximum single dose is 0.5 ml (0.5 mg). If there is no improvement after 5 minutes the same dose should be repeated.

If shock, bronchospasm or laryngeal oedema occur in addition to above

1. Maintain an adequate airway by suction, oropharyngeal airway, or intubation.
2. Repeat the subcutaneous adrenaline injection.
3. Give oxygen.
4. Establish an intravenous line for continued adrenaline infusion (0.05–0.5 mg/kg/min).
5. Give plasma or 0.9% sodium chloride 20 ml/kg over 10 minutes. If shock persists further fluid administration should be guided by CVP.
6. Antihistamine drugs – give one of the following:
   (a) Chlorpheniramine (Piriton) – available in ampoules containing 10 mg/ml. Dilute to 1 mg/ml with sterile water. Give 0.25 mg/kg up to total of 20 mg IV.
   (b) Promethazine (Phenergan) – available as 25 mg/ml ampoules. Dilute to give a solution of 1 mg/ml. IV doses: up to 1 year of age, 0.5 mg/kg; 1–7 years, 5 mg; 7–14 years, 10–25 mg; adults, 25–50 mg.
7. Give hydrocortisone 100 mg IV.

Later management

1. If response is poor, resuscitation should continue with volume replacement guided by CVP monitoring.
2. Hydrocortisone should be given; 100 mg every 4 hours.
3. Further doses of antihistamines should be given at 6–8 hourly intervals for up to 48 hours.
4. Sensitive patients should be given information bracelets. Highly sensitive children may require an adrenaline inhaler or an adrenaline injection kit, supplies of antihistamines for immediate use, and their families must be fully educated on immediate management (*see* page 560).

Referral

Severe shock, with multi-organ failure, is best managed in a paediatric intensive care unit, by a team experienced in the monitoring and circulatory support required. However, many shocked patients are either too ill to be transferred to an intensive care unit, or are seen in areas where these facilities are not available. In the absence of intensive care facilities, shock can generally be managed without the use of sophisticated equipment, by careful clinical assessment, and the use of simple non-invasive monitoring. *Patients should never be transferred to an intensive care unit without a secure airway and (if necessary) ventilation.* Initial resuscitation should always be performed before attempting transfer, to correct volume deficits and acidosis, replace blood loss, and establish vascular access. Patients are more likely to survive transfer if circulating volume and metabolic derangements are corrected before the journey. Hypoglycaemia and hypothermia are common during transfer of shocked children (especially neonates) and the child should be well insulated during the journey, and a glucose-containing infusion maintained. If shock and organ failure persist following initial resuscitation, the patient should be transferred to a paediatric intensive care unit if one is available. With modern intensive care techniques, even patients with severe shock and multi-organ failure may recover, and are most likely to do so in an intensive care unit.

References

ANTONACCIO, M. J. (ed.) (1977) *Cardiovascular Pharmacology, pp. 346–348.* New York: Raven Press

BONE, R. D. (1980) Treatment of severe hypoxemia due to the adult respiratory distress syndrome. *Archives of Internal Medicine,* **140,** 85–89

COHN, J. N. and FRANCIOSA, J. A. (1977) Vasodilator therapy of cardiac failure. *New England Journal of Medicine,* **297,** 27–31

CRONE, R. K. (1980) Acute circulatory failure in children. *Pediatric Clinics of North America,* **27,** 525–537

FULTON, D. R. and GRODIN, M. (1983) Pediatric cardiac emergencies. *Emergency Medicine Clinics of North America,* **1,** 113–123

GUYTON, A. C., JONES, C. E. and COLEMAN, T. G. (1973) *Circulatory Physiology: Cardiac Output and its Regulation, pp. 253–254.* Philadelphia: W. B. Saunders

HACKEL, D. B., RATCLIFF, N. B. and MIKAT, E. (1974) The heart in shock. *Circulation Research,* **35,** 805–811

HARMS, B. A., KRAMER, G. C., BODAI, B. I. and DEMLING, R. H. (1981) Effect of hypoproteinemia on pulmonary and soft tissue oedema formation. *Critical Care Medicine,* **9,** 503–508

HAZARD, P. B. and GRIFFIN, J. P. (1980) Sodium bicarbonate in the management of systemic acidosis. *Southern Medical Journal,* **73,** 1339–1342

HILBERMAN, M. and OSBORN, J. (1976) Monitoring of the patient in shock. In Ledingham, I. McA. (ed.), *Shock,* pp. 11–138. Oxford: Excerpta Medica

LEDINGHAM, I. McA. (1976a) Pathophysiology of shock. In Ledingham, I. McA. (ed.), *Shock,* pp. 1–20. Oxford: Excerpta Medica

LEDINGHAM, I. McA. (1976b) Management of septic shock. In Ledingham, I. McA. (ed.), *Shock,* pp. 272–295. Oxford: Excerpta Medica

LEVIN, D. L. (1984) Shock. In Levin, D. L., Morris, F. C. and Moore, G. C. (eds.) *A Practical Guide to Pediatric Intensive Care,* (2nd edn.) St Louis: C. V. Mosby

MILNOR, W. R. (1975) Arterial impedance as ventricular afterload. *Circulation Research,* **36,** 565–570

MORSE, T. S. (1983) The child with multiple injuries. *Emergency Medicine Clinics of North America,* **1,** 175–185

ORLOWSKI, J. P. (1983) Pediatric cardiopulmonary resuscitation. *Emergency Medicine Clinics of North America,* **1,** 3–25

PERKIN, R. M. and LEVIN, D. L. (1982a) Shock in the pediatric patient. Part I. *Journal of Pediatrics,* **101,** 163–169

PERKIN, R. M. and LEVIN, D. L. (1982b) Shock in the pediatric patient. Part II. *Journal of Pediatrics,* **101,** 319–332

SHOEMAKER, W. C. and HAUSER, C. J. (1979) Critique of crystalloid versus colloid therapy in shock and shock lung. *Critical Care Medicine,* **7,** 117–124

STORSTEIN, L. and TAYLOR, S. H. (eds.) (1984) New and old inotropic drugs. *Clinical Cardiology,* **7,** 119–124

SYKES, M. K. (1976) Pulmonary disturbances in shock. In Ledingham, I. McA. (ed.) *Shock,* Oxford: Excerpta Medica

TAYLOR, S. H., SILKE, B. and NELSON, G. I. C. (1982) Principles of treatment of left ventricular failure. *European Heart Journal,* **3,** Suppl. D: 19–43

TODRES, I. D., CRONE, R. K., ROGERS, M. C. and SHANNON, D. C. (1979) Swan–Ganz catheterization in the critically ill newborn. *Critical Care Medicine,* **7,** 330–335

WEIL, M. H. and HENNING, R. J. (1979) New concepts in the diagnosis and fluid treatment of circulatory shock. *Anesthesia and Analgesia,* **58,** 124–132

Further reading

PERKIN, R. M. and LEVIN, D. L. (1980) Common fluid and electrolyte problems in the pediatric intensive care unit. *Pediatric Clinics of North America,* **27,** 576–586

Chapter 11

Acidosis and electrolyte disorders

G. B. Haycock and J. A. Black

Acidosis

Acidosis may present as part of an acute, fulminating emergency, or be discovered during the investigation of a sick, deteriorating child. In either case, urgent action must be taken to correct the acidosis, while the underlying cause is identified and treated.

When acidosis should be assumed or suspected

1. Acute respiratory insufficiency. The acidosis is of mixed respiratory and metabolic type (CO_2 retention causes carbonic acidaemia: hypoxia leads to lactic acidosis). Correction of the respiratory problem is the definitive treatment.
2. Cardiac arrest. The mechanism is similar to that in (1). Restoration of cardiac output is the definitive treatment.
3. Shock from any cause (e.g. sepsis, severe dehydration, haemorrhage). The acidosis is metabolic. Improvement in tissue perfusion is the definitive treatment.
4. Increased depth and rate of respiration without cardiac or pulmonary cause (Kussmaul respiration).
5. Unexplained lethargy, cessation of weight gain or vomiting, especially in the newborn.

Acidosis in the acute emergency (a single reversible incident)

Pathophysiology

1. Acute respiratory acidosis. Complete cessation of all pulmonary gas exchange causes the pH to fall at the rate of 0.1 units/min and the PCO_2 to rise by 2.6 kPa/min (20 mm Hg/min): oxygen stores are completely depleted by 3–4 minutes (Swyer, 1975).
2. Acute metabolic (lactic) acidosis. Tissue hypoxia or poisoning (e.g. cyanide) causes rapid anaerobic glycolysis and the production of lactic acid at a rate far greater than the kidney can excrete the resulting hydrogen ion. The production of organic acids in diabetic ketoacidosis is analogous but less fulminant.
3. Some consequences of acute acidosis are given in *Figure 11.1;* certain specific conditions are shown in the notes.

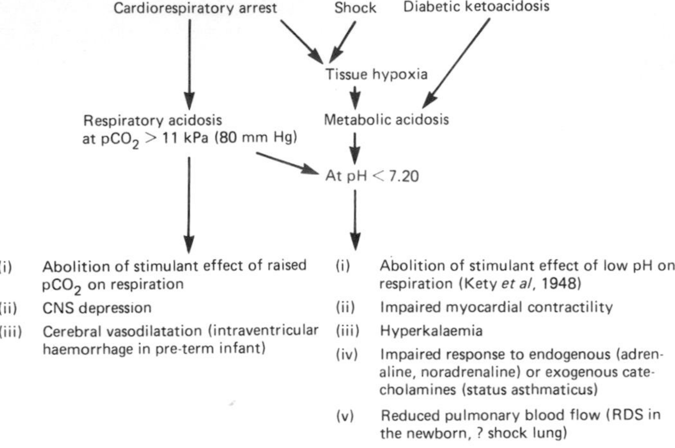

(i) Abolition of stimulant effect of raised pCO_2 on respiration
(ii) CNS depression
(iii) Cerebral vasodilatation (intraventricular haemorrhage in pre-term infant)

(i) Abolition of stimulant effect of low pH on respiration (Kety *et al*, 1948)
(ii) Impaired myocardial contractility
(iii) Hyperkalaemia
(iv) Impaired response to endogenous (adrenaline, noradrenaline) or exogenous catecholamines (status asthmaticus)
(v) Reduced pulmonary blood flow (RDS in the newborn, ? shock lung)

Figure 11.1 Acute acidosis

4. Acidosis impairs the response to resuscitation, and correction should therefore be attempted. Acute correction with alkali buys a little time only; a progressive acidosis of this kind can only be corrected by reversing the primary cause.
5. It follows that the dose of alkali should be calculated to raise the pH to a level at which normal responses are restored. This is equivalent to a pH of 7.25–7.30. Complete correction is unnecessary and may risk the production of a metabolic alkalosis when the primary condition is treated simultaneously.

The choice of alkali in acute progressive acidosis

Irrespective of the type or cause of the acidosis, intravenous sodium bicarbonate is the alkali of choice. More stable organic sodium salts (lactate, citrate, acetate) are only effective upon conversion to bicarbonate by the liver, which is likely to be impaired under the conditions described; excessive lactate is already present in acute metabolic acidosis. THAM has no advantage in practice and should be considered obsolete.

The use of sodium bicarbonate in metabolic acidosis

Sodium bicarbonate has its own disadvantages unless correctly used:

1. Molar (8.4%; i.e. 1 ml = 1 mmol $NaHCO_3$) and other commonly available concentrated bicarbonate solutions are hyperosmolar and locally irritant. They should be diluted in 5 or 10% glucose (1 part molar bicarbonate: 3 parts glucose; proportionately less for weaker solutions) and injected slowly over at least 1 minute.
2. Rapid injection of concentrated solutions of sodium bicarbonate may cause a bolus of hyperosmolar fluid to reach the brain, precipitating intracranial haemorrhage in the newborn. According to Finberg (1967) the maximum safe change in osmolality is 25 mosmol/kg body water over 4 hours, but other data

suggest that infants can tolerate smaller increases in osmolality over short periods; an IV injection of $NaHCO_3$ given over 5 minutes at a dose of 3–4 mmol/kg body weight will cause a rise of between 7.5 and 20 mosmol/kg body water within 5 minutes of completing the injection (Siegel *et al.*, 1973; Baum and Roberton, 1975).

3. The correction of a metabolic acidosis may cause coma from cerebral acidosis due to rapid transfer of CO_2 across the blood–brain barrier, particularly in diabetic ketoacidosis.

Calculation of the dose of sodium bicarbonate in metabolic acidosis

It is better to undercorrect than to overcorrect a metabolic acidosis, since overcorrection, particularly if accompanied by reversal of the underlying cause of the acidosis, may cause metabolic alkalosis, possibly with tetany, which is dangerous and difficult to correct. Appropriate undercorrection may be achieved either by (1) correcting to a standard bicarbonate of 15 mmol/ℓ; or (2) half-correcting the calculated base deficit – in either case giving no more bicarbonate than is calculated to raise the standard bicarbonate by 10 mmol/ℓ. On the assumption that the injected bicarbonate is distributed solely within the extracellular fluid (probably correct in the circumstances), the dose of bicarbonate is arrived at as the product of the desired degree of elevation of the plasma bicarbonate in mmol/ℓ, and the estimated extracellular fluid volume in litres. Extracellular fluid volume should be taken as 0.3 × body weight (kg) in infants below 1 year and 0.25 × body weight (kg) in older children.

The number of mmols of bicarbonate required to produce the necessary correction in an infant is either:

1. 15 minus the actual standard HCO_3 × weight in kg × 0.3 = mmol $NaHCO_3$ required: give the whole amount.

or,

2. Base deficit × weight in kg × 0.3: give ½ the calculated amount initially. (substitute 0.25 for 0.3 in the equations if the patient is over 1 year of age).

Examples:

1. Newborn infant with a birth weight 3.3 kg, standard HCO_3 10 mmol/ℓ; it is desired to correct to 15 mmol/ℓ.
ECF = 3.3 × 0.3 ℓ = 1.0ℓ.
Therefore, to raise the plasma bicarbonate by the desired 5 mmol/ℓ requires 5 mmol sodium bicarbonate, i.e. 5 ml of molar (8.4%) sodium bicarbonate solution. Hence the more general rule: *to raise the plasma bicarbonate of a newborn by 5 mmol/ℓ requires 1.5 ml of 8.4% sodium bicarbonate/kg body weight* (given suitably diluted).

2. Child in septic shock, weight 20 kg, base deficit 18 mmol/ℓ.
Full correction would require
Base deficit × body weight × 0.25
= 18 × 20 × 0.25 = 90 mmol sodium bicarbonate.
Following the ½ correction rule, the initial dose should be *45 mmol.*

NOTE: The notations upon which non-respiratory deviations are frequently reported by laboratories are NOT in mmols or milliequivalents, and should NOT be used as a basis for calculation.

Empirical use of sodium bicarbonate in the acute emergency

Intravenous sodium bicarbonate can be given without previous estimation of the acid–base state in an acute emergency in which the diagnosis is known and when it can be assumed that a severe metabolic acidosis is present. For example: resuscitation of the severely hypoxic newborn infant (*see* page 615) or in cardiac arrest (*see* page 278). The initial empirical dose of bicarbonate should be 5 mmol/ℓ of extracellular fluid, i.e. 5 × body weight (kg) × 0.3 (or × 0.25, *see* above) or 1.5 ml/kg 8.4% $NaHCO_3$.

Calculation of the dose of sodium bicarbonate in acute respiratory acidosis

This is not a common problem but may arise in sudden deterioration in respiratory distress syndrome in the preterm infant. In most cardiorespiratory emergencies there is a coexistent metabolic acidosis due to tissue hypoxia. However, the situation may arise in which the high PCO_2 has contributed to a potentially lethal pH of under 7.00 which requires correction; obviously a reduction in the respiratory acidosis by improved ventilation is much preferable, but may not always

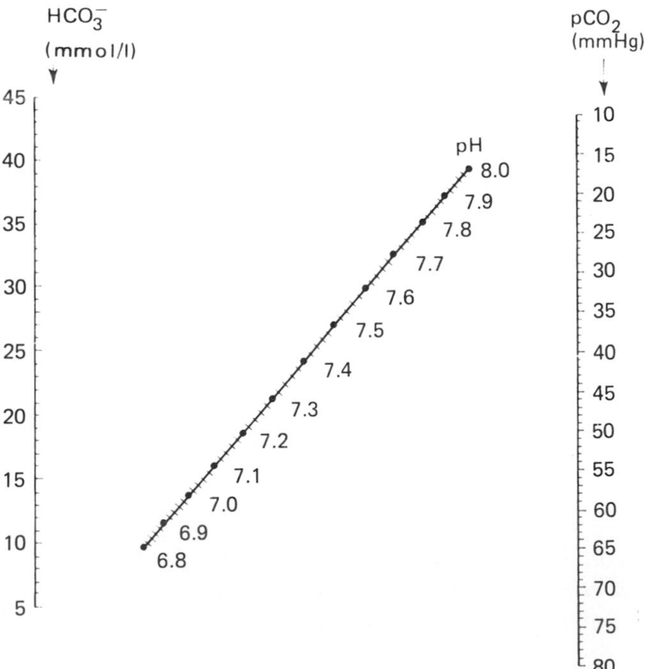

Figure 11.2 Nomogram to determine PCO_2 from pH and serum bicarbonate concentration (From Goldberg (1980a); reproduced by kind permission.)

be practicable if there is impaired gas exchange across the alveoli. Goldberger (1980a) suggests the following calculation, using the nomogram (*Figure 11.2*) to determine the plasma bicarbonate concentration which would be present if the pH were raised to 7.30 and the PCO_2 remained unchanged. If the actual standard bicarbonate level is known, the calculation becomes:

Desired standard HCO_3 (from nomogram) minus adult standard HCO_3 × weight in kg × 0.3 = mmol $NaHCO_3$ required.

Goldberger warns this correction should be done cautiously and therefore it is best to aim at a pH of 7.2 since a sudden reduction in PCO_2 after improved ventilation may leave a residual metabolic alkalosis.

Acidosis in the newborn

A metabolic acidosis may be seen in the newborn in the following conditions:

1. Late metabolic acidosis.
2. Proximal renal tubular acidosis.
3. Acute renal failure.
4. Neonatal chronic renal failure.
5. Inborn errors of metabolism.
6. Neonatal diabetes mellitus – *see* Chapter 50 (page 457).

1. Late metabolic acidosis

This is a disorder affecting preterm infants after the second week of life (Kildeberg, 1964). It is commonest in infants fed a diet high in cows' milk protein (and is therefore rarely seen nowadays). The precipitating event is probably an interruption in weight gain from some unrelated cause, upsetting the balance between hydrogen ion *intake* (dietary protein) and *utilization* (anabolism and growth). It must be distinguished from the low plasma bicarbonate level seen in *healthy* premature infants due to their physiologically low renal bicarbonate threshold (Schwartz *et al.*, 1979).

RECOGNITION

The infant shows an unsatisfactory weight gain despite an apparently adequate intake and becomes lethargic, with a greyish pallor, or apnoeic attacks. In the more severe cases there is vomiting and loss of weight. Hyperventilation is very rarely seen.

MANAGEMENT

1. The diagnosis is established by the finding of an uncompensated metabolic acidosis (normal PCO_2) in the absence of infection or other identifiable cause.
2. The protein intake should be reduced to physiological amounts and preferably changed to human or a 'humanized' (low protein) type of milk. Acute correction with a single dose of bicarbonate, calculated as above, is usually curative, and allows resumption of weight gain. The necessity for sustained alkali treatment calls the diagnosis into doubt.

2. Proximal renal tubular acidosis

Some infants have an unusually low renal threshold for bicarbonate reabsorption; they can acidify urine normally but only when the plasma bicarbonate is below this threshold value, i.e. at the cost of significant metabolic acidosis (Rodriguez-Soriano *et al.*, 1967). The disorder is self-limiting; the bicarbonate threshold rises with maturation and the acidosis resolves within 6–18 months.

RECOGNITION

Lethargy, poor feeding, vomiting and failure to gain weight, usually from the first week, in the absence of infection or other causes.

MANAGEMENT

1. Diagnosis: the finding of a hyperchloraemic metabolic acidosis with normal urinary acidification (urine pH <5.5) at abnormally low plasma bicarbonate concentration. *Hypokalaemia* is commonly present.
2. Treatment with alkali. Very large amounts of bicarbonate are needed (5–10 mmol/kg/day) to achieve sustained correction because massive urinary bicarbonate leakage occurs at plasma concentrations above threshold. A mixture of sodium and potassium citrate may be better tolerated.

3. *Acute renal failure*

Acute reversible renal failure is commoner in the neonatal period than at any other time. *It is rarely accompanied by oliguria* and is frequently misdiagnosed. For further discussion *see* Chapter 48.

4. *Neonatal chronic renal failure*

This may be due to a variety of congenital abnormalities of the renal tract. The commonest is bilateral renal dysplasia with reflux or obstruction. Infantile polycystic kidneys may present in this way. True renal hypoplasia occurs but is exceedingly rare.

RECOGNITION

Symptoms of acidosis (*see* above) usually precede other clinical features of uraemia. A history of predisposing insult (*see* Acute renal failure above) is absent, except by coincidence. *A history of oligohydramnios is common.*

MANAGEMENT

1. The finding of azotaemia (raised plasma creatinine) in an acidotic infant without a history of asphyxia or sepsis is strongly suggestive of chronic renal insufficiency. In the hands of a skilled examiner, ultrasound usually reveals the diagnosis.
2. Acidosis should be corrected with alkali in the usual way, and emergency treatment for hyperkalaemia should be given if necessary (*see* page 132). (In both acute and chronic renal failure volume overload may preclude treatment of acidosis with alkali. This is an indication for immediate dialysis.) The child should then be transferred immediately to a regional or supraregional unit for management of paediatric chronic renal failure.

5. *Inborn errors of metabolism (see also Chapter 91)*

RECOGNITION

Metabolic acidosis is common to many inborn errors of metabolism. Symptoms of acidosis are as described under Late metabolic acidosis. Associated signs and symptoms will depend on the individual disorder but commonly include jaundice, hepatosplenomegaly, neurological abnormalities (apnoeic attacks, seizures) and urine which is aromatic or contains reducing substances.

MANAGEMENT

The relevant diagnostic tests and dietary management are discussed in Chapter 91.

Hyponatraemia

A plasma sodium concentration of under 130 mmol/ℓ is abnormal, but symptoms are unusual at concentrations above 120 mmol/ℓ unless the plasma sodium falls unusually quickly. Symptoms are due to cerebral oedema; fall in the tonicity (effective osmolality) of the extracellular fluid causes osmotic water entry into brain cells, with consequent swelling. Movement of sodium into and out of brain cells takes place much more slowly than is the case with other cells, and compensatory adjustments in intracellular solute composition are therefore slow to occur.

Hyponatraemia occurs in five situations:

1. Pseudohyponatraemia. There is a low measured plasma sodium level but a normal sodium concentration in plasma water. It is due to expansion of the non-aqueous phase of plasma due to paraproteinaemia (virtually unknown in childhood) or gross hyperlipidaemia. The latter is occasionally seen, e.g. in the nephrotic syndrome, or untreated diabetes. Milky plasma is the clue; *plasma osmolality is normal.*
2. True hyponatraemia with normal osmolality. This is due to the presence of another osmotically active solute in abnormal amounts, usually glucose (Katz, 1973).
3. Hyponatraemia due to excess water administration (water intoxication). Specific causes include compulsive water drinking (rare in children) (Linshaw, Hipp and Gruskin, 1974), excessive oral or intravenous administration of hypotonic solutions (Dugan and Holliday, 1967), absorption of water through the respiratory tract during mechanical ventilation, or the use of mist tents with ultrasonic nebulizers. The use of water or hypotonic fluids for enemas, hopefully an obsolete practice, may also cause this type of hyponatraemia. It is extremely difficult, though possible, to produce dangerous dilution in this way if renal function is intact, but relatively easy if it is impaired.
4. Hyponatraemia due to abnormal sodium loss. The loss may be urinary, as in mineralocorticoid deficiency, diuretic abuse, the recovery phase of acute renal failure and 'salt-losing glomerulonephritis' (nephronophthisis is the commonest childhood cause of the last). Very immature newborn infants may become hyponatraemic owing to renal sodium loss, a consequence of renal immaturity (Al-Dahhan *et al.,* 1983). Alternatively the loss may be intestinal, as in hypotonic dehydration due to diarrhoea, or laxative abuse (rare in children). Losses in sweat may cause hyponatraemia in cystic fibrosis, especially during hot weather.

5. Hyponatraemia due to renal water retention:
   (a) Impaired renal function. The limited capacity to excrete solute-free water in acute or chronic renal failure may lead to dilutional hyponatraemia due to the continued *normal* intake of hypotonic or potentially hypotonic fluid.
   (b) Non-osmolar release of antidiuretic hormone (ADH) due to reduced effective arterial volume (Schrier and Bichet, 1981). This is seen in nephrotic syndrome, congestive cardiac failure, cirrhosis of the liver (rarely in childhood) and severe extracellular fluid volume contraction from any cause (*see* Burns, Chapter 4). Hyponatraemia due to water retention may be seen in hypothyroidism and glucocorticoid deficiency; in both it is probably due to impaired cardiac function.
   (c) The 'true' syndrome of inappropriate secretion of ADH (SIADH). This is seen when ADH is released in response to *neither* osmolar *nor* volume stimuli; it is much overdiagnosed. It is usually due to intracranial disease such as meningitis, tumours, or head trauma. The ectopic release of ADH from intrathoracic tumours has not been described in childhood.

Recognition

1. The cardinal symptoms and signs are neurological.
   (a) Early symptoms reflect altered brain function due to intracellular dilution. They include lethargy, headache, weakness, confusion and convulsions.
   (b) Late symptoms are those of raised intracranial pressure: severe headache and vomiting. Rarely, brainstem signs or decerebrate rigidity may be seen due to coning, *which may, however, be precipitated by a lumbar puncture* (*see* Chapter 26, page 744).
2. (a) Papilloedema and a tense or bulging fontanelle are inconstant signs, possibly because (in contrast to hydrocephalus) compression of the lateral ventricles allows considerable swelling to occur before the intracranial pressure rises.
   (b) Oedema or skin oedema (fingerprinting) may be present if there is a chronic water overload.
3. The urine (*see* Appendix 24 for urine specific gravity and osmolality).
   (a) In primary water overload states with normal renal function, ADH will be maximally suppressed and urine will be maximally dilute (<100 mosmol/kg water; specific gravity close to 1000). Urine sodium concentration is low (<20 mmol/ℓ).
   (b) In renal sodium losing states urine composition will vary according to the cause. In mineralocorticoid deficiency (e.g. salt-losing forms of adrenal hyperplasia) the urinary Na^+:K^+ ratio will be inappropriately high in relation to the blood values (low plasma Na^+, high plasma K^+). Generally, in the absence of renal failure, urinary sodium is high and the urine is moderately or well concentrated with respect to urea (urine:plasma urea ratio >20, plasma osmolality >450 mosmol/kg). Urinary chloride is particularly high in hyponatraemia owing to excessive use of loop diuretics (frusemide, ethacrynic acid, bumetanide).
   (c) In intestinal and sweat sodium-losing states, the urine is highly concentrated (osmolality >700 mosmol/kg) and virtually sodium and chloride free (urinary sodium and chloride <10 mmol/ℓ).

(d) In water retention due to non-osmolar release of ADH, the urine is disproportionately concentrated in relation to plasma osmolality. Sodium excretion is maintained despite its low plasma concentration, a consequence of ECF volume expansion. The urine is *not* necessarily more concentrated than plasma; e.g. if plasma osmolality is 250 mosmol/kg water, a urine osmolality of 200 is inappropriately high (it should be maximally dilute).

(e) In renal failure the urine is of similar osmolality to plasma (about 300 mosmol/kg water, specific gravity 1010). The sodium concentration is high, and that of urea low. The more severe the renal failure, the more closely does the urine resemble ECF in chemical composition.

Management

1. Pseudohyponatraemia requires no treatment except that of the causative condition.
2. Hyponatraemia associated with the presence of other osmotically active solutes is corrected by their removal (e.g. control of hyperglycaemia).
3. Hyponatraemia due to excessive water input:
   (a) *Without neurological symptoms.* Restriction of water intake will correct the abnormality.
   (b) *With cerebral symptoms.* Hypertonic saline (3 or 5%) should be given intravenously, while water input is restricted; 6 ml of 5% or 10 ml of 3% NaCl/kg body weight will raise the plasma sodium by approximately 10 mmol/ℓ. Half of this quantity should be given over the first 1–2 hours; if symptoms are not relieved, the remainder may be given over 12–24 hours (Goldberger, 1980b). *The minimum amount required to relieve symptoms should be given;* correction should be completed by water restriction.
4. Hyponatraemia due to sodium depletion:
   (a) With evidence of circulatory insufficiency. This is initially treated by volume expansion with plasma or equivalent. The quantity required is that needed to return the circulatory signs to normal including a rise in the peripheral (toe) temperature to within 2°C (4°F) of the central (rectal) temperature (Ibsen, 1967). Typically 20 ml/kg body weight will be required.
   (b) Without circulatory insufficiency (or after its correction). Treatment is by sodium replacement. In hypotonic dehydration due to diarrhoea, where potassium deficiency and acidosis are invariable, replacement is best achieved with an oral polyelectrolyte solution containing Na 90, K 20, Cl 80, HCO_3 30 mmol/ℓ and glucose 111 mmol/ℓ (20 g/l) (*see also* Chapter 46); most commercial preparations contain too much glucose and insufficient sodium (Hirschhorn, 1980). Intravenous isotonic (0.9%) sodium chloride is appropriate where the losses are non-alimentary. The quantity to be given should be calculated assuming a volume of distribution for sodium of 0.55 body weight (Dell, 1973). Thus, sodium deficit = $(Na_d - Na_e) \times$ weight $\times$ 0.55. (Na_d and Na_e = desired and existing plasma sodium concentration, respectively.) Confirmation of adequate extracellular fluid volume expansion is indicated by the return of significant urinary sodium and chloride excretion.
5. In non-osmolar ADH release:
   (a) Due to reduced effective arterial volume, the treatment is to correct the circulatory deficit, e.g. with albumin infusions in the nephrotic syndrome

and inotropic drugs in cardiac failure (*see* page 105). Water restriction may be employed *cautiously* since it may cause further circulatory volume contraction.

(b) Due to SIADH; water restriction is the treatment of choice, unless neurological symptoms are present, in which case treat as in 3(b) above. Attempts to force a water diuresis are self-defeating, since both chemical and osmotic diuretics promote large urinary sodium losses (and may themselves cause hyponatraemia). ADH release may be inhibited by the use of lithium carbonate or demeclocycline, but this should rarely be necessary.

Hypernatraemia

Hypernatraemia is defined as a plasma sodium concentration above 150 mmol/ℓ. It causes cellular dehydration due to osmotic loss of water from cells; the associated brain shrinkage causes acute neurological symptoms and may lead to brain damage. Chronic sodium retention (mineralocorticoid excess, liquorice or carbenoxolone ingestion, high-salt diet) *does not* cause hypernatraemia, but volume expansion, weight gain and hypertension, due to associated water retention.

Recognition

The symptoms of hypernatraemia are irritability, muscular hypertonia progressing to rigidity and often mimicking meningitis, and convulsions. Even when hypernatraemia is associated with dehydration, signs of extracellular volume depletion may be absent since the intracellular compartment is preferentially dehydrated.

Hypernatraemia may be seen in the following conditions:

1. Acute salt poisoning.
2. Hypernatraemic dehydration.
3. Diabetes insipidus.
4. Heatstroke – *see* Chapter 60.

1. Acute salt poisoning

This occasionally occurs in infants due to grossly inappropriate feeding, e.g. where feeds are accidentally made up with salt instead of sugar.

Recognition

Salt poisoning should be suspected in bottle-fed infants presenting with acute neurological symptoms and a plasma sodium level over 150 mmol/ℓ in the absence of evidence of water depletion or a history of diarrhoea. Confirmation requires elucidation of how the feed was prepared, and preferably laboratory analysis of a sample of the suspect milk. Recurrent salt poisoning has been described as a form of child abuse.

Management

Natriuretic agents such as frusemide should be given, with concomitant volume replacement with moderately hypotonic fluid (e.g. sodium chloride 0.45% in 2.5% glucose). Peritoneal dialysis may be required.

2. Hypernatraemic dehydration

This is seen in children with diarrhoeal dehydration in whom high-solute (especially high carbohydrate) feeds have been continued (Hirschhorn, 1980).

Recognition

It should be suspected in infants with a history of diarrhoea and appropriate neurological symptoms.

Management – *See Chapter 46 (page 410)*

3. Diabetes insipidus

This is due to deficiency of, or resistance to, ADH. The patient is in a state of continual water diuresis and becomes hypernatraemic unless copious water is taken. Thirst ensures this in older children, but infants are at great risk since they cannot indicate their need for water.

Recognition

Diabetes insipidus should be suspected in an infant or child with polyuria, recurrent pyrexias, and dehydration. It is confirmed by finding dilute urine (usually less than 200 mosmol/kg water) in the presence of concentrated plasma (plasma sodium over 150 mmol/ℓ, osmolality over 300 mosmol/kg). Unfortunately, brain damage is common in infants by the time the diagnosis is made.

Management

Copious water must be given by mouth in the first instance. The response to intranasal DDAVP (desmopressin) 10–40 μg will distinguish between 'pituitary' and 'nephrogenic' forms of the disease; the former responds by producing concentrated urine, the latter does not.

Hypokalaemia and potassium depletion

The correlation between the plasma potassium concentration and body (intracellular) stores is poor, and normal or high plasma levels may occur in haemoconcentration or metabolic acidosis even if total body stores are depleted; similarly, hyperkalaemia may occur without potassium overload, in renal failure. A low plasma potassium (<3.5 mmol/ℓ) usually indicates depletion, exceptions being metabolic alkalosis and hypokalaemic periodic paralysis. In this discussion hypokalaemia will be used as synonymous with potassium depletion.

Hypokalaemia should be suspected in the following situations:

1. Renal losses:
   (a) Mineralocorticoid excess: primary (virtually unknown in childhood), secondary, or iatrogenic.
   (b) Prolonged use of corticosteroids (most 'glucocorticoids' have some mineralocorticoid activity).
   (c) Loop diuretics (frusemide, ethacrynic acid, bumetanide) and thiazides.
   (d) Type I (distal) and type II (proximal) renal tubular acidosis.
   (e) Metabolic response to trauma (partly steroid induced).
   (f) Metabolic alkalosis.
   (g) High-output (polyuric) acute renal failure; recovery phase of oliguric renal failure.
   (h) Recovery phase of diabetic ketoacidosis.
   (i) Fanconi's syndrome (e.g. cystinosis).
   (j) Bartter's syndrome.
2. Gastrointestinal losses:
   (a) Vomiting or nasogastric suction.
   (b) Acute gastroenteritis.
   (c) Chronic diarrhoeal diseases.
   (d) Intestinal fistulae.
   (e) Purging (laxative abuse).
3. Inadequate intake:
   (a) Starvation, undernutrition.
   (b) Persistent vomiting (may be self induced and denied – *see* Anorexia Nervosa, page 521).

Recognition

In all conditions likely to be associated with hypokalaemia the plasma potassium level and ECG should be recorded frequently, or the ECG should be continuously visible.

Symptoms that suggest hypokalaemia are:

1. Lassitude, anorexia, abdominal distension, or ileus.
2. Muscle weakness, beginning in the legs and later affecting the respiratory muscles, does not usually develop until the plasma level is 2.5 mmol/ℓ or lower.
3. Cardiac arrhythmias include sinus bradycardia, prolonged P-R interval, A-V block, paroxysmal atrial tachycardia with A-V block (Goldberger, 1980c).
4. The ECG changes do not correlate with plasma levels. The usual abnormalities are shown in *Figure 11.3* (Goldberger, 1980c).

Management

1. Whenever possible, potassium salts should be given orally.
2. IV potassium should NEVER be given in:
   (a) Hyperkalaemia (plasma K >5.5 mmol/ℓ).
   (b) Oliguria or anuria.
   (c) Untreated adrenal failure.

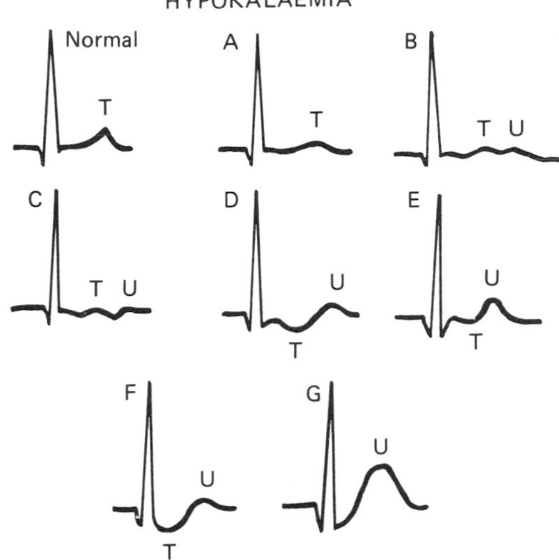

Figure 11.3 Electrocardiographic patterns of hypokalaemia.
(1) Lowering and broadening of the T wave. The Q-T interval is also slightly prolonged. Such a pattern may occur when the serum potassium is merely at a low normal level; for example, 3.5 mmol/ℓ (3.5 mEq/ℓ) (A).
(2) Low, broad T waves with a double summit, due to superimposition of the U wave on the T (B). The Q-T interval may appear markedly prolonged in such cases. However, the prolongation may be more apparent than real because it may be difficult to determine where the T ends and the U begins. Consequently, the Q-U interval, rather than the Q-T interval, is often measured.
(3) Downward T waves and prominent U waves. Such a pattern is best seen in precordial leads such as V_1 to V_4, which overlie the right ventricle and thus have an rS or RS pattern (D, E, F).
(4) Depression of the RS-T segment and slight lengthening of the Q-T interval (D, E). The RS-T may be slightly depressed, or may show several small undulations (C). D, E, F and G show more marked RS-T deviations. These RS-T segments have a sagging appearance, characteristic of hypokalaemia. (5) Increase in P-wave amplitude and widening of the QRS interval. (6) Numerous arrhythmias, including sinus bradycardia and prolonged P-R interval. Wenckebach type of A-V block, paroxysmal atrial tachycardia with A-V block (PAT with block). Arrhythmias due to digitalis toxicity may be precipitated or worsened (From Goldberger (1980c). Reproduced by kind permission.)

3. Estimation of the deficit:
   (a) In diarrhoeal dehydration, recovery balance studies have shown that the total potassium deficit is usually equal to or slightly greater than the sodium deficit (Darrow, 1946). The severity of the total body loss therefore varies with the type of dehydration (*Table 11.1*).
   (b) In diabetic ketoacidosis the deficit is usually of the order of 4–7 mmol/kg.
4. Replacement: this should normally be at the rate of 3 mmol/kg/24hr (2 mmol/kg/24 hr under 1 year). Potassium chloride is normally used but in renal tubular acidosis potassium citrate should be substituted.
   (a) Oral route: a 7.45% potassium chloride solution contains 1 mmol of potassium in 1.0 ml solution. Other alternatives are potassium chloride effervescent tablets (Sando-K tablets contain 12 mmol potassium and 8 mmol chloride; Kloral tablets contain 6.7 mmol potassium and 6.7 mmol chloride); potassium chloride slow tablets (Leo K, Slow-K tablets) contain 8 mmol potassium and chloride in a slow-release base).

(b) IV solutions should not contain over 40 mmol potassium/ℓ; a standard solution is potassium chloride and glucose which contains 5% glucose and potassium chloride 40 mmol/ℓ. A useful solution can also be made up by adding an ampoule of 2 mmol potassium chloride (0.15 g) in 5 ml to each 100 ml of IV fluid, giving a final concentration of 20 mmol/ℓ. The original IV solution must of course contain no potassium. It is useful to give potassium with glucose; the insulin response helps to repair intracellular potassium losses.

(c) In severe undernutrition, as in protein–energy malnutrition (*see* Chapter 69, page 603) large amounts may be required to replenish the deficit; it is safer to give the replacement at the normal rate but to continue for longer, rather than to increase the actual amount given in each 24 hours.

Table 11.1 Deficits of water and potassium in moderately severe dehydration*

	Water (ml/kg)	*Potassium* (mmol/kg)
Hypertonic	120–170	2–5
Isotonic	100–150	7–11
Hypotonic	40–80	10–14

* From Winters (1968).

Hyperkalaemia (*see also* Chapter 48, page 432 – Acute renal failure)

The clinical manifestations of hyperkalaemia, such as cardiac arrhythmias, or less commonly muscular weakness and paraesthesias are rare and should not occur if the clinician is aware of the commoner situations associated with hyperkalaemia and takes appropriate action before the plasma potassium reaches a critical level.

Causes of hyperkalaemia

If renal and adrenal function are intact, potassium loading is well tolerated and dangerous hyperkalaemia unusual. However, when potassium excretory capacity is impaired by acute renal failure, prerenal oliguria or mineralocorticoid deficiency, hyperkalaemia is to be expected whenever entry of potassium to the extracellular fluid exceeds this capacity. Such potassium entry may be exogenous (dietary or IV) or endogenous (catabolic states).

Contributory conditions which may accentuate or accelerate hyperkalaemia are:

1. Metabolic acidosis.
2. Cellular breakdown in trauma, burns, operation, haemolysis, infection, severe hypoxia, and acute starvation.
3. Potassium salts given inadvertently or as part of treatment:
   (a) Orally. Fruit and fruit drinks, especially citrus fruits, potatoes, chocolate, etc.; potassium salts given to alkalinize the urine; and drugs containing potassium (especially penicillins and other antibiotics).
   (b) Parenteral injections: antibiotics (as above); stored blood, especially when more than 5 days old.

(c) Potassium salts given too rapidly IV or in the presence of renal disease, oliguria or acidosis (*see* Appendix 8 for potassium preparation for IV use).

4. Mineralocorticoid deficiency: this may occur with any of the forms of acute adrenal failure in infancy or childhood (*see* Chapter 52, page 470).
5. Type IV renal tubular acidosis (hyperkalaemic RTA, pseudohypoaldosteronism).
6. Potassium-sparing diuretics (spironolactone, triamterene, amiloride), either alone or given with potassium-losing diuretics and potassium supplements (Cannon, 1973).

Recognition

1. Falsely high values may be due to haemolysed blood samples which are particularly common in capillary blood which has been obtained with difficulty. The laboratory should always indicate when the plasma or serum is sufficiently haemolysed to give a misleadingly high result.
2. In the immediate neonatal period (3 days) the plasma potassium may be as high as 8 mmol/ℓ in normal infants.
3. In all conditions in which hyperkalaemia can be expected, plasma potassium levels and ECG should be recorded at frequent intervals, or the ECG should be continuously visible.
4. The onset of a cardiac arrhythmia (sinus bradycardia, first-degree A-V block, nodal or idioventricular rhythm, ventricular tachycardia) in circumstances in which hyperkalaemia can be expected, requires urgent treatment to be started (*see* below) to reduce the plasma potassium level, without waiting for laboratory confirmation. Once an arrhythmia has become established the characteristics of hyperkalaemia (*Figure 11.4*) may not be easy to identify in the ECG.
5. The ECG changes correlate reasonably well with the plasma potassium level (*Figure 11.4*).
6. Less common symptoms are paraesthesias, and ascending paralysis.

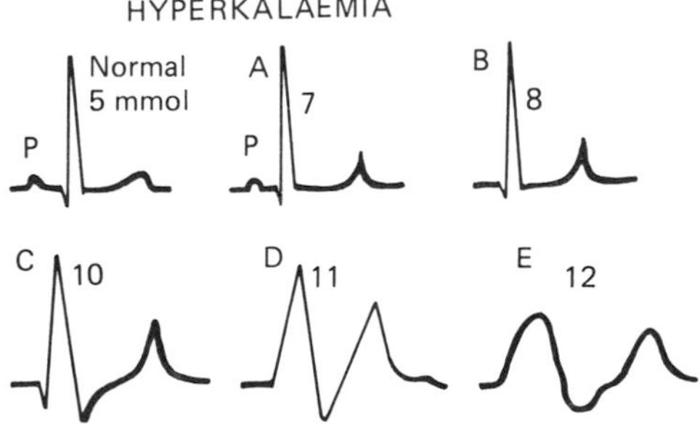

Figure 11.4 Electrocardiographic patterns of hyperkalaemia. At a concentration of about 6–7 mmol/ℓ (6–7 mEq/ℓ) tall peaked T waves with a narrow base and a normal or decreased Q-T occur (A). At about 8 mmol/ℓ (8 mEq/ℓ) the P waves may disappear or wander in and out of the QRS (B). At about 10 mmol/ℓ (10 mEq/ℓ) wide, aberrant QRS complexes appear (C). At about 11 mmol/ℓ (11 mEq/ℓ) biphasic deflections, caused by a fusion of the QRS complex, RS-T segment and the T wave appear (D). At 12 mmol/ℓ (12 mEq/ℓ), or even at 10 mmol/ℓ (10 mEq/ℓ), ventricular fibrillation and cardiac standstill and death may occur (E) (From Goldberger (1980d). Reproduced by kind permission.)

Management

1. In readily reversible conditions such as diabetic ketoacidosis or adrenocortical insufficiency, treatment of the primary condition will reduce the level of plasma potassium.
2. Immediate treatment is required in the presence of:
   (a) ECG changes such as disappearance of the P wave and widening of the QRS.
   (b) Cardiac arrhythmias associated with hyperkalaemia.
   (c) A plasma level of over 6.5 mmol/ℓ in the presence of renal failure, or over 8.0 mmol/ℓ in any circumstances.
3. Treatment should be given in the following order:
   (a) Stop all sources of exogenous potassium.
   (b) Inject IV 0.5 ml/kg of 10% calcium gluconate over 2–4 minutes with ECG control. Use a single dose only. This provides temporary protection of the cardiac conduction system, but does not change the level of plasma potassium.
   (c) Give $NaHCO_3$ IV in a dose of 1 mmol/kg over 5 minutes. This causes rapid movement of potassium into the cells. Give a further 1–2 mmol/kg by slow infusion over the next hour. Check acid–base status before giving further bicarbonate.
   NOTE: DO NOT mix calcium and bicarbonate in the same syringe: precipitation will occur.
   (d) Give 10% glucose in a dose of 40 ml/kg; this is followed by insulin (soluble, or monocomponent, such as Actrapid MC) in the proportion of 1 unit subcutaneously for every 3 g glucose (= every 30 ml of 10% glucose). If a suitable insulin preparation is not readily available, give glucose alone; an endogenous insulin response will occur (augmented by hyperkalaemia).

   NOTE: None of these measures will remove potassium from the body; (c) and (d) reverse the release of intracellular potassium.
4. In renal failure, potassium can be removed from the body using an ion-exchange resin. This should be given in the *calcium* phase (Calcium Resonium) in a dose of 1 g/kg up to three times daily. The resin can be given orally or by gastric tube in water (proportions as stated on the manufacturer's package), or by enema, in which case it should be mixed with sorbitol solution to prevent 'cast' formation, and removed after 4–8 hours with a 'cleansing' enema. In severe hyperkalaemia both routes may be used simultaneously.
5. In acute renal failure, dialysis is the definitive treatment, either peritoneal or extracorporeal. *Hyperkalaemia requiring the use of resin therapy in a child with acute renal failure is an indication for dialysis,* which should be started immediately after the above emergency steps have been taken (*see also* Chapter 48).

Hypocalcaemia

Symptoms of hypocalcaemia are unlikely at calcium levels over 1.9 mmol/ℓ (3.8 mEq/ℓ = 7.5 mg/100 ml; for calcium, 1.0 mg/100 ml = 0.5 mEq/ℓ = 0.25 mmol/ℓ).

ECG changes of hypocalcaemia – Prolongation of the Q-T interval with normal RS-T segment and normal T waves. ECG changes are difficult to interpret in the newborn.

The newborn

In the newborn, hypocalcaemia should be suspected in any infant with jitteriness, hyperirritability, or fits, for which no cause (hypoxia, hypoglycaemia, meningitis, cerebral haemorrhage) can be found.

Hypocalcaemia is relatively common in the newborn infant: hypomagnesaemia (*see* page 138) may accompany hypocalcaemia and in these circumstances the hypocalcaemia is resistant to the usual treatment but corrects itself or responds to treatment if the hypomagnesaemia is corrected first. For this reason, in the newborn, a request should always be made for estimation of both calcium and magnesium and laboratories serving neonatal medical and surgical units should routinely report both ions even if only one (usually calcium) is requested.

In many newborns hypocalcaemia is transient and asymptomatic and the calcium level returns to normal when the infant recovers from an episode of acute illness (e.g. severe hypoxia). Symptoms of hypocalcaemia in the newborn are usually non-specific and should only be attributed to hypocalcaemia after exclusion of other conditions (*see* below). There is no evidence that transient hypocalcaemia, whether symptomatic or not, causes cerebral damage, but persisting untreated or unrecognized hypocalcaemia is associated with mental retardation and it is therefore important to distinguish between transient and persisting hypocalcaemia.

Causes of hypocalcaemia

Transient hypocalcaemia

1. Onset during the first 48–72 hours of life. This is seen in the infants of low birth weight, and especially in preterm infants with respiratory distress syndrome, and also after birth hypoxia. The hypocalcaemia of the infant of the diabetic mother usually occurs after the first 48–72 hours. In none of these conditions does the hypocalcaemia last for more than 2–3 days and it is frequently asymptomatic.
2. During or immediately after exchange transfusion with citrated blood.
3. Between the 4th and 8th days of life (the exact time of onset depending upon the type of feeding schedule) in infants fed on unmodified (high-phosphate) cows' milk. Symptoms rarely last longer than 3–4 days even if untreated. Infants fed on human milk or modified (low-phosphate) cows' milk do not develop this form of hypocalcaemia. There is evidence that infants whose renal function lies in the lower part of the normal range are more at risk than others.
4. At the end of the first week up till the third week. Transient hypoparathyroidism may occur due to maternal hyperparathyroidism, whether primary or secondary.

Persisting hypocalcaemia

1. Severe vitamin-D deficiency in the mother, resulting in fetal or neonatal rickets, may cause hypocalcaemia with an onset at the 7th day onwards, which persists if untreated.
2. Idiopathic hypoparathyroidism and the 3rd and 4th pharyngeal pouch syndrome (Taitz–DiGeorge syndrome) may cause symptomatic hypocalcaemia as early as the first week, or not until the age of a few months.
3. Hypocalcaemia may be secondary to persisting hypomagnesaemia from any cause (*see* page 138).

Recognition

Symptoms

Symptoms attributable to hypocalcaemia are:

1. Clonic fits: focal, unilateral or generalized. The affected side may alternate. Tonic fits are rarely due to hypocalcaemia.
2. Hyperirritability, 'jitteriness' (repetitive jerking of the limbs either spontaneously or in response to any sort of stimulus, including loud noises).
3. Increased muscle tone.
4. Generalized oedema; rare.
5. Cardiac failure; rare.

NOTE: The absence or presence of Chvostek's sign is of no significance in the newborn.

Confirmation that hypocalcaemia is the cause of the symptoms

Since all the above symptoms can be due to other, more serious causes the diagnosis of symptomatic hypocalcaemia is one of exclusion and IV calcium gluconate should NOT be used as a therapeutic test (*see* below).

1. Fits. It is necessary to exclude hypoglycaemia, meningitis, intracranial haemorrhage, posthypoxic states, and hypomagnesaemia. In continuous or very frequent fits pyridoxine dependence must also be considered (*see* page 715).
2. Hyperirritability and 'jitteriness'. These occur in hypoglycaemia, posthypoxic states, and in hypomagnesaemia.
3. Increased tone is more likely in hypocalcaemia or hypomagnesaemia, and hypotonia in hypoglycaemia. The distinction is not a reliable one and increased tone alone is more likely to be due to one of the conditions given in (1) above.
4. Oedema and cardiac failure. Hypocalcaemia should be considered only when all the commoner causes have been excluded. A coexistent hypomagnesaemia may potentiate the effect of digoxin, as in potassium depletion.

Diagnostic levels of plasma calcium

In the newborn it is unlikely that levels above 1.9 mmol/ℓ (3.8 mEq/ℓ = 7.5 mg/100 ml) would cause symptoms though it must be recognized that the total plasma calcium gives no indication of the level of ionized calcium, which is really responsible for the symptoms. A fraction of the plasma calcium is bound to albumin. Hypoalbuminaemic states are associated with low total plasma calcium levels, but are *not* associated with low ionized calcium and symptomatic hypocalcaemia. It is therefore helpful to measure the plasma albumin concentration when hypocalcaemia is suspected.

Management

Asymptomatic

Even if hypocalcaemia, when discovered, appears to be asymptomatic, plasma calcium levels should be determined repeatedly until the level has returned to normal. If this is not done a persisting and potentially damaging hypocalcaemia will be missed.

Symptomatic

1. In all cases, the milk should be changed to a low-phosphate milk (human or modified cows' milk). Oral calcium supplements should be given (*see* below).
2. If fits are recurrent and severe an attempt should be made to control them with diazepam or phenobarbitone (*see* page 308) rather than with IV calcium gluconate, except in cases when conventional anticonvulsant treatment fails.

Oral preparations

1. Calcium gluconate 10%: this is the same preparation as is used IV; dose 15 ml (1.5 g) three or four times daily. 1.5 g of calcium gluconate contains 3.3 mmol (6.6 mEq) calcium.
2. Calcium lactate as a 6% suspension; dose 300 mg (5 ml) three or four times daily; 300 mg contains 2.0 mmol (4.0 mEq) calcium.
3. Calcium glubionate and galactogluconate syrup (Calcium-Sandoz Syrup): dose 5 ml 4–6 times daily. 5 ml contains 2.7 mmol (5.4 mEq) calcium.
4. Calcium chloride (*see* below).

Oral preparations of calcium should be used for all cases of symptomatic hypocalcaemia, except those with severe, very frequent, or continuous fits. The plasma level should be estimated after 12–24 hours on treatment, and earlier if necessary, and again 2–3 days after stopping treatment. If the hypocalcaemia is thought to be of the transient type, treatment is rarely necessary for longer than 3–4 days but it is necessary to demonstrate that a normal level can be maintained after stopping treatment.

Magnesium sulphate in the treatment of hypocalcaemic fits due to high-phosphate load (4th–8th day)

Turner, Cockburn and Forfar (1977) have suggested that even in the absence of symptomatically low levels of plasma magnesium, i.m. magnesium sulphate solution may be more effective than either phenobarbitone or oral calcium salts. They used 0.2 ml/kg of a 50% solution of magnesium sulphate in two (rarely three) doses at 12 hourly intervals (*see* page 139 for technique of injection).

The indications for vitamin D

1. Confirmed fetal or neonatal rickets.
2. Persisting hypocalcaemia which cannot be controlled by oral calcium salts.

Dose – Initially 1000 units (as calciferol) daily; the plasma calcium level should be estimated weekly. Large doses of vitamin D preparations given i.m. are not recommended because of the danger of hypercalcaemia.
Note – Hypoparathyroidism should be treated with hydroxylated derivatives of vitamin D_3;1,α-hydroxycholecalciferol ($1(OH)D_3$) (alfacalcidol, One-alpha, Leo Laboratories; capsules of 0.25 and 1.0 μg) or 1.25 dihydroxycholecalciferol (1.25 $(OH)_2D_3$) (calcitriol – Rocaltrol, Roche Products; capsules 0.25 and 0.5 μg). The dose of both preparations is similar: alfacalcidol, 0.05–0.08 μg/kg/24 hours, reduced to 0.025–0.05 μg/kg daily by the third or fourth day; and calcitriol, 0.1–0.5 μg *daily*, with similar reduction by the third or fourth day.

Drugs contraindicated

1. Injections of parathyroid hormone are of more use diagnostically than therapeutically since resistance soon develops if repeated doses are given.
2. Intravenous 10% calcium gluconate; this is contraindicated in all except the very rare cases of continuous or repeated hypocalcaemic fits, which are resistant to diazepam or phenobarbitone. If it must be given, a dose of 0.5–1.0 ml/kg should be used at each injection and given at the rate of 1 ml/minute, monitoring with ECG or stethoscope at the apex. The injection should be stopped if there is any slowing. The effect of intravenous calcium on the heart is said to be potentiated by digoxin and by hypokalaemia. The reasons against the use of IV calcium gluconate are that it is rarely indicated urgently and there is a danger of cardiac arrest; also leakage outside a vein causes severe tissue necrosis and calcification. Its effect is extremely brief and it is unnecessary in most cases of transient hypocalcaemia and is ineffective in persisting cases.
3. Calcium chloride: if given orally there is a risk of gastric perforation, and if given for more than 3–4 days a severe metabolic acidosis may result, particularly in pre-term infants. (For use of 10% calcium chloride IV in shock *see* Chapter 10, page 104).

Hypocalcaemia in the older child

Hypocalcaemia is relatively uncommon but should be considered as a possible cause of fits in the following situations:

1. In Asian children, particularly if there is clinical evidence of rickets, but even in its absence.
2. Children with known renal insufficiency, particularly if alkalis have been given.
3. In children who are dwarfed and mentally retarded (hypoparathyroidism, pseudohypoparathyroidism).
4. Any child with cataracts.
5. Children with heart disease and recurrent infections (3rd and 4th branchial arch, Taitz–DiGeorge syndrome).

Hypocalcaemia as a cause of tetanic manifestations such as carpopedal spasms, painful muscle cramps, and paraesthesias round the mouth and in the fingers and toes is relatively rare in childhood and is likely to be accompanied by clinical evidence which may point to the primary cause (*see* above). With increasing age the incidence of fits decreases and that of tetany increases. In adolescent girls hyperventilation tetany may occur with a respiratory alkalosis and a normal plasma calcium.

Management

In the older child the danger of extravasation of calcium gluconate outside the vein is small and there may be an indication for its use in continued or repeated hypocalcaemic fits or tetany until other and slower forms of treatment have taken effect (*see* above for precaution with IV injection). The maximum single dose at any age is 10 ml of the 10% solution.

On a long-term basis, treatment depends upon the primary cause.

Hypercalcaemia

Hypercalcaemia is defined as a plasma calcium level of more than 2.8 mmol/ℓ (5.5 mEq/ℓ = 11.0 mg/100 ml).

ECG changes in hypercalcaemia – shortening of the Q-T interval with rounded T waves and normal RS-T segments. Incomplete or complete A-V block or cardiac arrest may occur at levels of 4.5 mmol/ℓ (9.0 mEq/ℓ = 18.0 mg/100 ml) (Goldberger, 1980e).

This is a rare emergency in childhood. Nevertheless, levels of 3.8 mmol/ℓ (7.5 mEq/ℓ = 15 mg/100 ml) or higher carry a risk of renal damage and are seen in severe overdosage with vitamin D preparations and occasionally in severe idiopathic hypercalcaemia.

Recognition

In infants and children the usual signs are: muscular hypotonia, vomiting, thirst, polyuria, and constipation. In long-standing severe hypercalcaemia band-keratopathy may be present and nephrocalcinosis may be visible on a plain film of the abdomen. In vitamin D overdosage the long bones may show bands of increased density at the metaphyses with an area of reduced density just proximally. In idiopathic hypercalcaemia similar bands of increased density occur at the metaphyses but without the area of decreased density; in both cases there may also be increased bone density in the supraorbital region and in the base of the skull.

Management

Treatment is indicated when the plasma calcium level is over 3.8 mmol/ℓ (7.5 mEq/ℓ, >15 mg/100 ml), in the presence of severe signs such as vomiting, coma, or with a rising blood urea or oliguria.

1. Isotonic saline intravenously is said to be useful in a hypercalcaemic crisis but should be used with care because glomerular filtration may be impaired and there is therefore a risk of circulatory overload.
2. Frusemide is a powerful calciuretic drug, increasing calcium excretion even more than it does sodium. If used in combination with saline infusion (to replace the forced loss of salt and water) plasma calcium can be lowered rapidly. A suitable dose is 1–2 mg/kg orally or IV repeated 4–6 hourly if necessary. DO NOT use thiazides which *reduce* calcium excretion and *raise* plasma calcium.
3. If (1) and (2) are ineffective and the child is severely ill (usually in iatrogenic vitamin D poisoning), peritoneal dialysis with a calcium-free fluid should be considered (Selby *et al.*, 1984).
4. Large doses of corticosteroids will reduce hypercalcaemia but not in hyperparathyroidism.
5. Calcitonin (Calcitare, porcine) or Salcatonin (Calsynar, salmon). Preparations are available for subcutaneous or i.m. injection. Calcitonin, 160 units per vial, with gelatine diluent; Salcatonin, 100 units and 200 units per vial in saline acetate. The recommended dose is 4–8 units/kg daily subcutaneously or intramuscularly, the subsequent dose being adjusted according to the effect. Salmon calcitonin may be effective where the porcine preparation has failed; the maximum dose is up to 8 units/kg every 6–8 hours, subcutaneously or i.m. adjusted according to the clinical and biochemical effect. The effect of the

calcitonins is incomplete (producing a fall in serum calcium level of 0.6 mmol/ℓ; 1.2 mEq/ℓ, 2.4 mg/100 ml) and tends to decrease after 2–3 days even when treatment is continued (Wilkinson, 1984).

Hypomagnesaemia

Symptoms of hypomagnesaemia are unlikely to develop unless the plasma level is under 0.5 mmol/ℓ (1.0 mEq/ℓ = 1.2 mg/100 ml). ECG changes are rarely specific and are particularly difficult to interpret in the newborn.

The newborn

In this age group hypomagnesaemia may accompany hypocalcaemia, and when this occurs the hypocalcaemia is resistant to treatment with calcium salts or vitamin D. Correction of the hypomagnesaemia corrects the hypocalcaemia or renders it responsive to treatment. Isolated hypomagnesaemia is uncommon and is usually transient and asymptomatic.

Causes of hypomagnesaemia

1. Any of the usual causes of transient hypocalcaemia may also cause hypomagnesaemia.
2. Maternal magnesium depletion from malabsorption may produce symptomatic hypocalcaemia–hypomagnesaemia (Davis, Harvey and Yu, 1965).
3. A specific disorder of magnesium absorption (Strømme *et al.*, 1969; Nordio *et al.*, 1971) may cause symptomatic hypocalcaemia–hypomagnesaemia in the neonatal period, but more commonly at the age of a few months.

Recognition

It is usually impossible to distinguish, in this age group and on the basis of symptoms, between hypocalcaemia and hypomagnesaemia. Hypomagnesaemia should always be considered when hypocalcaemia is resistant to treatment, or in the investigation of hyperirritability or fits in which other causes have been excluded.

Management

Symptoms may be more severe and fits may be more frequent in hypocalcaemia–hypomagnesaemia than in isolated hypocalcaemia. Symptoms which are due to hypomagnesaemia will be completely relieved by magnesium salts, IV, i.m. or orally according to the degree of urgency.

Intravenous route

This should only be necessary when rapid relief of continuous or repeated fits is required, or when other routes are not practicable. A 1% solution of magnesium sulphate should be used (0.04 mmol = 0.08 mEq/ml), in a dose of 0.5–1.25 mmol (0.5–1.0 mEq) (12–36 ml) at a rate of not more than 1 ml/minute, using ECG controls since IV magnesium salts have similar effects on the heart to calcium salts, and should NEVER be injected rapidly: if practicable the blood pressure should be checked during and after the injection since magensium salts cause hypotension.

Intramuscular route

This is the usual route for the relief of acute symptoms, or when there is a possibility of failure of absorption from the gastrointestinal tract. The preparation normally used is a 50% solution of magnesium sulphate, given at 12 hourly intervals in a dose of 0.2–0.5 mmol (0.4–1.0 mEq) or 0.1–0.25 ml/kg. In transient hypomagnesaemia or in the treatment of phosphate-load hypocalcaemia (Turner, Cockburn and Forfar, 1977) two or occasionally three doses are adequate. Magnesium sulphate is a highly irritant solution and should be injected deep into the muscles of the mid-thigh. In very small infants a more dilute solution (25 or 12.5%) may be preferable.

Oral route

This is used in all non-urgent cases. The following preparations are available:

1. Magnesium sulphate can usually be tolerated in therapeutic amounts without producing diarrhoea, but should be diluted to 25 or 12.5% before use.
   Dose – 0.25–1.0 mmol (0.5–2.0 mEq) of magnesium (0.125–0.5 ml)/kg of 50% solution in divided doses.
2. If there has been recent diarrhoea, or large amounts are required to maintain magnesium balance or replace a large deficit, magnesium hydroxide (milk of magnesia) may be better tolerated than magnesium sulphate. The standard magnesium hydroxide preparation contains 8% of magnesium hydroxide, or 6.8 mmol (13.6 mEq) in 5 ml.
   Dose – 1–2 ml three times daily initially.
3. Other preparations available are magnesium citrate, lactate, gluconate (adult dose 3–6 g/24 hours; 1 g contains 4 mmol magnesium) and glycerophosphate.

Hypomagnesaemia in the older child

Infancy

Hypomagnesaemia, with or without hypocalcaemia may develop after extensive resection of the small intestine, and also in the various forms of cirrhosis in infancy. In the rare, probably genetically determined form of magnesium malabsorption (Strømme *et al.*, 1969; Nordio *et al.*, 1971) hypocalcaemia–hypomagnesaemia fits usually occur at the age of a few months, but occasionally as early as 2 weeks.

Other age groups

Hypomagnesaemia has occasionally been found to accompany hypocalcaemia in most of the conditions in which hypocalcaemia occurs. Probably the most important type of hypomagnesaemia occurs with the severe magnesium depletion seen in protein–energy malnutrition (protein–calorie malnutrition) (*see* page 604); in such cases hypocalcaemia is uncommon.

Recognition

Recurrent fits are the commonest presenting symptom, but, particularly in the older child, hyperirritability, carpopedal spasms, increased muscle tone, increased tendon reflexes and coarse tremors or squirming movements of the limbs may occur. Symptoms are unlikely above a level of 0.5 mmol/ℓ (1 mEq/ℓ = 1.2 mg/100 ml).

Management

Treatment is as for the neonatal period. In the magnesium malabsorption syndrome much larger quantities than usual are required to maintain a normal or near normal level of plasma magnesium and a total daily intake (*not* per kg) of 10–15 mmol (20–30 mEq) may be required even in small children or infants: treatment has to be maintained indefinitely.

In protein–energy malnutrition the acute symptoms may be relieved by i.m. magnesium sulphate (*see* above), followed by oral treatment until repletion has occurred (*see* page 604).

Hypermagnesaemia

Hypermagnesaemia exists when plasma magnesium level is over 1.25 mmol/ℓ (2.5 mEq/ℓ = 3.0 mg%).

ECG changes – prolonged P-R interval, prolonged QRS interval, tall T-waves, various degrees of A-V block or ventricular premature contractions (Goldberger, 1980f).

The newborn

1. In infants born after a hypoxic delivery a transient and symptomless hypermagnesaemia may occur, but requires no treatment.
2. Treatment of pre-eclampsia in the mother by injection of magnesium sulphate just before delivery may cause symptomatic hypermagnesaemia in the newborn, with drowsiness, hypotonia, and respiratory paralysis.

In the older child

1. Magnesium sulphate enemas in Hirschsprung's disease have caused hypermagnesaemia from retention of the enema fluid.
2. Magnesium sulphate purgative or the use of magnesium-containing antacids in renal failure have also caused symptomatic hypermagnesaemia.

Recognition

Hypermagnesaemia should be considered when drowsiness or muscle weakness develops in any of the situations described above. Clinically the progression of symptomatology is given in *Table 11.2*.

Table 11.2 Symptoms of hypermagnesaemia in relation to plasma level*

Symptom	*Plasma levels*		
	mg/100 ml	mmol/ℓ	mEq/ℓ
Hypotension, peripheral vasodilatation	3.6–6.0	1.5–2.5	3.0–5.0
Drowsiness	6.0–8.5	2.5–3.5	5.0–7.0
Loss of tendon reflexes	8.5	3.5	7.0
Depression of respiration	12.0	5.0	10.0
Coma	14.0–18.0	6.0–7.5	12.0–15.0
Cardiac arrest	18.0–24.0	7.5–10.0	15.0–20.0

* After Goldberger (1980f). Reproduced by kind permission.

Management

1. In the newborn, weakness or incipient paralysis of the respiratory muscles may require an exchange transfusion and assisted ventilation.
2. In the older child the plasma magnesium level may be lowered by increasing the fluid intake provided that renal function is normal.
3. IV calcium gluconate has been suggested as an antagonist to the acute effect of magnesium on the heart.
4. At any age respiratory weakness due to hypermagnesaemia may require mechanical ventilation, and other symptoms of acute intoxication (*Table 11.2*) with ECG changes may require peritoneal dialysis or exchange transfusion according to the age of the child.

References

AL-DAHHAN, J., HAYCOCK, G. B., CHANTLER, C. and STIMMLER, L. (1983) Sodium homeostasis in term and preterm neonates. I:Renal aspects. *Archives of Disease in Childhood,* **58,** 335–342

BAUM, J. D. and ROBERTON, N. R. C. (1975) Immediate effects of alkaline infusion in infants with respiratory distress syndrome. *Journal of Pediatrics,* **87,** 255–261

CANNON, P. J. (1973) Diuretic therapy in patients with renal disease. In Winters, R. W. (ed.) *The Body Fluids in Pediatrics,* pp. 514–517. Boston: Little, Brown and Company

DARROW, D. C. (1946) The retention of electrolyte during recovery from severe dehydration due to diarrhoea. *Journal of Pediatrics,* **28,** 515–540

DAVIS, J. A., HARVEY, D. R. and YU, J. S. (1965) Neonatal fits associated with hypomagnesaemia. *Archives of Disease in Childhood,* **40,** 286–290

DELL, R. B. (1973) Pathophysiology of dehydration. In Winter, R. W. (ed.) *The Body Fluids in Pediatrics,* pp. 134–154. Boston: Little, Brown and Company

DUGAN, S. and HOLLIDAY, M. A. (1967) Water intoxication in two infants following the voluntary ingestion of excessive fluids. *Pediatrics,* **39,** 418–420

FINBERG, L. (1967) Dangers to infants caused by changes in osmolal concentration. *Pediatrics,* **40,** 1031–1034

GOLDBERGER, E. (1980) *A Primer of Water, Electrolyte and Acid–Base Syndromes,* 6th edn. (a) p. 143, 171; (b) p. 64; (c) p. 298; (d) p. 269; (e) p. 344; (f) p. 362. Philadelphia: Lea and Febiger

HIRSCHHORN, N. (1980) The treatment of acute diarrhoea in children. An historical and physiological perspective. *American Journal of Clinical Nutrition,* **33,** 637–663

IBSEN, B. (1967) Treatment of shock with vasodilators, measuring skin temperature on the big toe. Ten year's experience in 150 cases. *Diseases of the Chest,* **52,** 425–429

KATZ, M. A. (1973) Hyperglycaemia-induced hyponatraemia; calculation of expected serum sodium depression. *New England Journal of Medicine,* **289,** 943–944

KETY, S. S., POLIS, B. D., NADLER, C. S. and SCHMIDT, C. F. (1948) The blood flow and oxygen consumption of the human brain in diabetic ketoacidosis and coma. *Journal of Clinical Investigation,* **27,** 500–510

KILDEBERG, P. (1964) Disturbances of hydrogen ion balance occurring in premature infants: II. Late metabolic acidosis. *Acta Paediatrica Scandinavica,* **53,** 517–526

LINSHAW, M. A., HIPP, T. and GRUSKIN, A. (1974) Infantile psychogenic water-drinking. *Journal of Pediatrics,* **85,** 520–522

NORDIO, S., DONATH, A., MACAGNO, F. and GATTI, R. (1971) Chronic hypomagnesaemia with magnesium-dependent hypocalcaemia. *Acta Paediatrica Scandinavica,* **60,** 441–448

RODRIGUEZ-SORIANO, J., BOICHIS, H., STARK, H. and EDELMANN, C. M., Jr. (1967) Proximal renal tubular acidosis. A defect in bicarbonate reabsorption with normal urinary acidification. *Pediatric Research,* **1,** 81–98

SCHRIER, R. W. and BICHET, D. G. (1981) Osmotic and non-osmotic control of vasopressin release and the pathogenesis of impaired water excretion in adrenal, thyroid, and edematous disorders. *Journal of Laboratory and Clinical Medicine,* **98,** 1–15

SCHWARTZ, G. J., HAYCOCK, G. B., EDELMANN, C. M., Jr., and SPTIZER, A. (1979) Late metabolic acidosis: a reassessment of the definition. *Journal of Pediatrics,* **95,** 102–107

SELBY, P. C., PEACOCK, M. and MARSHALL, D. H. (1984) Hypercalcaemia: management. *British Journal of Hospital Medicine,* **31,** 186–197

SIEGEL, S. R., PHELPS, D. L., LEAKE, R. D. and OH, W. (1973) The effects of rapid infusion of hypertonic sodium bicarbonate in infants with respiratory distress. *Pediatrics,* **51,** 651–654

STRØMME, J. H., NESBAKKEN, R., NORMANN, T., SKJÖRTEN, SKYBERG, D. and JOHANNESSEN, B. (1969) Familial hypomagnesaemia. *Acta Paediatrica Scandinavica,* **58,** 433–444

SWYER, P. R. (1975) *The Intensive Care of the Newly Born,* p. 36. Basle: S. Karger

TURNER, T. L., COCKBURN, F. and FORFAR, J. O. (1977) Magnesium therapy in neonatal tetany. *Lancet,* **1,** 283–284

WILKINSON, R. (1984) Treatment of hypercalcaemia associated with malignancy. Leading article. *British Medical Journal,* **288,** 812–813

WINTERS, R. W. (1968) Disorders of electrolyte and acid–base metabolism. In Barnett, H. L. (ed.) *Pediatrics,* 14th edn. Englewood Cliffs, New Jersey: Appleton-Century-Crofts

Part III

Emergencies Involving the Face and Neck

Chapter 12

Emergencies involving the eyes

David Taylor*

Except in the neonatal period, ophthalmic emergencies are little different in children from those in young adults as far as immediate management is concerned, though the long-term results may be influenced by any interruption of the development of vision and binocular co-ordination in a child. Any situation therefore which calls for prolonged covering of an eye or any possibility of interference with vision, however minor, should be referred to an ophthalmic surgeon promptly after immediate treatment has been given.

Mechanical trauma

Orbit

Orbital haemorrhage

RECOGNITION

The common black eye will usually resolve without treatment, the haemorrhage being subcutaneous and largely in front of the orbital septum, but haemorrhage inside the obit itself may produce proptosis and interference with ocular movements, giving double vision. Orbital haemorrhage rarely leads to any long-term visual deficit, but early evidence of this in preverbal children can be an afferent pupil defect, in which the pupil of the affected eye fails to contract to light as readily as the unaffected eye.

MANAGEMENT

No specific treatment is required; it is usual to cover with a light pad or shade. Admission for observation is advised if the intraorbital pressure is obviously high. It is important to exclude orbital fracture and ocular injuries.

Orbital fracture

RECOGNITION

Fracture of the floor of the orbit may lead to depression of the bone and trapping of orbital tissue and extra-ocular muscles in the fracture line. This 'blow-out' fracture

* Alan Stanworth died on May 17th, 1981. Mr David Taylor kindly agreed to revise Mr Stanworth's chapter for the second edition.

can be produced by relatively minor trauma even in the absence of much bruising, and if untreated is likely to lead to permanent interference with ocular movement and troublesome diplopia.

It is important to remember the possibility of this condition after any blunt trauma to the orbit; diplopia should be asked about, vertical and horizontal eye movements examined, and the lids separated if they are closed by the swelling, to permit examination. Radiography is essential if there is any doubt; the fracture may not be shown by straight radiographs and may require tomography.

MANAGEMENT

Treatment is not an emergency, the eye movements being observed for a few days before deciding whether exploration and repositioning of the orbital contents and support of the orbital floor by an implant is necessary.

Penetrating wounds of the orbit

RECOGNITION

These can injure the extra-ocular muscles and their nerves, blood vessels and even the optic nerve if the penetration is to the apex of the orbit.

MANAGEMENT

No treatment should be given other than a simple pad, and referral to an ophthalmic surgeon. Protruding foreign bodies should not be removed in the casualty department since this may produce unnecessary trauma and haemorrhage.

Lids

Trauma

RECOGNITION

Trauma to the lids is usually obvious but the possibility of additional injury to the eye, orbit, and head must be remembered.

MANAGEMENT

Blunt trauma without rupture of the skin or conjunctiva, with bruising will resolve without treatment. Wounds of the lid heal well if sutured early with preservation of as much injured tissue as possible. Involvement of the lid margin needs suturing with fine sutures to restore the margin and is best done by an ophthalmologist; the margin is sutured first with a fine suture which slightly everts the wound edges, using the grey line which runs between the lash line and the openings of the tarsal glands as a landmark. The main substance of the lid is then sutured in layers from back to front using buried absorbable sutures for the deep layers and fine non-absorbable sutures for the skin.

Lacrimal involvement in trauma

RECOGNITION

Any laceration at the inner end of the lower lid should be carefully examined to assess the possibility of canaliculus damage. A lacrimal probe passed through the lower canaliculus after dilating the punctum will demonstrate whether the canaliculus is involved; this manoeuvre is best carried out by an ophthalmologist since false passages are easily produced.

MANAGEMENT

A torn lower canaliculus is best repaired by an ophthalmologist familiar with microsurgery.

Conjunctiva

The conjunctiva heals remarkably well and small lacerations of 3 mm or so can be left without stitching. Larger gaping lacerations require stitching with fine catgut.

Foreign bodies

These can usually be lifted off with a moist swab but if embedded may require to be picked up with fine forceps and snipped off leaving a small hole in the conjunctiva which easily heals without a suture. Foreign bodies can be easily missed in the upper fornix and they are best detected by lifting the lid away from the eye and looking under the lid with bright illumination.

Subconjunctival haemorrhage

This produces a localized bright red patch which obscures the vascular markings. No treatment is needed but it is important to find out how it arose and exclude an underlying penetrating injury.

Cornea

Corneal abrasions

RECOGNITION

These can be delineated by fluorescein drops which stain the loss of surface a bright green colour.

MANAGEMENT

Small abrasions will normally heal rapidly if given antibiotic drops (e.g. chloramphenicol) to prevent secondary infection. Large abrasions may need the addition of a short-acting mydriatic such as cyclopentolate 1%, and a light pad may make the patient more comfortable.

Foreign bodies

These may be gently wiped off with a moist piece of cotton wool; if embedded they are best removed under topical anaesthetic by someone with experience, using a fine needle to minimize trauma, followed by antibiotic drops; if a large abrasion remains, mydriatic drops such as cyclopentolate 1% or homatropine 2% are needed.

Corneal lacerations

These need expert treatment; if gaping, they may require suturing even if they do not penetrate the full thickness of the cornea.

Xerophthalmia

This is seen as a 'dullness' of the eye, a white corneal opacity or a 'cheesy' appearance of the conjunctiva in an eye that may be somewhat inflamed, in a child who has other evidence of malnutrition and who may have some difficulty in seeing, especially in the dark. It is treated by oral retinol acetate (vitamin A) (100 000 units daily for the first 2 days, then repeat one dose in 2 weeks; if over the age of 2 years, give twice the dose (King, King and Martodipoero, 1978)), a protein-rich diet and topical antibiotics. Severe xerophthalmia especially with serious superimposed infection is known as keratomalacia which requires vigorous and urgent treatment with topical and systemic antibiotics and improvement in general nutrition (in severe cases or when there is a possibility of malabsorption, give 100 000 units of retinol palmitate (Ro-A-Vit) i.m., followed by oral treatment, as above).

Perforating wounds of the globe

Recognition

After injuries to the lids and surface of the eye a careful examination should be made for evidence of perforating wounds. These may include obvious lacerations of the cornea and sclera, protrusion of the ciliary body or choroid through the sclera; a hole may be visible in the iris. The pupil may be distorted. Blood may be seen on the iris or in the anterior chamber; blood in the vitreous may appear as opacities or prevent a view of the fundus. A foreign body, if large, may be seen inside the eye but most foreign bodies are too small or too obscured by blood to be visible.

Management

Any suspected perforating wound should be treated by no more than prevention of the child rubbing the eye and *immediate referral to an ophthalmic department.*

Non-perforating injury to the globe

Recognition

Contusions involving the interior of the eye may produce haemorrhage into the anterior chamber (hyphaema), distortion of the pupil, tears in the iris, vitreous haemorrhage, and injury to the choroid and retina.

Management

Any evidence of these conditions requires admission of the patient to an ophthalmic department.

Chemical injuries and burns

Recognition

Such injury is usually obvious from the history, swelling of the lids, congestion of the conjunctiva, and opacity of the cornea. The severity of the injury may be underestimated if the blood vessels of the conjunctiva have been destroyed, leading to a white appearance rather than to congestion; the extent of the damage to the cornea can be shown by a green staining with fluorescein drops.

Management

Immediate treatment is vital in cases of chemical injury. Copious irrigation with any bland fluid that is available should be started at once, and kept up for at least 10 minutes. The fluid used for irrigation is of little consequence; saline is as good as anything and water can be used if saline is not available. The volume of the fluid used is more important than its nature. Any obvious pieces of foreign matter such as lime can be removed with moist cotton wool or a swab, but force to do this should not be exerted. Meanwhile arrangements should be made for treatment in an ophthalmic department since thorough cleansing of the burnt area requires skilled nursing and even general anaesthesia. The use of antibiotic drops is worth while if there is any delay. (Burns – *see* page 31).

Acute inflammation

Orbital cellulitis

Recognition

Infection entering the orbit from the nasal sinuses or bloodstream may produce signs of cellulitis, with swelling, redness, and closure of the lids, pain and tenderness, and pyrexia; the orbital pressure may reach such a degree as to obstruct circulation and so lead to visual loss, though this is rare in children.

Management

Firstly an assessment by an ENT surgeon and sinus X-rays are carried out. If there is any discharge it is cultured. Then wide-spectrum systemic antibiotics are used and the patient admitted to an ophthalmic department.

Acute dacryocystitis

Recognition

In infancy this is a rare complication of congenital blockage of the nasolacrimal duct, giving rise to tenderness and swelling at the inner canthus.

Management

A systemic antibiotic will be necessary in the severe cases, with subsequent treatment of the underlying cause by probing.

Styes and inflamed tarsal cysts

Recognition

These produce localized tender swellings on the margin (styes) or in the substance (tarsal cyst) of the lids.

Management

Antibiotic drops or ointment hourly are usually sufficient to control the acute attack, together with simple toilet to remove any debris and dried mucopus from the lid margins.

Rapid onset of lid swelling

This may be due to one of the preceding infections, to allergies to drops or ointments or associated with generalized allergies, or to bee or wasp stings. The management is that appropriate to cause.

Acute conjunctivitis

Recognition

This is characterized by redness and discharge; it is uncomfortable but not painful. Most cases will respond well to cleansing of the eye with moist cotton wool to remove discharge, together with antibiotic drops in frequencies varying from every few minutes in the acute type of gonococcal ophthalmia neonatorum to every 2 hours in the less acute inflammations. Padding of the eye is contraindicated. Severe ophthalmia neonatorum should be seen by an ophthalmologist and transferred to an ophthalmic department if necessary (*see* page 652 for antibiotic treatment); i.m. benzyl penicillin should always be given in addition to local treatment.

Corneal ulceration related to acute conjunctivitis

Recognition

This may follow or accompany acute conjunctivitis; the redness is more marked around the edge of the cornea, the condition is painful, and discharge is produced only by the accompanying conjunctival irritation. Vision will be blurred unless the ulcer is confined to the periphery of the cornea. Pyogenic corneal infections usually produce obvious opacity in the cornea, but herpes simplex infections may be difficult to see even with the use of fluorescein drops; the primary infections with herpes simplex often show as punctate corneal staining but secondary infections may show the typical dendritic figure. *Fluorescein drops should be used in any eye in which corneal ulceration is a possibility*. Treatment is by referral to an ophthalmic surgeon with atropine and appropriate antibiotic drops for pyogenic infections or idoxuridine drops (1% solution) hourly by day and two hourly at night or other antiviral agents for herpes simplex infection. Steroid drops should NOT be used.

Infantile glaucoma (buphthalmos)

Recognition

The condition may be already present at birth but more commonly becomes obvious at the age of a few months. Infantile glaucoma may lead to an increased size of the eye with stretching of the cornea and rupture of the corneal endothelium. This can give rise to corneal oedema which causes irritable eyes with photophobia and watering. Discharge is not a feature. The eye may not be so obviously enlarged as to attract attention unless the possibility is considered. Any unduly photophobic baby should be referred to an ophthalmologist. Any child with a 'portwine stain' (naevus flammeus) (Sturge–Weber syndrome) on the face should be followed up by an ophthalmologist for life because of the risk of glaucoma.

Management

Urgent referral to an ophthalmologist skilled in the management of this condition is essential.

Acute iridocyclitis

Recognition

This produces a painful eye with circumcorneal injection, variable diminution in vision, and usually an irregular small pupil. This last sign indicates that atropine drops should be given four hourly, but an ophthalmic assessment is urgent. Do NOT use steroid drops unless it is certain that there is no corneal ulceration from herpes simplex infection.

Subacute iridocyclitis

This occurs in Still's disease (juvenile rheumatoid arthritis) and is usually asymptomatic. Patients with the pauciarticular form of Still's disease should have regular eye checks even in the absence of any symptoms.

Sudden loss of vision

Sudden loss of vision in children is not common and there may be little obvious evidence of ocular disease. Investigation should be started urgently. Chronic and even congenital diseases affecting mainly or entirely one eye may present as sudden loss of vision since the early stages of visual loss may not be noticed, especially by the young patient. Hysteria may also have to be considered (*see* page 525).

Retinal detachment

This may occur apparently spontaneously as a result of congenital or old inflammatory defects in the retina; it may also follow blunt trauma to the head or any trauma to the eye after an interval of days, weeks or months. Operation is urgent unless the detachment is of long standing.

Optic neuritis

This is rare in childhood but when it occurs it is often bilateral, with loss of acuity and colour vision and with a central visual field defect. Referral to a neurologist or neuro-ophthalmologist should not be delayed.

Optic nerve compression

Tumours affecting the anterior visual system may present with unilateral or bilateral visual loss.

Papilloedema

In its early stages this does not cause more than transient episodes of blurring of vision, but when prolonged may lead to visual loss and secondary optic atrophy.

Double vision

A squint leading to double vision is not common in childhood but the sudden onset of 6th nerve palsy may herald a blocked valve in hydrocephalus or other cause of acutely raised intracranial pressure. A 3rd nerve palsy in an older child may be due to an aneurysm and all patients with acquired diplopia require urgent investigation.

Neonatal emergencies

Ophthalmia neonatorum

This is dealt with under conjunctivitis (*see* above; also *see under* Acute Infections in the Newborn, page 652).

Watering of the eyes

This is usually due to lacrimal blockage and is not usually obvious in the first 2 to 3 weeks since tear production is low, but it may be the basis of chronic redness and discharge in infancy, requiring antibiotic drops three times daily, repeated digital pressure over the lacrimal sac to try to empty it into the nose, and probing of the lacrimal ducts at the age of 4–6 months if the condition does not settle. Photophobia and watering should alert the clinician to the possibility of glaucoma.

Corneal opacity

This may be due to:

1. A developmental anomaly of the anterior eyeball.
2. Infantile glaucoma (*see* above).

3. Rupture of the posterior layers of the cornea during birth particularly after the misapplication of forceps; this produces corneal oedema which gradually subsides over a few days; no treatment is indicated in the acute stage but the potential visual loss needs ophthalmic management.
4. One of the mucopolysaccharidoses.
5. Corneal infection.

All require an ophthalmic opinion.

Large eyes

An obviously large eye requires an ophthalmic opinion.

Cataracts

Cataracts and other opacities in the refractive media of the eye can be detected in seconds by the correct use of the ophthalmoscope. With the ophthalmoscope set so that the observer can clearly see the eye looking at it from 2 feet (0.6 m) through the aperture the normally red reflection from the fundus is observed. If this is not clearly seen then the baby should be referred to an ophthalmologist immediately. Patients with Down's syndrome, congenital rubella, and any other syndrome associated with cararact should be referred to an ophthalmologist. The suggestion by parents that their child has an unusual appearance in the pupil, whether this is described as grey, white, bluish, or 'a haze', even only seen in certain light, calls for an urgent referral to an ophthalmologist. It can be caused by retinoblastoma, developmental anomalies, and retrolental fibroplasia; the prognosis of retinoblastoma is greatly improved by early diagnosis.

References

KING, M., KING, F. and MARTODIPOERO, S. (1978) *Primary Child Care, A Manual for Health Workers,* Book One, p. 191. Oxford Medical Publications

Further reading

HARTLEY, R. D. (ed.) (1983) *Pediatric Ophthalmology,* Philadelphia: W. B. Saunders

SHAFFER, R. N. and WEISS, D. I. (eds) (1970) *Congenital and Pediatric Glaucoma.* St. Louis: C. V. Mosby

WYBAR, K. C. and TAYLOR, D. (eds) (1983) *Pediatric Ophthalmology – Current Aspects.* New York: Marcel Dekker

Chapter 13

Traumatic injuries of the head, face and neck

R. C. W. Dinsdale

In all cases presenting it should be remembered that:

1. Treatment of an acute neurosurgical emergency has priority over other injuries.
2. Accurate assessment and treatment is essential in all cases to prevent permanent deformity, whether or not they present as an acute emergency in the first place.
3. The injury may be non-accidental.

The injuries which may result from trauma to the bones and soft tissues of the head, face and neck are considered briefly under the following headings:

1. The skull.
2. Eyes and ears.
3. The bony complex of the mid-face: maxilla, malar, nasal bones and the palate.
4. The mandible and soft tissues of the lower face and neck.

The skull (acute brain injury)

This is dealt with in greater detail under 'Acute Neurosurgical Emergencies' (*see* Chapter 25). Briefly, it is important to look for evidence pointing to:

1. Destructive injury to the brain which may be indicated by limb weakness, hemiparesis, irregularity of the pulse, or inequality of the pupils (*see* page 284).
2. Deterioration of consciousness due to continuing intracranial bleeding, extradural haemorrhage or traumatic cerebral oedema (*see* pages 285 and 288).

The eyes and ears

1. 'Blow-out' fractures with depression of the orbital floor are easily missed and may lead to diplopia and occasionally result in blindness if not recognized at the time (*see* page 145).
2. Penetrating injuries of the cornea, orbit and globe are also serious and should be looked for carefully (*see* pages 146–148).
3. Direct injury to the nose or ear including the mastoid area require careful assessment by an ENT surgeon (*see* pages 197 and 203).

The bony complex of the mid-face: maxilla, malar, nasal bones and the palate

The maxilla complex may be detached from the skull by fracture of its thin leaf-like plates of bone. The detached portion as a whole, or in pieces, may be driven backwards and downwards towards the sphenoid body, taking the nasal bones, palate, alveolar process and attached soft tissue with it. A common single 'piece' injury consists of an in-fracture of the malar bone, with the occasional involvement of the structures in the orbital cavity. Avulsed teeth may be inhaled and will require removal by bronchoscopy (*see* Ear, Nose and Throat Emergencies, page 196).

The possible effects of this type of injury are:

1. The nasopharyngeal airway may be narrowed or completely obliterated by displacement of the bony complex.
2. As a consequence, there is reduction in the alternative (oral) airway by encroachment upon the tongue space.
3. The brisk bleeding from torn blood vessels in the nasal and pharyngeal region into the tissues and pharynx, and the impaired efficiency of the muscles of the nasopharyngeal sphincter due to displacement of the palate, are both likely to cause further obstruction of the airway.
4. Where the fractures extend into bony fissures and across foramina, important structures may be damaged directly by compression and tearing, or indirectly by pressure from clotted blood. These structures may include:
   (a) The olfactory nerve and dura mater by involvement of the cribriform plate.
   (b) The optic and ophthalmic nerves, retinal artery and other structures in the foramen lacerum.
   (c) The chorda tympani nerve as it leaves the temporal bone.
   (d) The maxillary division of the 5th nerve as it passes through the foramen rotundum and its branch in the infraorbital canal.

The mandible, soft tissues of the lower face and neck

The mandible, to a large extent, protects the tongue, hyoid bone and larynx from direct injury, and involvement of these structures in the absence of damage to the mandible is unusual, the exception being strangulation. In most fractures of the mandible in the child, there is little displacement but where a segment is detached carrying the muscles attached to the genial process, control of the tongue can be lost with obstruction of the airway. This is more likely to happen when the patient is supine.

The airway may also be at risk from swelling of the soft tissues under the tongue and in the laryngeal region, in particular after an attempt at strangulation. If larger vessels are ruptured in the neck or floor of mouth, a haematoma may cause a similar embarrassment.

The lip may be insensitive if the inferior dental nerve has been damaged, and less commonly the tongue if the lingual nerve is involved.

An indirect fracture at the neck of one or both mandibular condyles may follow a blow or fall on to the chin.

When the patient arrives

1. Ensure that:
   (a) The mouth and pharynx are clear of blood and foreign bodies.
   (b) Aspiration of blood is not taking place. This is best achieved by placing the patient on the right side. Insert an oral airway if required.
   (c) Major haemorrhage is under control.
   (d) A note is made of the size, response to light, and position of each pupil.
   (e) An assessment is made of the degree of shock by reference to the blood pressure, pulse and respiration rates. The accessory muscles of respiration are used both in the 'air hunger' which follows acute blood loss and also when the airway is partly obstructed.
   (f) The site of an accessible vein for infusion is marked or noted.
   (g) Heat loss is reduced to a minimum; a metal foil blanket is ideal, but make sure that the face, neck and upper thorax are visible.
2. Each case should now be written up. The notes should include:
   (a) An account of the circumstances of the injury from a witness, if available. This should record the time, place and cause of accident, if known, with a clear description (including the duration) of any episode of loss of consciousness.
   (b) A medical history (especially of bleeding tendency) should be obtained from the parents or guardian if they are with the child, or *a note made to do this when they arrive.*
   (c) The result of symptomatic enquiry (if the level of consciousness permits). Many questions to a confused and crying child with a severe injury are unlikely to elicit useful information; instead it is advisable to make a positive or negative record of evidence for loss of vision, or double vision, and changes in hearing.

Clinical and radiographic examination

Before proceeding to a detailed examination of an injury apparently limited to the face, the patient should be reviewed to exclude:

1. Injury to the skull (acute brain injury).
2. Other injuries, particularly bleeding into the thorax, peritoneal cavity, pelvis and tissues surrounding the long bones (*see also* Chapter 3).

The mid-face, mandible and neck

General

Engorgement of the neck veins with use of the accessory muscles of respiration suggests a possible obstruction of the airway. There may also be a stridor if there is laryngeal involvement.

Extra-oral examination

The shape of the face may be considerably changed following the set-back of the bony complex of the mid-face with widening in the malar area. Downward displacement will produce an apparent lengthening of the face, and the mouth may be propped open upon the molar teeth. A similar appearance may result from a bilateral fracture of the mandibular condyles with shortening of the ascending ramus.

The systematic examination should look specifically for:

1. A leak of cerebrospinal fluid from the ear or nose. In the case of a nasal leak this may be difficult to see because of mixtures with blood, or because the fluid is lost as a postnasal drip.
2. Bleeding from the ear, nose or mouth, and the presence of clotted blood.
3. The presence and distribution of subconjunctival haemorrhage. This examination may not be possible owing to extensive soft-tissue swelling, and this fact *should be recorded* so that there is a reminder in the notes to do it later (*see* page 147).
4. Evidence of sensory loss of the skin of the forehead, the cheeks, lips or tongue.
5. Evidence of motor nerve injury (e.g. 7th cranial).

It is important to remember that, as time passes from the moment of injury, the mid-face tissues swell quickly and the presence of a step or gap that would indicate a fracture is often difficult to detect by palpation. The extent of swelling which could mask a considerable displacement must therefore be taken into account.

Examination is best carried out standing behind the patient and 'crawling' with the fingers around the orbital margins and nasal bones feeling for defects and comparing left with right. The less obviously injured parts should be examined first so that the child, if conscious, may gain confidence from this selective approach. It is normally possible to feel the head of the condyles on jaw movement and also the whole of the lower border of the mandible. The presence of surgical emphysema and its distribution, especially any extension into the cervical and mediastinal spaces, should be noted.

Intra-oral examination

The facial soft tissues and lips may be torn (degloved) from the underlying bone of the jaws in falls, particularly from bicycles, horses or moving vehicles. Impacted material from the ground may be present. In road traffic accidents, non-radiopaque foreign bodies such as wood, plastic or glass may be in the tissues. Fractures of the underlying bone will be seen through the wound. With closed fractures, the presence of an ecchymosis into the soft tissues on the alveolus or into the floor of the mouth will prompt a search for an underlying fracture. The teeth should be checked, looking especially in either jaw for groups of loose teeth attached to the alveolar process (in the younger child a detached segment may contain the forming permanent teeth). A search should be made for loose tooth fragments in open wounds, e.g. in the lip. If empty sockets are present, the missing teeth may still be in the mouth, lying in the sulcus or under the tongue and obscured by blood.

Radiographic examination

If radiographs can be obtained, two plain film views at least should be requested and should include preferably an occipito-mental and lateral view of the skull and jaws. Fractures of the facial bones are difficult to diagnose and an expert opinion on the films should be obtained before discharge.

A tooth, or foreign body lying in the pharynx will be difficult or impossible to see, therefore a request for airway radiographs should state that teeth are missing; a dislodged tooth may be seen on a chest radiograph (*see* Ear, Nose and Throat Emergencies, page 196).

Management of injuries to the mid-face, mandible and neck

It is important to ensure that *further* episodes of airway obstruction do not occur, particularly where there has been an earlier loss of consciousness through obstruction, throttling or injury to the brain. A second obstruction may well change a prognosis for complete recovery to one of permanent brain injury through hypoxia. The same effect may also result from an episode of obstruction in the presence of a continuous severe blood loss, particularly in the small (under 2 years of age) child with relatively small blood volume (*see also* Chapter 3).

Immediate arrangements (for the severe case)

1. A regular routine of observation in a *good light*, preferably natural lighting, should be established to detect and treat:
   (a) Changes in the level of consciousness (*see* Acute Head Injuries, page 283).
   (b) Changes in the adequacy of the airway.
   (c) Changes in the colour of the patient. The development of cyanosis will be more obvious in natural light than artificial, as the normal skin tones will be preserved.

   Whenever there is a possibility of obstruction to the airway and especially in mandibular fractures, a suture of 2/0 black silk should be passed through the dorsum of the tongue as far back as possible. The thread should be long enough to reach the chest. In the deeply unconscious patient or where a downward displacement of the maxillary complex has occurred, an oropharyngeal airway should be inserted. The passage of an orotracheal tube in a severely injured child is not easy, but it is life saving if it can be managed. If these measures do not ensure an adequate airway, a tracheostomy must be carried out immediately (*see* page 327).
2. The patient should be reviewed from time to time to detect any effect that continuing blood loss might have upon the airway. It is difficult to detect silent postnasal or pharyngeal bleeding into the respiratory tract, especially where the cough or swallowing reflex is impaired. An adequate aspiration routine should be established. Continuing nasal haemorrhage demands treatment, and a pack of ribbon gauze should be inserted. The time of insertion *should be recorded* with an instruction in the notes that it should be removed or replaced within 24 hours (*see also* Ear, Nose and Throat Emergencies, page 201).
3. It is wise at this stage to set up an IV line before collapse of veins in shock makes this difficult. Blood should be taken at this stage, if this has not been done before, for baseline haemoglobin estimation.
4. Where a cerebrospinal fluid leak is suspected, ampicillin or amoxycillin should be given intramuscularly or intravenously. The use of these antibiotics should also be considered in extensive open fractures of the facial bones, or where the viability of soft tissues is in doubt (for dosage *see* Appendix 11).
5. The fluid balance should be monitored.

Medium-term arrangement (In the first 24 hours, assuming an Intensive Treatment Unit is not available for transfer)

1. If a tracheostomy has been performed, a regular nursing routine of observation should be established.
2. If an anaesthetic is to be given to cover some other urgent surgical procedure, the opportunity should be taken to secure and tie the accessible bleeding vessels in the soft tissues. Care should be taken to avoid the inclusion of the larger sensory nerves in the forceps. An effort should be made to obtain coverage of exposed bone, preserving as much soft tissue as possible. Quite large sections of jaw bone with teeth attached and teeth inside will survive.
3. Tetanus toxoid should be given if the wound is open or contaminated.
4. Provided that the airway is clear and haemorrhage is under control, all other maxillo-facial procedures can be deferred, if necessary for several days, *but the next step* must be planned at the earliest opportunity as part of the overall surgical management, in order to reduce deformity.

Mistakes in management

1. In the early stages, no case of head, face or neck injury should be given:
   (a) Drugs which depress the central nervous system or the respiratory centre.
   (b) A general anaesthetic, except to cover a life-saving operation such as tracheostomy or craniotomy.
   (c) Any solution containing adrenaline or noradrenaline for local analgesia by injection, particularly if a general anaesthetic might be required later. (A preparation containing prilocaine 3% with felypressin would be acceptable.)
2. The manipulation of loose fragments is unwise, as this can cause further bleeding. If a dental or maxillofacial specialist is available a continuous haemorrhage can sometimes be controlled by *the stabilization* of the larger fragments.
3. A repair of a penetrating injury of the palate, common in children, should not be undertaken until an *ENT or plastic surgical opinion* has been obtained.

Chapter 14

Dental emergencies: oral haemorrhage and traumatic injury to the teeth

R. C. W. Dinsdale

Oral haemorrhage

This is considered under three headings:

1. Secondary haemorrhage (post-extraction and traumatic).
2. Recurrent haemorrhage.
3. Spontaneous haemorrhage.

Secondary haemorrhage (post-extraction and traumatic)

In the normal child, persistent haemorrhage from a tooth extraction socket (or accidental injury to the mouth) is uncommon. Occasionally a dental case may present as a true emergency, which must be distinguished from the emotionally charged minor problem that arises occasionally in all accident and emergency departments.

History

A clear history of the extraction or injury sustained should be secured. The following questions will help with the diagnosis and also with assessment of suitability for anaesthesia if required later:

1. Where and when were the extractions carried out?
2. Why were the teeth removed? For drainage of an abscess, or as a part of a routine treatment plan? (The hyperaemia of acutely inflamed tissue may be a factor in continued haemorrhage.)
3. How many deciduous, and more important, permanent teeth were removed? (The latter will have a larger root surface area with a greater potential for blood loss.)
4. How were the teeth removed? With local analgesia or general anaesthetic?
5. Were any tablets taken for pain before or since the extraction, in particular those containing aspirin or narcotic drugs?
6. Has the bleeding ever stopped?
7. Has the patient been rinsing excessively?
8. Has the patient been overactive, restless or crying?
9. What measures have already been tried?

10. Was there a period of reduced fluid intake on account of toothache before the extraction?
11. When was the last meal taken?
12. Have there been any previous episodes of post-extraction dental bleeding or of spontaneous nasal bleeding? Any history of bruising, or any known family history of a bleeding or coagulation disorder?

Examination

GENERAL

The pallor of a child with a stomach full of swallowed blood must not be confused with the pallor associated with excessive blood loss. Therefore, an assessment of blood loss and degree of dehydration should be made. The record should include the blood pressure, pulse and respiration rates, making an allowance for the effects of apprehension.

LOCAL EXAMINATION

This should be carried out in a good light, as follows. Using a small swab applied gently and intermittently to the bleeding site and an aspirator fitted with a small tip (a large aspirator with a vigorous sucking action is frightening) the following observations should be made:

1. Is there bleeding from one or more than one socket?
2. Is there evidence of local trauma? A forceps laceration should be obvious; a laceration is less easily seen on the lingual side of the lower teeth.
3. Is any unsupported tissue present which can be moved by cheek or tongue?
4. Is there evidence of an ecchymosis or haematoma by extension from the extraction site into adjacent tissues? (The presence of a large haematoma may be the first manifestation of a previously unsuspected bleeding diathesis.) A haematoma may also indicate the presence of a jaw fracture.
5. Have the sockets already been sutured?

From the history and these observations, an estimate of total and continuing rate of blood loss should be made. The significance of this must be considered in relation to the blood volume and age of the child (*see* page 21).

It should also be possible to suggest a likely cause for the bleeding, usually due to local factors, but impairment of platelet function from aspirin intake must also be considered, particularly in the absence of any previous personal or family history of bleeding.

Management

IMMEDIATE TREATMENT

The emphasis should be on control by local means, making use, in one form or another, of applied pressure.

As an interim measure, the patient should be encouraged to close lightly on a *small swab* trimmed to cover the tooth socket and to fit between adjacent teeth.

Provided that the bleeding is not copious and the cardiovascular system is stable, treatment may then be deferred for up to 2 hours until the services of a dental surgeon can be obtained. If this is not feasible, the following routine should be followed:

1. Smear a little lignocaine surface anaesthetic paste on two small pledgets (0.5 cm) of cotton wool. Place one each side of the tooth socket in the sulcus.
2. Two minutes later, using a short fine needle, preferably 25–27 gauge, inject 0.5 ml 3% prilocaine with felypressin slowly under the lax mucosa on either side of the tooth socket. (Avoid any local analgesic solution containing adrenaline or noradrenaline in case a general anaesthetic is required later.)
3. It should now be possible to place one or two across-the-socket sutures using 4/0 or 5/0 black silk or 4/0 catgut on a curved 22 mm preferably reverse-cutting needle. If catgut is used, it should be 'triple'-tied.
4. A second, tailored swab, of a height just greater than the crown of the extracted tooth, can then be placed over the newly stabilized socket. The patient closes gently on this for 15 minutes.
5. Next, remove the swab and wait. If there is no fresh bleeding after a further 15 minutes, it can be assumed that a stable clot has formed and syneresis has commenced.

In the small child, or where co-operation is not forthcoming, the administration of a general anaesthetic in order to place the sutures accurately must be considered. Intubation is essential because of the risk of a sudden reflux of swallowed blood from the stomach. (The opportunity can also be used to gain access to a vein for any subsequent infusion that may be needed.)

IF BLEEDING CONTINUES

The site should be re-examined carefully and the placement of further sutures (possibly under a general anaesthetic) should be considered. If the bleeding is from *more than one* tooth socket and sutures have failed to control it, a systemic cause should be suspected. Should facilities for the assay of clotting factors and study of platelet function not be immediately available, an injection of either hydrocortisone hemisuccinate 100 mg (subcutaneously or IV) or dexamethasone phosphate 4 mg (IV) may be tried. If effective, the bleeding will stop spontaneously in approximately half an hour. These drugs appear to reduce capillary permeability (Robson and Duthie, 1952) and increase their resistance to trauma (Dinsdale, Dixon and Figures, 1980). The short-lived elevation of the serum cortisol level will not interfere with subsequent coagulation studies should these be required later. If bleeding still continues and the services of a dental specialist or a haematologist are not available, the case should be transferred to the nearest centre known to provide these services.

NOTE – Intramuscular injections SHOULD NOT BE GIVEN until the presence of a coagulation disorder has been excluded.

Recurrent haemorrhage

Infection of a soft-tissue wound in the mouth, occurring perhaps a week after an extraction or soft-tissue injury, is the most usual cause. The bleeding is brisk and difficult to control, the tissues being swollen and friable. Several episodes of bleeding may have occurred prior to referral with considerable blood loss, and the patient may also be dehydrated.

Management

1. A dental specialist should be called immediately or the patient transferred.
2. Interim treatment; apply pressure as for secondary haemorrhage to reduce total blood loss.
3. A transfusion with whole blood or equivalent may be required to treat shock and anaemia, and to cover the further blood loss that will occur during treatment.
4. A general anaesthetic is often necessary to provide the best conditions for a detailed examination. This should be given by an experienced anaesthetist who will take into account the state of the cardiovascular system and previous drug therapy.
5. The principles of treatment. A series of sutures, taking deep bites of tissue, should be inserted across the socket and the adjacent soft tissues undersewn. A specific bleeding point may be secured with a fine artery forceps and tied off. Exuberant granulation tissue may also be removed at this stage and an impression taken for the construction of an acrylic splint to cover the site.
6. An antibiotic, preferably benzylpenicillin, should be given.

Spontaneous haemorrhage

Spontaneous haemorrhage from the gums or continued haemorrhage from some trivial injury, for example an accidental bite of the tongue or cheek, or frenal tear, is unusual in the normal child. A systemic cause or *non-accidental injury* must be suspected.

An abnormal tendency to bleed may be revealed at the time of eruption of the teeth or when the change from the deciduous to the permanent dentition is taking place. The deciduous teeth will be loose and there is often a hyperaemia at the point of attachment.

Spontaneous bleeding from the gums will most often be associated with a severe anaemia, leukaemia or other blood disorder, but may also follow the treatment of some of these conditions with chemotherapeutic agents. Suspicion that a blood disorder is present or that the child may be scorbutic will be supported by the presence of small petechial haemorrhages on the soft palate and cheeks, especially if there is evidence of bruising elsewhere on the body.

Management

Whereas in the treatment of post-extraction dental haemorrhage the emphasis was upon control by local means using pressure, the successful management of this type of bleeding depends more upon the correct diagnosis and treatment of the underlying disorder, e.g. infusion of blood, the administration of desmopressin (DDAVP) or concentrates such as Factors VIII or IX appropriate to the diagnosis, and stabilization of the clot using oral aminocaproic acid (ϵ aminocaproic acid, EACA) or tranexamic acid. In such cases a haematologist should be consulted and the services of an experienced dental surgeon obtained. Should this not be feasible, the case should be considered for transfer to the nearest centre known to provide such a service.

Local treatment must be co-ordinated with general treatment. The local measures will include suturing to stabilize soft tissue, removal of loose teeth and excision of soft tissue where necessary. Occasionally acrylic splints may be specially constructed to fit over and protect exposed sites from trauma until healing can take place. An antibiotic will be required, especially for those patients on immunosuppressive or chemotherapeutic drugs.

Traumatic injuries to the teeth

Whilst accidental damage to the teeth cannot be regarded as life threatening, doctors in accident and emergency departments are frequently asked by anxious parents to provide advice and treatment. These injuries may be broadly classified as follows:

1. Direct damage to crown, pulp or root.
2. Indirect damage to the developing tooth resulting in enamel hypoplasia or root dilaceration (a tooth with a deformed root).
3. Avulsion, with or without attached alveolar bone.

For general reference *see* Andreason (1972).

Direct damage to crown, pulp or root

It is customary to describe injuries to the teeth numerically (the classification by Ellis (1960) is much used):

Class I – Traumatized tooth. No crown or root fracture.
Class II – A fracture confined to the enamel or including both enamel and dentine but not exposing pulp.
Class III – A fracture involving enamel with pulp visible as a pink spot through a thin layer of dentine.
Class IV – A fracture involving enamel, dentine and exposing the pulp.
Class V – A fracture involving dentine, cementum and pulp (root fracture).

Radiographic examination

Dental radiographs will exclude root fractures (Class V) and damage to adjacent and opposing teeth. Soft-tissue films will detect fragments in the lip and tongue.

Management

All patients with a history of trauma to the teeth should be seen by a dental surgeon, preferably within 24 hours, even if no obvious injury has been sustained. In Class I injuries, the pulp may degenerate gradually, and therefore regular examination is required to detect change and start treatment.

Class I, II and V injuries require no immediate treatment. Class III and IV injuries require treatment within 24 hours to offer the best prospect of retaining the vitality of the pulp tissue. This is important if the root is still forming. If possible, a dental surgeon should be called to these cases as materials are now available to provide immediate protection to the exposed pulp tissue (Watkins and Andlaw, 1977).

Indirect damage to developing teeth, enamel hypoplasia and root dilaceration

Both types of injury may follow from the impaction of the root of a deciduous incisor tooth into the follicle of the permanent successor. The permanent central incisor is unfortunately the tooth most frequently involved.

Management

Depending upon a number of factors (the most important being the age of the child) it will occasionally be possible, after the impacted deciduous tooth has been removed, to reposition the displaced permanent crown by firm pressure upon the displaced buccal plate of bone. This will realign the crown of the permanent tooth and give the dentine papilla a chance to continue the process of root formation and so reduce the degree of dilaceration. As this should be done within 24 hours, the case should be referred to a dental surgeon as soon as possible.

Avulsion

Replantation may be tried. The chances of a successful result are reduced if:

1. More than 2 hours have elapsed since the tooth was lost.
2. The root surface has been allowed to dry out.
3. The root cementum has been damaged by instrumentation or excessive handling.
4. The root is not fully formed.

Management

In response to a telephone enquiry: what should be done with a completely displaced tooth? Answer: immerse the tooth in cold milk from a refrigerator, or less good, in iced isotonic saline (1 teaspoon of salt to a tumbler of water). Try to arrange for a dental surgeon to be present when patient arrives. If not available:

1. Immerse the tooth in sterile normal saline immediately.
2. Smear a little lignocaine surface anaesthetic paste on two small (0.5 cm) pledgets of cotton wool. Place one each side of the tooth socket in the sulcus.
3. Two minutes later, using a short fine needle, inject 0.5 ml 3% prilocaine with felypressin into the lax tissues on either side of the socket.
4. Completely aspirate the blood clot and irrigate with normal saline until the socket is clean.
5. Reinsert the tooth and hold it in place for at least 10 minutes. Many teeth will stay in place even if protruding slightly from the socket. It will usually be possible to realign the tooth by orthodontic means at a later date. If the tooth will not stay in the socket, while the local analgesic is still effective, try moulding several layers of thin aluminium (kitchen) foil or foil from a dental X-ray film packet over the crown of the tooth and of the teeth each side; trim with scissors.
6. Refer to dental surgeon within 24 hours. An assessment can then be made as to whether to proceed with treatment, which may include fixation, or to remove the tooth and compensate for the loss in some other way.
7. An antibiotic, amoxycillin or benzylpenicillin in standard dose, should be given.
8. Tetanus toxoid should be given.

References

ANDREASON, J. D. (1972) *Traumatic Injuries to the Teeth.* Copenhagen: Munksgaard

DINSDALE, R. C. W., DIXON, R. A. and FIGURES, K. H. (1980) ACTH and resistance of small blood vessels to trauma: use of mucosal petechiometry. *British Journal of Oral Surgery,* **18,** 97–101

ELLIS, R. G. (1960) *The Classification and Treatment of Injuries to the Teeth of Children,* 4th edn. Chicago: Yearbook Publishers

ROBSON, H. N. and DUTHIE, J. J. R. (1952) Further observations on capillary resistance and adrenocortical activity. *British Medical Journal,* **i,** 994–996

WATKINS, J. L. and ANDLAW, R. J. (1977) Restoration of fractured incisors with an ultra-violet light polymerised composite resin. *British Dental Journal,* **142,** 249–252

Chapter 15

Acute swellings of the face

R. C. W. Dinsdale

Most rapidly enlarging swellings of the facial tissues, including the floor of the mouth and the tongue, are caused by an acute spreading infection; a few may be due to a drug allergy (*see* page 559) or follow bee or wasp stings. A patient may present with extensive swelling resulting from accidental or non-accidental injury, or as a sequel to dental and surgical treatment. This kind of swelling may represent either the diffuse products of injury, the inflammatory exudate from a supervening infection, or the accumulation of blood in the tissues as a haematoma. A haematoma can develop after the injection of a local anaesthetic; it may form rapidly and result in an urgent referral to hospital. Occasionally the development of a large haematoma is the first manifestation of a previously unsuspected bleeding diathesis in a young child.

The management of a swelling arising from accidental injury is dealt with in Chapter 13 (page 155).

The management of the rare condition of hereditary angio-oedema – in which oedema can arise either spontaneously or unexpectedly from a minor injury, a dental injection, or surgery – is discussed on pages 515–516.

Complications

It should be remembered that death may result from one or more of the following complications associated with the acute swellings described:

1. Obstruction of the airway due to an extension of the swelling into the lax tissues around the larynx.
2. An acute pulmonary oedema as part of an acute anaphylactic response, or from a secondary chest infection.
3. A cavernous sinus thrombosis by the extension of an acute infection via the communicating veins.
4. The development of septicaemia.

Acute infections of the face

With modern antibiotic therapy, spreading infections of the facial tissues rarely become life-threatening emergencies. However, an acute infection in a patient with any condition where it is known that the ability to respond is impaired should be treated with respect. Examples are severe diabetes, patients taking immunosuppressive drugs, and genetically determined disorders such as the Wiskott–Aldrich syndrome. Less often, in a malnourished or medically compromised patient, cancrum oris and acute osteomyelitis of the facial bones from secondary invasion may follow a viral infection such as measles.

Finally, it is important to remember that:

1. In the differential diagnosis of acute swellings in the cervical and submandibular region, parotitis and the submandibular adenitis of infancy must be considered.
2. Irrespective of the origin of the infecting organism, whether from the teeth, skin surface or tonsil, the lymph node draining the area may swell suddenly and this, not the primary source, becomes the chief presenting feature of the case.

Causes

The most common source of organisms leading to inflammatory swellings of the face are the teeth, their supporting structures, and the skin surface.

Dental disease

Extension into the soft tissues by direct spread usually occurs:

1. Through a perforation in the alveolar process, buccally (or labially), lingually (or palatally) and arises from a lesion at the apex of a tooth, the pulp of which has become necrotic, usually from caries, or sometimes as a result of traumatic damage to the tooth (*see* Chapter 14).
2. From an infection of the soft tissues around the crown of an erupting tooth (pericoronitis) or the supporting structures (periodontitis). The tooth crown may not be visibly decayed.

From maxillary anterior teeth, the spread may be upwards into the lip and between the muscles of facial expression, to involve the lax tissues in the infra-orbital region or from posterior teeth, backwards to the infra-temporal fossa. From mandibular teeth, the spread may be inwards to involve the floor of the mouth and the submandibular spaces, or outwards and downwards to involve the cervical spaces. (*Note* – The skin over a large abscess may rupture spontaneously leading to the development of a chronic dentocutaneous sinus.)

Skin surface

Extension by direct spread may occur via an infected lesion at the ala of the nose or the angle of the mouth, leading to facial swelling, a cellulitis or an abscess. There is a small risk of cavernous sinus thrombosis if the swelling arises in the vicinity of the upper lip, the nose or the inner canthus of the eye. (*Note* – The lymph node draining the face situated anterior to the facial artery as it passes over the mandible is often enlarged and may be confused with a swelling arising from the mandibular teeth by direct extension.)

Assessment of a case for drainage:

1. It is sometimes difficult to decide whether pus is present. A swelling may be too small, too tense or too painful to obtain the classical sign of fluctuation. The

presence of a soft, exquisitely tender spot is sufficient evidence of pus formation and will indicate a suitable point for drainage.

2. It is important to determine whether access to the mouth and throat will be possible if an anaesthetic is required. Four observations are important:
   (a) Can the mouth be opened? Trismus usually signifies a dental condition, but acute tonsillar infections and parotitis can also be responsible.
   (b) Are the tissues in the floor of the mouth and around the base of the tongue swollen?
   (c) Is the tongue fixed or elevated?
   (d) Is there evidence of airway obstruction?

Management

1. A child with a rapidly enlarging inflammatory swelling of the face or neck, who is pyrexial, should be admitted for observation, especially if the airway is considered to be at risk.
2. Seek a dental opinion to assist with the diagnosis.
3. As surgical intervention will often be necessary, the anaesthetist should also be informed in good time as these cases carry a high risk of an airway complication.
4. The extraction of the causative tooth will provide drainage and the rapid resolution of most swellings of dental origin. An intraoral incision in the sulcus (avoiding the mental nerve), the floor of mouth or the palate (avoiding the greater palatine artery) may occasionally be required.
5. An incision along the line of a natural skin crease, designed to avoid damage to the facial nerve, should be made to drain an abscess pointing externally. At this time it is preferable to extract the causative tooth if the swelling is of dental origin; the pus can be sent for culture.
6. No attempt at surgical decompression of a brawny swelling should be undertaken until there are positive signs of localization of pus. The policy should be to concentrate instead upon intensive antibiotic therapy and the preservation of the airway, if necessary by tracheostomy (Holland, 1975).
7. Where there is toxaemia with an elevated temperature suggesting septicaemia or there is a possibility of subacute bacterial endocarditis (in a child with a possible cardiac lesion, blood should be taken for culture *before* an antibiotic is given. Provided that the patient is not sensitive to penicillin, this is the antibiotic of choice. If oral penicillin has already been started, this should be supplemented by an intramuscular injection of benzylpenicillin with the addition of cloxacillin when there is reason to suspect a resistant staphylococcal infection. No change should be made with this regimen until the results of culture and sensitivity tests are available. If the patient is known to have had a sensitivity reaction to penicillin, the choice is more difficult, for there is no one antibiotic as effective as penicillin.
8. Dehydration should be corrected by IV fluids (*see* page 409).
9. Hyperpyrexia should be treated by cooling.
10. With a mid-face swelling, on the appearance of the earliest sign of a possible cavernous sinus thrombosis, anticoagulant and parenteral antibiotic therapy should be started.

The management of facial swelling due to a large haematoma

1. If the airway is thought to be at risk, admit the patient for observation, being ready to perform a tracheostomy if necessary.
2. Assess the effects upon the cardiovascular system of blood loss into the tissues.
3. Seek a dental opinion to assist with the diagnosis.
4. Prescribe an antibiotic in standard dose, avoiding the *intramuscular* route.
5. If a disorder of coagulation is thought to be present, a haematologist should be consulted as soon as possible.
6. Surgically, leave a haematoma alone; aspiration or incision to drain is rarely necessary except where the airway is in jeopardy.

Reference

HOLLAND, C. S. (1975) The management of Ludwig's angina. *British Journal of Oral Surgery,* **13,** 153–159

Part IV

Intensive Treatment and Emergency Anaesthesia

Chapter 16

An intensive treatment unit for children

A. M. Wilson

Organization

There can be no more precise definition of an intensive treatment (or care) unit than 'an area where there is a concentration of skills, expertise and equipment for the treatment of those who are seriously ill or whose physical state is liable to change rapidly'. This covers all units from those where the equipment per bed costs many thousands of pounds to more modest areas designated for the ill child. The paramount features are in the skills of the staff and their preparedness to act quickly.

An intensive treatment unit is a meeting point for many disciplines. Usually the beds are undesignated, thus allowing any doctor to admit to the unit. Nevertheless, there must be one person in charge to co-ordinate the functions of the unit. He does not look after the patients, but is in administrative charge. It is important to understand his function to achieve the best use from an Intensive Treatment Unit (ITU).

Functions of the administrative leader

1. Decisions on admission and discharge policy. He will make them in consultation with all staff, medical and nursing.
2. Decisions on operational policies. Although many individuals are admitting patients there must be standard routines.
3. Liaison with nursing, radiology and laboratory staff.
4. Support for unit nursing and junior staff.
5. Availability for consultation on any of the above points and, if of the appropriate speciality, offering of specialist opinion.
6. Training of nursing and junior staff in new techniques, new equipment and resuscitation.
7. Co-ordination of the purchase and use of equipment ensuring cost effectiveness.
8. Supervision of emergency services for the remainder of the hospital.
9. Involvement in any major accident plan.

The administrative leader need not be involved in the practical management of each patient, but acts as a co-ordinator. To be able to do this he will:

1. Follow the progress of each child.
2. Ensure equipment is being used correctly and to maximum advantage.

3. Attempt to co-ordinate treatment if more than one clinical firm is involved.
4. Ensure that the whole aspect of the child's care is being considered.
5. Ensure that the case notes are adequate to achieve continuity of care between firms and at staff changeover.
6. Ensure that instructions to nursing staff are of correct standard.

Any physician or surgeon admitting a child retains independent medical care of the patient but must sacrifice some control of the technical and practical management. The overriding principle must be communication so that each member of the therapeutic team knows exactly what he is expected to do and not to do.

Suggested rules for practical administration

1. Patients remain under the primary care of the admitting consultant.
2. Emergency treatment will be undertaken by unit staff and the admitting firm is to be informed as soon as possible.
3. Where many firms are concerned with one patient they should formally decide on the allocation of responsibilities, e.g. control of respiration, fluid balance, etc., and communicate this to the nursing staff.
4. No treatment to be changed *by anyone* without informing the house officer of the admitting firm.
5. All changes of condition to be recorded in the case-notes.
6. All changes of treatment to be recorded, together with the reason for the change. Thus the next person can understand the reasoning behind any management.
7. No verbal messages to be accepted.
8. All settings of apparatus, drip rates, ventilators and monitor alarm limits to be recorded.
9. Only ITU standard records to be kept.
10. On admission a summary similar to that of Problem Orientated Medical Records is to be completed as follows: (a) Diagnosis; if necessary provisional. (b) Reason for ITU admission, e.g. nursing, monitoring or ventilation; and the facilities of the unit required. (c) Indications for change of treatment, or for summoning medical help. (d) Expected course of progress; to help in booking 'planned' admissions as after major surgery. (e) Destination on discharge.

Everything done to a child must be prescribed including not only drugs, but:
1. Diet.
2. IV therapy.
3. Oxygen therapy.
4. Physiotherapy.
5. Monitoring (type and alarm limits).
6. Humidification, ventilation, and suction.
7. Turning, sponging, etc.

This rigid approach is necessary when so many are working in one area to avoid conflict and omissions.

Indications for admission to an intensive treatment unit

No rigid criteria can be applied as the size of the unit will determine what type of cases shall be admitted. The ability of other wards in the hospital to handle very ill children will affect the case load of an ITU. The admission of a child to ITU is traumatic to the parents and should be used like any drug, i.e. prescribed only when genuinely indicated. Equally the ITU should not be seen as an area of last resort, more interested in machines than patients, and separated from the 'ordinary' hospital. A flexible ITU can offer many services apart from the management of the desperately ill.

Indications for admission include:

1. Support of depressed vital functions by the use of special equipment.
   (a) Respiratory system: intubation, ventilation, accurate control of the inspired atmosphere, inhalation therapy, blood gas analysis, lung function testing.
   (b) Cardiovascular system: intra-arterial monitoring for pressure and analysis, continuous ECG monitoring, implanted pacemaker.
   (c) Renal system: control of fluid balance, dialysis.
   (d) Central nervous system. Clinical, and intracranial pressure monitoring.
2. When a sudden change in condition is anticipated or possible.
   (a) Respiratory system: especially applicable to obstructive disease, where intervention may be necessary, and to post-operation cases where respiratory failure may occur due to tiring or the necessary use of analgesics.
   (b) Poisoning: when the drug cannot be identified, or the nature of its action is unknown a child should be admitted to an ITU. When changes are expected it is always better to transfer a child early. This can be done in a planned unhurried manner, placing the child near the staff and equipment which may be required, and so avoiding emergency intervention under unsuitable conditions.
3. When special skills may be necessary. The ITU offers the opportunity for a concentration of monitoring both by nursing staff and by machine. The routine monitoring of basic vital signs, e.g. pulse, temperature, respiratory rate, non-invasive blood pressure, can be performed without handling the child, advantageous for the smaller patient. In an incubator the measurements can be obtained without disturbing the constant warmth, humidity and oxygen. Machines have the advantage of not tiring, and being accurate over a wider range than human observation. Modern trend recorders can be used in a prognostic sense by projecting the recorded trace.

   Such monitoring is best carried out in an ITU as the most effective use of these expensive machines can only be achieved with the experience of regular use; but machines assist nursing care, not replace it.
4. Uncommon procedures may usefully be concentrated in an ITU so allowing a few staff to build up considerable experitse.
   (a) Intravenous nutrition. Care of the long-catheter central line, and of the IV solutions require strict attention to asepsis. Liaison with the dietician and with the pharmacy is facilitated where IV nutrition is performed or at least commenced in one site.
   (b) Exchange transfusion and peritoneal dialysis. Children undergoing these procedures require temperature control, pulse and ECG monitoring. Since

these are available, with control of inspired oxygen and humidity in addition, the ITU is well equipped to handle such procedures.

5. Within the limits of an ITU some nurses may be trained to undertake duties outside their normal range, such as intravenous injections. Children who must receive such treatment include those having administration of analgesia after surgery. There are good arguments that children undergoing surgery late at night should remain in ITU until the following day. Thus they receive analgesia with no delay and without upsetting their sleep.

Attention to the child as well as the disease

We prefer the term intensive CARE unit, emphasizing the need for loving care of the child. ITU nurses are encouraged to nurse, and play with, the children as part of the treatment. After extubation, where the airway is still partially obstructed, it may be necessary to sit and cuddle a child for a long time to avoid worsening of stridor by struggling and increased oxygen consumption. This treatment, waiting for oedema to settle, does not look like intensive care but may be just what is needed to avoid reintubation.

Parents must be thought of as patients of the intensive care unit when their child is admitted. They need support and explanation to be able to be of assistance. A booklet or leaflet outlining the function of the unit is useful, especially for an emergency admission, rather than post-operation when explanation and a visit to the unit is possible beforehand. Parents should be fully informed and an everyday-language version of (10) (p. 174) is a good basis for explanation. Frequent short visits should be encouraged. Most parents understand the need to leave when the medical staff wish to speak freely, particularly if an updating explanation is given subsequently.

Toys also should be welcomed, even a favourite cuddly toy which looks bacteriologically suspect. The child has lived with this for a long time and its psychological benefits outweigh any danger. We have on occasion autoclaved a teddy bear but do not recommend it.

Care after the acute emergency

Children frequently recover quickly, resulting in an apparently well child being in the ITU. Patients should not be discharged too soon, in case of relapse. Having to be re-admitted to ITU is very frightening for the child and worrying for the parents. It upsets the morale of the unit staff and loses the confidence of the rest of the hospital. Also, and most importantly, ITU nursing is very wearing with many disappointments. Being able to talk to and play with a cured child is therapy for the staff.

Specialized equipment

Much anxiety in treating seriously ill children, whether in an area of a general ward or in an adult intensive treatment unit, comes from unfamiliarity with their size and reaction to therapy. Anxiety can be reduced by the preparation of packs for various procedures. Thus the equipment, although infrequently needed, is kept together and readily presented. Most packs will fit into an A4 size box file for tidy storage.

Paediatric intensive treatment packs:

1. *Intubation* – Laryngoscopes, including infant straight bladed. Complete sets of endotracheal tubes, 2.5 mm to 8 mm. Sets should include one for immediate oral use, and one or more for long-term nasotracheal intubation. Sterile scissors for shortening tubes. All equipment for securing a long-term tube. Depending on the method preferred this will include orthopaedic felt or foam, Elastoplast, needles, thread and needle holder. Set of assorted connectors and tubing for attachment to humidifier and ventilator.
2. *IV equipment* – Sets of needles (27G and larger) and cannulae (24G and larger). Administration sets including burettes for liquid and for blood. Three-way taps, low-volume connector and T-piece injection ports. Ready-made small splints and fixing materials. Plaster of Paris for scalp vein fixation.
3. *Drug pack* – To contain the few drugs used in resuscitation but in lower doses and with diluting liquids. The pack should be sealed and marked with its expiry date. Most importantly the pack should contain a schedule of doses for various ages and weights (*see* pages 6–9).
4. *Ventilation* – Paediatric self-inflating bag and masks. Paediatric size tubing for adult ventilators. Also instructions for the setting of ventilators, and for any alterations to be made to a ventilator, including its attached humidifier, when used for children.
5. *Monitoring* – Contains ECG electrodes of different sizes and kits for other forms of monitoring in use such as complete intra-arterial and CVP lines. The use of local anaesthesia before inserting an arterial cannula is welcomed in children. If it is available in such a kit, time is saved.
6. *CHECK LISTS.* Reference has been made to instructions on drug doses, and ventilator settings. Each unit can develop its own check lists which might include:
   (a) Length and diameter of endotracheal tubes.
   (b) Ventilator settings.
   (c) Drug dose regimens.
   (d) Intravenous regimens: (i) fluid intake; (ii) intravenous drug therapy; and (iii) slide rules for IV infusions.
   (e) Chart of electrolyte and energy content of intravenous solutions.
   (f) Oxygen mixing flow/concentration chart.
   (g) Instructions on construction of breathing systems, e.g. CPAP, IMV circuits.
   (h) Simple resuscitation plan, and resuscitation record chart.
   (i) Brain death and organ transplantation protocols.
   (j) Instructions for infrequent procedures, e.g. peritoneal dialysis.
   (k) Contents list of all paediatric packs.
   (l) List of other useful equipment, e.g. infusion controllers, and their location in the hospital.

Ethical problems of turning off a ventilator (*See also* Cardiac Arrest, page 276)

Although the decision to stop ventilator treatment in the presence of a beating heart is never easy, recent writing has clarified the position. The key question is whether there is brain death. If brain death is diagnosed it follows that the patient is dead and *that there is no point in continuing treatment*. This concept is directly analagous to any disease process where, when death supervenes, all therapy is withdrawn. It helps by defining death and so avoiding such illogical episodes as 'keeping a patient alive until his family have seen him'. If he is dead then treatment is pointless and should be discontinued. It places the responsibility for the determination of brain death directly on the medical staff who must make a diagnosis of brain death.

Diagnosis of brain death (*See also* Chapter 27, Brain Death)

Before proceeding to the formal tests for Brain Death the doctor in charge of the case must:

1. Be certain that all possible forms of treatment have been tried.
2. Be convinced that an adequate time has elapsed since the accident or disease for a steady state to have been reached. There are many reports of unexpected recovery after severe damage, but, in fact, this is rare. Nevertheless, the possibility must be considered.
3. Feel that no survival is possible off the ventilator. If survival without the ventilator is possible the problem for the doctor is resolved whatever the cerebral state. Ventilation may be stopped and the child allowed to take his chance as a self-supporting if not self-sufficient individual.
4. Also feel that survival on the ventilator will *never* result in conscious awareness. There is no objective test to ascertain whether this last point holds true. Use is made of clinical observations, experience of similar cases, and the formal tests of brain death.

Brain death tests

Doctors should refer to any national guidelines. In the UK these are contained in the DHSS Code of Practice concerning Cadaveric Organs for Transplantation.

In summary the guidelines require:

1. Initial exclusions. The state of coma must not be due to depressant drugs, primary hypothermia or metabolic or endocrine disturbances. The respiratory failure for which the patient is on a ventilator must again not be due to the above causes or due to relaxant (neuromuscular blocking) drugs. 'There should be no doubt that the patient's condition is due to irremediable structural brain damage. The diagnosis of a disorder which can lead to brain death should have been fully established.'
2. Tests performed under ideal conditions:
   (a) No sign of conscious awareness.
   (b) Loss of all pupillary and corneal reflexes.
   (c) Absence of vestibulo-ocular reflexes.
   (d) Loss of all cranial nerve response.
   (e) No response to bronchial stimulation.
   (f) No respiratory movements in the presence of a normal or raised pCO_2.

In some countries further tests such as electroencephalography or cerebral angiography are required.

Whoever makes the decision must consider the parents. It is not fair to their future life to try to give parents this decision to make but many will wish to participate. It is usually the parents who first suggest that treatment is no longer of any use. Others seem to prefer to be told some such formula as 'We will have to try him without the ventilator', and later to be told that the attempt has failed. In this way treatment is seen to be continued until the very end.

The nursing staff on an ITU will have spent day and night working for the child and a sudden reversal from full treatment to abandonment can leave them hurt and confused. The sister-in-charge must be involved in the decision with full explanation so that she can support her nurses in their understanding of the situation.

With the ever-present risk of litigation only a consultant may switch off a ventilator. This can never be a delegated duty. He must record accurately why the action was taken and personally certify death.

Further reading

DIAGNOSIS OF BRAIN DEATH (1976). *British Medical Journal*, **ii**, 1187–8

DEPARTMENT OF HEALTH AND SOCIAL SECURITY. Health Notice HN(83)3. *Introduction of Brain Death Checklist*

Chapter 17

Emergency anaesthesia

A. M. Wilson

All children undergoing anaesthesia must be considered to be at some small, but definite, risk. Although the normal child does not present an increased anaesthetic risk compared with adults, when the preoperative preparation must be reduced, as for emergency anaesthesia, any risk will be increased. Before anaesthesia the resident should take a brief history and examine the points of importance to the anaesthetist. Ideally, the anaesthetist will do this for himself, or repeat it. A resident should consider the possibility of anaesthetic difficulties at an early stage in the management of emergency patients, as this may materially affect treatment. For example, a child with airway abnormality would require admission after anaesthesia for an operation that would normally be performed on an out-patient.

The features of importance to anaesthesia can be elicited by a few questions, a brief examination, and essential investigations which will rarely exceed a basic two or three.

The history will usually be included in the admission of the patient. Even when the history is limited, as in a limb fracture in a previously healthy child, or for an extremely urgent case, the following questions must be asked specifically.

1. Was the child well until this present illness?

2. Is there any sign of cough or cold?

The presence of even mild upper respiratory disease complicates all inhalation anaesthetics. Nasal discharge may initiate laryngeal obstruction, either mechanically or by causing spasm during induction and awakening. The infection may be developing or be caused to develop into postoperative bronchopneumonia. Any sign of a cough or cold should cause the child to be admitted, following an emergency anaesthetic. Treatment by physiotherapy should be started, and antibiotics given if indicated.

3. Does the child suffer from asthma or have any other allergic disease, e.g. eczema?

Some anaesthetic drugs, such as curare, cause histamine release and are better avoided. Certain induction agents have a higher incidence of hypersensitivity response which may be increased in patients already showing such reactions.

4. Is there any history of heart or chest disease?

Particularly, one is looking for a history of congenital cardiac abnormality, especially a shunt which may reverse with the alteration of intrathoracic pressure during anaesthesia. Any patient in whom there is such a history must be admitted so that anaesthesia can be performed in a theatre fully equipped for cardiac monitoring and resuscitation, and with adequate assistance for the anaesthetist. As so many procedures produce a transient bacteraemia, all patients with known congenital heart disease should be given prophylactic antibiotics. Currently, a single dose of amoxycillin 3 g given orally 1 hour beforehand is adequate for dental procedures. Where gastric absorption is delayed, or the anaesthetist prefers no oral material, intramuscular antibiotics must be used.

The problems of respiratory disease are largely those of secretion production. Their presence may influence the technique of anaesthesia. Lung function tests are rarely of material help in an emergency case.

5. Is there any current renal disease?

Renal disease may present problems due to electrolyte disturbance or to inability to excrete some of the drugs given. Electrolyte disturbances, particularly of potassium balance, can cause problems with muscle relaxants, e.g. suxamethonium. This same problem can occur at some stages in the management of burned patients, particularly if they become infected.

6. Is there any history of jaundice or hepatitis?

Although many anaesthetic drugs are metabolized in the liver, it is rare for liver disease, unless severe, to cause a prolonged effect. However, where liver disease exists, barbiturates should be given sparingly. These drugs are not now used for premedication but thiopentone is still popular for induction. Liver disease, whether obstructive or parenchymal, is an absolute contraindication to the use of halothane and trichloroethylene. In obstructive jaundice opiates should be avoided because of their effect on the sphincter of Oddi. All jaundiced patients should be regarded with great suspicion. Where active hepatitis B, or the carrier state, is suspected there is a duty to warn all staff handling the patient and any laboratory to which samples are sent.

7. What drugs is the patient taking or has taken in the last year?

Fortunately, children are prescribed few drugs that affect or may interact with anaesthesia. Nevertheless this question must be asked to reveal the following groups of drugs.

Corticosteroids

Many children receive steroids for asthma and eczema. The regular administration of steroids can suppress the output of endogenous steroids stimulated by the stress of operation and anaesthesia. There is then the risk of hypotension or 'adrenal crisis' which is most likely to occur just before anaesthesia or in the early postoperative period. Most emergency conditions involve a strong emotional stimulus, so the steroid requirement will be very high. Under ideal conditons adrenocortical function can be tested by giving artificial ACTH (the synacthen test) (*see* page 472) and increased steroids given if the response is diminished. Where there is any doubt, even if the last course of steroids was up to 9 months previously, it is best to err on the safe side, and to give hydrocortisone over the period of the operation and for the next day. For a standard course of steroid cover *see* page 473. There is no harm in such a short course, and it avoids the risk of an unnoticed hypotensive episode during the night after the operation.

Cardiac glycosides (digoxin etc.)

Children taking these drugs must be admitted and fully monitored with an ECG during the operation. Routine administration of these drugs should not be stopped.

Insulin in diabetes mellitus (*see also* page 454)

Patients with diabetes mellitus present little anaesthetic difficulty, but the anaesthetic and operation upset the control of the diabetes, by requiring starvation, and because the stress of the procedure changes insulin requirements.

If the patient is controlled by oral hypoglycaemic drugs or by diet alone (unlikely in children), the hypoglycaemic drug is omitted until the patient is able to take food again. Where the child is taking insulin the aim of management is as simple a regimen as possible. For emergency surgery there is not time to stabilize the diabetes on soluble insulin. The overriding principle is to ensure that the blood glucose is high rather than low. The time of the last dose, the amount given and the type of insulin should be noted. An infusion of 5% glucose should be set up and the blood glucose level estimated as quickly as possible. The naked-eye examination of Dextrostix is adequate to prevent the more dangerous hypoglycaemia. The time taken to resettle the patient on his original insulin dose will depend on the severity of the operation, and whether food can be taken soon after. If there are problems getting control it is wise to ask a more experienced paediatrician for assistance.

8. Has he attended hospital recently?

Any disease may be of importance to the anaesthetist. A child with porphyria is equally likely to break a limb as a normal child and his disease may go unmentioned in a busy casualty department when the diagnosis of the injury is obvious. An induction dose of thiopentone can be fatal in porphyria.

9. Has he been given an anaesthetic previously?

This is to reveal previous anaesthetic problems. Parents and children rarely know details, only that there was difficulty. On most occasions the problem is related only to the one anaesthetic, but should suggest an examination of previous case-notes. Points to record are difficulty in breathing, delayed or slow awakening, an unplanned transfer to an Intensive Treatment Unit, or admission after a day case booking. If there has been any problem, ask whether a card or identity disc was issued. Investigation of the rest of the family suggests a genetically linked disorder (*see* below). Certain units have a specific interest in one disease and this can be a useful clue. All intravenous induction agents have on occasion caused hypersensitivity reactions. In the absence of the case-notes, questioning may elicit a comment made by a previous anaesthetist.

Adverse reactions may occur with any agent, and local anaesthetics should be remembered. Lignocaine in excessive dosage, or accidentally injected intravenously, can cause epileptiform seizures requiring control by intravenous thiopentone. Although the addition of adrenaline allows the use of larger doses, adrenaline itself may cause fainting in susceptible individuals.

10. Is there a family history of anaesthetic difficulties?

This question often causes raised eyebrows but it may reveal life-threatening disorders, as there are a few familial conditions causing anaesthetic problems.

Malignant hyperpyrexia (MH) (autosomal dominant)

Recognition

The incidence of this condition is 1:60 000 anaesthetics but where a parent or grandparent suffered an attack the risk for children is greatly increased. Some cases described as 'ether convulsions' were suffering from MH. The cause is an enzyme-uncoupling which allows metabolism to proceed unrestrained, resulting in stiff muscles and the production of heat. The temperature can rise by 4° C (8°F) in 10 minutes which can be fatal if unchecked. Numerous drugs act as a trigger; halothane, suxamethonium, nitrous oxide and lignocaine have all been implicated. It is only recognized early enough to be treated by approaching every anaesthetic with suspicion. The routine monitoring of temperature from the induction of anaesthesia onwards is recommended. The onset of MH may be recognized by difficulty in achieving relaxation and efficient ventilation at the beginning of an anaesthetic. The patient is noticed to be very hot, and cyanosed despite high inspired oxygen concentration.

There is no certain blood test for this condition although a raised serum creatine phosphokinase activity is suggestive. A muscle biopsy is the definitive test but takes a long time and can be performed in only a few centres.

Management

PREVENTIVE

Where there is any suspicious history of MH, admit the child so that anaesthesia can be given in ideal conditions where monitoring and treatment are available. A minimum of drugs is used, if possible being limited to thiopentone and oxygen. Local anaesthesia using prilocaine should be considered.

EMERGENCY

If the condition is suspected then action must be prompt.

1. All anaesthetic agents are withdrawn and ventilation continued with oxygen alone. Intubate if possible to obtain better control of the airway.
2. Give large dose of steroids, e.g. 4 mg dexamethasone IV.
3. START COOLING – Every effort must be made to lower the temperature. Cooling children is easier than cooling adults because of their relatively large surface area. Cold-water blankets are effective, as are ice-filled bags packed into groins, axillae and around the neck. Core temperature, rectal or nasopharyngeal, should be monitored continuously with an electric thermometer.
4. DANTROLENE – All operating theatres should have a 'Malignant Hyperpyrexia Pack' containing the drugs currently thought to be of use. Dantrolene 1 mg/kg IV is given and repeated at 5–10 minute intervals up to 10 doses as required to control the temperature rise.
5. Take an arterial sample of blood for analysis of acid–base state for control of the severe metabolic acidaemia which always occurs.
6. After resuscitation, transfer the patient to an Intensive Treatment Unit for temperature and acid–base monitoring, as the rise in temperature can recur.

Pseudocholinesterase deficiency (autosomal recessive)

This occurs in 1:2000 anaesthetics and is due to inability to break down the normally short-acting muscle relaxant suxamethonium. The defect may be an absolute absence, or reduction, in the amount of pseudocholinesterase, or an abnormal enzyme. This difference, demonstrated by laboratory tests, is irrelevant clinically.

Recognition

After a dose of suxamethonium, the respiration, instead of returning to normal after 5–7 minutes, fails to return and, depending on the pseudocholinesterase level, may take up to 48 hours to return. This is an acutely embarrassing situation but not dangerous in a well-prepared hospital. When suspected, confirmation is by:

1. Nerve stimulator to demonstrate complete neuromuscular blockade.
2. A blood enzyme level.

Management

The only treatment is to continue ventilation of the sedated patient. Efforts to stimulate by use of drugs should be avoided. Enzyme levels should be measured a few days later. If positive, as the condition is transmitted as an autosomal recessive other members of the family, starting with brothers and sisters, should be investigated. Many departments of anaesthesia provide this service and issue identification cards or discs.

Other muscular disorders

Disorders such as myotonia congenita can cause unexpected reactions to the neuromuscular blocking drugs.

11. When did he last eat or drink?

This is the most important single question of interest to an anaesthetist. A patient with a full stomach may vomit and inhale the vomitus, causing respiratory obstruction, bronchopneumonia, or the acid-inhalation syndrome. In fact, the stomach is never empty and the risk of regurgitation during induction is always a possibility. For medico-legal reasons it is often assumed that the stomach will be empty by 4 hours after the last meal, and it is customary to wait this time before anaesthesia. Many factors found in emergency conditions – e.g. pain, shock, hypotension and fear – delay gastric emptying. The classic case is the child breaking an arm while running out to play after a large fatty meal. For all the above reasons his stomach will not empty for many hours. Enquiry must be made of the interval between eating and the injury, and also the nature of the last meal.

When a patient is known to have a full stomach the operation should be delayed for some hours, or done under local anaesthesia. If this is not possible, precautions must be taken to prevent inhalation of vomited or regurgitated material. The anaesthetist may chose to induce anaesthesia on the side with head-down tilt. Alternatively he may prefer to use Sellick's manoeuvre (cricoid pressure). Everyone should know how to do this, as it requires assistance. The cricoid cartilage, the only complete tracheal ring, is pushed back to compress the oesophagus against the vertebral bodies. Identify the cricoid with an index finger, press back with the thumb and middle finger steadying it in the midline. Apply pressure as soon as anaesthesia is induced and release only when the anaesthetist is satisfied that the airway is secure. If vomiting occurs, prompt tipping of the trolley may prevent inhalation. Small children can be elevated by the legs and held upside down.

Inhalation syndromes

Obstructive

Total respiratory obstruction due to inhalation of solid material is uncommon. Under anaesthetic conditions the foreign body may be visible with a laryngoscope and can be removed with Magill forceps. If it is in the trachea a Heimlich manoeuvre may eject it. Bronchoscopy will be necessary to remove large quantities of partly solid material.

Postoperative bronchopneumonia

Treat as for bronchopneumonia (*see* page 235).

Acid-inhalation syndrome, the gravest risk

Inhalation of small quantities of strong acid, pH 4.0 or less, causes severe bronchospasm, cyanosis, and increased pulmonary secretion, and can be fatal. Treatment should be by immediate artificial ventilation with oxygen, support of the circulation with IV fluid, isoprenaline if necessary, and IV steroids. Bronchoscopy to remove solid material may be useful but not at the expense of adequate oxygenation.

Examination of the patient for emergency anaesthesia

The examination before anaesthesia starts with a quick look at the shape of the head, face and neck, and the mobility of the neck. The most common problems of anaesthesia are related to difficulty with the airway. Facial abnormalities such as asymmetry may make it impossible to obtain a fit with an anaesthetic mask, and so indicate intubation. Difficulty in maintaining an airway may occur with a large tongue, as found in Down's syndrome, if there is pharyngeal swelling or enormous tonsils or even just a blocked nose. Intubation problems can occur with a small jaw, best seen in a profile view. If neck movements are restricted laryngoscopic view is limited. The child should be asked to open his mouth wide so that the teeth can be examined for any likely to be dislodged. If any are obviously loose a note should be made so that there is no doubt later, should an extraction prove necessary.

Routine examination of the respiratory system concentrates on finding signs of infection, or of bronchospasm. The presence of cardiac murmurs requires a search of the child's history for previous investigation or treatment, and the need for prophylactic antibiotics.

Investigations

Some units require numerous routine pre-anaesthetic investigations. For emergency anaesthesia haemoglobin estimation and sickle test are all that is necessary. The haemoglobin (or PCV) is needed for the management of fluid and blood balance. An arbitrary level of 10 g/100 ml is accepted as that below which anaesthesia for *routine* surgery should not be performed. A sickle test (Sickledex) should be performed in all children of coloured races. As a general rule if the haemoglobin level is over 9.5 g/100 ml with a positive sickle test the child has almost certainly sickle-cell trait and should present no anaesthetic problem. Nevertheless, precautions to avoid even mild hypoxia should be taken.

Investigations such as plasma electrolytes, and chest X-ray, are indicated for anaesthetic purposes only where clinical examination reveals abnormalities in the appropriate system.

Fitness for anaesthesia

The final decision must rest with the anaesthetist but it will often fall to the resident, in an emergency, to decide this in order to make the arrangements for anaesthesia and operation. In the absence of obvious disease of the cardiorespiratory, renal or hepatic systems a patient whose exercise tolerance is equal to or approaches that of his peers in size should be considered fit for anaesthesia. Each resident should decide his own exercise tolerance criteria.

Having taken the appropriate history and examined the patient the resident should communicate his findings to the anaesthetist as concisely as possible, but should always ask for assistance in deciding on fitness for anaesthesia or the need for further investigations if he is in any doubt.

Administration of emergency anaesthesia

It is unlikely that the paediatric resident will be asked to give an anaesthetic without having received the necessary further training. However, where circumstances require anaesthesia to be given, each doctor should learn a simple, safe anaesthetic technique, understanding the dangers and difficulties. Modern anaesthesia has become so safe that it is often forgotten that every anaesthetic carries many risks, including fatality.

The description given below would be suitable for children aged 2 years upwards for manipulation of fractures, incision of abscesses or even, if nothing else is available, emergency abdominal surgery. It must be emphasized that the doctor who has not received postgraduate training in anaesthesia should attempt the administration *only* if there is no one else available.

Table 17.1 Cases at risk, to be excluded by history and examination

Mechanical	Poor airway:
	  Facial abnormality
	  Restricted neck movement
	  Restricted jaw movement
	  Large tongue
	  Loose teeth or dental bridges
	  Enormous tonsils
	  Blocked nose
	  Pharyngeal infection
	  Known laryngeal abnormality
	  Airway narrowing due to infection
	Full stomach
	Marked obesity
	Severe scoliosis
	Hydrocephalus

Intercurrent illness	Respiratory infection Asthma Cardiac abnormalities Anaemia Renal disease Electrolyte disturbance Jaundice Hypovolaemia
Drug therapy	Steroids Diabetes mellitus Cardiac glycosides (digoxin usually)
Untoward reactions	Pseudocholinesterase deficiency Malignant hyperpyrexia Hypersensitivity to anaesthetic agents Porphyria

Pre-operative assessment

The doctor should decline all small patients and babies, and any whose history and examination reveal serious abnormality (*Table 17.1*). The child should be known to have been starved for 4 hours. It is most dangerous to anaesthetize a hypovolaemic patient; blood or fluid loss should have been replaced before induction.

Pre-anaesthesia check

This cannot be over-emphasized. Those who regularly, but infrequently give anaesthetics can prepare written check-lists. Every doctor should be sufficiently familiar with the standard Boyle's anaesthetic apparatus to be able to give oxygen by positive pressure ventilation, as resuscitation may be needed at any time.

Before starting the anaesthetic the following points should be checked:

1. *The patient*
   (a) The above criteria are met, and anaesthesia for the patient is within the competence of the doctor.
   (b) Consent for operation has been obtained.
   (c) A needle or cannula has been placed in a vein.
2. *Equipment:*
   (a) Table. Facilities for tipping the table or trolley must be available.
   (b) Suction. Must be of sufficient power and flow to be able to remove regurgitated material quickly. Check that it is working and how to turn it on.
   (c) Anaesthetic machine. Check that there are two sources of oxygen, whether from two cylinders or from wall-supply and one cylinder, and similarly for nitrous oxide. Note the position and functioning of the 'oxygen flush' control. Ensure that all vapourizers and other gases are turned *off*.
   (d) Ancillary equipment. The breathing system, often known as the 'anaesthetic circuit' consisting of bag, tube, valve and mask should be checked by occluding the outlet with a thumb, inflating the bag with gas, and then compressing it to demonstrate the ability to produce positive pressure. Leave the expiratory valve wide open after this test. A working laryngoscope together with suitable sized tubes must be available.
   (e) Drugs. Atropine, suxamethonium, and saline for dilution of drugs, together with syringes and needles.

Administration of anaesthesia

The principal points are:

1. At least 33% oxygen should be used throughout.
2. A clear airway is essential at all times.
3. A slightly too deep anaesthetic is safer than a slightly too light anaesthetic.
4. The minimum number of alterations and adjustments should be made.
5. Atropine should be given to all patients during the anaesthetic, either 0.3–0.6 mg i.m. 1 hour before or 0.2–0.4 mg IV just before induction.
6. The child is placed on his left side on a level table.
7. The position of the table tilting control is checked with the patient in position.
8. Oxygen is turned on at 3 ℓ/min, nitrous oxide at 6 ℓ/min and halothane (Fluothane) at 1/2%.
9. While talking to the child, gradually approach his face with the mask, encouraging him until the mask can be applied to the face. When the mask is applied lightly to the face the reservoir bag can be seen moving, showing respiration without obstruction. This must be monitored continuously throughout the anaesthetic, as should the pulse.

10. Increase the concentration of halothane by ½% steps up to 3%.
11. Hold the chin forward to ensure unobstructed respiration. With a child on his side respiratory obstruction is less likely.
12. If laryngeal stridor develops decrease the halothane by 1% and then gradually increase the concentration again.
13. When there is steady unobstructed respiration at 3% halothane the patient can be turned onto the back and/or the operation commenced.
14. Turning onto the back may make the maintenance of the airway more difficult. The introducing of an oro-pharyngeal airway, passed over the tongue, may help.
15. Once the operation has started, if there is no response to surgical stimuli, the halothane concentration is reduced to 1.5% and maintained at this level for the whole operation. Adjust upwards if the patient appears light, and downwards if respiration seems to be depressed as seen by decreasing respiratory bag movements.*
16. At the end of the operation the anaesthetic is continued until the child is turned onto the side again. Halothane and nitrous oxide are turned off. Oxygen is given at 5 ℓ/min until there are signs of returning consciousness.
17. It is essential to remain with the child until he wakes.

Where halothane is to be avoided, enflurane (Ethrane) may be substituted in the above scheme, starting at ½% but doubling the concentrations quoted for halothane thereafter.

What can go wrong?

Vomiting at induction and awakening

If vomiting occurs during induction, immediately tilt the table and give oxygen. Suck out the mouth and pharynx. While head-down on the side, inhalation is most unlikely. When the vomiting stops anaesthesia is continued. Vomiting during emergence is more common, but less dangerous, and, provided the position is maintained and oxygen is given, is unlikely to cause difficulty, but the child must be kept close to a suction apparatus.

Laryngeal stridor during induction

This is due to secretions irritating the vocal cords in the half-anaesthetized child. At the first sign of stridor the halothane which is somewhat irritant should be reduced by 1% and the nitrous oxide turned off. This is in case the stridor becomes worse. As the stridor decreases the halothane is increased by two steps before reintroducing nitrous oxide. The too-early introduction of an airway is a likely cause of stridor; if so it should be removed.

(* The comment about deep and light anaesthesia is to be treated carefully. With too light anaesthesia, vomiting and laryngeal spasm can be lethal. With careful monitoring the commonest risk of a slightly deeper anaesthetic, respiratory depression, can be treated by ventilation while the halothane concentration is reduced.)

Cessation of respiration due to halothane

Turn off the halothane, screw down the expiratory valve until nearly closed, and control respiration by regularly squeezing the bag until respiration returns. Re-start halothane at a lower concentration than before. Remember to re-open the expiratory valve.

Cardiac arrest

Unlikely to occur in the absence of previous hypoxia, so prevention is paramount. Overdose of halothane will first produce respiratory arrest which if treated correctly will not go on to cardiac arrest.

If cardiac arrest, or profound bradycardia, occurs inform the surgeon immediately, turn off all anaesthetic agents and give oxygen alone by positive pressure ventilation. The surgeon should start external cardiac massage at once; *see* page 276.

An intravenous infusion of sodium bicarbonate 8.4% (1 ml contains 1 mmol) is set up and a dose of 1 ml/kg is run in.

If the pulse had been diligently monitored and the arrest, due to anaesthetic causes, was noticed immediately, these measures will result in a rapid recovery and return of heart beat.

Ketamine

It is suggested that ketamine is particularly safe for short procedures in children because there is retention of muscular tone, so protecting the airway. It may be used for painful procedures such as bone marrow or liver biopsies, or for sedation for diagnostic and therapeutic radiology.

It must be stressed that ketamine is an anaesthetic with all the dangers of an anaesthetic. A paediatrician who wishes to use this drug must prepare himself by ensuring that he is able to manage the airway, including intubation, of the age of child he is treating. Ketamine may be used only when there is adequate equipment for resuscitation. The child must be prepared as for conventional anaesthesia.

Method of use

Intravenous administration

A needle or cannula is securely placed in a vein. Atropine is not essential but is usually recommended to control salivation. An initial dose of ketamine 2 mg/kg is given over at least 45 seconds. Rapid injection will cause respiratory arrest which must be treated with oxygen by mask and assisted ventilation. Further doses of 0.5 mg/kg are given as the anaesthesia lightens. For short procedures small movements should be expected unless rather deep anaesthesia has been achieved. Laryngeal spasm is most unlikely despite ‘light’ anaesthesia. Try to keep the patient on the side; this is particularly suitable for lumbar punctures.

Intramuscular route

If a vein is not available, 10 mg/kg may be given. Onset of anaesthesia takes up to 5 minutes and lasts for about an hour. With either administration, but especially i.m., the child must not be left unsupervised until consciousness has fully returned.

Ketamine is a useful agent in suitably qualified hands and seems not to produce psychological effects in children aged under 10 years, even when repeated frequently.

Intravenous anaesthesia (Bier block)

For local anaesthesia of the upper limb the technique of intravenous anaesthesia is very successful in those children who will accept it. Although a simple technique, it carries risks and has been associated with a number of deaths in children. Those intending to use this technique should seek expert tuition in the finer details, but some points stand out. Bier block should never by performed by an operator working alone; there must always be someone whose duty it is to watch the patient. The double cuff equipment must be checked to see how it works, as there are many different designs of inflation apparatus. The doctor must be familiar with the local anaesthetic agent used, including its toxic reactions, as the dose approaches the maximum permitted.

Part V

Respiratory Tract Emergencies

Chapter 18

Ear, nose and throat emergencies

J. T. Buffin

Accidents

Foreign bodies

Ear and nose

RECOGNITION

A history of insertion may or may not be given. In the ear there may be no symptoms. In the nose, their continued presence causes a unilateral foul-smelling discharge. Diagnosis is easily confirmed by inspection.

MANAGEMENT

Inexpert attempts at removal may implant the foreign body (FB) deeper, and are to be avoided. A hook or ring probe passed beyond the FB may be used to roll it out of the ear. In the nose (and occasionally in the ear), it may be retrievable with nasal dressing forceps. Once in the nasal vestibule, prevent back-sliding by fixing it with a finger pressed in the groove at the side of the nose.

Pharynx

RECOGNITION

Fish bones or other sharp objects may implant in the pharynx, causing a pricking sensation and pain on swallowing. Older children should localize the site of impaction accurately. Impaction is commonest at the lower pole of the tonsil and posterior third of the tongue. Inspection with a good light and spatula may reveal the FB. A laryngeal mirror can show the back of the tongue.

MANAGEMENT

Occasionally direct removal is possible. More commonly removal under general anaesthesia is necessary.

Oesophagus

RECOGNITION

FBs stick in the oesophagus because of their size or because of their sharp edges. At the narrowest site, the cricopharyngeal sphincter, there is acute discomfort and profuse salivation. Lower down, symptoms are less dramatic, though there will be a moderate or complete dysphagia.

MANAGEMENT

At the cricopharyngeal level urgent removal under general anaesthesia is necessary. Preliminary radiography causes unnecessary discomfort and delay. At a lower level radiography will define smooth opaque objects (such as coins), whose removal is less urgent, and which will often navigate the alimentary tract uneventfully. Sharp or impacted FBs require prompt removal to minimize the risk of perforation and mediastinitis. Their removal at oesophagoscopy is often difficult and should be done by an expert.

Larynx *(See also* Upper Airway Obstruction, pages 205–209)

RECOGNITION

Persistent and sometimes severe stridor which follows an episode of coughing or choking while food or some other object is in the mouth must be taken to indicate the possibility of an impacted FB in the larynx.

MANAGEMENT

Immediate direct examination of the larynx and removal of the FB under general anaesthesia is required. Where removal is traumatic or where laryngeal oedema is present, subsequent intubation will be necessary. Where the diagnosis is presumed and the patient is *in extremis,* direct examination and removal will be justified without anaesthesia, followed by intubation and resuscitation.

Bronchus

RECOGNITION

A history of choking and cyanosis while eating, (especially peanuts) or the unaccountable loss of teeth during a facial injury must alert the clinician to the possibility of inhalation into the lower respiratory tract. Following the accident, there may be a symptom-free period, or there may be an expiratory whistling or wheeze which could be mistaken for asthma.

MANAGEMENT

Radiography in full inspiration and full expiration should be performed whenever a bronchial FB is suspected. The FB itself will rarely be visible, but impaction in a main or segmental bronchus often causes a valvular obstruction with over-distension of the affected lung or lobe, which is well seen in the expiratory film. Later segmental collapse and consolidation may occur. Bronchoscopic removal by an expert under general anaesthesia is essential.

Local trauma

The ear

Acute trauma

RECOGNITION

Although normally accidental, the possibility of non-accidental injury to the ear (and nose) should always be considered. The lesion itself is obvious, with local pain, and bleeding if the integrity of the skin has been broached. The pinna, ear canal, and tympanic membrane may be involved separately or in combination.

MANAGEMENT

The meatus is filled with blood which is best left untouched because of the risk of introducing infection. Analgesics and systemic antibiotics should be given. Later referral to an ENT unit is advisable. More serious injuries with vertigo or facial palsy require immediate transfer to a specialist unit.

Otitic barotrauma

A difference in pressure between the air on either side of the tympanic membrane may cause pain and deafness or even rupture, with bleeding and tinnitus.

RECOGNITION

Sudden pressure changes are due to: a box on the ear, explosion, diving or falling into water, or sudden decompression accidents in aircraft. Slower pressure changes occur in aircraft during take-off and descent and are especially likely when the Eustachian tube is blocked by an acute or chronic catarrhal condition. Again, pain and deafness result with occasional rupture if the tympanic membrane has been previously damaged or perforated.

MANAGEMENT

If rupture occurs, secondary infection is likely and should be prevented by antibiotics.

The nose

Recognition

The history of injury is obvious. Fracture of the nasal bones is rare in young children but common in older ones. Displacement of the nasal bones is apparent unless obscured by bruising. X-rays of the nose have limited value except as medico-legal evidence. Submucosal haematoma of the nasal septum may also occur and cause considerable obstruction. There is a risk of infection of the haematoma with abscess formation and also of necrosis of fragments of cartilage with subsequent deformity.

Management

Manipulation and reduction of the displaced nasal fragments must be completed within 3 weeks of the accident.

Reduction of displaced septum or cartilages must await resolution of the haematoma. For a haematoma of the septum antibiotic cover should be started immediately and the clot should be drained by a curved incision anteriorly and inferiorly on the septal mucosa: unattached fragments of cartilage should be removed.

Pharynx and palate

Recognition

Laceration may result when a stick, or some similar sharp object in the mouth is pushed into the palate while running and falling. Occasionally the soft palate may be perforated completely and partially detached from the bony palate. Deeper injuries may involve the region of the great vessels at the base of the skull.

Management

The area heals rapidly, usually without any intervention. Indications for surgery are continued bleeding, possible presence of the lacerating agent in the wound, and extreme detachment of the soft palate. Exposure under general anaesthesia will be required.

Insect stings

Recognition

A bee or wasp sting in the mouth may produce rapidly extending oedema involving the supraglottic region, with severe airway obstruction.

Management

1. Assessment of degree of obstruction and maintenance of airway (*see* page 205).
2. Prevention of further oedema. *See also* Venomous Bites and Stings (page 560) and Anaphylactic Shock (page 113).

Drugs which are of use are, in order of potency and speed of action:

Adrenaline 1:1000 Hydrocortisone Antihistamine drugs	Doses in section of Anaphylactic Shock (*see* page 114).

Antibiotics should also be given.

Swallowed corrosives (*see also* Acute Poisoning, page 74)

As with other poisons one must know exactly what has been swallowed, how much, and how long ago.

Recognition

The history is usually self-evident: burns round the mouth, face and neck and inside the mouth are likely, but the oesophagus may be burned without lesions in the mouth. Pain is usually present except with phenolic compounds such as cresols (e.g. vaporizers): salivation is usually marked. Oedema of the pharynx may occur, spreading to cause laryngeal obstruction. When there has been vomiting, there is the possibility of inhaled corrosive with lower-respiratory obstruction. In severe cases there may be perforation of oesophagus or stomach within a short time.

Management

LOCAL

As soon as the child's general condition permits, a nasogastric tube should be passed under general anaesthesia: this allows nasogastric feeding and will prevent complete occlusion of the lumen of the oesophagus by adhesions. Where respiratory obstruction is present, a tracheostomy should be performed. The nasogastric tube should be retained for 3 weeks.

GENERAL

Antibiotics: a wide-spectrum antibiotic such as ampicillin should be given parenterally and later down the nasogastric tube. Corticosteroids i.m. or IV (hydrocortisone, 25 mg 6 hourly) should be continued for 3 weeks.

Major trauma to head and neck

This is considered in detail under Emergencies Involving the Face and Neck (page 155). However, the following additional points are of particular importance:

1. Haemorrhage from major arteries in the facial region may show itself as epistaxis: local pressure may stop the bleeding but surgical haemostasis may be required.
2. Direct injury to the larynx may fracture the cartilage. Crepitus should be looked for by palpation of the larynx; there may be excessive bruising of the neck or surgical emphysema of the neck. Exploration of this area is for the specialist.
3. Local haematoma causing airway obstruction may necessitate tracheostomy.
4. Dislodged teeth may be inhaled: they can usually be identified on a chest radiograph and should be removed by bronchoscopy.
5. Torn mucosal lining of the airway may cause air to track into the mediastinum with resulting pneumothorax.
6. Loss of cerebrospinal fluid (CSF) from the nose or ears implies a fracture of the skull and tear of the meninges. Close observation in hospital is required and the opinion of a neurosurgeon should be obtained. When CSF leaks from the ear the lesion is usually self-sealing.
7. All patients with craniofacial injuries who have a facial palsy or weakness should be seen by an otologist.

Symptomatic emergencies

It is important that the parents' anxieties should be appreciated and allayed as far as possible. This will reduce the child's anxiety and increase co-operation.

Painful conditions

Earache

Infants cannot complain of earache but they may scream, rub their ears or bang their head. The ears of an infant (or non-communicating child) who appears to be in pain should always be examined. Otitis media should be suspected in a child who has had a cold and wakes screaming during the night.

Apart from otitis media, tonsillitis, oral infection, or disease in the teeth especially in the lower jaw may all cause pain referred to the ear.

OTITIS MEDIA

Recognition
In actual inflammation of the middle ear the tympanic membrane may show appearances ranging from slight indrawing, with congestion of vessels, to a grossly distended bulging membrane.

Management
Simple analgesics may be necessary: antibiotics should be given, either penicillin, ampicillin or amoxycillin. In most cases oral treatment is adequate but an inadequate response within 24 hours suggests a failure of the oral route and intramuscular benzylpenicillin should be started. Myringotomy is very rarely needed.

Note: Haemophilus influenzae is a common infecting organism under the age of 5 years. In this age group, ampicillin or amoxycillin may be preferred to penicillin.

ACUTE MASTOIDITIS

Recognition and management
There is evidence of otitis media, and in addition pain and tenderness over the mastoid bone which must be distinguished from painful deep cervical lymph nodes. In late cases the child may be very ill and there will be redness and oedema or even fluctuation over the mastoid region. In babies the clinical picture is sometimes less severe, and an otitis media may progress relatively silently to mastoiditis and present as an emergency with a well-established post-aural periosteal abscess. Full doses of antibiotics should be given immediately. Cortical mastoidectomy will be indicated for most patients.

FURUNCULOSIS OF THE EXTERNAL MEATUS

Recognition
This is a very painful condition. The swelling of the ear canal sometimes spreads behind the ear, with redness and oedema over the mastoid region. The pre-auricular gland is sometimes enlarged and tender. The characteristic finding is acute pain on touching or attempting to move the pinna or on introducing an aural speculum into the meatus. The distinction from mastoiditis is not always easy: radiography may show loss of definition in the mastoid air cells in mastoiditis. In difficult cases the opinion of an otologist should be obtained.

Management
The infecting organism is invariably a staphylococcus. Antibiotics may be withheld if the diagnosis is certain and the infection is localized. A wick soaked in glycerine and ichthyol will reduce the pain. Analgesics and local heat are also helpful.

Painful throat conditions

TONSILLITIS

This is the most likely cause of pain on swallowing.

Recognition
The red fauces and tonsils are easily recognized; an exudate does not necessarily indicate a bacterial infection and may occur in glandular fever or other viral infections.

Management
Viral infections should be treated symptomatically, while clear-cut bacterial infections will respond to penicillin, ampicillin or amoxycillin; a throat swab should be taken if antibiotics are to be used.

Bleeding

The nose

RECOGNITION

Normally this is obvious, but it may not be obvious when the blood is swallowed. The first sign of trouble may be vomiting of blood.

Local causes
Physical agents, trauma (picking or rubbing the nose) coughing and sneezing. Drying of the nasal mucosa produces crusts whose separation causes bleeding: this is sometimes aggravated by central heating. Congestion occurs in colds, chronic sinusitis and allergic rhinitis.

Vascular abnormalities
Haemangioma of the face involving the nose may bleed heavily; occasionally a capillary abnormality may be the cause. Hereditary telangiectasia should also be considered.

Disorders of haemostasis
Normally there will be other evidence of blood disorder, such as petechiae or bruising. Epistaxis may be the presenting symptom in idiopathic thrombocytopenic purpura or other causes of thrombocytopenia, including leukaemia. Coagulation disorders such as haemophilia rarely cause epistaxis unless as a result of direct trauma.

MANGEMENT

Assessment of blood loss

A description should be obtained: 'steady drip', 'continuous stream', 'constant ooze', etc. It is also important to discover whether bleeding is still continuing, and to ask if there have been previous episodes, and if so how many, at what intervals and how long ago was the last one. This will give some idea of an anaemia present before the epistaxis. The pulse rate and blood pressure must be recorded at regular intervals if there is evidence of shock.

Investigations

A base-line haemoglobin estimation should be obtained.

Transfusion

If transfusion may be required, blood is taken for grouping and cross-matching at the same time as the Hb estimation.

Local treatment

The local lesion is usually a single point on the antero-inferior part of the septum. Suction may be necessary to obtain a clear view of the bleeding point. Local pressure can be applied to the side of the nose which is bleeding, close to the face and pressing on to the nasal floor as well as the septum. The child's own thumb can be used to apply this pressure. If local pressure fails or bleeding recurs whenever pressure is released or if a blood disorder is suspected, packing the nose will be necessary. In a child 1–2.5 cm (½–1 inch) ribbon gauze lubricated with glycerine or liquid paraffin should be used (or Bismuth Iodoform Paraffin Paste – BIPP). Gauze impregnated with a vasoconstrictor can be used, but with care, since considerable absorption may occur, with systemic effects.

As a preliminary to cauterization, ribbon gauze soaked in a mixture of 5 ml of 10 per cent cocaine with two or three drops of 1:1000 adrenaline is used to produce anaesthesia and vasoconstriction.

Packing the nose is unpleasant and must be done firmly, packing on to the floor of the nose first and folding the gauze on itself in layers until the roof of the nose is reached. The pack is retained by an adhesive dressing on the nostril. In small or frightened children, packing should be done under general anaesthesia. If bleeding persists in spite of packing the nasal cavity, the nasopharynx may also be packed. Various methods are available: using an inflatable balloon catheter of the Foley type or a gauze swab secured by thread stays passing round the nasal columella. If bleeding persists in spite of these measures, division of the external carotid artery or the anterior ethmoid artery in the orbit will be necessary unless the haemorrhage is accepted as the terminal phase of malignant disease or leukaemia.

The throat

RECOGNITION

Bleeding from a tonsillar vessel occurs sometimes in acute tonsillitis but rarely requires treatment. Postoperative bleeding after tonsillectomy usually occurs within the first few hours after surgery and is the responsibility of the surgeon. Secondary haemorrhage, after return home, is due to infection and may occur from several days, up to 3 weeks, after operation.

MANAGEMENT

Secondary haemorrhage: the child should be readmitted to hospital and observed. Mild sedation and antibiotics should be given. The occasional case in which bleeding does not settle will require examination under general anaesthesia and diathermy coagulation.

The ear

Bleeding from the ear generally induces a disproportionate amount of parental anxiety: blood loss is usually trivial.

RECOGNITION

Traumatic laceration may be obvious. Spontaneous bleeding followed by a purulent discharge may occur after rupture of the drum in otitis media and is normally preceded by the characteristic pain: however this may not have been recognized in the young child. In influenza epidemics blisters containing blood or blood-stained serum are sometimes found on the tympanic membrane; a small amount of bleeding occurs if these blisters rupture. In chronic otitis media brief episodes of bleeding may occur.

MANAGEMENT

For lacerations, *see* Trauma. Bleeding from the other causes described above requires treatment of the primary condition though the bullous influenzal condition needs no specific treatment; however, if this diagnosis is uncertain it is safer to treat as for acute otitis media.

Acute loss of function

The ear

RECOGNITION

Acute loss of function in the ear may be indicated by one or more of the following: deafness, vertigo, facial paralysis.

MANAGEMENT

None of these symptoms constitute a threat to life but all require prompt referral to a specialist.

The nose

RECOGNITION

The two important symptoms are anosmia and inability to breathe through the nose. Anosmia as an acute presenting symptom must be extremely rare.

Nasal and Nasopharyngeal Obstruction in the Newborn (see page 669).

Acute dysphagia

For oesophageal atresia and tracheo-oesophageal fistula in the newborn *see* page 249.

Dysphagia is a rare cause of urgent trouble in children except as a result of an impacted foreign body (*see* page 196) or from food impacted above a stricture due to previous surgery, or trauma, or stricture at the lower end of the oesophagus in hiatus hernia.

RECOGNITION

In the older child, food impaction causes sudden difficulty in swallowing; treatment is the same as for a foreign body.

Aphonia

Loss of voice may develop suddenly as a result of acute laryngitis or extreme over-use of the voice from shouting, singing or screaming. In older children hysterical aphonia may occur.

RECOGNITION

The circumstances in which aphonia occurs are usually obvious. In the newborn, lack of cry may be due to paralysis of the vocal chords from birth trauma; this is usually unilateral; bilateral cord paralysis presents with severe inspiratory stridor.

MANAGEMENT

Aphonia alone is not an emergency but accompanying inspiratory stridor from inflammation in the young child ('croup', epiglottitis, laryngotracheobronchitis) or bilateral cord paralysis in the newborn may require urgent relief by tracheostomy. Hysterical aphonia require prompt attention since the longer it is allowed to persist the more difficult is its cure.

Chapter 19

Upper airway obstruction

A. W. Boon

Acute upper airway obstruction may proceed rapidly to complete airway occlusion, respiratory arrest, and death. It is frightening for the child and his parents, and calls for skilful management based on clinical judgement. The overriding principle is the maintenance of an adequate airway.

Recognition

Upper airway obstruction presents with stridor, a harsh sound caused by obstruction to airflow in the larynx or trachea. Inspiratory stridor suggests an extrathoracic obstruction to the airway. Expiratory stridor indicates involvement of the intrathoracic airway.

Assessment of severity of airway obstruction

1. *Stridor* (for Stridor in the newborn, *see* Chapter 80).
   (a) Inspiratory and expiratory stridor generally indicates severe obstruction *except* in *chronic* conditions such as the tracheal compression due to a vascular ring; an acute upper respiratory infection may, however, precipitate severe obstruction.
   (b) A sudden decrease in the intensity of the stridor suggests physical exhaustion and impending collapse.
2. *Recession.* The degree of chest wall recession is a good reflection of the severity of the airway narrowing. Suprasternal recession ('tracheal tug') and sternal recession are seen in severe stridor.
3. *Hypoxia.* Initially this is manifested by pallor, tachypnoea, tachycardia, restlessness, and anxiety. Cyanosis is a late sign indicating the need for urgent intervention.
4. *Lethargy.* Lethargy and confusion are due to physical exhaustion and hypoxia. There is a grave risk of sudden collapse and death.

Acute laryngotracheobronchitis ('croup')

This is the commonest cause of acute stridor in childhood. The term 'croup' is usually used synonymously with laryngotracheobronchitis, although the term is sometimes wrongly used for any form of stridor. It is nearly always viral in origin with the parainfluenza viruses being the commonest pathogens. The respiratory syncytial virus, influenza, rhinoviruses, and measles are also important causes. The inflammatory oedema of the mucosa and submucosa causes narrowing of the airway especially in the subglottic area. It usually affects pre-school children, with a peak incidence in the second year of life.

Recognition

There is usually a history of an upper respiratory tract infection for one or two days before the illness. The child then develops a barking cough, a hoarse voice, and inspiratory stridor. The child is not usually particularly ill and a high fever is unusual. Typically the stridor first occurs at night. If there is only mild narrowing of the airway, the stridor will occur only when the child is upset and hyperventilating. With increasingly severe stridor there may be the signs listed previously. The diagnosis is usually clear (*see Table 19.1* for differential diagnosis of acute stridor). *If there is any possibility of acute epiglottitis the throat should not be examined because of the risk of precipitating complete airway obstruction.* A lateral X-ray of the neck may demonstrate subglottic narrowing, but the danger that the disturbance of obtaining the X-ray may precipitate respiratory arrest outweighs any diagnostic advantage.

Table 19.1 Differential diagnosis of acute inspiratory stridor

	Laryngotracheobronchitis	*Epiglottitis*	*Foreign body*
Causative organism	Viral	H. influenzae	–
Age	6 months to 3 years	Over 3 years	1–4 years
Preceding URTI	Yes	25% of cases	No
Onset	Gradual	Rapid	Sudden
Dysphagia	No	Severe with drooling	No
Cough	Barking	Absent	Frequent
Stridor	Inspiratory	Inspiratory and expiratory	Inspiratory and expiratory
Voice	Hoarse	Muffled	Normal
Fever	Low grade	High	Absent
White cell count	Normal	Neutrophil leucocytosis	Normal
Blood culture	Negative	H. influenzae	Negative
Treatment	Symptomatic Intubation rarely required	Chloramphenicol* Intubation usually necessary	Laryngoscopy and removal

* See page 208 for chloramphenicol resistant organisms

Management

At home

Many children with mild stridor can be managed at home. The traditional remedy is to put the child in the bathroom and run the hot taps, or to boil a kettle of water. *All* children under the age of 1 year should be admitted to hospital. Severe stridor or a progression of symptoms despite treatment also warrant hospital admission.

In hospital

1. *Frequent observations.* The child should be observed closely but with minimal disturbance, as any upset will increase the stridor. Good hydration is important so that sticky secretions do not aggravate the airway obstruction.
2. *Humidity.* Traditionally, children with 'croup' have been nursed in mist tents or 'croupettes'. There is, however, no evidence that cold mist in any way influences the course of the disease. The nebulizers are frequently noisy so that the stridor cannot be heard and the dense mist makes observation difficult. A further disadvantage is that many children find them very frightening.
3. *Drugs:*
   (a) Antibiotics are not indicated because the disease is viral in origin.
   (b) Steroids have been claimed to be of benefit, but there is no evidence to support their use (Tunnessen and Feinstein, 1980).
   (c) Nebulized racemic adrenaline has been popular in the United States (Taussig *et al.*, 1975). However, its effect is short lived and it should not be used as definitive treatment.
   (d) Sedation should be avoided as restlessness is due to hypoxia until proved otherwise.
4. *Oxygen.* Hypoxia in a child with severe obstruction is an indication for intubation or tracheostomy. It should only be given while preparations are in hand for relief of the obstruction.
5. *Relief of obstruction.* About two per cent of children admitted to hospital with acute laryngotracheobronchitis will require mechanical relief of the obstruction. The decision to intervene and overcome the obstruction must be made on clinical evidence (*see* Chapter 22 on Acute Respiratory Failure). Blood gas analysis is of no help in making this decision.
6. *Intubation. This must be done by a skilled paediatric anaesthetist* under a general anaesthetic. The tube can usually be removed after 2–5 days once the oedema has resolved.
7. *Tracheostomy.* Facilities for immediate tracheostomy must be available when intubation is attempted (for techniques *see pages 223 (Intubation) and 327 (Tracheostomy)*.
8. *As a first-aid measure,* insertion of a wide-bore intravenous cannula through the cricothyroid membrane into the trachea may be life saving.

Acute epiglottitis

This is a severe, life-threatening septicaemic illness caused by *Haemophilus influenzae* type B. Gross oedema of the epiglottis and aryepiglottic folds causes rapidly progressing airway obstruction. It tends to occur in a slightly older age group than acute laryngotracheobronchitis, usually over the age of 3 years.

Recognition

There is usually a brief history of the child becoming increasingly feverish and ill over a few hours. Older children may complain of a sore throat, and refuse to eat or drink. The breathing becomes increasingly noisy and the voice is muffled.

The child looks pale and ill, and often has an anxious expression. There is typically a high fever of 39° C (102° F). Most children prefer to sit up leaning forward and breathe through the mouth with the chin elevated to maintain a patent airway. Drooling of saliva because of dysphagia is characteristic. There is often both inspiratory and expiratory stridor.

The diagnosis should be apparent from the history and typical appearance of the child. *If acute epiglottitis is suspected, the throat must* NOT *be examined because of the risk of precipitating respiratory arrest.* Furthermore, lying the child down or moving the child may have a similar effect. For these reasons, in general, a lateral X-ray of the neck should NOT be obtained. Occasionally, the investigation may be helpful if the diagnosis is in doubt. Blood culture will almost invariably yield a growth of *H. influenzae.*

Management

1. *Relief of obstruction.* The majority of children with epiglottitis will require intubation. This must be performed by a skilled paediatric anaesthetist under general anaesthesia. On direct laryngoscopy the diagnosis is confirmed by seeing the oedematous epiglottis, looking like a red cherry. The child is then intubated using a nasotracheal tube, and can usually be extubated after 24–48 hours.

   In an emergency, insertion of a wide-bore intravenous cannula through the cricothyroid membrane into the trachea may be life saving.
2. *Antibiotics.* Many strains of *H. influenzae* type B are now resistant to the β-lactam antibiotics (e.g. ampicillin and amoxycillin). For this reason chloramphenicol intravenously in a dose of 100 mg/kg/day in four divided doses is the antibiotic of choice. Strains of Haemophilus resistant to chloramphenicol as well as to ampicillin and amoxycillin are being reported increasingly. If this is suspected, cefotaxime (Claforan) 200 mg/kg/day IV or i.m. or latamoxef (Moxalactam) 50 mg/kg/day IV or i.m. should be used.

Foreign body

Recognition

A foreign body lodged in the larynx may present acutely as a severe attack of choking or coughing leading rapidly to complete airway obstruction and respiratory arrest. In many children, however, the choking episode may be overlooked and the child will present with inspiratory and expiratory stridor. It is therefore important to consider the diagnosis in any small child with stridor of sudden onset. The voice is usually unaffected.

Although a radiograph of the neck may be helpful, many foreign bodies, such as plastic buttons and tiddly-winks, are radiolucent.

Management

Acute presentation with complete airway obstruction

1. The child should be placed head down and four sharp blows should be delivered between the scapulae (Melker, 1978).
2. If this fails the Heimlich manoeuvre or the chest thrust should be attempted. The Heimlich manoeuvre is performed by putting one's arms around the patient's waist from behind, grasping one's fist with the other hand against the

epigastrium and compressing the abdomen with a quick upward thrust (Heimlich, Hoffman and Canestri, 1975). The chest thrust is similar except the low-chest and mid-chest positions are used.
3. If the above are ineffective, digital removal should be attempted.
4. Instrumental removal of the foreign body with Magill forceps may be possible.
5. Cricothyroid membrane puncture with a large-bore cannula is usually effective if all else fails, as large foreign bodies do not usually impact below the vocal cords.

Delayed presentation with stridor

Treatment is by laryngoscopy and instrumental removal of the foreign body.

Diphtheria (*see* page 210)

Although very rare, the possibility of this disease must be considered in a child who has not been immunized against diphtheria.

References

HEIMLICH, H. J., HOFFMAN, K. A. and CANESTRI, F. R. (1975) Food-choking and drowning deaths prevented by enteral subdiaphragmatic compression. *Annals of Thoracic Surgery,* **20,** 188–95

MELKER, R. J. (1978) Removal of aspirated tracheal foreign bodies. *Journal of Pediatrics,* **93,** 722–723

TAUSSIG, L. M., CASTRO, O., BEAUDRY, P. H., FOX, W. W. and NUREAU, M. (1975) Treatment of laryngotracheobronchitis (croup). Use of intermittent positive-pressure breathing and recemic epinephrine. *American Journal of Diseases of Children,* **129,** 790–793

TUNNESSEN, W. W. and FEINSTEIN, A. R. (1980) The steroid–croup controversy: An analytical review of methodological problems. *Journal of Pediatrics,* **96,** 751–756

Chapter 20

Diphtheria

B. Heyworth

Diphtheria is caused by infection with virulent strains of *Corynebacterium diphtheriae.*

Diphtheria varies in severity and toxicity depending on the type of organism, site of infection, and immunity of the host. Nasal infections are usually less severe than laryngeal or pharyngeal infections and mitis organisms less toxic than intermedius or gravis. Superficial cutaneous, conjunctival, auditory meatal canal, or vulvo-vaginal lesions, although causing little toxaemia, produce some toxin and can give rise to complications. The conjunctiva is oedematous, inflamed and may show membrane formation. Even superficial skin fissures or impetiginous lesions may contain virulent diphtheria strains. The typical skin lesion is a circumscribed, punched-out skin ulcer with an undermined, thickened edge and greyish membranous base, the so-called desert or veldt sore.

Laryngeal infection is more common in infants and may produce severe illness, particularly because of laryngeal obstruction. Although pharyngeal infection is less common in those under 6 years of age, it carries a higher mortality. Diphtheria is now rare in most temperate countries but can be imported. In tropical countries it has been said to be rare but is being increasingly reported and may occur all year round.

The incubation period is short, varying from 2 to 5 days. Dipththeria may cause four emergencies;

1. Laryngeal obstruction.
2. Haemorrhagic and severe toxic pharyngeal diphtheria.
3. Cardiovascular involvement.
4. Paralysis.

Laryngeal diphtheria

This usually presents early in children but in adults it occurs 1–2 weeks after the onset, by extension from the pharynx. It is worse in patients under 3 years of age. Infection with mitis strains often causes laryngeal diphtheria, especially in the tropics.

Recognition of symptoms

The onset of symptoms is gradual and they are initially 'dry', in contrast to croup or measles. There is a change in voice and cry. A croupy cough 'like the distant bark of a young dog' progresses to stridor. The child loses appetite and develops a fever, usually slight (37–38°C; 98.6–100.4°F).

Signs

Tachypnoea and increasing dyspnoea develop with suprasternal, epigastric, subcostal and intercostal indrawing, and accessory muscles are used. Restlessness, a weak rapid pulse, rising blood pressure, and cyanosis indicate severe respiratory failure with hypoxia and hypercapnia.

Management (immediate treatment)

A patent airway must be obtained by endotracheal intubation or tracheostomy. This should be done preferably *before* signs of respiratory failure are present. Humidification is essential while the tube is in place. Antitoxin and benzylpenicillin are given (*see* below).

Other complications

Secondary bronchopneumonia occurs in laryngeal and pharyngeal diphtheria in children. Continued fever, rising pulse and blood pressure in a restless child in the presence of an adequate airway indicate extension of the membrane to the lower respiratory tract. This is grave, but repeated aspiration, humidification and physiotherapy may allow expectoration of the bronchial cast and recovery. Toxaemia is less than in pharyngeal diphtheria, paralysis is rare and heart failure occurs late or secondary to pulmonary pathology.

Haemorrhagic diphtheria

This occurs early, mainly in children.

Recognition

1. Severe toxaemia, restlessness or apathy, usually with obvious nasopharyngeal diphtheria.
2. A thin, usually blood-discoloured membrane on the tonsils and throat is associated with marked oedema and lymphadenopathy, the 'bull-neck' appearance.
3. Petechiae and small ecchymoses, particularly over pressure points and bony prominences. Epistaxis and occasionally mucosal bleeding may occur. Most children die from toxaemia. Many of those who recover will suffer severe myocardial damage in the second and third week and almost all survivors suffer paralysis. The mortality is over 80 per cent without early antitoxin treatment.

Management

Antitoxin } *See* below
Penicillin }

Cardiovascular complications

Peripheral circulatory failure (early)

This usually occurs in the first few days of illness in a severely toxic child.

Recognition

The signs are hypotension, tachycardia with a weak pulse, pallor, apathy, and often hypothermia. Vomiting may occur and may be persistent. There may be little cardiac enlargement but the heart sounds are faint and the ECG usually shows low voltage QRS complexes, with flattened or inverted T waves, prolonged or depressed S-T segment and sometimes conduction defects. Nevertheless the ECG is sometimes entirely normal.

Management

Rest is essential. Attempts to treat 'shock' with corticosteroids have not been encouraging but they may help with conduction defects. ECG monitoring should be continuous if possible. Intravenous fluids should be given with care since they may precipitate heart failure.

The use of an α-blocker, such as phenoxybenzamine, may be helpful but careful monitoring of the central venous pressure is essential and its use in diphtheria has not been reported. Catecholamine support may also be necessary.

Late cardiovascular complications

These occur in the second or third week in about 10 per cent of cases with a mortality of about 60 per cent.

Recognition

Many ECG abnormalities occur, not always with clinical manifestations. Serious heart disease is due to myocardial damage with conduction defects.

Right or left-sided failure can occur, sometimes together. Almost all cardiac arrhythmias have been described and repeated examination is necessary to detect arrhythmia early. Serial chest X-rays will detect early cardiomegaly and a raised serum aspartate aminotransferase level is suspicious. Continuous ECG monitoring avoids disturbing the child. The following arrhythmias are associated with a bad prognosis:

1. Atrial fibrillation and flutter. These are unusual.
2. Complete heart block.
3. Bundle-branch block, right, left or alternating, in combination with A-V dissociation or nodal rhythm.
4. Ventricular paroxysmal tachycardia leading to ventricular fibrillation.

Mural endocarditis can occur and give rise to emboli and hemiplegia. Valvular endocarditis and pericarditis are rare.

Management

1. Rest in an upright position.
2. Digitalization at the first sign of heart failure.
3. The treatment of cardiac arrhythmias is conventional (Gellis and Kargan, 1980; Morgan, 1863).

Digitalization can been carried out prophylactically but may unnecessarily complicate the picture and is of unproved value.

Paralysis

Palatal paralysis

This can occur in the first week with severe pharyngeal diphtheria, probably by direct spread of toxin. It is not itself usually serious but may indicate serious disease and future complications.

Other paralyses

These normally occur 3–5 weeks after the onset of the disease, in about 20 per cent of cases of pharyngeal diphtheria, less commonly in laryngeal and nasal disease. In about 10 per cent of cases it is severe and in about 3 per cent it is fatal. Most affected are children aged between 2 and 10 years. Emergencies occur owing to paralysis of the muscles of the pharynx and larynx, intercostals and diaphragm.

Recognition

'Nasal' speech and regurgitation or reluctance on the part of the child to drink are signs of palatal paralysis. For the presentation of signs and symptoms of respiratory paralysis *see* Poliomyelitis (page 321).

Management

As there is usually a combination of swallowing and respiratory difficulty, the best treatment is probably tracheostomy with or without intermittent positive-pressure ventilation. Paralysis may last a few days or a few weeks. Although recovery is usually complete, paralysis may cause an increased mortality during the 6th to 9th week of the disease due to respiratory failure. For treatment of acute respiratory failure *see* page 222. Other paralyses occur but do not cause emergencies.

Drug therapy

Antitoxin

Before antitoxin was used the overall mortality in diphtheria was about 20 per cent. It is now 5–10 per cent, even when antitoxin is not given until the 4th day or later. The dose of antitoxin varies with the site, extent and toxicity of the infection, but not with the age of the child. *Table 20.1* shows a suggested regimen.

Before giving diphtheria antitoxin, enquiry should be made as to whether the child has previously received serum, or suffers from allergies (such as asthma or eczema). If the history is negative, intramuscular antiserum can be given.

Table 20.1 Regimen for antitoxin in diphtheria

Site	*Toxicity*	*Dose (units)*	*Route*
Nasal, conjunctival, cutaneous	Usually slight	2 000–10 000	i m
Faucial	Usually moderate	10 000–30 000	i m
Laryngeal with respiratory symptoms	Usually slight	30 000–50 000	i m or i v
Nasopharyngeal, faucial–nasopharyngeal	Usually severe	50 000–100 000	i v

If the history is positive or doubtful, sensitivity testing must be done. A subcutaneous injection of antiserum 0.2 ml of a 1 in 10 solution will give a generalized reaction within 30 minutes in a sensitized patient. If no reaction occurs give undiluted antiserum 0.2 ml subcutaneously and observe for a further 30 minutes before giving the intramuscular dose.

Following any dose of antiserum the patient should be observed closely for at least 30 minutes. If antiserum is required intravenously, a dose of 10 000 i.u. should first be given intramuscularly, and after 30 minutes if no generalized reaction has occurred, the antiserum may be given in full dosage intravenously by SLOW injection. The patient is then observed for at least a further 30 minutes.

If the sensitivity testing is positive, rapid desensitization can be carried out. This is done by the administration of increasing quantities of antiserum by subcutaneous injection at half-hourly intervals until no sensitivity response occurs. It is best to begin with 0.2 ml of a 1 in 100 dilution and to increase the dose tenfold until 2 ml of undiluted antiserum can be given. The therapeutic dose can then be given intramuscularly.

Adrenaline (1:1000 solution) must *always* be on hand (*see* Anaphylactic shock, page 114). In a sensitized person, because of the rapid production of antibody, the therapeutic effect of antiserum will be reduced and short lived.

Penicillin

This is the antibiotic of choice. The usual dose is benzylpenicillin 300–600 mg (500 000–1 million units) 6 hourly for 7–10 days. Soluble penicillin can be replaced by procaine penicillin after the initial toxic symptoms have subsided or where toxicity is slight. Erythromycin is best reserved for carriers or in patients known to suffer from penicillin sensitivity.

References

GELLIS, S. S. and KARGAN, B. M. (1980) *Current Pediatric Therapy* Chapter 9, p. 134. Philadelphia: W. B. Saunders

MORGAN, B. C. (1963) Cardiac complications of diphtheria. *Pediatrics,* **32,** 549–557

Further reading

CHRISTIE, A. B. (1980) *Infectious Diseases* (3rd edn.) p. 868. Edinburgh: Churchill-Livingstone

KRUGMAN, S. and WARD, R. (1981) *Infectious Diseases of Children* (7th edn.) p. 13. St. Louis: Mosby

MARTINDALE'S EXTRA PHARMACOPOEIA (1977) (27th edn.) Diphtheria Antitoxin, p. 1631. London: Pharmaceutical Press

Chapter 21

Haemoptysis

J. O. Warner

Introduction

Massive, life-threatening blood loss from the respiratory tract is very rare after the neonatal period. Furthermore, it is unusual to elicit a history of expectoration of sputum in an infant or young child, as any secretions reaching the pharynx and mouth are promptly swallowed. From the history there may be difficulty in distinguishing the origin of blood which may have arisen from an epistaxis, haematemesis, or a true haemopytsis.

Neonatal pulmonary haemorrhage (*see also* page 251)

Recognition

Extravasation of blood from the lungs of neonates, occurring in 1/1000 live births, is usually a sign of serious underlying disease and is often rapidly fatal. Pulmonary haemorrhage may rarely be an isolated phenomenon, usually in premature infants, but is more commonly found as a complication of bacterial pneumonia, generalized sepsis, severe birth asphyxia, hypothermia, rhesus isoimmunization, congenital heart disease or defective coagulation. The underlying common denominators in most cases are shock, disseminated intravascular coagulation (DIC) with consumption coagulopathy, and pulmonary oedema. Presentation is usually obvious, with collapse accompanied by outpouring of large amounts of blood-stained frothy fluid from the trachea, mouth, and nose, in a premature or small for dates and often previously sick neonate.

Management

There is no time to await the results of investigation, but coagulation studies including a search for fibrin degradation products and screening for sepsis should be initiated. Vigorous resuscitation using intermittent postive pressure ventilation (IPPV) with positive end expiratory pressure (PEEP), correction of anaemia and hypovolaemia preferably by fresh blood transfusion (or initially fresh frozen plasma) and a broad-spectrum combination of intravenous antibiotics must be commenced immediately.

Minor post-neonatal haemopytsis

Recognition

Though frightening to patients and parents, most haemoptyses are minor, but they may indicate serious underlying disease. Blood streaking of sputum may occur with acute infections such as tonsillitis, pertussis or pneumonia. It may also be a feature in patients with chronic suppurative lung disease such as cystic fibrosis or bronchiectasis from other causes.

Management

No specific treatment is required but investigation and treatment of the possible underlying condition must be initiated.

Major post-neonatal haemoptyses

Recognition

Frank haemoptysis requires more rigorous investigation and there are several important and potentially life-threatening causes.

Inhaled foreign body

Chronic or recurrent cough with lobar collapse or overinflation on chest radiograph should lead to suspicion of an inhaled foreign body. Direct questioning may elicit a history of choking on peanuts or a bone, etc.

Tuberculosis

Primary tuberculosis occasionally presents with haemoptysis but the additional features of cough, weight loss, fever, chest radiographic abnormalities, and positive Mantoux test will also be found.

Gastro-enterogenous duplication cyst

Ulceration of the mucosa in a gastric duplication cyst may produce severe life-threatening haemoptysis, but most cases are asymptomatic and are detected incidentally on chest radiographs, or present with symptoms of compression of the oesophagus and large airways.

Cystic fibrosis

Major haemoptysis with bright red fresh blood may occur in cystic fibrosis patients with severe pulmonary involvement. It is almost always a late symptom in known cases. Occasionally it is associated with an intra-cavity aspergilloma.

Pulmonary haemosiderosis

This is a rare condition characterized by recurrent intra-alveolar haemorrhage. It begins in infancy or childhood with recurrent iron-deficiency anaemia and attacks of fever, dyspnoea, wheeze, tachycardia, and sometimes haemoptysis. This may form part of Goodpasture's syndrome, and occurs in other immunologically mediated conditions such as systemic lupus erythematosus, Henoch–Schönlein purpura, and allergic broncho-pulmonary aspergillosis.

Hydatid cyst

Occasionally a hydatid cyst ruptures into a bronchus producing haemoptysis and expectoration of a watery fluid. It may also lead to dyspnoea and an acute allergic reaction. Preceding features may include vague ill health and symptoms of bronchial compression.

Pulmonary arteriovenous fistula (A-V fistula)

This usually presents with haemoptysis in adults. In children it is more likely to be associated with dyspnoea, cyanosis and finger clubbing, when there is a large shunt through single or multiple fistulae. Some occur in patients with hereditary haemorrhagic telangiectasia.

Bronchial tumours

Benign hamartomas, adenomas, and angiomas are very rare but may present with haemoptysis. Malignant tumours such as fibrosarcoma and carcinoma are even rarer.

Thromboembolism

Pulmonary infarction may complicate sickle cell anaemia, bacterial endocarditis or infected atrial cannulae (i.e. V-A shunts for hydrocephalus).

Management

Most cases will have other features which render the diagnosis obvious, and management will be for the underlying disorder. Basic investigation would include a chest radiograph and a Mantoux test. Arteriography may aid diagnosis in duplication cysts, A-V fistulae and cystic fibrosis (bleeding from bronchial artery). Bronchoscopy will be required to remove foreign bodies and surgery to excise tumours, A-V fistulae, and duplication cysts. Major bleeding in cystic fibrosis patients can occasionally be treated by embolization of the offending bronchial artery. Acute haemorrhage in pulmonary haemosiderosis may be controlled by a course of high-dose steroids.

References

CHANG, S. H., MORRISON, L., SHAFFNER, L. and CROWE, J. E. (1976) Intrathoracic gastrogenic cysts and haemoptysis. *Journal of Pediatrics,* **88,** 594–596

FAIRFAX, A. J., BALL, J., BATTEN, J. C. and HEARD, B. E. (1980) A pathological study following bronchial artery embolization for haemoptysis in cystic fibrosis. *British Journal of Diseases of the Chest,* **74,** 345–352

PHELAN, P. D., LANDAU, L. I. and OLINSKY, A. (1982) In *Respiratory Illness in Children (Pulmonary Haemosiderosis).* pp. 383–387. Oxford: Blackwell Scientific Publication

Further reading

TROMPETER, R., YU, V. Y. H., AYNSLEY-GREEN, A. and ROBERTON, N. R. C. (1975) Massive pulmonary haemorrhage in the newborn infant. *Archives of Disease in Childhood,* **50,** 123–127

FIRTH, J. R., McGREADY, S. J., SMITH D. S. and MANSTMANN, H. C. (1983) Pulmonary haemorrhage and massive haemoptysis. In (E. L. Kendig and V. Chernick, eds.) *Disorders of the Respiratory Tract in Children* (4th edn.). pp. 923–932. Philadelphia: W. B. Sanders

Chapter 22

Acute respiratory failure

A. M. Wilson

Acute respiratory failure is life threatening. Action is required within minutes to prevent brain damage and death. It is those diseases which present with a gradual worsening of respiration that pose the greatest difficulty in management. Knowing when to interfere by the introduction of an artificial airway or by assistance with ventilation must often be a purely clinical decision based on repeated observations. These conditions may result in an acute-on-chronic state of hypoxia; when ventilation finally becomes inadequate the body has very little oxygen stores from

Table 22.1 Causes of acute respiratory failure in children

Respiratory arrest and inadequacy failure (PCO_2 is diagnostic)	*Obstructve failure (no test of severity)*	*Oxygenation failure (PO_2 is most helpful. PCO_2 level depends on many aspects)*
Cerebral	ANY LEVEL !! FOREIGN BODY !!	Pneumothorax
Coma from any cause		Pleural effusion
Head injury	Upper airway	Pulmonary collapse
Poisoning	Facial trauma	Pneumonia
Anaesthesia		Pulmonary embolism
Meningitis or encephalitis	Enlarged tonsils and adenoids	Fat embolism
Tumour		Diffuse intravascular coagulation
Hypothermia	Epiglottis	
	Acute epiglottitis	
Spinal cord		
Cervical cord injury	Larynx	
Poliomyelitis	Laryngeal spasm	
Tetanus	Laryngeal oedema	
	Laryngeal trauma, including intubation	
Neural	Acute laryngitis	
Polyneuritis (Guillain–Barré)	Acute laryngotracheobronchitis	
Neuromuscular junction		
Myasthenia gravis	Small airways	
Anaesthetic relaxants	Acute bronchiolitis	
Nerve gas poisoning	Asthma	
Defoliant weed killers	Pulmonary oedema	
	Inhalation of liquids and drowning	
Musculoskeletal		
Flail chest injury	Pleura	
Porphyria	Tension pneumothorax	

which to draw. Survival after total apnoea or anoxia depends on the oxygen stored in the body, of which an adult has approximately 1800 ml, mainly in the lungs (450 ml) and in the circulating blood. Thus an adult consumes about one-sixth of his oxygen stores per minute. A child has a higher metabolic rate and the neonate consumes just under a third in the same time. The smaller the child the more rapid must be the relief of respiratory failure. The only store that can usefully and quickly be increased is that in the lungs by administering high concentrations of oxygen. Patients with limited respiratory reserve should be given oxygen before performing any manoeuvre that might either inhibit breathing or cause an increased oxygen consumption. These include examination of the pharynx and even painful things like intravenous infusions.

Respiratory failure has many causes (*Table 22.1*). However, the first principle in management must be to assess the degree of failure, and determine whether this needs treatment, rather than to make a definitive diagnosis. Thus treatment will

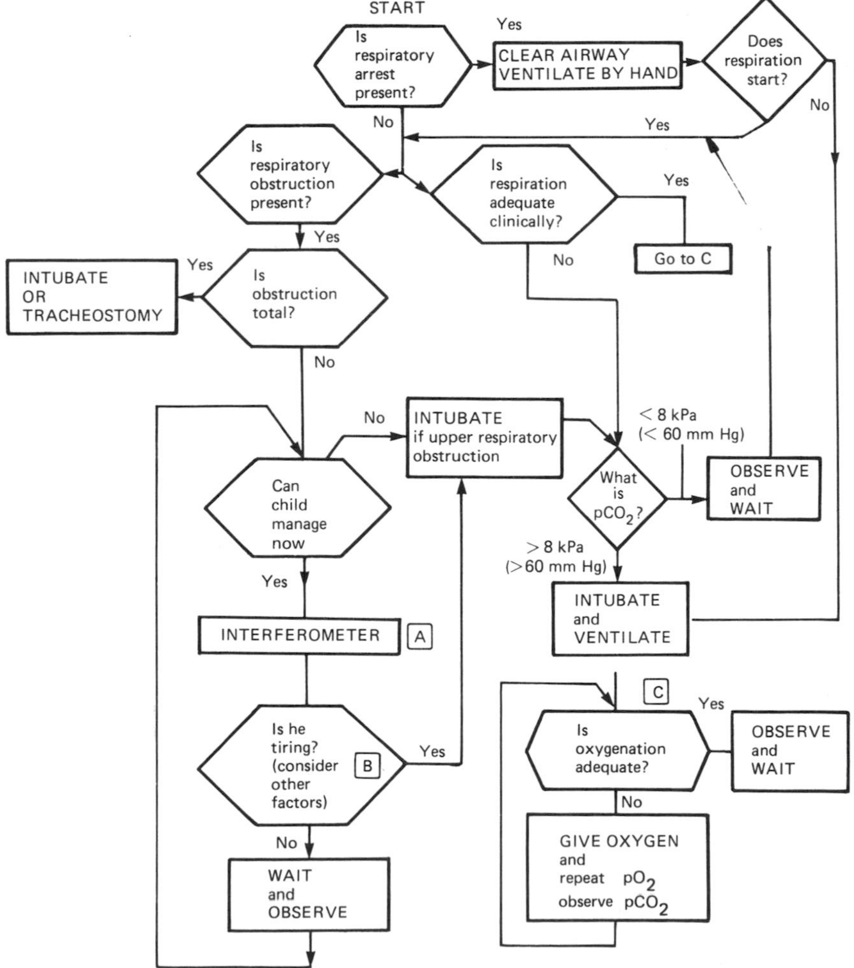

Figure 22.1 Scheme for management of acute respiratory failure. For explanations of A and B refer to text.

frequently precede diagnosis. *Figure 22.1* shows a scheme suggesting the urgent approach to respiratory failure from any cause. This is preceded by some definitions, and succeeded by notes referred to in the scheme (*see* page 221).

The diagnosis of respiratory failure is surprisingly difficult despite the availability of lung function and blood gas analysis. Total failure is obvious and requires little clinical acumen to recognize. The possibility of respiratory failure, either present or anticipated, should be considered in all children who have noisy breathing. However well a child appears, 'noisy breathing is obstructed breathing'. Other signs such as visible contraction of the sternomastoids, and indrawing of the intercostals or suprasternal notch are equally worrying, as is cyanosis, despite apparently adequate respiration. More difficult are the children who are reaching a late stage in an obstructive disease and whose respiration becomes quiet. Here the absence of noise may indicate an inability to continue breathing against a severe obstruction. Cyanosis suggests a serious situation but the absence of cyanosis is compatible with severe hypoxia. *Anxiety, pallor and restlessness can all indicate hypoxia which needs urgent relief.*

Definitions

Respiratory arrest

There is no respiratory effort and therefore no mechanical exchange of gas between the lungs and the atmosphere. The patient becomes cyanosed within 2 minutes and the PCO_2 level of the blood rises steadily. This is an absolute, easily diagnosable state; survival is dependent upon the 'stored oxygen'. the patient needs both maintenance of the airway and ventilation.

Respiratory failure

Respiratory activity is present but is ineffective. This is divisible for diagnostic and therapeutic purposes into three categories.

Inadequacy failure

Here there is no obstruction to the airway but mechanical gas exchange is reduced by some extra-pulmonary part of the respiratory system, neural or muscular. The level of depression is difficult to assess clinically but it can be quantified by measuring the arterial PCO_2. The normal value is 5.3 kPa (40 mm Hg). Thus a value of 8.0 kPa (60 mm Hg) represents 50 per cent depression and would be a strong indication for ventilation. The PCO_2 level, when divided into 5.3 gives an indication of the adequacy of ventilation. 1 is normal, less than 1 indicates hypoventilation or inadequacy. If the peripheral circulation is unimpaired a capillary PCO_2 will give a meaningful result.

Obstructive failure

There is noisy respiration and obvious respiratory difficulty. Noise will be absent if the obstruction is total, or if the respiration is also depressed. Respiratory effort is seen by in-drawing of the thoracic wall and the use of accessory muscles. The child may sit up and clutch at the bed or a table in an effort to breathe. Respect this;

forcing him to lie down to be examined may reduce his ability to breathe. This patient requires relief, either medical or surgical, of the obstruction. It is important to realize that there is no test to determine the degree of obstruction or the moment to intervene. The point of intervention will be a clinical judgement based on the investigations listed below and must be before an element of inadequacy is overlaid on the obstruction.

Any decision on when to intubate balances the need to relieve unresolving obstruction and the known risks and complications of intubation (*see* later).

Oxygenation failure

This occurs when pulmonary pathology results in a reduction of transport of oxygen across the alveolar membrane. Ventilation will be normal or even increased by hypoxia. At first sight the child appears not to be in respiratory failure, but may be overbreathing; only the signs of incipient hypoxia and later cyanosis point to the diagnosis. An arterial PO_2 will be diagnostic. The management is to give oxygen in controlled concentrations, and to repeat the blood gas analysis to achieve an adequate PO_2. The PCO_2 is also measured for evidence of inadequacy.

Scheme of management (*see Figure 22.1*)

The scheme is presented as a logical approach to the immediate management of respiratory failure. In most cases the answers at the hexagonal decision points are a clear yes or no, or the result of a test. However tests are not always helpful and the management is based very much on clinical impressions, especially at points labelled A and B.

A. Interferometer (*see Figure 22.1*)

The name given to a set of signs to aid the clinical decision when to intervene and intubate a child to overcome an upper respiratory obstruction, which include:

1. Both inspiratory and expiratory stridor – a grave sign indicating severe obstruction.
2. Cyanosis; only seen when the obstruction is severe or when there is also pneumonic involvement.
3. Decreasing awareness, loss of interest in toys, etc., suggestive of hypoxia.
4. Failure to take food and drink. The child who cannot take time off breathing to drink and swallow has little reserve.
5. Rising pulse rate.
6. Varying respiratory rate. As though the child is trying to find the optimum breathing pattern.
7. Obvious tiring, especially with inability to sleep.
8. A rising PCO_2. This is a *too late* sign, and shows that inadequacy of ventilation has occurred. In acute respiratory obstructive disease, including asthma in children, the PCO_2 remains at near-normal levels even in the presence of cyanosis. A high PCO_2 means that the child is unable to compensate, is severely ill and close to respiratory, and possibly cardiac, arrest.

B. (*see Figure 22.1*)

The above list of signs cannot give an absolute answer as the significance of the observations will be affected by other factors which include:

1. Length of history. If respiratory obstruction has lasted for many hours with no improvement, intubation may be preferred.
2. Time of day.
3. Availability of staff.
4. Availability of ancillary services.

Consideration of the last three factors may suggest a planned intubation at the end of the day, to forestall an emergency procedure at night when X-ray and laboratory services are at a minimum.

Practical management of respiratory failure

Respiratory arrest and inadequacy

Ensuring a clear airway

The patient should be placed on his side (the left makes for easier intubation later), to allow secretions, vomit and blood to drain away from the larynx, and to encourage the jaw and tongue to fall forward. The jaw is held forward by pressing from behind the angle of the mandible. In small children 'holding the jaw up' by pressing below the chin causes obstruction by raising the tongue against the palate. The mouth is inspected for any debris including dislodged teeth which can be cleared with a finger or by suction. Respiratory efforts should be watched to see if they return or are obstructed.

Artificial ventilation

Artificial ventilation is started as soon as the airway is clear. In hospital it should always be possible to perform this with oxygen from an anaesthetic or resuscitation circuit, or from an 'Ambu' or similar self-inflating bag.

All doctors should make themselves familiar with the equipment available locally, but it may be necessary to perform air resuscitation by the mouth-to-mouth or mouth-to-tube methods.

During any resuscitation the highest available concentration of oxygen should be used. Children, unlike bronchitic adults, rarely depend on an hypoxic drive. *Oxygen does not depress ventilation.*

BAG AND MASK

The mask is applied over the mouth and nose, and the head held to maintain a clear airway. The use of a rubber or plastic airway passed over the tongue may help. The bag of the apparatus is squeezed regularly to inflate the lungs. As a practical rule the rate per minute of inflation is 32 minus the age in years. The volume expelled can only be assessed by watching the movement of the chest. The aim is to produce more movement than is seen in normal respiration. A baby needs only 20–40 ml per breath and over-inflation can cause pneumothorax.

MOUTH-TO-MOUTH (EXPIRED AIR) RESUSCITATION

Expired air resuscitation relies on the 14.5% oxygen in expired breath being sufficienct to sustain life in an apnoeic person. Mouth-to-mouth ventilation is performed after clearing the airway. A watch should be kept on chest movement as this is the only way to know that artificial ventilation is effective. The use of a barrier such as a porous sheet designed for the purpose or even a pocket handkerchief, or tubes such as double-ended airway make the process more efficient and acceptable.

Endotracheal intubation

Endotracheal intubation should be within the ability of all doctors. Visualization of the larynx with a direct laryngoscope is easier when there is anoxia and loss of tone. There are two main designs of laryngoscope which are used in different ways. The curved 'adult' Macintosh type can be used for children down to, and often less than, 6 months, while a straight type is more useful in smaller babies.

Technique

POSITION

Intubation is easiest with the patient flat on his back, but to avoid tracheal soiling by secretions it may have to be performed on the side. A pillow under the head, *but not the shoulders,* helps greatly. The head is then extended on the neck to obtain the position described as 'sniffing the morning air'.

LARYNGOSCOPY

The curved laryngoscope is then introduced into the right of the mouth and passed directly back until the uvula is seen. Then it is rotated across the tongue until the tip of the epiglottis comes into view. When the tip of the blade lies in the fossa between epiglottis and tongue (*Figure 22.2a, b*) traction in the direction of the handle (arrowed) will make the laryngeal opening visible.

The straight-bladed laryngoscope (*Figure 22.3*) is passed (after correct positioning of the patient) over the tongue and into the upper end of the oesophagus. Under vision it is then slowly withdrawn until the larynx comes into view. This approach is preferred because of the large floppy epiglottis of neonates obscures the view of the larynx when a curved blade is used.

INTUBATION

Choosing a tube of the correct length and size can be difficult in an emergency. The sizes of tube most likely to be suitable at various ages are shown in Appendix 23. These refer to children with no abnormality, and it may be that the recommended size will not pass through the cords. An endotracheal tube should never be forced into position, and if tight, a smaller one should be tried so that a loose fit is obtained. Care must be taken not to advance the tube into a main bronchus; normally the tube should be passed 2–3 cm past the cords. Where obstruction is present, such as that of acute laryngotracheobronchitis, the tube should be advanced until the obstruction is relieved. The tube should be firmly fixed to prevent any further movement or displacement.

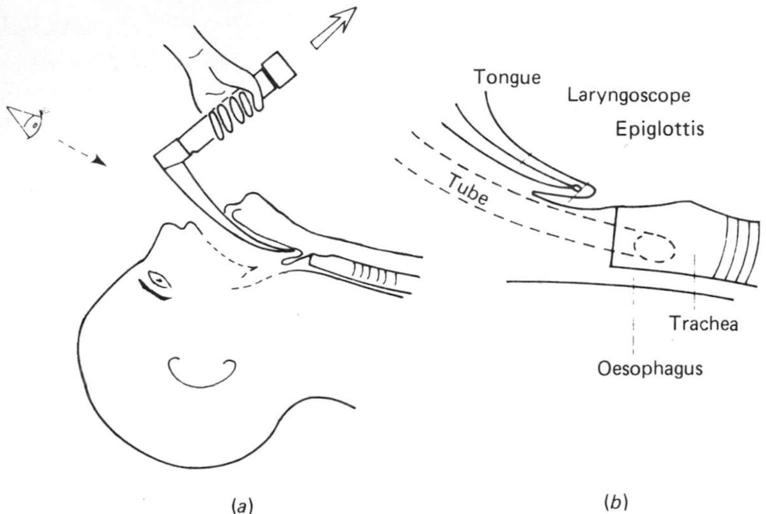

Figure 22.2 Laryngoscopy using the curved-blade laryngoscope.

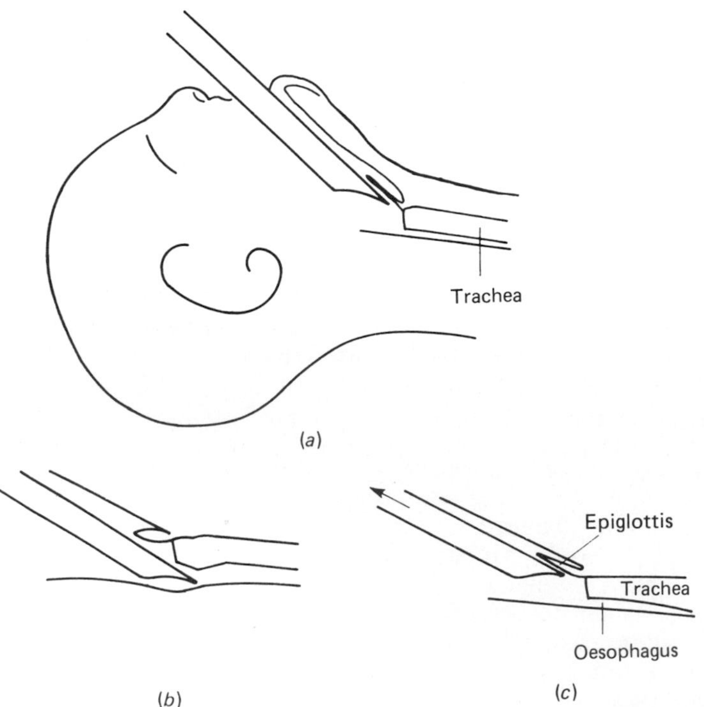

Figure 22.3 Laryngoscopy using the straight-bladed laryngoscope (for children aged under 6 months).

After intubation, artificial ventilation may be continued with the resuscitation circuit connected directly to the tube. Some form of escape valve is incorporated in the circuit as direct connection of the oxygen supply to an intubated patient can be fatal.

Conditions requiring specific treatment

Tetanus, strychnine poisoning, status epilepticus and other convulsive episodes

The spasms prevent adequate ventilation and also increase oxygen consumption. These patients need paralysis and heavy sedation in an intensive treatment unit. In tetanus there are often sympathetic activity episodes, with wide swings in pulse and blood pressure which require sympathetic blocker therapy. (For treatment of tetanus *see* Chapters 33–35.)

Myasthenia gravis

Respiratory crises may be precipitated by failure to take treatment, by overtreatment or intercurrent infection. Emergency treatment is, in addition to control of airway and ventilation, to give edrophonium chloride 0.5–1 mg IV or i.m. as a test. If this short-acting anticholinesterase is effective, neostigmine 0.04 mg/kg may be given for more prolonged action. The patient should be treated where there are facilities for artificial ventilation if there is no response to treatment, or in the case of a neostigmine crisis which requires withdrawal of therapy.

Post-anaesthesia

Patients who have received non-depolarizing anaesthetic relaxants e.g. curare, pancuronium, or alcuronium may show prolonged or renewed effect after return from the operating theatre. The initial treatment is neostigmine 0.04 mg/kg IV with atropine 0.2–0.6 mg IV to counteract the cardiac-slowing effect of neostigmine.

Transfer of a child with respiratory problems

Make an assessment of the likely progress of the disease during the transfer, taking into account all factors, including the fright of an ambulance journey and the effects of vibration. Many procedures are impossible in a moving ambulance, including the use of a mercury sphygmomanometer and tracheostomy. Even effective ventilation by bag and mask is awkward. Maintenance of temperature is difficult, particularly when making frequent observations. Try to secure an airway before setting out as this will obviate the need to intubate on the way, and ensure connection of ventilating equipment to the child. Establish a venous cannula and secure all apparatus firmly. Seek advice from the receiving hospital and have them informed of your departure. Attention to such details will make the journey less fraught. If transferring a baby for possible surgery have a consent form signed if the parents are not accompanying you, and take a sample of the mother's blood for cross-matching.

Complications of intubation and ventilation

(See also under IPPV treatment with tracheostomy in tetanus, page 327).

Intubation removes the protective function of the nose in warming and humidifying the inspired gases, and of the cough in removing secretions or foreign matter. It also removes the ability of the child to cry and attract attention. The psychological trauma of intubation must be remembered and an intubated child can never be left alone if he is confined to bed. The following list outlines many of the possible complications of intubation and ventilator therapy.

Dangers of intubation

1. *Obstruction. Passing a tube does not guarantee a clear airway.*
   (a) The tube may be obstructed owing to:
      Kinking;
      Movement in trachea;
      Secretions and crusting;
      Dislodgement.
   (b) Bronchial obstruction due to the above causes and unilateral bronchial intubation.
2. Damage to structures involved in intubation.
   (a) During insertion of tube, damage to:
      Lips;
      Teeth;
      Frenulum of tongue;
      Pillars of fauces;
      Posterior pharyngeal wall;
      Larynx.
   (b) Structures on which the tube and allied apparatus rests and in which pressure necrosis is possible:
      Skin of face and head;
      Upper lip;
      Nasal septum;
      Pharynx;
      Vocal cords and arytenoids;
      Subglottic region, especially cricoid ring;
      Tracheal mucosa.
3. As a consequence of sedation:
   (a) Corneal damage (open eyes).
   (b) Pressure sores.
   (c) Intestinal ileus.
   (d) Dehydration.
   (e) Constipation.
4. As a consequence of bypassing the nose and larynx:
   (a) Tracheal dehydration and crusting of secretions.
   (b) Loss of tracheal ciliary action.
   (c) Entry of infection.
   (d) Inability to cough effectively.

5. Additional dangers of ventilator therapy:
   (a) Failure of the machine.
   (b) Accidental disconnection.
   (c) Pneumothorax or pneumomediastinum.
   (d) Hyper- or hypoventilation.
   (e) Oxygen toxicity.
   (f) Results of using neuromuscular blocking drugs.
   (g) Alteration of cardiac status by changing intrathoracic pressures.

Management of long-term intubation

The list of complications given above demonstrates how necessary is a scrupulous approach in the treatment of an intubated child.

Technique

The traumas of intubation are minimized by careful technique. Seize every opportunity to practise intubation whether in theatre or on a stillborn infant. Trauma, to everyone, is less when intubation is performed in a planned manner, rather than at the last minute. With a deteriorating child request a consultation with the department responsible for managing airway problems as early as possible. This allows planning and a move to an ITU while still fit for transfer. Intubation is an operation, usually requiring anaesthesia, and an operation consent form should be completed. Arrange for this to be done before the parents leave the hospital.

Type of tube

For long-term use (over 4 hours) a plastic tube should be used. Red rubber tubes cause hyperaemic reactions if left in place. The nasotracheal route is favoured for children as fixation is easier and the child is able to eat and drink when ready to do so. The initial intubation should be through the mouth using the type of tube with which the operator is most familiar. When the airway and oxygenation have been secured a change can be made to the long-term tube, or transfer can be arranged. The child will now probably require an anaesthetic because oxygenation has been restored, even if the first tube was passed under emergency conditions.

Tube diameter

The correct diameter is crucial in a tube that will remain in place for many days. Pressure necrosis of the vocal cords with subsequent granuloma formation can occur. In children the cricoid ring is the narrowest part of the airway. Too large a tube may result in oedema, or even necrosis with fibrosis at this site. At best this will result in inspiratory stridor at the time of extubation and require reintubation; at worst subglottic stenosis may develop. The diameter of the tube may be chosen from formulae or tables (*see* Appendix 23), but these will not give the correct result in the presence of either congenital or acquired abnormality. A tube which will pass with ease through the external nares will usually pass the cricoid ring. Repeated trial of different diameter tubes should be made to find one that just fits. The use of uncuffed tubes is usual in children and a small air leak between tube and trachea is expected.

Tube length

The length of the tube is equally important. There are tables of length-against-age but the practical way of determining the correct length is when exchanging the initial oral tube for a nasal tube. The end of the tube can be seen entering the cords and is advanced until the midpoint of the trachea, as judged from the size of the child, or until the obstruction is passed. The nasal end of the tube is then marked to avoid further insertion. As the patient moves, the inner end of the tube slides up and down the trachea so positioning must avoid the two dangers of dislodgement and bronchial intubation.

Fixation

Adequate fixation is necessary for the reasons given above and because the child will become restless. There are many forms of headband described, on which the tube and its fittings are fixed, to avoid movement. A common complication of the *Jackson–Rees* tube is necrosis of the nasal septum, which is completely avoidable by correct positioning. Less common is mid- or lower tracheal stenosis resulting from movement of the tube end on the tracheal wall. When designing and applying a headband care must be taken not to obscure the child's vision with apparatus, as this is an anxiety-inducing factor. The headband must be capable of supporting the weight of ventilator and humidifier tubing, both in the horizontal position and when the child is sitting. Occasionally the adhesive plaster used in a headband causes a reaction of the underlying skin of sufficient severity to be an indication to change to a tracheostomy.

Sedation

Children tolerate intubation and ventilation remarkably well, and settle very quickly, after an initial period of sedation. The need for sedation should be foreseen as a child *in extremis* from say, acute epiglottitis, will, within minutes of being intubated, be very lively. His first action will be to attempt extubation. A safe regimen is to give intravenous doses of diazepam 0.05 mg/kg, and pethidine 0.2 mg/kg. *SUCH A CHILD MUST BE WATCHED CONTINUOUSLY TO OBSERVE THE EFFECT OF THESE DRUGS WHICH DEPRESS RESPIRATION.* There is a need for frequent sedation at first but this diminishes rapidly until none is required in a rational child. Where continuous PCO_2, and other monitoring is in routine use infusions of sedatives may be used.

A ventilated child has greater need for sedation and even neuromuscular-blocking drugs. During this period of immobility many protective reflexes are abolished. These patients need full neurosurgical nursing including eye and mouth toilet, regular turning, treatment of pressure areas, and routine physiotherapy.

Sedation of children with respiratory difficulties is potentially dangerous, and may be given only when there is competent continuous observation.

The child's general comfort should be given careful attention. All painful procedures, IV lines and nasogastric tube, should be passed while the child is asleep for the intubation. The intubated child does not have to lie down and often wants to play an active part in what is happening. Parental visiting will be a great distraction from his problems. A full stomach (*see* later) is a good sedative.

Tube care: Obstruction, humidification and suction

Tube obstruction is a common complication. Breathing dry gas, especially of a high oxygen concentration, rapidly stops ciliary activity in the tracheal mucosa in the region of the end of the tube. This results in interruption of the normal upward sweep, and a build-up of secretions which gradually encroaches on the lumen and eventually blocks the tube. If allowed to dry the secretions become encrusted and may be impossible to remove.

Recognition

A child with a totally obstructed tube will become very restless, with intercostal and suprasternal indrawing and increasing cyanosis. Listen to the open end of the tube and if there is no movement of air do not waste time trying to suck out the tube but PULL IT OUT. *The child with respiratory obstruction and no tube stands a chance. The child with a blocked tube stands no chance.* Prevention is less dramatic. Although the accumulation of secretions is the most common cause of obstruction, if the child is restless or if the ventilator pressure is high look for mechanical obstruction due to kinking or to the rotation of the bevel of the tube against the tracheal wall. Both sides of the chest must be examined with a stethoscope to exclude a main bronchus intubation due to too long a tube.

Humidification is provided by gas warmed to 34–37°C (93–98.4°F) and fully saturated with water vapour. The temperature of the inspired gas should be measured close to the patient to ensure that there is neither risk of scalding of the airway nor of inadequate water vapour. Ultrasonic nebulizers provide an unmonitored concentration of water which can, by absorption in the airways, result in overhydration and hyponatraemia. Air fully saturated at body temperature contains 42 mg water per litre of air. If a hot-water humidifier is not available, bubbling the gas supply through cold water is much better than nothing, by producing about 20 mg/ℓ. Both humidification and suction are facilitated by the instillation of saline 0.1–1 ml into the tube before suction. Instillation is additonal to humidification and cannot replace it.

Suction is the other essential in preventing blockage of the tube by secretions. Production of secretions is marked in some diseases and requires aspiration every 15 minutes. The catheter should be about one-third of the diameter of the lumen. A large catheter will subject the lung to negative pressure, with possible collapse. It should not be passed more than 0.5 cm beyond the tube for routine suction. When stiff catheters are necessary for sucking small tubes, greater projection will result in the taking of ‘suction biopsies’ of the tracheal mucosa. Suction technique must be gentle and aseptic. Suction traps for sputum specimens should be available when a child is first intubated. Oxygenation is impaired during suction, so the inspired oxygen should be increased for a few minutes beforehand.

Ventilation

The use of mechanical ventilators cannot be covered in detail here, but some practical points must be made. A patient receiving artificial ventilation runs the risks not only of intubation, but also those of the machine. All machines must be expected to fail. Nursing instructions should include details of the action to be taken in such event. There must be a separate method of ventilating by hand, such as a self-filling bag, immediately available. If there is any doubt about the machine's function the rule is 'Disconnect the ventilator and ventilate by hand using the simplest system while the problem is diagnosed'.

Ventilator observations include the peak airway pressure, synchrony of ventilator and chest movement as well as the usual nursing observations. Common problems are leaks, low pressure, obstructions and high pressure. Tube obstruction has been mentioned, but signs of ventilating difficulty, rising ventilator pressure, uneven chest movement, and unexplained cyanosis may point to pneumothorax. Pneumothorax is not uncommon and cannot be clinically diagnosed with certainty in a patient on a ventilator. If suspected, an X-ray must be taken. Failing this, a needle should be inserted into the pleura in the mid-axillary line. If there is no air leak this should be repeated on the opposite side, and followed by a chest drain if necessary.

Most patients are moderately hyperventilated to assist in the control of spontaneous respiratory efforts. Restlessness suggests hypoventilation which is frequently due to leaks in the circuit or accidental alterations of the ventilator controls. A check should be made for leaks at every joint especially at those restrained by sticky tape. The control settings should be recorded so that accidental movement can be rectified.

Oxygen toxicity

Pulmonary oxygen toxicity occurs whenever the inspired oxygen value is above 21% given enough time. The inspired oxygen should always be monitored, and where possible its effect should be monitored by direct measurement of arterial PO_2. The tendency to increase oxygen 'just to be safe' must be resisted.

Fluid intake

All intubated patients have an intravenous line and a nasogastric tube. After intubation gastric emptying and absorption is inhibited for a time, which can be as short as 6 hours in children. During this period IV fluids are needed to maintain intake, to replace intake lost during the early phase of the disease and to ensure adequate hydration for 'internal humidification'. Due to the changed intrathoracic pressures hypovolaemia is tolerated badly by ventilated patients. Fluid intake is calculated and given at first intravenously, gradually reducing this as gastric absorption permits increased intake. The taking of food, and a full stomach, is a potent sedative and keeps children happy. If there is any doubt about the competence of the vocal cords around the tracheal tube a small drink of brightly coloured liquid is given. Providing the colour is not recovered by endotracheal suction further food may be given.

The dangers of intubation and ventilation are many. The above procedures should be practised only when there are adequate staff and facilities. Only under these conditions and with scrupulous attention to detail can good results be obtained.

Chapter 23

Respiratory emergencies

A. W. Boon

Respiratory disorders are among the commonest childhood illnesses and are the major cause for paediatric hospital admission. As a result of the respiratory problem there is frequently respiratory embarrassment or insufficiency. The aim of management is to prevent respiratory failure or to treat it promptly if it develops.

Respiratory failure

The function of the respiratory system is to oxygenate the blood and to eliminate carbon dioxide. Respiratory failure will therefore result in a fall in the PaO_2 (less than 8 kPa or 60 mm Hg) and a rise in $PaCO_2$ (greater than 6.5 kPa or 50 mm Hg).

Mechanism

Ventilatory inadequacy

Central respiratory depression, neuromuscular, or rib-cage defects may produce inadequate ventilation and respiratory failure. A rising $PaCO_2$ is an early feature. Although the accompanying hypoxia can be relieved by increasing the inspired oxygen concentration (FiO_2) the CO_2 retention can only be corrected by intermittent positive-pressure ventilation (IPPV).

Upper airway obstruction

Initially, the child's hyperventilation will maintain normal blood gases. With increasing resistance to airflow, the alveolar ventilation decreases, resulting in hypoxia and hypercapnia. Only by relieving the obstruction will the blood gases return to normal.

Ventilation–perfusion inequalities

This may be secondary to a variety of respiratory disorders including acute asthma, pneumonia, bronchiolitis, and pneumothorax. Whenever there are inequalities of ventilation and perfusion there will be an increase in the alveolar–arterial oxygen tensions. The PaO_2 falls, but initially there is compensatory hyperventilation which maintains a normal or low $PaCO_2$. If there is a substantial amount of poorly ventilated lung, even hyperventilation will not prevent the development of hypercapnia.

Hypoxia and cyanosis resulting from perfusion of poorly ventilated lung can be distinguished from hypoxia resulting from shunting (e.g. cyanotic heart disease) by giving the patient 100% oxygen to breathe. In hypoxia secondary to pulmonary disease, the PaO_2 will eventually rise to high levels, but not with shunting.

Recognition

Respiratory failure should be anticipated if there is severe dyspnoea, stridor, wheezing, or marked chest wall recession, together with the use of accessory muscles of respiration. Pallor, anxiety and restlessness often indicate hypoxia. Cyanosis is a fairly late sign. Subsequently, there is impairment of the level of consciousness and eventually coma.

Management

Oxygen

Hypoxia can usually be corrected by increasing the FiO_2. Neonates and young infants can be given oxygen via a Perspex headbox. Younger children can be nursed in an oxygen tent. Older children will usually tolerate a light, plastic face mask or nasal cannulae. Whatever the means of oxygen administration, the gas should be humidified.

Children rarely lose their CO_2 respiratory drive. There is therefore little danger in giving up to 100% oxygen for short periods. Nevertheless, prolonged inspiration of increased oxygen concentrations may produce lung damage. It is therefore important to monitor the FiO_2 at regular intervals. The aim of therapy should be to maintain the PaO_2 above 6.5 kPa (50 mm Hg), which represents 80 per cent saturation at pH 7.40

Humidification

Apart from humidification of inspired gases, the use of humidity in respiratory disorders is declining. Although the use of a warm moist atmosphere is traditional in the management of laryngotracheobronchitis ('croup') its value is unproven. Most cold water vapour condenses out in the upper airway. Furthermore, many children are frightened by mist tents; and the dense mist and sound of the nebulizer make observation very difficult.

Sedation

As restlessness is so often a symptom of hypoxia, sedation of the child in respiratory failure is best avoided. Although restlessness and distress aggravate stridor and asthma, it is much better to use a calm, reassuring manner to allay anxiety. Often the admission of the child to the relatively calm environment of the hospital ward will produce a marked improvement.

Endotracheal intubation

See pages 223–225.

Tracheostomy (*see* page 327)

Endotracheal intubation by a skilled anaesthetist usually avoids the need for emergency tracheostomy. Tracheostomy is usually indicated for long-term maintenance of an artifical airway, e.g. for prolonged ventilation, laryngeal web, etc.

Blood gases in the management of respiratory failure

Measurement of PaO_2 and pH on arterial blood samples should be routine in any child with impending or established respiratory insufficiency. (For details of technique *see* Practical Procedures, page 726.)

In the neonate, monitoring of the transcutaneous PO_2 and PCO_2 are very useful, although the equipment requires regular calibration and checking against arterial blood gas determinations. In older children ear oximeters enable cutaneous non-invasive measurement of oxygen saturation.

Oxygen

A PaO_2 of less than 11 kPa (85 mm Hg) is probably abnormal in most children outside the neonatal period.

Carbon dioxide

The $PaCO_2$ provides the best guide to the adequacy of ventilation. Elevation of the $PaCO_2$ above 6 kPa (45 mm Hg) indicates significant respiratory depression, airway obstruction, or ventilation–perfusion imbalance.

Acid–base balance

CO_2 retention is associated with respiratory acidosis. An acute episode of CO_2 retention will lead to a fall in pH. In chronic CO_2 retention, there is renal compensation, the kidneys' excretion of hydrogen ion rises so that the base excess increases and the pH returns to normal. A chronic respiratory acidosis is therefore characterized by a high $PaCO_2$, normal pH and high base excess.

Acute asthmatic attack

An acute asthmatic attack presents with respiratory insufficiency due to severe airway obstruction. The term 'status asthmaticus' has no real scientific meaning.

The airway obstruction is produced by a combination of smooth muscle spasm, mucosal oedema, and plugging of the airways by mucus. Dynamic compression of the airways by the high intrapleural pressure on expiration adds to the expiratory airway resistance. As a result the lungs become hyperinflated.

Recognition

In younger children, the attack will usually be preceded by an upper respiratory tract infection followed by coughing and wheezing. Some suddenly develop very severe wheezing, triggered by emotion, exercise, coughing, or exposure to an allergen.

Indications of severity include:

1. Cyanosis.
2. Pulsus paradoxus.
3. A silent, hyperinflated chest.
4. Drowsiness.
5. Pallor and restlessness.
6. Peak expiratory flow rate (PEFR) less than 25 per cent of that expected for height.
7. Use of accessory muscles of respiration.

Chest X-rays are not routinely indicated in most acute asthmatic attacks and should, in any case, be deferred until after the initial therapy. Blood gas estimations are useful in the management in very severe cases, where there is typically a low PaO_2, a raised $PaCO_2$ and a metabolic acidosis. Ideally blood gas sampling should be via an indwelling radial or brachial arterial catheter (*see* Chapter 93, Practical Procedures).

Management

Before initiating treatment it is important to determine what drugs the child has already received. This is particularly important if the child is receiving treatment with a theophylline derivative or inhaled steroid therapy.

Oxygen

Correction of hypoxia is the first aim of treatment. Oxygen can most conveniently be given via a face mask while the child is receiving nebulizer therapy. Normally 40 per cent oxygen is adequate but in severe illness 70 per cent oxygen may be required.

Bronchodilators

A β_2 agonist via a nebulizer, e.g. salbutamol 2.5 mg for children under 12 years to 5.0 mg for older children, diluted to 2 ml with normal saline. The nebulizer can be driven by a pump, from a pressurized cylinder, or from a wall supply. This therapy can be repeated 2–4 hourly, providing there is close medical supervision of the patient.

If the child shows no response or a rapid relapse, IV aminophylline is usually effective. Providing the child is NOT receiving therapy with a theophylline-type drug, a loading dose of 5 mg/kg is given by slow IV infusion via the burette of a giving set over 15–20 minutes. More rapid administration may cause fatal cardiac arrhythmias. The loading dose is followed by a slow IV infusion of aminophylline at a rate of 1 mg/kg/hour. *The loading dose of aminophylline must not be given to a child already receiving treatment with oral theophylline.*

Steroids

Most children requiring intravenous therapy for asthma should be given steroids. Additionally, if the child is receiving inhaled or oral steroid therapy he should be given systemic steroid therapy. Corticosteroids are given as intravenous hydrocortisone (100–200 mg 3–4 hourly). It should be noted that steroids take 4–6 hours to act. Once intravenous therapy is stopped intravenous hydrocortisone can be replaced by oral prednisolone (2 mg/kg/day to a maximum of 60 mg/day) for 3 days or so.

Hydration

Although the child with an acute asthmatic attack will have increased respiratory water loss, care should be exercised in rehydration as there may be inappropriate ADH secretion. For this reason intravenous fluids in the form of 0.18% NaCl in 4% glucose should be limited to the child's normal fluid requirements.

Sedation

Sedation of the child in incipient respiratory failure should be avoided, as restlessness is frequently a sign of hypoxia. A calming, reassuring manner is a much better way of allaying anxiety.

Physiotherapy

This has no place during the acute attack as it merely disturbs and tires the child. Once the attack is resolving, a normally active child will clear any residual mucus plugs very rapidly.

Mechanical ventilation

The decision to ventilate may be based on clinical criteria, particularly the level of consciousness, or on blood gas evidence of respiratory failure (a $PaCO_2$ greater than 8 kPa (60 mm Hg)). Very high peak airway pressures up to 70 cm H_2O may be required. A volume-cycled ventilator should be used if available because of the rapid changes in airway resistance during recovery, which may predispose to a pneumothorax developing. Fortunately, the need for ventilation is rare.

Bronchial lavage

If the child is intubated and ventilated, instillation of 0.9% sodium chloride 1–2 ml/kg may facilitate the clearing of mucus plugs and debris. However, its value is disputed.

Antibiotics

As over 95% of acute asthmatic attacks in children are triggered by viral infections, antibiotics do not form part of the routine therapy.

Acute pneumonia

The incidence of pneumonia is highest in the pre-school years, especially in the first 2 years of life. Thereafter it becomes increasingly rare.

The infecting agent varies with the child's age. Viruses are the major aetiological agents in childhood pneumonia, with the respiratory syncytial virus, parainfluenza, influenza, and adenovirus being the major pathogens.

In neonates and infants with impaired immunity, Gram-negative organisms such as *E.coli, Pseudomonas aeruginosa,* Klebsiella and proteus are important pathogens. The Group B β-haemolytic streptococcus and *Staphylococcus aureus* are the main Gram-positive pathogens at this age. Additionally, *Pneumocystis carinii* and *Chlamydia trachomatis* are important rarer pathogens in this group.

Outside the neonatal period the pneumococcus is the commonest bacterial pathogen. *Staphylococcus aureus* is a relatively rare, but important cause of pneumonia in the first year of life. *Mycoplasma pneumoniae* predominantly affects the older child between the ages of 5 and 15 years.

Recognition

Viral pneumonia

After prodromal upper respiratory symptoms, the child becomes increasingly feverish, listless and anorexic, with a cough, tachypnoea, and tachycardia. On auscultation there may be only a few scattered fine crackles, but patchy consolidation is visible in the chest X-ray.

Pneumococcal pneumonia

The onset may be very rapid, with a high fever in an ill, delirious child. There may be a dry cough and tachypnoea with an expiratory grunt, but physical signs of consolidation may be completely absent. Meningism may occur with upper lobe pneumonia and lower lobe pneumonia may present with abdominal pain. The chest X-ray classically reveals lobar consolidation, although it may be patchy in infants.

Staphylococcal pneumonia

This presents acutely as a toxic, possibly shocked infant. The chest X-ray reveals widespread, circumscribed patchy consolidation. Additionally, there may be pneumatocoeles, large thin-walled cavities containing air.

Mycoplasma pneumonia

This usually has an insidious onset, with malaise, headache, fever, myalgia, and sore throat. Subsequently, a persistent cough and mucoid sputum are characteristic. Scattered fine crackles may be the only chest signs and the X-ray findings of diffuse infiltrates frequently seem out of proportion to the physical signs.

Investigations

Other investigations, in addition to the chest X-ray, which may be helpful include:

1. *Differential white count.* A neutrophil leucocytosis and increase in immature forms suggests a bacterial infection.

2. *Blood culture.* This is the only practicable method of isolating a bacterial pathogen.
3. *Nasopharyngeal aspirate.* The respiratory syncytial virus can be rapidly identified using the immunofluorescent antibody test.
4. Acute and convalescent viral antibody titres may enable a retrospective diagnosis to be made. Similarly, viral cultures are available only after a long delay.
5. Lung tap. This is a hazardous procedure and rarely justified now. Pneumocystis pneumonia can usually be diagnosed on a clinical response to cotrimoxazole rather than by lung biopsy.

Management

The ill child will require careful monitoring and supportive measures. Cyanosis should be corrected with oxygen. In infancy, bottle feeding may not be possible and nasogastric feeding or intravenous fluids will be required.

Although pneumonia in childhood is usually viral in origin, in practice viral pneumonia cannot be clearly distinguished from bacterial pneumonia. Therefore antibiotic therapy is almost always indicated.

In neonates, a broad spectrum of antibiotic cover should be provided using a combination of penicillin, gentamicin, and cloxacillin. In the seriously ill infant the antibiotic combination of amoxycillin and cloxacillin is usually adequate. If there is lobar pneumonia, suggesting a pneumococcal infection, penicillin is the drug of choice. Erythromycin is the antibiotic of choice for mycoplasma pneumonia.

Acute bronchiolitis

This is the major lower respiratory tract infection of infancy. Every year it occurs in epidemics from late autumn until early spring. By far the most important pathogen is the respiratory syncytial virus (RSV), but the parainfluenza, influenza, rhino- and adenoviruses are responsible for some cases.

Recognition

The illness begins with increasing nasal discharge, poor feeding, and a cough. The cough has a typical vibrant character which is often a helpful diagnostic sign. After 3 or 4 days, the baby develops increasing breathlessness and difficulty with feeding. At this stage the infant may be pale or cyanosed with tachypnoea, recession, and a hyperinflated chest. An audible wheeze is often present, and on auscultation widespread high-pitched expiratory wheezes and fine crackles are present throughout the chest. Hepatomegaly is a frequent finding, due to a combination of downward displacement of the diaphragm and swelling secondary to viraemia. Cardiac failure is very rare in bronchiolitis. Despite the severity of the illness, the child is frequently afebrile. In early infancy and debilitated children apnoeic attacks are a potentially fatal complication. The chest X-ray shows hyperinflation of the lungs with patchy areas of segmental collapse and consolidation. A particularly helpful investigation is the identification of the RSV from a trap sputum.

Management

Oxygen

Oxygen should be given to correct hypoxia. In small babies this may be via a headbox in an incubator or cot. In older infants an oxygen tent can be used. Most babies with severe bronchiolitis benefit from being nursed sitting up, or with a head-up tilt in the cot or incubator.

Hydration

Most infants admitted to hospital with bronchiolitis will be unable to take oral feeds adequately. Nasogastric feeding is usually tolerated, but the increased airway resistance produced by the feeding tube, and the effects of gastric distention on the diaphragm, may lead to further respiratory embarrassment. In this case intravenous fluids should be given instead. Inappropriate ADH secretion may occur in severe bronchiolitis, and it is therefore important to monitor the baby's fluid balance, electrolytes, and weight.

Mechanical ventilation

Respiratory failure (indicated mainly by a $PaCO_2$ greater than 8.5 kPa (60 mm Hg) and severe apnoea are the indications for mechanical ventilation. The need for ventilation usually arises in babies less than 3 months old, in whom a neonatal ventilator should be used.

Antibiotics

Antibiotics are of no value in bronchiolitis. In practice, however, it may sometimes be difficult to distinguish between bronchiolitis and pneumonia although the identification of the RSV in a nasopharyngeal aspirate provides reassuring evidence that antibiotics are not indicated. If bronchopneumonia cannot be excluded it is prudent to commence antibiotic therapy. Secondary bacterial infections following bronchiolitis are rare.

Bronchodilators

Bronchodilators are in general ineffective under the age of 1 year (Lenney and Milner, 1978). Steroids also have not been shown to be effective in this disorder.

Cardiac failure

This is overdiagnosed in bronchiolitis. It usually occurs in a child with pre-existing congenital heart disease in whom a diuretic and possibly digoxin are of benefit.

Acute laryngotracheobronchitis, epiglottitis and 'croup' *See* pages 205–208

Aspiration

Milk or gastric contents

Aspiration of milk or gastric contents occurs in infancy due to gastro-oesophogeal reflux, and in older children with cerebral palsy and incoordinated swallowing. It is frequently difficult to distinguish between recurrent episodes of aspiration and asthma. Examination of the sputum for fat-laden macrophages and a 'milk scan' using technetium and a gamma camera should provide confirmation of the diagnosis. Individual episodes are treated as pneumonia.

Foreign bodies

See page 208.

Chemicals

Paraffin, white spirit, and other hydrocarbons are frequently accidentally ingested by children. Such episodes may be accompanied by aspiration during swallowing or vomiting. Respiratory symptoms usually occur within a few hours if there has been significant inhalation. Radiological changes mainly affecting the lung bases often precede clinical evidence of aspiration.

Supportive treatment may be required for a large aspiration. Emetics or gastric lavage are contraindicated. Fortunately, most episodes are very mild and complete recovery is the rule.

Pneumothorax

Spontaneous pneumothorax is rare in children outside the neonatal period. Occasionally it may accompany a severe asthmatic attack. Usually there is an underlying pulmonary disorder such as cystic fibrosis, lung cysts, or a staphylococcal pneumonia.

Recognition

Pneumothorax usually occurs abruptly with pain, breathlessness, and sometimes cyanosis. The child is frequently distressed, with tachypnoea and chest-wall recession. In a tension pneumothorax the trachea and mediastinum will be shifted away from the affected side. The percussion note is hyper-resonant and there are decreased breath sounds on the affected side. The diagnosis is confirmed radiologically.

Management

A small pneumothorax may not require treatment unless the child's condition is deteriorating. A large pneumothorax, tension pneumothorax, or pneumothorax complicating cystic fibrosis should be drained using a drain attached to an underwater seal inserted in the 3rd or 4th interspace in the anterior or mid-axillary line.

Smoke inhalation and respiratory burns

See Chapter 5, page 35

Whooping cough

Because of relatively low uptake of pertussis immunization, whooping cough continues to occur in epidemics every couple of years. Nearly all cases are caused by *Bordetella pertussis*.

Recognition

The illness starts with upper respiratory symptoms of a watery nasal discharge and a dry non-specific cough lasting about 1 week. This is followed by the paroxysmal cough. The clinical presentation is by no means uniform:

1. Some children develop the classical paroxysmal cough of increasing pitch, followed by an inspiratory whoop due to inspiration through adducted vocal cords.
   During the paroxysms the child has facial congestion and may be cyanosed. The coughing paroxysms may be followed by vomiting. Crying, feeding, or any other disturbance often provoke the paroxysms which are usually more frequent at night.
2. Infants and some older children do not whoop. The diagnosis should be considered in any child with a paroxysmal cough but clear lungs on auscultation.
3. In infants the coughing paroxysms are frequently followed by apnoea. Apnoeic attacks may also occur without a preceding coughing paroxysm.

The chest X-ray is usually normal. A lymphocytosis of 20 000/mm^3 or more is a strong pointer towards the diagnosis. *B.pertussis* can be cultured from a pernasal swab.

Management

Management of paroxysms

During severe paroxysms the infant should be given oxygen to relieve hypoxia. The excessive secretion should be gently aspirated. Over-vigorous suction may precipitate further paroxysms.

Apnoeic attacks or severe hypoxia will require immediate endotracheal intubation. Usually the child can be extubated after a few minutes once spontaneous respiration resumes.

Prevention of paroxysms

No pharmacological agent seems to make much difference to the course of the illness. Cough suppressants and sedative drugs have little or no effect on the paroxysms. However, steroids in high dosage (e.g. prednisolone 4–5 mg/kg/day) may be helpful for young infants with very severe symptoms.

Antibiotics

Although *B.pertussis* is usually sensitive to erythromycin, the use of antibiotics makes little or no difference to the clinical course of the condition. Nevertheless, antibiotics will render the child non-infective. Contacts can also be protected by prophylactic erythromycin.

Neonatal respiratory emergencies

Respiratory disorders in the neonatal period usually present with signs of respiratory distress:

1. Tachypnoea (respiratory rate > 60/min).
2. Chest wall recession.
3. Expiratory grunting.
4. Cyanosis.

It is important to note that respiratory distress is *not* a diagnosis in itself. The underlying aetiology can only be determined from the history, a chest X-ray, and further investigations.

Causes of respiratory distress

1. Pulmonary:
   (a) Hyaline membrane disease (idiopathic respiratory distress syndrome).
   (b) Transient tachypnoea of the newborn ('wet-lung disease').
   (c) Neonatal pneumonia.
   (d) Pneumothorax.
   (e) Meconium aspiration.
   (f) Congenital lobar emphysema.
   (g) Pulmonary haemorrhage.
   (h) Congenital lung cyst (rare).
2. Extra-pulmonary:
   (a) Diaphragmatic hernia.
   (b) Tracheo-oesophageal fistula.
   (c) Phrenic nerve palsy.
3. Non-respiratory:
   (a) Cardiovascular:
      Cyanotic congenital heart disease;
      Persistent fetal circulation (persistent pulmonary hypertension of the new born);
      Blood loss.
   (b) Neurological disorder.
   (c) Metabolic disorders.

Pulmonary causes of respiratory distress

Hyaline membrane disease (HMD) (Idiopathic respiratory distress syndrome (IRDS)

This affects preterm infants and is due, at least in part, to surfactant deficiency. As a result there is a failure of adequate lung expansion and the work of breathing is increased. Ventilation/perfusion mismatch is frequently present. Consequently the baby becomes increasingly hypoxic, with a metabolic acidosis due to tissue hypoxia.

RECOGNITION

Signs of respiratory distress develop at or soon after birth, and certainly by the age of 4 hours. A chest X-ray shows a uniform 'ground-glass' appearance of the lungs and an air-bronchogram caused by the normal air-filled bronchi silhouetted against the relatively underexpanded lungs.

MANAGEMENT

The aim is to support the neonate until adequate surfactant production occurs and the disease resolves. This usually takes 3 or 4 days, although the condition may be more prolonged in very preterm infants.

MINIMAL NECESSARY INTERVENTION

This remains one of the corner-stones of management. Any handling or disturbance may produce a fall in the PaO_2 and a worsening of the baby's condition. Nevertheless, the infant should be closely monitored as follows:

Blood gases
There is no absolutely safe level of inspired oxygen (FiO_2) especially in the very preterm baby. Certainly, if the baby requires an FiO_2 of over 0.3 (30% oxygen) at 2–3 hours of age either an umbilical arterial or right radial arterial catheter should be inserted (*see* Chapter 93, Practical Procedures). Arterial 'stabs' invariably disturb the baby and produce often meaningless values of PaO_2. Transcutaneous (Tc) monitoring of PaO_2 and $PaCO_2$ is now widely available, but the equipment requires regular checking against arterial blood gases, and the monitors are therefore best used as trend recorders. Alternatively the PaO_2 may be continuously recorded using an electrode at the tip of an umbilical arterial catheter.

Temperature
The temperature should be monitored with a skin or rectal probe. Alternatively, the axillary or rectal temperature should be measured regularly with a thermometer.

Heart rate
An ECG monitor, preferably with an audible signal, and alarms to detect bradycardia (<100/min) or tachycardia (>180/min) provides continuous measurement of the heart rate.

Respiration
A basic minimum level of respiratory monitoring may be provided by an apnoea monitor. However, a continuous visual display on a scope with preset upper and lower alarm limits is preferable.

Blood pressure
An indwelling arterial catheter attached to a pressure transducer enables continuous recordings of the infant's blood pressure to be made.

THERMOREGULATION

Maintenance of a normal body temperature increases the baby's chances of survival. Conversely, hypothermia increases the oxygen requirements, with detrimental results. Heat loss may be reduced by putting a bonnet on the baby, using a double-walled incubator, humidifying the incubator, or putting the infant in a polythene bag.

OXYGEN

Initially, the baby should be given sufficient oxygen to keep him pink. This is most conveniently administered using a Perspex headbox. The FiO_2 should be measured using an oxygen analyser. An FiO_2 of over 0.3 (>30%) at 2–3 hours of age indicates the need for blood gas monitoring (*see* pages 233 and 242).

The aim of oxygen therapy is to maintain the PaO_2 between 8 and 12 kPa (60 and 90 mm Hg). Hyperoxia should be avoided because of the risk of retrolental fibroplasia.

VENTILATORY SUPPORT

Continuous positive airway pressure (CPAP)
CPAP reduces the tendency of the surfactant-deficient lung to collapse at end-expiration, and improves oxygenation. CPAP should be considered in a baby who fails to maintain adequate oxygenation with FiO_2 of over 0.5 (50% oxygen). In the baby of less than 1500 g it is usually preferable to proceed straight to mechanical ventilation.

CPAP may be applied either via an endotracheal tube or via a nasal prong. A suitable distending pressure is 5 cm H_2O. The FiO_2 should be the same as that in the headbox. Most infant ventilators are now equipped to provide CPAP.

Intermittent positive pressure ventilation (IPPV)
Improvements in the design and performance of infant ventilators, with an increased awareness of factors preceding periventricular haemorrhage, have resulted in earlier mechanical ventilation for hyaline membrane disease. IPPV is applied through a naso-tracheal or oro-tracheal tube.

Indications for IPPV:

1. A PaO_2 under 6 kPa (45 mm Hg) with an FiO_2 over 0.7 (>70%).
2. A $PaCO_2$ over 8 kPa (60 mm Hg).
3. A pH under 7.2 secondary to respiratory failure.
4. Collapse or apnoea.

Using conventional ventilator therapy, initial settings as follows would be appropriate:

Peak airway pressure	: 20–25 cm H_20.
Positive end-expiratory pressure (PEEP)	: 3–5 cm H_20.
Respiratory rate	: 30/min.
Inspiratory:Expiratory (I:E) ratio	: 1:1.
FiO_2	: 0.7 (70%).

Subsequent ventilator settings should be adjusted in accordance with regular blood gas determinations. (For further details, *see* page 242).

Recently, alternative ventilator regimens have been used including high-frequency ventilation (60–120/min) and high-frequency oscillatory ventilation (800–1800/min) (Marchak *et al.*, 1981).

FLUIDS AND NUTRITION

Severe respiratory distress precludes oral feeding, and even nasogastric feeding may cause respiratory embarrassment. An IV infusion of 10% glucose should therefore be set up starting at 60 ml/kg/day. Supplements of NaCl and KCl at 2–3 mmol/kg/day should be added after 24 hours. In babies of over 1500 g birthweight it is usually safe to delay feeding until ventilatory support is no longer required. For the smaller baby, the need for ventilation may be more prolonged; therefore, total parenteral nutrition (TPN) should be started at about 48–72 hours of age.

CORRECTION OF ACIDOSIS

Ideally, adequate ventilation should avoid respiratory acidosis and enable at least a partial correction of a metabolic acidosis by improving oxygenation. There is now evidence (Levene, Fawer and Lamont, 1982) that acidosis may predispose to periventricular haemorrhage. Therefore, the pH should optimally be kept over 7.2 with a base excess of less than −10. In the underperfused, shocked infant an infusion of plasma or plasma protein fraction (PPF) 10–20 ml/kg run in rapidly will restore the blood pressure and correct the acidosis. Bicarbonate 8.4% should be used with care, remembering that it is very hypertonic. The aim should be a half-correction of the acidosis. The dose of bicarbonate can be calculated from the following formula:

$$\frac{\text{Body weight (kg)}}{3} \times \text{Base deficit} \times \frac{1}{2}$$

The bicarbonate should be infused over 1 hour (for further discussion of the treatment of acidosis, *see* pages 118–121).

SURFACTANT THERAPY

Initial experience with endogenous surfactant (dipalmitoyl lecithin) introduced into the lungs of babies with HMD was disappointing. Recently, encouraging results have followed the instillation of a surfactant solution into the trachea (Fujiwara *et al.*, 1980).

Acute complications of HMD

PULMONARY AIR LEAK

Although 1 per cent of normal vaginally born infants develop a spontaneous pneumothorax at birth, the incidence is greatly increased in HMD requiring ventilatory support; 20–40 per cent of babies being ventilated for HMD develop a pulmonary air leak.

PULMONARY INTERSTITIAL EMPHYSEMA (PIE)

Pulmonary interstitial emphysema (PIE) results from alveolar rupture leading to extravasated gas tracking along the perivascular sheaths into the interstitial tissues.

Recognition

PIE occurs almost exclusively in preterm babies being ventilated for HMD. The air-leak may be asymptomatic or may be associated with clinical evidence of deterioration with worsening blood gases. The chest X-ray shows either multiple small cystic lucencies or streaky linear radiolucencies radiating from the hila.

Management

1. Avoidance of further barotrauma to the lungs; reducing the peak airway pressure and positive end-expiratory pressure may prevent extension of PIE and encourage spontaneous resolution.
2. *High-frequency ventilation.* Increased ventilation frequency may enable adequate gaseous exchange to occur with much lower inflation pressures (Ng and Easa, 1979). Alternatively, this may be an indication for high-frequency oscillatory ventilation.
3. Selective intubation. If PIE is localized to one lung, selective intubation of the contralateral main bronchus may allow the PIE in the affected lung to resolve. Alternatively, the bronchus to the affected lung may be selectively obstructed.
4. *Surgery.* Lobectomy has been advocated for PIE under tension affecting a single lobe.
5. *Pulmocentesis.* In the infant with extensive severe PIE there may be a place for needling of the affected lung followed by insertion of a drain directly into the lung.

PNEUMOTHORAX (*see* also page 239)

Pneumothorax may be preceded by PIE or occur on its own, usually in a baby receiving ventilatory support.

Recognition

A pneumothorax should be suspected in any baby being ventilated or on CPAP who deteriorates suddenly or becomes more difficult to ventilate. Clinical signs are frequently lacking, but there may be a displaced apex beat due to mediastinal shift. Occasionally, the diaphragm is displaced downwards, resulting in apparent hepatosplenomegaly.

Differences in transillumination between the two sides of the chest using a cold-light source and fibreoptic system is a useful and rapid method of diagnosing moderate to large pneumothorax. If there is doubt and the baby's condition allows it, a chest X-ray will confirm the diagnosis.

Management

Nearly all pneumothoraces require drainage. This is best achieved using a plastic cannula inserted through the lateral chest wall, connected to an underwater seal or Heimlich flutter valve. Blind needling of the chest is to be avoided as it is more likely to produce a pneumothorax than to treat it.

PNEUMOMEDIASTINUM

Apart from the rare complication of surgical emphysema, pneumomediastinum is a generally benign disorder in neonates.

PNEUMOPERICARDIUM

This should be suspected in a child who becomes hypotensive, with a poor cardiac output and muffled heart sounds. Chest X-ray shows gas completely surrounding the heart and limited by the pericardial sac.

Pericardiocentesis (*see* page 276) using a needle introduced under the xiphisternum aimed towards the left shoulder may be necessary in some cases, with catheter drainage if the air accumulates again.

PERSISTENT FETAL CIRCULATION (PERSISTENT PULMONARY HYPERTENSION OF THE NEW BORN)

See page 250

INFECTION

Increasing signs of respiratory distress or difficulty in ventilation, with fine crackles in the lungs should suggest infection. Additionally there may be non-specific signs of infection (*see* page 655).

After a full infection screen and chest X-ray, the infant should be started on penicillin, gentamicin, and cloxacillin.

PERIVENTRICULAR HAEMORRHAGE (*see* Chapter 72, page 626)

Large bleeds may lead to hypotension, peripheral circulatory failure, metabolic acidosis, and fits. Occasionally, the fontanelle is tense and bulging. Sclerema is associated with massive haemorrhage. Most haemorrhages are asymptomatic and only detected on head-scanning using real-time ultrasound with a sector scanner.

Treatment should be aimed at prevention, avoiding pre-disposing factors such as hypoxia, hypercapnia, or acidosis, and maintaining stable cerebral perfusion. Ethamsylate, phenobarbitone and vitamin E have all been claimed to be of benefit in prevention.

TECHNICAL PROBLEMS ASSOCIATED WITH MECHANICAL VENTILATION

Sudden deterioration during ventilation is frequently associated with blockage or displacement of the endotracheal tube. An important sign is absence of chest movement during ventilation.

Suction through the endotracheal tube may unblock the tube. In some instances this is ineffective and the tube will need to be changed. Copious mucoid secretions may require bronchial lavage with 1–2 ml of 0.9% NaCl.

Finally, it is important to consider the possibility of a fault in the ventilator or leaky connections in the ventilator circuit.

Transient tachypnoea of the newborn ('wet-lung disease')

This condition is believed to be caused by delayed clearing of lung liquid.

RECOGNITION

The diagnosis should be considered particularly in babies delivered by elective caesarean section. It is often seen in full-term infants. The infant presents with signs of respiratory distress with tachypnoea often the dominant feature.

The chest X-ray shows streaky shadowing radiating from the hila and fluid in the horizontal fissure.

MANAGEMENT

The condition is self-limiting and usually resolves within 24 hours. Occasionally resolution takes longer and persistent fetal circulation may be a complication. There is no specific treatment other than oxygen and supportive management.

Neonatal pneumonia

Pneumonia is the commonest severe infection in newborn infants. Predisposing factors include prolonged rupture of the membranes, preterm labour, and excessive obstetric manipulation. The commonest pathogen is now the Group B streptococcus. Gram-negative organisms such as *E.coli, Pseudomonas aeruginosa* and Klebsiella are also important, together with *Staphylococcus aureus* and occasionally *Listeria monocytogenes.*

RECOGNITION

Pneumonia should be suspected in any baby with antecedant risk factors presenting with signs of respiratory distress. The early form of Group B streptococcal disease may be clinically and radiologically identical with HMD. Apnoeic attacks are a particularly ominous sign.

A full infection screen should be carried out. The ratio of immature to total neutrophils (the I:T ratio) (Manroe, *et al.*, 1979) and a gastric aspirate, looking for white cells and organisms are useful.

MANAGEMENT

Antibiotic therapy should be initiated as soon as cultures have been taken. High-dose penicillin therapy (250 000 units/kg/day) should be combined with an aminoglycoside such as gentamicin. Antibiotics should be continued for at least 10 days.

Pneumothorax

Although this usually occurs as a complication of HMD, it may occur following a normal delivery, and especially active resuscitation; in this case, signs of respiratory distress will be present from birth. Pneumothorax may also result from attempts to resuscitate or ventilate infants with hypoplastic lungs, as in diaphragmatic hernia, hydrops fetalis or renal agenesis (Potter's syndrome); or after prolonged leakage of amniotic fluid. Meconium aspiration carries a greatly increased risk of pneumothorax, due to the ball-valve effect of inspissated meconium. HMD is also associated with an increased incidence of pneumothorax, especially if the baby is treated with CPAP or IPPV (*see also* page 243). Lung perforation can occur with over-vigorous endotracheal suction, especially if the catheter is pushed beyond the carina. Insertion of a chest drain may also perforate the lung (*see also* page 239).

Meconium aspiration

Intrapartum asphyxia frequently leads to the passage of meconium during labour and delivery. This in turn leads to the possibility of aspiration of meconium into the trachea and bronchi. Cerebral hypoxia is therefore a frequent association of meconium aspiration.

RECOGNITION

This usually occurs in a term or post-term infant with signs of intrauterine growth retardation. Meconium staining of the skin and nails is usually present. Signs of respiratory distress are present from birth. Additionally, the chest is barrel shaped. The chest X-ray shows hyperinflation of the lungs with flattening of the diaphragms. Coarse patchy areas of radiodensity are interspersed with areas of radiolucency. Pneumomediastinum and pneumothorax are complications.

MANAGEMENT

Prevention by active tracheal suction at birth before the baby has breathed is the ideal treatment.

Treatment of the established condition is essentially supportive. Oxygen is given to correct hypoxia. Mechanical ventilation tends to be difficult as high inflation pressures are required. The infant should be started on prophylactic treatment with penicillin and gentamicin because of the increased risk of pneumonia.

Congenital lobar emphysema

This rare condition may present as respiratory distress soon after birth. Wheezing and cyanosis are often associated, with mediastinal shift away from the affected side. The breath sounds may be diminished over the area of involvement. Chest X-ray shows an overexpanded hyperlucent lobe.

MANAGEMENT

Urgent bronchoscopy is required if the symptoms are severe. If the airway obstruction cannot be readily relieved, lobectomy is indicated.

In the milder case, bronchoscopy may be curative. Lobectomy is not always required as the abnormal lobe represents a progressively diminishing percentage of the total lung volume with increasing lung growth.

Pulmonary haemorrhage

see ***pages 215 and 251***

Congenital lung cysts

These very rare malformations may occur as solitary or multiple lesions. Peripheral cysts are more common than the central bronchogenic cysts. They may present with wheezing and stridor, especially during crying when the cysts tend to distend. Another presentation is a picture very similar to lobar emphysema due to partial bronchial obstruction and air-trapping.

MANAGEMENT

Cysts causing respiratory symptoms should be resected urgently. Even asymptomatic cysts should probably be resected because of the possibility of enlargement, compression of normal lung or infection.

Extra-pulmonary causes of respiratory distress

Diaphragmatic hernia

This results from a defect in the pleuroperitoneal canal. The left side is most commonly affected.

RECOGNITION

The onset of symptoms depends on the amount of abdominal viscera in the chest and the degree of pulmonary hypoplasia. The most severely affected infants present with signs of neonatal asphyxia. The clue to diagnosis is a shift of the apex beat to the right, with diminished or absent breath sounds over the left chest. The abdomen may be scaphoid because of displacement of the bowel.

Less severely affected babies present with signs of respiratory distress especially with feeding. The presence on chest X-ray of gas-filled bowel shadows in the hemithorax confirms the diagnosis. However, even though the infant has developed symptoms, a chest X-ray taken within a few hours of birth may show a uniformly opaque hemithorax because air has not yet filled the bowel; under these circumstances the apex beat will not yet be displaced.

MANAGEMENT

The severely affected infant should be resuscitated using endotracheal intubation and IPPV. FACE MASK VENTILATION IS ABSOLUTELY CONTRAINDICATED as it is likely to produce increasing gaseous distension of the stomach and intestine. The stomach should be kept deflated by a nasogastric tube with free drainage.

Traditionally, immediate surgical closure of the defect has been advocated. Recently, some centres have delayed surgery while attempting to improve the baby's condition. Postoperative ventilation is almost invariably required. Vasodilators such as tolazoline may be helpful in preventing the common complication of persistent fetal circulation (PFC).

Tracheo-oesophageal fistula

This diagnosis must be excluded whenever there is a history of polyhydramnios. An 8 FG stiff catheter with a radio-opaque line should be passed down the oesophagus. If it cannot be passed into the stomach, a chest X-ray with the catheter *in situ* will show the lower end of the pouch.

The infant produces copious oral secretions which provides a further important diagnostic sign. If the condition remains undetected, the first feed produces choking, cyanosis, and often aspiration.

The rare H-type fistula may require a cine-swallow or endoscopy to reveal the diagnosis.

MANAGEMENT

The treatment is surgical. While awaiting surgery, the saliva should be aspirated using a Replogle tube. If possible a primary repair is performed. In some cases a gastrostomy may be required before definitive surgery.

Phrenic nerve palsy

A traumatic delivery is the usual cause of this disorder (*see also* page 621).

RECOGNITION

Phrenic nerve palsy is usually associated with a brachial paralysis (Erb's palsy). The baby presents with signs of respiratory distress and sometimes apnoeic attacks. Chest X-ray shows elevation of the affected diaphragm, and screening will demonstrate paradoxical diaphragmatic movement on the affected side.

MANAGEMENT

Most infants require no treatment. The severely affected infant may require IPPV. Occasionally, plication of the diaphragm may be required.

Non-respiratory causes of respiratory distress

Cardiovascular

CYANOTIC CONGENITAL HEART DISEASE (*see also* Cardiac Emergencies, page 263)

Cyanotic congenital heart disease can usually be differentiated from HMD. This is particularly true in a term baby with transposition of the great vessels in whom there may be a murmur with well-expanded lungs on chest X-ray. The presence of cardiac failure may make the distinction much more difficult. A nitrogen wash-out test (*see* page 261) is usually helpful, although HMD complicated by persistent fetal circulation (*see below*) may produce a very small rise in PaO_2.

PERSISTENT FETAL CIRCULATION (PFC) (PERSISTENT PULMONARYHYPERTENSION OF THE NEWBORN) (*see also* page 259)

This may occur in the absence of any pulmonary disorder. Usually, however, PFC is associated with another disorder, such as HMD, meconium aspiration, diaphragmatic hernia, or severe perinatal asphyxia. The cause is a failure of the pulmonary vascular resistance to fall. As a result there is pulmonary hypertension and right-to-left shunting through the foramen ovale and ductus arteriosus.

Recognition
The presentation may be indistinguishable from certain forms of congenital heart disease or severe pulmonary disease such as Group B streptococcal pneumonia. There is a severe hypoxia which is not correctable with 100% oxygen. Cardiac ultrasound is helpful in excluding a structural heart lesion and in demonstrating a right-to-left intracardiac shunt at atrial level by observing microbubbles produced by a 2 ml injection of intravenous saline.

Management
Ideally one should aim at prevention, by avoidance of intra-partum or postnatal asphyxia.

1. *Ventilatory support.* A period of mechanical ventilation is nearly always required for this condition. Initially, hyperventilation with respiratory rates of

100–120 per min may help to lower the $PaCO_2$ and correct an acidosis. The aim should be to maintain a PaO_2 above 10 kPa (75 mm Hg) and a $PaCO_2$ below 3 kPa (22.5 mm Hg). Paralysis with pancuronium or curare may facilitate ventilation; furthermore, the resulting histamine release may lead to pulmonary vasodilatation.

2. *Pulmonary vasodilators.* If hyperventilation fails to improve the shunting, a pulmonary vasodilator may be of help. Tolazoline is the most commonly used agent. Unfortunately, it also produces systemic vasodilatation, and therefore continuous measurement of the arterial blood pressure is essential while giving the drug. The drug is normally given as a bolus of 1–2 mg/kg, followed by an infusion of 1–2 mg/kg/hour if a response is achieved. Hypotension should be treated by an infusion of plasma.

   Nitroprusside and prostacyclin have also been used although there are few controlled studies.
3. *Blood loss* (*see also* page 671). Overt blood loss (from a haemorrhage) or inapparent blood loss (from a feto-maternal or twin–twin transfusion) may present as respiratory distress. Correction of circulatory failure and anaemia usually leads to prompt resolution of the respiratory distress.

Neurological causes

Severe perinatal asphyxia, cerebral trauma, and intracranial haemorrhage are frequently associated with signs of respiratory distress. The diagnosis is usually obvious, both from the history (fetal distress, difficult instrumental delivery, low Apgar score) and from the examination (hypotonia, absent primitive reflexes, and convulsions). Treatment is directed towards the intracranial cause.

Metabolic causes

Hypoglycaemia, hypothermia, and acidosis may each cause signs of respiratory distress. Treatment is that of the underlying disorder.

Bleeding from the upper airway and haemoptysis

Massive pulmonary haemorrhage (*see also* page 215)

No complete explanation has been found for this, which occurs particularly in small-for-dates low birthweight infants. It may be an extreme form of pulmonary oedema secondary to hypoxia.

RECOGNITION

The affected infant usually deteriorates rapidly, with signs of increasing respiratory distress leading to cyanosis, bradycardia, and hypotension. Bright red, frothy blood is seen issuing from the trachea or up an endotracheal tube. Chest X-ray shows changes ranging from diffuse granularity to patchy or widespread opacities.

MANAGEMENT

Rapid progression of the condition frequently precludes any effective therapy and treatment is largely supportive to provide adequate oxygenation using mechanical ventilation. Positive end-expiratory pressure seems to limit further bleeding. Correction of anaemia and any coagulation defect is also of benefit. Antibiotic therapy (penicillin, gentamicin and cloxacillin) is indicated if associated infection is a possibility.

Staphylococcal pneumonia

This may mimic massive pulmonary haemorrhage. A history of staphylococcal skin sepsis may precede the onset of respiratory symptoms. Treatment is with cloxacillin and gentamicin.

Intrathoracic gastrogenous cyst

This form of neurenteric cyst may ulcerate and rupture into a bronchus causing haemorrhage and haemoptysis. Technetium scanning is a useful diagnostic procedure as the isotope is taken up by the gastric mucosa lining the cyst. Treatment is by surgical removal.

Apnoea

The high incidence and serious consequences of apnoeic attacks make this one of the most important of neonatal respiratory emergencies.

Recognition

APNOEA OF PREMATURITY

Although this is the commonest cause of neonatal apnoea it is essentially a diagnosis by exclusion. The apnoeic attacks are a consequence of immaturity of the respiratory centre. Nevertheless, the attacks do not usually commence until the baby is 48–72 hours old. Between attacks the babies appear to be quite well. They usually cease spontaneously once the baby has reached 2 kg or the equivalent of 36 weeks gestation.

SECONDARY APNOEA

Apnoeic attacks are frequently symptomatic of some other disorder in the neonate. These are as follows:

Infection
Any severe infection may precipitate apnoea, e.g. urinary tract infection, pneumonia, meningitis, or septicaemia. Apnoea complicating actual or apparent HMD should always raise the possibility of a Group B streptococcal pneumonia.

Biochemical disturbance
Hypoglycaemia, hypocalcaemia, and hypo- or hypernatraemia may present as apnoea. Hyperbilirubinaemia also predisposes to apnoeic attacks, although the combination of apnoea and jaundice is suggestive of sepsis.

CNS disorders
Intracranial haemorrhage, asphyxial or traumatic CNS damage may all be associated with apnoea. There are usually other signs of neurological disturbance such as abnormality of tone and absence of the primitive reflexes. Convulsions may present as recurrent apnoea.

Gastro-oesophageal reflux
Some studies have demonstrated an association between gastro-oesophageal reflux and apnoea (Herbst, Minton and Book, 1979). Nevertheless, the presence of milk in the nasopharynx is probably secondary to the apnoeic attack rather than its cause.

Management

All babies at risk of developing apnoeic attacks should have continuous monitoring of respiration. The machine should give an audible alarm after 15 or 20 seconds of apnoea. Additionally, there should be a continuous record of the heart rate, as obstructive apnoea will not be associated with an absent respiratory effect, but promptly produces a profound bradycardia.

ENVIRONMENTAL TEMPERATURE

Maintenance of incubator temperature at the lower end of the neonatal thermal environment is said to reduce the frequency of apnoeic attacks.

OXYGEN

A small increase in FiO_2 to 0.25–0.3 (25–30%) may produce a marked reduction in the frequency of apneoic attacks. *In the very preterm baby who has normal gas transfer this therapy carries with it a considerable risk of retrolental fibroplasia.* The FiO_2 must be continuously monitored, although there is no 'safe' level of inspired oxygen. Therefore the PaO_2 and $TcPO_2$ should also be monitored in order to avoid hyperoxia.

METHYLXANTHINES

Intravenous aminophylline (loading dose of 6 mg/kg followed by 4 mg/kg/day in three divided doses) or oral theophylline (4 mg/kg/day) are both effective in reducing the number of apnoeic attacks. As the half-life of the methylxanthines is variable, it is important to monitor blood levels, aiming for a level of 5–15 μg/ml. Alternatively, caffeine citrate with a loading dose of 10 mg/kg followed by a daily dose of 2.5 mg/kg/day (Aranda *et al.*, 1979) aiming to achieve a level of 5–20 μg/ml is also effective.

CONTINUOUS POSITIVE AIRWAY PRESSURE (CPAP)

CPAP delivered by a nasal prong also reduces the frequency of apnoea. A pressure of 2–5 cm H_20 is usually sufficient to abolish apnoea.

VENTILATION

If all else fails the infant must be ventilated. As the lungs are normal, low peak airway pressure can be used (12–14 cm H_20). Inspiratory time should be limited to less than 1 second. It is frequently possible to ventilate at rates as low as 5–10 per minute (slow Intermittent Mandatory Ventilation, IMV). Nasal prong ventilation may avoid the risks of endotracheal intubation.

Upper airway obstruction

See also Nasal and Nasopharyngeal Obstruction (Chapter 81)

Choanal atresia

This is caused by a partial or complete failure of canalization of the posterior nares. Complete obstruction presents with severe respiratory distress from birth, although the infant is able to cry normally. In partial obstruction, symptoms may only be apparent during feeding. For further details of recognition and management *see* page 669.

Pierre–Robin syndrome

Associated with micrognathia and cleft palate is the tendency of the tongue to obstruct the nasopharynx and oropharynx (glossoptosis).

MANAGEMENT

The upper airway obstruction may be relieved by nursing the baby face down so that gravity displaces the tongue forward. If the baby continues to show signs of respiratory distress and cyanosis or fails to thrive, the obstruction may be bypassed using a long nasopharyngeal prong. Occasionally, tracheostomy may be required. The problem gradually improves spontaneously with the growth of the mandible.

Neonatal stridor (see also **Chapter 80***)*

Neonatal stridor may be caused by compression of the upper airway or by intrabronchial occlusion of the airway.

Causes of airway compression include vascular rings and tumours. Intrabronchial occlusion of the airway may be due to a subglottic haemangioma (often associated with cutaneous cavernous haemangiomata) or a laryngeal web. Laryngeal spasm may accompany hypocalcaemic tetany or convulsions.

A relatively common cause of neonatal stridor is laryngomalacia or floppy larynx. Subglottic stenosis is fortunately a rare complication of prolonged endotracheal intubation. The diagnosis is made by direct laryngoscopy.

MANAGEMENT

Floppy larynx requires no treatment. Other causes of mechanical obstruction should be dealt with surgically. Occasionally, careful tracheal dilatation may be possible. Laryngeal webs and haemangioma usually require a tracheostomy followed by surgical excision of the lesion.

Vocal cord paralysis

See page 668.

References

ARANDA, J. V., COOK, C. E., GORMAN, W., *et al.* (1979) Pharmacokinetic profile of caffeine in the premature newborn infant with apnea. *Journal of Pediatrics,* **94,** 663–668

FUJIWARA, T., CHIDA, S., WATABE, Y., MAETA, H., MORITA, T. and ABE, T. (1980) Artificial surfactant therapy in hyaline-membrane disease. *Lancet,* **i,** 55–59

HERBST, J. J., MINTON, S. D. and BOOK, L. S. (1979) Gastroesophageal reflux causing respiratory distress and apnoea in newborn infants. *Journal of Pediatrics,* **95,** 763–768

LENNEY, W. and MILNER, A. D. (1978) At what age do bronchodilator drugs work? *Archives of Disease in Childhood,* **53,** 532–535

LEVENE, M. I., FAWER, C-L. and LAMONT, R. F. (1982) Risk factors in the development of intraventricular haemorrhage in the preterm neonate. *Archives of Disease in Childhood,* **57,** 410–417

MANROE, B. L., WEINBERG, A. G., ROSENFELD, C. R. and BROWNE, R. (1979) The neonatal blood count in health and disease. Reference values for neutrophilic cells. *Journal of Pediatrics,* **95,** 89–98

MARCHAK, B. E., THOMPSON, W. K., DUFFTY, P., *et al.* (1981) Treatment of RDS by high-frequency oscillatory ventilation: A preliminary report. *Journal of Pediatrics,* **99,** 287–292

NG, K. P. K. and EASA, D. (1979) Management of interstitial emphysema by high-frequency low positive-pressure hand ventilation in the neonate. *Journal of Pediatrics,* **95,** 117–118

Further reading

AVERY, M. E., FLETCHER, B. D. and WILLIAMS, R. G. (1981) The lung and its disorders in the newborn infant. London: W. Saunders

PHELAN, P. D., LANDAU, L. I. and OLINSKY, A. (1982) *Respiratory Illness in Children* (2nd ed.). Oxford: Blackwell Scientific Publications

Part VI

Cardiac Emergencies

Chapter 24

Cardiac emergencies

James L. Wilkinson

Perinatal cardiac emergencies

First 24 hours

Cyanosis

Cyanosis in the first few hours of life may be due to a wide variety of conditions. As a general rule non-cardiac causes considerably outnumber cardiac causes at this age. The importance of looking for and, if possible, identifying the cause cannot be overstressed, however. For non-cardiac causes of cyanosis in the newborn, *see* pages 665–666.

'PERSISTENT FETAL CIRCULATION' (PERSISTENT PULMONARY HYPERTENSION) (*see also* page 250)

Occasionally, an infant with no apparent other disease, respiratory or otherwise, may show severe central cyanosis due to persistent right–left shunting via the foramen ovale and the ductus. The condition may be difficult to distinguish from cyanotic heart disease, without cardiological investigation. The same physiological disturbance is frequently seen in infants with respiratory or neurological problems and is probably the reason why they may appear to have cyanosis out of proportion to their degree of respiratory distress.

Investigations should include a hyperoxia test (*see* page 261) and, in cases where doubt persists, two-dimensional echocardiography. Cardiac catheterization is now rarely needed.

Treatment involves correction of acidosis, nursing in increased oxygen in an incubator and in some cases positive pressure ventilation or use of CPAP. If cyanosis and hypoxia are severe the use of vasodilators such as tolazoline or prostaglandin E may be beneficial in lowering pulmonary resistance and pressure, though in some infants systemic hypotension may contraindicate such therapy and dopamine infusion may be considered as an alternative.

Prognosis is variable. Some infants recover completely over a few days while others become progressively more hypoxic and acidotic and deteriorate steadily despite treatment.

Cardiac failure

Obvious cardiac failure, which is apparent from birth or within the first few hours is rare. The commoner non-cardiac causes include severe haemolytic disease of the newborn or intrapartum fetal haemorrhage. Cardiac causes are discussed under 'first week' (*see* below). Treatment depends upon the cause which must be identified urgently. Diuretics and digitalization play an important secondary role, immediate transfusion or exchange transfusion being necessary in appropriate cases.

Heart block

Congenital heart block is discussed under 'arrhythmias'. It is unusual for an infant with isolated congenital heart block to develop severe symptoms in the first few days of life but any infant with evidence of coexisting cardiac defect or developing heart failure should be referred immediately to a cardiac centre.

First week

Cyanosis

Cyanosis persisting beyond 24 hours or appearing after the first day of life, in the absence of other apparent cause (*see* above), is likely to be due to cardiac disease. The commoner conditions which present with cyanosis include:

1. Transposition of the great arteries.
2. Pulmonary atresia.
3. Tricuspid atresia.
4. Total anomalous pulmonary venous return.

The assessment of the infant with suspected heart disease is discussed below.

Cardiac failure

Development of cardiac failure at this age is usually due to severe congenital heart disease. An important early sign is failure of the infant to lose weight in the first few days of life, or even gain weight from birth. Cardiac failure may develop in babies with non-cardiac problems such as respiratory distress syndrome or severe infection, particularly septicaemia.

The cardiac conditions presenting at this age include:

1. Hypoplastic left heart syndrome.
2. Persistent ductus arteriosus of prematurity.
3. Infantile coarctation syndrome.
4. Complex anomalies.

Cyanosis with heart failure

The development of both cyanosis and evidence of cardiac failure in the first week of life is almost always due to severe congenital heart disease such as:

1. Transposition of the great arteries.
2. Total anomalous pulmonary venous return.
3. Complex anomalies.

Emergency assessment

The emergency assessment of infants with suspected congenital heart disease should include the following investigations.

Chest X-ray

For evidence of cardiac enlargement, abnormal cardiac shape or position, pulmonary plethora or oligaemia, etc.

ECG

For abnormalities of rate or rhythm, atrial or ventricular hypertrophy.

Electrolytes

Especially calcium and glucose.

Blood gas analysis

Estimation of pH, PCO_2, standard bicarbonate, and base deficit on arterial or capillary blood and estimation of arterial PO_2 in cyanosed patients (*see* below).

Hyperoxia test (cyanosed infants)

If significant cyanosis is present this is a useful test and helps to distinguish between cyanosis due to cardiac disease and that due to non-cardiac problems.

Arterial oxyten tension (PO_2) is measured either transcutaneously (TcO_2) or from an arterial sample. The latter should be obtained from the right radial artery, as this eliminates desaturation due to persistent right–left ductal shunting, and if a transcutaneous probe is used this should be placed on the right upper chest for the same reason. A sample should be taken at rest while the infant is breathing air or 30% O_2. The infant is then nursed in a headbox in 100% O_2 (or as close to 100% as can be obtained) for 20 minutes and the sample is repeated. Failure of the PO_2 to rise above 13 kPa (100 mm Hg) on this test is strongly indicative of cyanotic heart disease. In most infants with non-cyanotic heart defects or respiratory disease the level will rise in excess of 20 kPa (150 mm Hg) (Jones *et al.*, 1976).

If the infant is ventilating poorly due to neurological disease or severe respiratory problems the test may be carried out with the infant intubated and hand-ventilated with 100% O_2.

A cruder method of performing this test is to observe the baby's colour without taking arterial samples. If the degree of cyanosis diminishes very markedly in high O_2 concentration it is unlikely that the cyanosis is due to cardiac disease.

When these investigations have been done a decision should be made whether the infant should be referred for specialized cardiological assessment. At the same time emergency treatment should be commenced if indicated.

Emergency treatment may include:

1. Diuretics if cardiac failure is present.
2. Digoxin; again if cardiac failure is present.
3. Intravenous fluids; in sick infants, but keep volume low ($\simeq$60 ml/kg/24 hours).

Prostaglandin therapy

Institution of prostaglandin therapy should be considered in those severely cyanotic neonates who are likely to have a ductus-dependent pulmonary circulation. It may also be considered in neonates presenting in severe and rapidly progressive congestive cardiac failure and who are thought on clinical grounds to have hypoplastic left heart syndrome or coarctation of the aorta (with ductus-dependent systemic circulation) (*see* page 266).

Correction of metabolic acidosis

See pages 118–200.

Correction of hypocalcaemia with oral or intravenous calcium gluconate

See page 136 for dosage and dangers of IV calcium gluconate.

Correction of hypoglycaemia with intravenous glucose

See page 462.

Persistent ductus arteriosus of prematurity

The small premature infant (less than 1500 g) is prone to show signs of a persistent ductus arteriosus in the early weeks of life. In many cases the infant will have evidence of cardiorespiratory distress and such signs, in conjunction with bounding pulses and a precordial or basal systolic or continuous murmur, are highly suggestive of a significant ductus.

Initial management should include diuretic therapy (but probably avoiding frusemide – *see* page 264), and fluid restriction. If cardiorespiratory distress persists indomethacin should be given in a dose of 0.1 mg/kg intravenously (or orally). If signs of a significant ductus still persist the dose may be repeated 8 hourly to a total of three doses. Indomethacin is most effective when given in the first 7–10 days of life, but is probably best avoided in asymptomatic infants and in those where symptoms can be controlled effectively by fluid restriction and diuretic therapy (Gersony *et al.*, 1983).

Infants who are in severe cardiorespiratory difficulties and in whom symptoms fail to improve after appropriate treatment, including indomethacin, present a difficult therapeutic problem. These patients, especially if ventilator dependent and where attempts to wean from respiratory support are unsuccessful, will usually require urgent surgical ligation of their ductus.

Indications for referral to a special unit

Cyanotic infants

Cyanotic babies require immediate referral for cardiological assessment if there is other evidence of cardiac disease (abnormal X-ray, ECG or presence of loud murmur, etc.) or if the hyperoxia test fails to raise the arterial PO_2 above 13 kPa (100 mm Hg).

Acyanotic infants

Babies without cyanosis but with evidence of heart disease (other than premature infants with signs of a persistent ductus arteriosus) require urgent referral if evidence of cardiac failure appears or if the femoral pulses are reduced or absent, whether or not cardiac failure is present.

If a decision is made to transfer a baby to a cardiac unit, it is important to ensure that the parents are informed of the reasons for transfer and the gravity of the situation. If one or both parents is not accompanying the child, consent for cardiac catheterization and possible Rashkind septostomy should be obtained at the referring hospital and a signed consent form should accompany the referral letter, notes and X-rays, which should, if possible, accompany the patient.

Cardiac failure

Causes

The commoner conditions, which may lead to cardiac failure, vary at different ages. The following list contains some of the commoner diseases or abnormalities which are likely to present with heart failure in each age group.

First 2 weeks:
- Hypoplastic left heart syndrome.
- Persistent ductus of prematurity.
- Coarctation of the aorta.
- Complex anomalies.
- Neonatal myocarditis.

2–4 weeks:
- Coarctation of the aorta.
- Complex anomalies.
- Ventricular septal defect.

4–12 weeks:
- Ventricular septal defect (large).
- Persistent ductus arteriosus (large).
- Coarctation.

3–12 months:
- Onset of failure less common. May occur in many defects; often precipitated by superimposed chest infection. May be due to acquired heart disease (*see* below).

After 12 months:
- Myocarditis (rheumatic or non-rheumatic). (Acute rheumatism and new cases of rheumatic carditis are now relatively uncommon in Western countries.)
- Bacterial endocarditis.
- Rheumatic carditis.
- Terminal feature of complex congenital heart lesions.

Recognition

The main symptoms in infants are respiratory, with dyspnoea on feeding or at rest, and tachycardia. Physical signs include tachycardia, tachypnoea, intercostal and subcostal recession, Harrison's sulci and hepatomegaly. Peripheral oedema, in infancy, is usually mild and easily overlooked. Such oedema, if present, is best seen over the dorsum of hands and feet and in the periorbital areas. It is usually non-pitting and can be mistaken for subcutaneous fat. Crepitations in the lung fields are a late manifestation, and may be due to superimposed infection. Longstanding heart failure is frequently associated with failure to thrive and an abnormal tendency to chest infections. In the first week of life cardiac failure may cause an early increase in weight, the expected initial drop failing to occur. This should always raise suspicion of cardiac disease.

Acute distension of the liver, also due to cardiac failure, may mimic an acute abdominal emergency.

Management

Diuretics (Table 24.1)

In severe heart failure in infancy the first choice diuretic should usually be frusemide, though recent work suggests that this drug promotes prostaglandin release and may inhibit ductal constriction in the newborn period, and for this reason frusemide should probably not be used as the diuretic of first choice in premature infants with suspected persistent ductus arteriosus (Green *et al.*, 1983). In other circumstances frusemide may be given initially intramuscularly in a dose of 1–1.5 mg/kg (up to 5 mg). The child should have a urine bag on and may be weighed before and 4 hours after the dose. If an inadequate diuresis is obtained further doses may be given, increasing the amount by 1–2 mg at each injection. Frusemide may be given intravenously but the initial dose should not exceed 1 mg/kg, as a very rapid diuresis may occur.

Maintenance oral diuretics should be started as soon as the infant's condition is improving.

In children over a year initial intramuscular frusemide should be given in a dose of 5–10 mg. Even quite large children may have a good diuresis on doses of 5 or 6 mg, so it is safer to start with a relatively small dose and repeat with increasing amounts of drug at 4 hourly intervals if the response is poor.

In less severe cardiac failure chlorothiazide is a satisfactory alternative to frusemide.

When administering loop diuretics, such as frusemide or chlorothiazide, over a prolonged period, it is important to prevent the development of potassium depletion, by giving potassium supplements (e.g. potassium chloride 50 mg/kg every 6 hours), or by adding a potassium retaining diuretic such as amiloride or spironolactone.

Table 24.1 Oral diuretic doses in infancy: to be given once or twice daily

Drug	*Initial dose* (mg/kg)	*Increased dose if ineffective* (mg/kg)
Chlorothiazide	25	40–50
Frusemide	2	4–6
Amiloride (given *with* another diuretic)	0.2	–

Digitalization (Table 24.2)

The role of digitalis, in the treatment of heart failure, has been changing in recent years. Most cardiologists now consider that diuretic therapy is of much greater importance and that digitalis should be used with caution, if at all.

While it is traditional to commence treatment by 'digitalization' it should be appreciated that the main purpose of this in earlier times was to provoke a diuresis fairly quickly. As the diuresis is now induced by specific diuretic drugs, it is doubtful whether traditional 'digitalization' is essential and it is undoubtedly safer to commence treatment with maintenance doses and allow the effect to develop over several days.

Various dosage regimens are used and there is little agreement between different units. In general infants tolerate higher doses, weight for weight, than older children and adults.

Table 24.2 Suggested doses of digoxin

Weight (kg)	*24 hr digitalizing dose* (mg/kg)		*24 hr maintenance* (mg/kg)	
	Oral	*i.m.*	*Oral*	*i.m.*
0–7	0.06	0.04	0.015	0.01
Above 8	0.04	0.03	0.01	0.005

The digitalizing dose may be given in three or four equal parts at 6 or 8 hourly intervals. In sick infants rapid digitalization by the intramuscular route may be employed. In less severe situations oral digitalization is to be preferred unless the child is vomiting.

In small premature babies and in newborns, who often tolerate digoxin less well than more mature infants, the doses should be reduced to two-thirds of those recommended above.

DIGITALIS INTOXICATION

The development of persistent bradycardia, A-V dissociation or ectopic beats, are indications to stop digoxin for 24–48 hours and, if possible, to obtain an estimation of digoxin level. Vomiting should be regarded with suspicion in a child on digoxin and if repeated or unattributable to other causes, the dose of digoxin should be reduced and a digoxin level performed if possible.

In any child, where digitalis toxicity is suspected, the serum potassium should be checked and, if low, oral potassium supplements should be given.

Other measures

OXYGEN

Sick infants in heart failure should be nursed in an incubator or a tent in 30% O_2.

HUMIDIFICATION

Adequate humidification prevents drying out of respiratory secretions and reduces insensible fluid loss. It is desirable for small infants nursed in incubators and should also be used when a larger child is nursed in a tent.

SEDATION

Sedation is desirable if the child is distressed or agitated. Chloral hydrate may be adequate as an initial measure but if more regular sedation is required trimeprazine or promethazine are preferable. For doses *see* pages 832 (trimeprazine) and 828 (promethazine). The severely ill child may benefit from a single dose of morphine (*see* below; pulmonary oedema).

POSITION

The infant is best nursed head up. This may easily be achieved by tipping the incubator tray. Older infants may be nursed in a chair inside a tent.

FEEDING

Small, frequent feeds are better tolerated than large ones. A total fluid intake of 150 ml per kg should not be exceeded and a lower intake (120 ml per kg) is desirable in the severely ill infant until failure is controlled. If the child is vomiting, reduced strength feeds or clear fluids may be better tolerated. Low sodium milk is not necessary with current diuretics.

Severe congestive cardiac failure in the early newborn period

Severe or rapidly progressive congestive failure appearing in the first 2 weeks of life is a common feature of infants with hypoplastic left heart syndrome or coarctation of the aorta. While the former condition is not amenable to surgery, it is always important to establish the diagnosis with certainty (usually by cross-sectional echocardiography) before abandoning vigorous treatment. In both conditions, lower limb pulses are usually obviously reduced or absent at the time of presentation with cardiac failure (though they may have been palpable in the early neonatal period). In hypoplastic left heart syndrome upper limb pulses are also weak or impalpable, while in coarctation, the right arm pulse (and often the left arm pulse) is usually easily felt and a discrepancy between upper and lower limbs is obvious. In such infants, the lower segment of the systemic circulation (and in hypoplastic left heart syndrome the upper segment as well) is to some extent ductus dependent and increasing symptoms are related to closure of the ductus in the early days of life. For this reason, in those infants where manifestations of congestive failure do not respond quickly to diuretic therapy (and especially where severe oliguria or anuria persist) institution of prostaglandin therapy is desirable. Prostaglandin E_1 should be administered by an intravenous infusion using a motorized syringe pump and in an initial dose of 100 ng/kg/min dropping to 10–20 ng/kg/min after half an hour. Complications of prostaglandin therapy include pyrexia, hypotension and apnoeic attacks. In infants whose condition still remains critical, additional measures may be required including ventilatory support, correction of metabolic acidosis, and infusion of an inotropic agent such as dopamine 5 μg/kg/min (by motorized syringe pump).

Pulmonary oedema

Frank pulmonary oedema is a relatively uncommon problem in paediatric practice. It may develop in infants and children with severe untreated heart failure due to the previously listed conditions. Characteristically it occurs in lesions associated with severe pulmonary venous obstruction, such as the hypoplastic left heart syndrome and some cases of total anomalous pulmonary venous return. In older children it may be seen in association with severe carditis, either rheumatic or non-rheumatic and is most often seen after major surgery. Occasionally severe fluid overload due to excessive transfusion or large volumes of IV fluids may, in a sick child, produce pulmonary oedema, even in the absence of underlying heart disease.

Recognition

Increasing dypsnoea with marked intercostal and subcostal recession and crepitations in the lung fields are the clinical signs of developing pulmonary oedema. Tachycardia, increasing cyanosis and rising PCO_2 are usually present. The diagnosis is confirmed by the chest X-ray appearance of diffuse hazy shadowing with marked perihilar opacifications and upper lobe venous distension. Differentiation from diffuse bronchopneumonia may be difficult.

Management

Intramuscular frusemide (1.5 mg/kg: up to 6 mg) should be given on diagnosis and digitalization commenced if the child is not on digoxin already (*see* previous section). The child should be sedated with morphine (0.2 mg/kg) and nursed in 30% O_2 sitting up in a chair or tilted head up in an incubator. Antibiotics should usually be given, even if no definite evidence of infection exists, as infection is a common precipitating factor. An intravenous infusion should be commenced so that a ready route for administration of drugs is available, but the rate of infusion must be carefully controlled to prevent further fluid overload, and should not exceed 60 ml per kg per 24 hours until the situation is under control.

If the situation is deteriorating or the PCO_2 exceeds 12 kPa (90 mm Hg) positive pressure ventilation should be considered and is the simplest and surest method of controlling severe pulmonary oedema.

Venesection may be tried if the above measures fail, but should not be necessary unless facilities for positive pressure ventilation are not available. Up to 10 ml per kg of blood may be removed by aspirating blood via a tap connected between the IV infusion tubing and the intravenous cannula. Insertion of a central venous line makes removal of blood much easier.

Cyanosis and cyanotic attacks

Cyanosis in the newborn period

Rapidly progressive cyanosis in the early newborn period is a feature of infants with transposition of the great arteries or with cyanotic defects associated with low pulmonary blood flow (e.g. pulmonary atresia). In most such infants worsening cyanosis is related to gradual closure of the ductus arteriosus in the early days of life. This can be halted or reversed by therapy with intravenous or oral prostaglandin (E_1 or E_2). Oral prostaglandins may be given in a dose of 62.5 μg hourly initially. Intravenous prostaglandins should be given by a motorized syringe pump to maintain constancy of rate and the initial dose should be 50–100 ng/kg/min reducing to 10–20 ng/kg/min after half an hour. Complications of prostaglandin therapy include pyrexia, hypotension, and apnoeic attacks. The latter may be of sufficient severity to require positive pressure ventilation, but are rare if the dose is kept to 20 ng/kg/min or lower.

Prostaglandin therapy in cyanotic infants with ductus-dependent pulmonary circulation is an effective short-term palliative measure. It should be considered in any severely cyanotic and hypoxic neonate, especially if his condition is deteriorating and acidosis is present or developing (*see* emergency treatment of neonate with heart disease, page 266).

Cyanosis and cyanotic attacks in later infancy and childhood

The cyanosed infant is prone to develop several complications which may need urgent treatment and which can often be prevented if foreseen in time.

Acidosis

Severe hypoxia with cyanosis frequently leads to the development of a metabolic acidosis. If this results in the blood pH falling below 7.2 or the base deficit exceeding 10 mmol per litre this indicates severe hypoxia requiring urgent treatment.

Any child with severe cyanosis should have an estimation of his blood gases to assess the degree of acidosis resulting from hypoxia. Capillary blood gives satisfactory values in most cases.

Correction of acidosis, in severe cases, is best achieved by intravenous sodium bicarbonate according to the standard formula (*see* page 119).

In milder degree of acidosis, bicarbonate (8.4%) may be given orally or by nasogastric tube in a dose of 1–2 ml per kg. The dose may be repeated at ½ hourly intervals until adequate correction has been achieved.

In any infant, with cyanotic heart disease, who becomes severely acidotic it is important to seek and treat any precipitating cause (e.g. infection, dehydration, etc.). If acidosis persists or recurs despite adequate treatment then urgent consideration should be given to the need for surgery to relieve the hypoxia (e.g. palliative systemic–pulmonary shunt or balloon atrial septostomy).

Polycythaemia

Secondary polycythaemia in the cyanotic child is an important cause of cerebral vascular thrombosis and resulting cerebral infarction or death. Such catastrophies occur if dehydration becomes superimposed, as may occur in febrile illnesses of any kind in which fluid loss is increased and intake reduced. Maintenance of an adequate fluid intake is therefore of vital importance to the cyanosed child who has a febrile illness. If oral fluids (by mouth or nasogastric tube) are not tolerated intravenous fluids should be given at a rate of 100–150 ml per kg per 24 hours.

Any cyanosed and polycythaemic child, who is having his oral fluids restricted before surgery or dental extractions, should have intravenous fluids to prevent dehydration.

Cyanotic attacks (hypoxic 'spells')

Severe cyanotic attacks, sometimes leading to loss of consciousness, are a characteristic feature of Fallot's tetralogy, but may ocur with other cyanotic lesions.

Attacks are usually precipitated by exertion, feeding or crying, although intercurrent infection and dehydration may play a part. The attacks are extremely distressing to the child, who usually becomes increasingly agitated until consciousness is lost. Continued crying and struggling tend to worsen the attack.

Management

The first-aid treatment of the attack is to quieten the child and stop him crying. This may often be achieved, if attempted early in the episode, by picking him up, cradling and soothing him. Failing this, or if the attack is already well established, morphine 0.2 mg/kg i.m. should be given. Nursing in the knee–chest position may be helpful. (This is equivalent to the squatting position adopted by the older child.) Oxygen (100%) may be given by face mask, but as the benefit achieved by this is slight, there is little to be gained by persisting with it if the face mask causes further distress, which may in itself prolong the attack.

Severe acidosis may develop during the attack, requiring correction by sodium bicarbonate. In most cases, however, acidosis will resolve spontaneously once the attack has been terminated and attempts at intravenous injection (or even blood gas determination by heel prick) may, by distressing the child further, prolong or worsen the attack.

The use of intravenous propranolol or other β-adrenergic blocking drugs in the acute management of cyanotic attacks should only be undertaken by specialized cardiac units, as they can lead to severe myocardial depression. However, in children who have started to experience such attacks it is often possible to reduce both frequency and severity by giving oral propranolol (0.5–1 mg/kg 8 hourly). Such therapy is highly effective in many cases as a short-term expedient to reduce the risk of death or cerebral damage during an attack. None the less, the development of cyanotic attacks is an indication for urgent surgical intervention in most cases, and referral to a specialized unit is then a matter of urgency.

Arrhythmias

Paroxysmal supraventricular tachycardia

In paroxysmal supraventricular tachycardia a severe tachycardia (rate usually between 180 and 300 per min) develops suddenly, and the attack may last from a matter of a minute or two to several days. The paroxysm ends as suddenly as it started, although there may be a period of sinus tachycardia following its cessation. Attacks may recur frequently (even several in a day) or they may subside for months or years with only very occasional bouts. Between episodes the rhythm is usually normal. Some patients only ever have one attack.

Recognition

Older children complain of palpitations and sometimes dizziness or faintness. Abdominal pain or chest pain may also occur. In infants, pallor, dyspnoea, and the development of cardiac failure indicate an attack.

The pulse is very rapid, of small volume, and regular. Cough, dyspnoea and hepatomegaly are signs of developing cardiac failure. The ECG shows a regular tachycardia with a rate of 200–300 per minute. The complexes are usually relatively normal in configuration but P waves are difficult to see.

After cessation of tachycardia the ECG may be normal but in a proportion of cases ventricular pre-excitation is apparent. This may be manifest as Wolff–Parkinson–White syndrome or merely as a short PR interval (Lown–Ganong–Levine syndrome).

Management

It is often worth trying a variety of vagotonic manoeuvres as initial treatment. Traditional measures include carotid sinus massage and eyeball compression but more effective and safer is use of the so-called 'diving response'. This may be evoked by sudden application of an ice bag over the upper face (including the nose) for 15–20 seconds (Bissett, Guam and Kaplan, 1980). A plastic bag containing ice-cold water is suitable for this purpose.

Digitalization with intramuscular digoxin should usually be commenced and will frequently bring about the end of an attack within an hour or two.

If the child is distressed or cardiac failure is developing, rapid termination can usually be achieved with intravenous verapamil. This should be given by slow intravenous injection in a dose of 0.1–0.2 mg/kg over 10 minutes, with continuous electrocardiographic monitoring. The dose may be repeated after half an hour if the attack still persists, though in most cases the episode will terminate during or shortly after the initial injection. There have been reports of prolonged asystole after use of verapamil in the neonatal period (Radford, 1983), but this is unlikely if the drug is given by slow injection rather than as a rapid 'bolus'.

If verapamil is unavailable, and rapid termination of the attack is desired, this may also be achieved by the use of d.c. cardioversion. This is a quick and sure way of stopping the tachycardia but necessitates general anaesethesia or sedation with intravenous diazepam (0.2 mg/kg). The latter, if used, should be given over 2–3 minutes and a further period of 2–3 minutes should be allowed to elapse before application of the shock.

The initial charge used should not exceed 1 j/kg. It is undesirable to use an unsynchronized defibrillator as this can precipitate ventricular fibrillation. However, where synchronization is not available and the situation demands urgent treatment use of a non-synchronized shock may be justifiable.

After the attack the child should usually be maintained on oral digoxin. If bouts are frequent and disabling further antiarrhythmic drugs such as propranolol (0.5–1 mg/kg 8 hourly) may be added, but, in general, failure to control the arrhythmia with digoxin alone usually indicates the need for referral to a specialist cardiac unit.

Heart block

Heart block, in childhood, may be congenital or acquired. If acquired it is usually due to myocarditis or to surgical damage to the conducting pathways.

Congenital heart block is, in the majority of cases, an isolated abnormality, unassociated with other congenital cardiac anomalies. The rate is usually faster than that seen in acquired block; Adams–Stokes attacks are rare and most patients are asymptomatic and require no treatment. When congenital heart block is associated with other cardiac defects, these tend to be complex (e.g. corrected transposition).

Recognition

The slow heart rate, which accelerates inadequately in response to exercise, may cause dyspnoea or dizziness on exertion or even at rest. Cardiac failure seldom develops with uncomplicated congenital heart block unless the rate is below 50 per minute, but may occur when other congenital cardiac defects are also present, or in the course of myocarditis. Loss of consciousness or convulsions occurring due to prolonged periods of asystole or other associated arrhythmias (Adams–Stokes attacks) should be viewed very seriously and indicate the need for urgent artificial pacing.

Physical examination shows a slow, but usually regular, pulse with a rate in infants below 100 per minute and in older children of 40–60 per minute. The pulse is of large volume. The apex is forceful and may be displaced. Cannon waves are frequently seen in the jugular venous pulse. An ejection systolic murmur maximal at the base of the heart is common and is due to the large stroke volume. An apical diastolic murmur or third sound is frequently heard and may also be 'functional'.

Diagnosis

The ECG shows heart block, which is usually complete (third degree). Occasionally second degree block may be seen.

Chest X-ray shows some cardiac enlargement in most cases, even if no other cardiac lesion exists. This results from the large stroke volume.

Management

Treatment is usually only required if heart failure is present or when Adams–Stokes attacks occur.

Cardiac failure should be treated initially with diuretics, digoxin should be withheld unless cardiac failure is severe as it is apt to cause instability of the idioventricular rhythm, which may result in Adams–Stokes attacks. When failure does not respond to diuretics alone, however, digitalization may be carried out cautiously.

Adams–Stokes attacks demand immediate consideration of artificial pacing and this will usually involve transfer to a cardiac unit. Intravenous isoprenaline (1–2 μg/kg) may be given as an emergency measure to restore the cardiac rhythm if asystole is present.

In patients whose rhythm is obviously unstable, and in whom episodes of profound bradycardia or asystole are producing recurrent loss of consciousness, an infusion of isoprenaline at a starting rate of 0.075 μg/kg/min may be commenced, pending placement of a transvenous endocardial pacing catheter.

Sick sinus syndrome

Persistent sinus bradycardia (rate less than 60 per minute) associated with periodic sinus arrest or sinoatrial block and/or short-lived paroxysms of supraventricular tachycardia characterize this syndrome. The condition is rare in childhood but should be remembered as an occasional cause of unexplained syncopal attacks or convulsions.

Recognition

The condition is asymptomatic except for bouts of dizziness or syncope, which may be accompanied by convulsive movements. The attacks occur irregularly with little or no warning. Physical examination during an attack may show severe bradycardia or asystole. Between attacks the pulse is usually slow (50–60 per minute) and may be irregular with runs of very slow rhythm interspersed with short runs of tachycardia.

Diagnosis

The diagnosis depends on the characteristic ECG features of sinus bradycardia with runs of tachycardia and periodic severe slowing. In some cases the rhythm may be normal at rest and the arrhythmia may be evoked by exercise. The ECG should therefore include a long lead II both at rest and after exercise.

Management

Patients who experience dizziness should be encouraged to lie down if symptoms develop or place the head between the knees. Only with recurrent and disabling syncope should insertion of an artificial pacemaker be considered.

Ventricular tachycardia

This sinister arrhythmia is occasionally seen in children with myocarditis, or following surgery. It may rarely be due to digitalis intoxication. The rate may vary between 120 and greater than 300 per minute. When the rate is rapid the cardiac output is severely impaired and consciousness may be lost. There is a very high risk of progression to ventricular fibrillation.

The ECG shows bizarre, wide QRS complexes, and the form of the complexes and the rate may vary.

Management

Immediate cardioversion with d.c. shock is the treatment of choice. Synchronization is desirable, but not essential. If the arrhythmia recurs lignocaine (1 mg/kg) should be given intravenously and the shock repeated. If tachycardia recurs repeatedly or frequent extrasystoles remain after conversion, a continuous infusion of lignocaine at a rate of 1–2 mg/kg/hour may be given, while specialist cardiological advice is sought.

Carditis and pericarditis

Acute myocarditis

Acute myocarditis may be rheumatic or non-rheumatic in aetiology. Rheumatic carditis (now rare in many parts of the world) is usually accompanied by other manifestations of acute rheumatic fever such as arthritis. Viral myocarditis may be preceded or accompanied by other manifestations of viral infection, such as coryzal symptoms, fever or gastrointestinal upset. Non-rheumatic carditis, occurring without clinical or pathological evidence of viral infection, is usually presumed to be viral.

Recognition

Dyspnoea, tachypnoea, tachycardia, and signs of cardiac failure in a previously well child with no known heart defect are the major indications of myocarditis. In rheumatic fever murmurs of mitral or aortic incompetence or an apical mid-diastolic (Carey–Coombs) murmur may appear. A pericardial rub is sometimes heard.

Investigations

Chest X-ray; ECG; Hb; WBC; ESR; blood culture; viral studies; ASO titre; throat and nose swabs.

Recognition

Chest X-ray usually shows generalized cardiac enlargement with pulmonary venous congestion and sometimes pulmonary oedema.

ECG will often show T wave flattening or inversion and reduced voltage of QRS complexes. Conduction defects, such as first degree block (common in rheumatic carditis), bundle branch block, or more severe degrees of block, may occur. Extrasystoles or paroxysmal tachycardia are sometimes seen.

Management

Diuretics and digitalization form the basis of management of cardiac failure (*see* Cardiac Failure). The management of arrhythmias may be difficult but digoxin should not be withheld unless it is likely that the rhythm disturbance is digitalis induced. Patients with myocarditis are, however, more than usually sensitive to digitalis and the development of any arrhythmia in a patient who is fully digitalized should give rise to suspicion of digitalis toxicity.

Bed rest should be enforced in the acute phase of carditis and if necessary the patient may be sedated. In the acutely ill patient, especially if there is evidence of anxiety or pulmonary oedema, morphine (0.2 mg/kg) may be used.

Antibiotics should be given if there is evidence of associated lung infection and in rheumatic carditis penicillin should be given to eliminate any residual streptococcal infection.

Corticosteroids are of little proven value in the treatment of acute carditis except when it is rheumatic in origin (and even then, though the effect may be dramatic at the time, they probably do not influence the long-term outcome). If heart block develops, however, a short course of steroids is probably justified. In infants hydrocortisone 50 mg 6 hourly i.m. or IV is satisfactory. In older children larger doses will be required.

Kawasaki's disease

The development of a picture resembling acute myocarditis during the acute phase (first 2 weeks) of the illness in a patient who has the features and fulfills the diagnostic criteria for acute mucocutaneous lymph node syndrome (Kawasaki's disease) is a rare but serious problem. Such a complication, usually manifested by gallop rhythm, muffled heart sounds and evidence of cardiac failure (which may show features of cardiogenic shock in severe cases) suggests severe coronary angiitis.

Recognition

The diagnosis rests on clinical criteria as no diagnostic test exists. Chest X-ray may show cardiomegaly and pulmonary congestion. The electrocardiographic changes include diminished R wave voltages, flat T waves, prolonged PR or QT intervals and occasionally Q waves or ST segment changes suggestive of myocardial infarction. Definite evidence of coronary angiitis and aneurysm formation is dependent on two-dimensional echocardiography or coronary arteriography, but there is probably no place for the latter, a highly invasive investigation, in the acute phase of the illness. However, in patients who survive the acute stage an aortogram and/or selective coronary arteriograms may be performed with little hazard and may be desirable, at least in those patients who have clear clinical or ECG evidence of cardiac involvement.

Management

During the acute illness all patients should be given aspirin in a dose of 30 mg/kg/day and this should be continued for at least 6 months in patients with evidence of coronary aneurysm formation. *Steroids are contraindicated.* Other measures are supportive e.g. anti-congestive drug therapy. Surgery, such as coronary artery bypass grafting, may be considered in selected patients after the acute illness has subsided and where coronary occlusion has occurred as a late phenomenon, or when symptoms of myocardial ischaemia are present.

Prognosis

Whilst mortality in Kawasaki's disease overall is low (2%), that in patients with coronary artery involvement is considerably increased and those who present with severe myocardial damage and cardiac failure carry a particularly grave outlook. Sudden death may occur during the acute phase of the illness and, rarely, may occur late, after apparent clinical recovery (Yanagihara and Todd, 1980).

Infantile beri-beri

The development of acute congestive cardiac failure in an infant living in an area of the world where gross malnutrition is common should always arouse suspicion of infantile beri-beri. Whilst most such infants are breast fed by thiamine-deficient mothers (who may or may not have signs of beri-beri themselves) some are artificially fed.

Recognition

The infant is usually between 1 and 6 months old and has often appeared well and fed normally until a few days before the onset of cardiac failure. Initial symptoms including vomiting, poor feeding, restlessness, and sometimes drowsiness.

Examination shows evidence of dyspnoea, liver enlargement, tachycardia, and a gallop rhythm. Some oedema may be seen. Later hypotension, peripheral cyanosis and shock supervene.

Non-cardiac findings include hoarseness or aphonia, absent tendon reflexes and, in some cases, meningism or convulsions.

ECG shows right ventricular preponderance and chest X-ray some cardiomegaly and pulmonary congestion.

Management

Though differentiation from acute myocarditis or congenital heart disease may be difficult, the suspicion of infantile beri-beri should be enough to justify immediate thiamine therapy, which acts as a diagnostic test. A dose of 25 mg may be given by i.m. injection; in very ill children an IV injection gives an almost immediate response. Response to treatment is usually rapid and improvement will be seen within an hour in most cases. Other treatment will include general measures such as oxygen, diuretic or antibiotic therapy, where indicated.

Thiamine therapy should be continued for 1–2 weeks and measures should then be taken to modify the family diet (including treating the mother if she is breast feeding) to avoid further thiamine deficiency.

Acute pericarditis and tamponade

Acute pericarditis may be viral, bacterial or, rarely, fungal in origin. It may also occur in association with rheumatic carditis and collagen diseases. It seldom causes a large effusion with risk of tamponade except when of bacterial aetiology, and only then is it likely to require urgent treatment.

Cardiac tamponade, which occurs when a large effusion interferes with cardiac function, may be due to non-infective conditions such as malignant disease, including leukaemia.

Recognition

Retrosternal chest pain made worse by breathing or coughing, and often relieved by sitting up and leaning forward, is the characteristic pain of acute pericarditis. Fever and tachycardia are usually present and a pericardial friction rub may be heard unless a large effusion is present.

With the development of a large effusion dyspnoea, cough and abdominal pain are frequent. Tachycardia, small volume pulses with pulsus paradoxus and raised jugular venous pressure are the clinical signs and these, in association with a large, globular, heart shadow on X-ray, without other cause should suggest the diagnosis. Muffled heart sounds and an increase in the area of cardiac dullness to percussion are additional features, but are less reliable signs for the inexperienced.

Investigations

Chest X-ray; ECG; two-dimensional echocardiogram; Hb; WBC; blood culture; viral studies.

Chest X-ray shows a large, globular heart shadow with clearly defined edges. Occasionally it is possible to see a denser shadow within it, which is the heart itself.

The ECG may show signs of acute or chronic pericarditis with S-T segment elevation or T-wave flattening or inversion. In a large effusion low-voltage complexes may be seen in all leads.

Differentiation from myocarditis can be difficult and if in doubt a cardiological opinion should be sought. Two-dimensional echocardiography is diagnostic.

Management

If septic pericarditis is suspected antibiotic treatment should be started without awaiting results of cultures. It is desirable to get a sample of pericardial fluid for culture before starting treatment, but this is not always possible. A satisfactory initial antibiotic regimen is benzylpenicillin (50 mg/kg 6 hourly) and chloramphenicol (50 mg/kg per 24 hours) given IV.

Digoxin is contraindicated in the presence of tamponade, and diuretics should be used with caution.

Pericardial aspiration should, ideally, only be done by trained personnel with electrocardiographic monitoring and a defibrillator available.

If transfer to a cardiac unit is not possible and the patient's condition is critical the following technique for pericardiocentesis should be used.

PERICARDIAL ASPIRATION

The patient should be lying supine, propped up with head and shoulders at an angle of 45 degrees. A wide-bore lumbar puncture needle may be used with a 20 ml syringe and three-way tap. The needle is inserted to the left of the xiphisternum upwards and backwards, at an angle of 45 degrees, behind the sterum. If fluid is not readily found the procedure should be stopped.

The risks of pericardiocentesis are the production of ventricular fibrillation or laceration of the heart or a coronary artery, resulting in haemopericardium. These risks can be reduced by connecting the barrel of the aspirating needle via a sterile connector to the V lead of the ECG monitor. Contact between the needle and the ventricular myocardium produces sudden marked elevation of the S-T segment on the ECG thus obtained, and if this is seen the needle should be withdrawn.

An alternative approach is via the fifth intercostal space anteriorly. The needle is introduced just lateral to the mid-clavicular line but internal to the edge of the cardiac dullness. This method carries a greater risk of damage to coronary arteries and can also produce a pneumothorax.

Cardiac arrest (see also Chapters 1 and 2)

Cardiac and respiratory arrest are so closely interrelated, the one following the other rapidly whatever the cause, that their management must be considered together. The wide variety of circumstances and diseases which may lead to cardiorespiratory arrest need not be considered here except in so far as the immediate management involves, as it always must, an attempt to identify the cause.

Complete cardiorespiratory arrest, indicated by apnoea, pallor, or cyanosis, and absence of the carotid or femoral pulses is usually obvious.

If cardiac arrest or arrhythmia is the initiating factor, cyanosis and loss of consciousness precede respiratory arrest, which is itself preceded by transient hyperpnoea and then apnoea with occasional gasps before complete respiratory arrest.

When respiratory factors are the cause, the pulse is usually palpable after consciousness is lost and when respiratory efforts are feeble or absent.

Vomiting may occur, as a late feature, in a cardiorespiratory arrest from any cause, and aspiration of vomit is likely. While aspiration of vomit is occasionally the primary event in a cardiorespiratory arrest it is more often secondary and, for this reason, it should not be regarded as the initiating factor until other possibilities have been ruled out.

Drill (see also Chapter 1)

Initiation of treatment for a cardiorespiratory arrest is usually in the hands of the nursing staff. Adequate instruction and training of nurses are therefore vital.

An instruction sheet, as below, should be available in wards, casualty departments, etc., but the drill must be familiar to all staff so that reference to the chart during the emergency should not be necessary.

Cardiac and respiratory arrest procedure

On finding a patient collapsed or unconscious:

1. Shout for help.
2. If no pulse is palpable start external cardiac massage. (The femoral or carotid pulse is easier to feel than the radial in a collapsed child.)
3. Clear airway of vomit and mucus by suction or finger, extend neck and elevate chin (to prevent tongue occluding pharynx).
4. If no spontaneous breathing, ventilate with bag and face mask or commence mouth-to-mouth respiration. Ensure adequate chest movement occurs with each ventilation.
5. As soon as help arrives send someone to summon cardiac arrest team, by pressing emergency bell or telephoning.
6. Send someone to get emergency drugs and drip.

POINTS TO REMEMBER:

1. THE CHILD MUST BE ON A **FIRM** SURFACE IF CARDIAC MASSAGE IS TO BE EFFECTIVE (USE A BOARD IF NECESSARY).
2. IN INFANTS, PLACE ONE HAND BEHIND INFANT'S CHEST AND MASSAGE WITH FINGERS OF OTHER HAND.
3. APPLY FIRM PRESSURE TO CENTRE OF CHEST TO COMPRESS HEART BETWEEN STERNUM AND SPINE.

The following points merit amplification.

Cardiac massage

The object of external massage is to compress the heart between sternum and spine. Pressure should therefore be exerted over the sternum rather than the ribcage, which is ineffective in producing an output and tends to result in multiple rib fractures.

In infants pressure should be applied over the mid-sternum as depression of the lower third of the sternum can cause rupture of the liver.

An alternative method in infants, to that on the drill sheet, is to hold the chest between the hands with the fingers behind and compress with the two thumbs.

A compression rate of 100 per min is satisfactory for infants and children.

Ventilation

Adequate ventilation can only be achieved by intubation and ventilation with a bag. As an emergency measure ventilation with a bag and face mask may be performed, but it is vital to ensure that the chin is elevated and that an adequate seal is obtained.

Mouth-to-mouth respiration (*see* Acute Respiratory Failure, page 223) is a satisfactory alternative but requires training and some practice to be effective. Whatever method is used it is important to ensure that adequate chest movement is occurring and that the airway is kept clear of vomit, mucus, etc.

It is helpful to alternate external cardiac massage with ventilation, giving five compressions of the heart between each ventilation of the lungs.

Monitoring

As soon as cardiac massage has been commenced and ventilation is proceeding the patient should be connected to an ECG monitor. If this shows ventricular fibrillation then defibrillation should be attempted without delay as the likelihood of reversion to a stable rhythm is greater if this is done early. (An initial shock of 1 J/kg should be used.)

Intravenous infusion

While the ECG monitor is being obtained or connected a drip should be commenced for administration of drugs. Either percutaneous cannulation of a peripheral vein or a 'cut-down' may be used, the latter being indicated if peripheral veins are collapsed and cannot be entered percutaneously.

The long saphenous vein at the ankle is the easiest cut-down site, but it can be difficult to cannulate in small infants and occasionally the saphenous at the groin or an antecubital vein may be used. The latter techniques carry risks of inadvertent arterial damage and should preferably not be attempted by the inexperienced operator.

The infusion rate should be kept to a minimum until the situation is under control. It is easy to inadvertently run in large volumes of fluid if the drip is left unobserved!

Drugs

Correction of acidosis

Sodium bicarbonate 8.4% (molar) may be given by bolus injection over 1–2 minutes in a dose of 1–2 ml/kg. This will not correct a significant degree of acidosis but if larger doses are to be given the rate of infusion should not exceed 0.5 ml/kg/min as the solution is extremely hypertonic. If the patient has been hypoxic for a long period further bicarbonate may be given, up to a total of 5 ml/kg. This dose should not be exceeded until blood gas determination has been performed. Total correction of acidosis may be achieved by using the standard formula: *see* page 119.

Cardiac stimulants

If the ECG monitor shows bradycardia or asystole, or if no peripheral pulses are palpable despite an apparently satisfactory rhythm and rate, cardiac stimulants should be given:

1. Calcium gluconate (10% solution), 0.5–2 ml IV (≃0.1 ml/kg).
2. Adrenaline 1:10 000, 1–3 ml IV (100–300 μg)
   or
   Isoprenaline 10–50 μg IV.

These drugs may be repeated if no effect is obtained after 2–3 minutes.
Direct intracardiac injection is seldom, if ever, worthwhile except as a last resort.

3. Glucose 50%. In all infants under a year it is worth giving 2–3 ml 50% glucose.
4. Antiarrhythmic drugs. If ventricular fibrillation recurs repeatedly after defibrillation, ensure that adequate acid–base correction has been given; then give lignocaine 1–2 mg/kg.
   If severe bradycardia persists or recurs despite earlier measures, give atropine 0.15–0.6 mg.

When to stop (*see also* Chapter 27)

The decision to stop is seldom easy. It should always be left to the most senior member of the 'team', who should take into account the following points:

1. *Time elapsed before resuscitation started.* If this is likely to have exceeded 3 minutes then success is very improbable.
2. *Evidence of cerebral activity.* Fully dilated, fixed pupils, in the absence of any spontaneous respiratory efforts, and which fail to constrict despite adequate external massage for 10 minutes, are a strong indication of brain death.
3. *Underlying illness.* If the child's underlying condition is known and is unlikely to be compatible with recovery, or is likely to result in severe, permanent disability, a decision should be sought from the consultant responsible whether resuscitation should be abandoned. If a senior person, preferably the consultant, is not available to make this decision, then resuscitation should be continued.
4. *Duration of arrest.* If there is evidence of residual brain activity (respiratory efforts, small pupils) it is reasonable to continue with resuscitative efforts for at least an hour. Successful resuscitation without brain damage can certainly occur after 90 minutes or more of massage. On the other hand, failure to obtain an adequate cardiac output within an hour despite adequate acid–base correction and cardiac stimulants strongly suggests an irremediable situation.

When satisfactory respiration and circulation have been established, children in whom normal consciousness does not return, or in whom it is considered probable that neurological damage has been sustained, should receive appropriate treatment to limit cerebral oedema. This may include the use of mannitol, hyperventilation and/or steroids (*see* Chapter 27). The use of high-dose barbiturates and maintained hypothermia may also be considered (*see* page 296). It is important that consideration of such measures should occur early following cardiorespiratory arrest and should not be delayed in the hope that as the hours pass it will be clearer whether cerebral damage has occurred. By the time that clear evidence of neurological deficit is seen, it is likely to be too late to institute appropriate treatment with any real prospect of limiting permanent damage.

References

BISSETT, G. S., GUAM, W. and KAPLAN, S. (1980) The icebag: a new technique for interruption of supraventricular tachycardia. *Journal of Pediatrics,* **97,** 593–595

GERSONY, W. M., PECKHAM, G. J., ELLISON, R. C., MIETTINEN, O. S. and NADAS, A. S. (1983) Effects of indomethacin in premature infants with patent ductus arteriosus: results of a national collaborative study. *Journal of Pediatrics,* **102,** 895–906

GREEN, T. P., THOMPSON, T. R., JOHNSON, D. E. and LOCK, J. E. (1983) Frusemide promotes patent ductus arteriosus in premature infants with respiratory distress syndrome. *New England Journal of Medicine,* **308,** 743–748

JONES, R. W. A., BAWNER, J. H., JOSEPH, M. C. and SHINEBOURNE, E. A. (1976) Arterial oxygenation and response to oxygen breathing in differential diagnosis of congenital heart disease in infancy. *Archives of Disease in Childhood,* **51,** 667–673

RADFORD, D. (1983) Side effects of verapamil in infants. *Archives of Disease in Childhood,* **58,** 465–466

YANAGIHARA, R. and TODD, J. K. (1980) Acute febrile mucocutaneous lymph node syndrome. *American Journal of Diseases of Children,* **134,** 603–614

Part VII

Neurological emergencies

Chapter 25

Acute neurosurgical emergencies

D. N. Grant

Acute head injuries

Children, particularly babies and infants, are extremely labile in their response to brain trauma; and, though appearing initially to have suffered no harm from a head injury, may rapidly deteriorate while a life-threatening situation may arise. The severity of the damage is not always proportional to the apparent degree of trauma, and significant injury to the brain may result from an incident which might well have left an adult unscathed. It is often difficult to decide whether a child should be admitted to hospital. In case of doubt, one should always err on the side of safety.

Criteria for admission to hospital

1. Any child who has an injury sufficiently severe to cause loss of consciousness, even if only for several minutes.
2. Any child with a skull fracture.
3. Any child who remains or becomes drowsy following the injury.

An exception can sometimes be made in the case of children whose parents are sufficiently intelligent and level-headed to carry out the necessary observations through the night following the injury, with the proviso that there must be no delay in bringing the child back or getting in touch with the hospital at the first suspicion of deterioration.

Children selected for admission can be divided into those about whom there is no present worry, but who may develop complications; and those who are clearly seriously injured and in need of urgent attention.

Severe injury

Management

In a severe injury there are a number of essential observations which must be rapidly but carefully carried out, leading in turn to particular lines of action.

Airway and respiration

In the unconscious patient, particularly if supine, the airway is likely to be obstructed by the tongue; this is reversed in the semi-prone position with the lower jaw pulled forward. If this is inadequate, an oral airway may be effective provided it is of sufficient bore to prevent further obstruction, it is long enough to reach the back of the tongue, and is of rigid material or at least has a rigid portion opposite the incisor teeth to prevent its total obstruction by spasm of the jaw muscles. Accumulated vomitus, blood and mucus must be removed from the mouth and pharynx. If these manoeuvres are ineffective, as they would be for example in profuse haemorrhage into the mouth or nasopharynx, an endotracheal tube must be inserted.

All casualty officers and residents ought to be able to do this without waiting for an anaesthetist. Inadequate respiration demands intubation and ventilation. *It is difficult to over-stress the deleterious effect which airway obstruction, with its resulting accumulation of carbon dioxide in the bloodstream leading to cerebral vasodilation, has on a brain which may already be grossly swollen from traumatic oedema.*

Blood pressure

As soon as the airway is secure, the blood pressure is checked. It is often said that a head injury, unless it has caused catastrophic brain damage, is unlikely itself to cause low blood pressure. While this is true in adults and older children, babies can lose a significant fraction of their blood volume into a scalp haematoma or from a scalp laceration. However, in the absence of such an explanation, the cause of low blood pressure must be sought elsewhere. Bleedings into the thorax, peritoneal cavity, pelvic tissues or around long bone fractures are the likeliest possibilities. Resuscitation is aimed at restoring the blood pressure according to the cause.

Assessment of vital functions

1. The pattern and frequency of respiration previously observed.
2. The blood pressure and pulse.
3. The conscious level in terms of response to stimuli of increasing intensity such as ordinary conversation appropriate to the age, shouting, non-painful and, finally, painful stimulation if required. During this stimulation the presence of any obvious limb weakness will be detected.
4. The size, equality or otherwise, and reaction of the pupils.

These observations form a baseline for later comparisons; *the use of vague terms such as stupor and semi-coma is to be deprecated.* A change from the baseline will indicate the onset of complications sufficiently early to treat them before irreparable damage is done. Deterioration is usually due to intracranial bleeding and traumatic oedema.

Radiography

Good quality plain radiographs of the skull should be taken, for fractures, sprung sutures, and intracranial air indicative of a compound fracture; but X-ray of the skull is not necessarily an essential emergency investigation.

Warning signs of complications

1. Progressive deterioration in level of consciousness.
2. Progressive dilatation and sluggish response to light in a previously normal pupil.
3. The appearance or worsening of a neurological deficit in the limbs.
4. All these may be accompanied by bradycardia, rising blood pressure and altered respiratory pattern.

In children there may be a misleading phase of increased activity and irritability with a rising pulse rate during the onset of rising intracranial pressure. However dramatic the onset of signs indicative of complications, there must be time which can profitably be spent in telephoning the nearest neurosurgeon before making the next move.

Extradural haematoma

Recognition

1. Extradural bleeding may be anticipated even after mild trauma such as a kick on the head while playing football or a fall against the pavement. There may be loss of consciousness for a short period although this is by no means always the case. After this, there is apparent recovery for a few hours, although, during this so-called lucid interval, there is often increasing headache and drowsiness.
2. By the time of examination in hospital there may be sufficient extravasation of blood outside the skull to result in a boggy swelling in the scalp. One pupil may already be larger, usually on the side of the haematoma. Plain radiographs of the skull may be helpful in showing a fracture crossing the markings of the middle meningeal vessels or one of the major venous sinuses.
3. It is possible for extradural bleeding to occur, particularly in children, without the presence of a fracture. The temporoparietal suture may be temporarily separated at the time of injury, rupturing the middle meningeal artery and returning immediately to its normal configuration.

Management

1. When some or all of the danger signs are present, and particularly when the situation has deteriorated to the extent of one pupil being fixed and dilated, the child's brainstem may be about to undergo irreversible damage, *and there may be minutes in which to initiate effective treatment.*
2. Ideally the haematoma should be evacuated without transfer to a more distant hospital and without more specialized and time-consuming investigation. In a desperate situation shaving the head can be omitted.
3. Assuming that the situation, although critical, is not desperate, the following sequence should be followed:
   (a) An endotracheal tube is inserted, for anaesthesia if necessary, but more importantly, to ensure an adequate airway.
   (b) Blood is taken for emergency cross-matching because, although the quantity of blood in the haematoma is unlikely to be significant in relation to total blood volume (except in the very young), profuse haemorrhage which is difficult to control may be encountered when the haematoma is evacuated.

(c) *Preparation*. While a theatre and basic instruments are prepared, the head is shaved. If time permits the shave shoul be complete to allow further burrholes through an uncontaminated field if the first is unproductive.

(d) *In theatre*. The patient should be placed on the operating table with a 10-degree head-up tilt to diminish the venous pressure in the head. The relevant side of the head, that on which the pupil first became dilated (or in the absence of that sign, the side with the skull fracture or external evidence of trauma) is turned to face upwards, any tension in the neck being minimized by placing a large sandbag under the shoulder.

(e) *Operative technique* (*Figure 25.1*). A linear incision about 4 cm (1½ in) in length is made over the fracture site at the point of external trauma or, failing these indicators, midway between the external auditory meatus and the posterior limit of the orbital margin. The lower end of this incision must extend down to the zygomatic arch. The incision is carried at one stroke

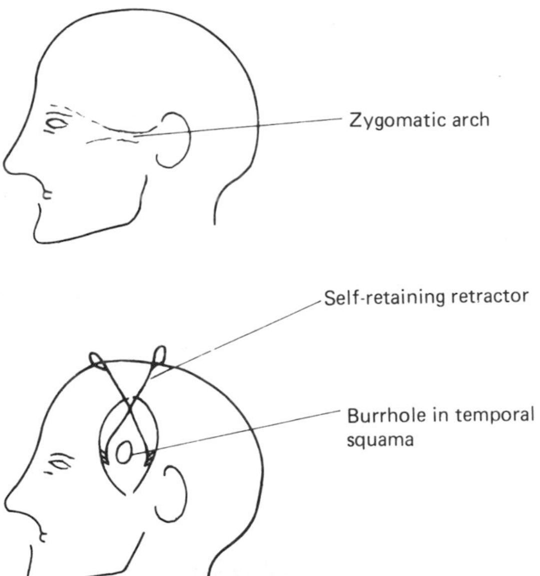

Figure 25.1 Site of skin incision for evacuation of acute extradural haematoma

down to the pericranium. A self-retaining retractor, such as a mastoid retractor, is then inserted, both to separate the edges of the incision and to arrest bleeding from the scalp. The pericranium is then incised and scraped aside. A burrhole is made preferably with a brace and bit, but if this is not available, a suitable opening can be made with hammer and gouge or chisel. If the diagnosis is correct, the dura will not be seen at this stage, as it is covered by haematoma which will begin to extrude through the opening. Gentle suction will assist the evacuation of the clot. As soon as a significant quantity of the haematoma has emerged, the pressure upon the brainstem is relieved and the situation is no longer acutely life-threatening. *If expert assistance is expected, it is probably advisable to proceed no further*. If, however, help is not at hand, the scalp incision should be extended sufficiently widely to allow the burrhole to be enlarged with bone-nibbling instruments into an oval craniectomy some 6 cm (2–2½ in) in diameter. Through this the remainder of the haematoma can be evacuated, allowing the surface of the dura to be exposed. The ruptured middle meningeal artery may be visible and can be coagulated with diathermy or underrun with a stitch. Occasionally the artery is torn as it emerges from the foramen spinosum. Haemorrhage from this site may be controlled by plugging the hole in the bone with wax, gelatin sponge or muscle. The exposed dura is usually hyperaemic and produces a troublesome amount of blood from multiple sites, which, if not controlled, would result in reaccumulation of the extradural haematoma. This reaccumulation is most readily limited by hitching the dura at a number of points around the edges of the craniectomy to the adjacent pericranium, using sutures which are passed through avascular areas of dura and which ideally penetrate only the outer layer of the dura, thus avoiding puncturing underlying cortical vessels. The wound may then be closed in several layers, including a simple drain if there is doubt about the efficacy of the haemostasis. If the site first selected for the burrhole does not reveal the expected extradural blood two further burrholes should be made, one over the frontal pole and another in the posterior parietal region. If none of the sites show extradural blood and the situation remains critical there is little to be lost in opening the dura, particularly if it appears to be dark blue in colour. Should the lesion in fact be an acute subdural haematoma, sufficient blood may be released to relieve the distortion of the brainstem. It is unfortunately more probable that a thin film of blood will be encountered over a contused cerebral cortex.

Acute subdural haematoma

Acute subdural bleeding usually results from laceration of dural venous sinuses, from cerebral laceration or from tearing of bridging veins from the surface of the brain to the dural sinuses. Usually the deterioration is less rapid than in extradural bleeding. A rapidly compressing haematoma can arise from a tear in a major venous channel. Whereas in extradural haemorrhage the underlying brain is often intact, in subdural bleeding there is commonly associated damage to the cerebral hemisphere.

Recognition

The clinical picture is less stereotyped and the site of the haematoma less predictable.

Management (Figure 25.2)

The patient should, if possible, be transferred to hospital for neuroradiological investigation, ensuring an adequate airway, if need be, by inserting an endotracheal tube. *If the deterioration is rapid and transfer of the patient is not practicable, the haematoma should be sought via multiple burrholes as for extradural bleeding*. The initial exploration should be at the site of a fracture or external trauma. Three

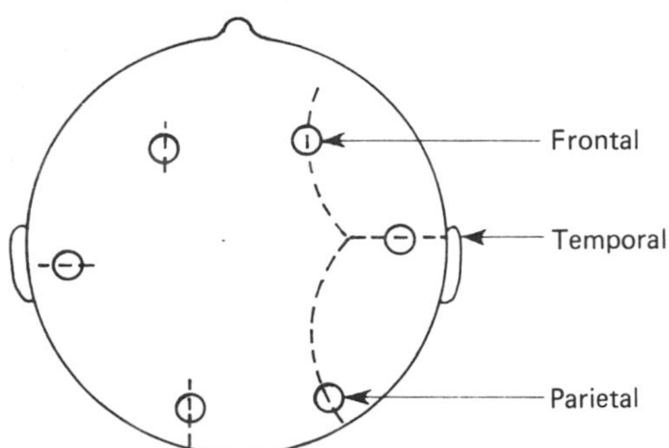

Figure 25.2 Site of burrholes for acute subdural haematomas. The frontal and temporal or temporal and parietal incisions can be connected as shown by the dotted lines in order to turn a formal craniotomy flap with the help of additional burrholes if wider exposure is required

burrholes situated frontally, temporally, and in the posterior parietal region are the minimum requirement to cover the surface of one cerebral hemisphere, and it is possible to miss a significant haematoma in spite of such a search. The possibility of a contrecoup injury makes it necessary to explore the surface of the second hemisphere, if the first side is found to be free from haematoma. Posterior fossa subdural haemorrhage is fortunately rare; this should be considered where a fracture line is seen to pass into the foramen magnum. *Such a patient may deteriorate suddently with respiratory irregularity or arrest and should preferably be sent for observation to a neurological centre.* Posterior fossa burrholes are technically more difficult for the inexperienced operator.

Extradural and acute subdural bleeding and the general surgeon

The operations described for the relief of extradural or acute subdural bleeding should be within the capabilities of every general surgeon. If the child's condition is judged to be deteriorating rapidly and transfer time to a neurosurgical unit is measurable in hours rather than minutes, the surgeon on the spot should proceed, encouraged by the fact that prompt evacuation of a haematoma results in a normal child, whereas undue delay all too commonly results in death or severe and irreversible brainstem damage.

Traumatic cerebral oedema

This is much more common as a cause of deterioration than a surface haematoma. The oedematous area is usually circumscribed and therefore limited in the clinical effect it produces. However the process may be progressive, involving both hemispheres widely, particularly if exacerbated by an inadequate airway. If it is not feasible to transfer the patient for neuroradiological study, the deterioration must be assumed to be due to accumulating haematoma until proved otherwise. Having established that there is no haematoma, cerebral oedema is assumed by exclusion to be the reason for the patient's deterioration and is treated by the measures described in the next section.

Acutely raised intracranial pressure (see also Chapter 26)

Recognition

This occurs when a space-occupying lesion, e.g. a neoplasm, abscess or haematoma, reaches such dimensions that compensation by venting of cerebrospinal fluid or venous blood from the intracranial compartment is exhausted.

Cerebral oedema

More diffuse increase in brain bulk by cerebral oedema as in trauma, encephalitis, and lead poisoning, or increase in cerebrospinal-fluid volume in hydrocephalus, has the same ultimate ill effects. These are impaired respiration and finally cardiovascular activity from interference with brainstem centres either by mechanical distortion, impaired arterial-blood supply or haemorrhagic infarction.

Intracranial tumours

Intracranial tumours in childhood rarely present as life-threatening emergencies without some clue in the history such as alteration in personality, deterioration in school performance, increasing complaint of headache, clumsiness of limbs or gait, or impaired vision.

Cerebral abscess

Intracerebral abscess is found in association with cyanotic heart disease, chronic sepsis in middle-ear or nasal sinuses, following compound skull fracture or associated with dermal cysts or sinuses.

Recognition

When a neoplasm or abscess finally results in an acute rise in intracranial pressure, there is depression of consciousness, eventually leading to unconsciousness. There is likely to be papilloedema, although its absence, particularly when the lesion has evolved rapidly, does not exclude the presence of raised intracranial pressure. The pulse rate is likely to be slow and the blood pressure high. When the brainstem is in danger there is pupillary inequality or gaze palsies and periodic or irregular gasping respiration.

Management

Relief of brainstem compression

It is necessary to relieve brainstem compression without waiting for expert assistance. If in doubt about the efficacy of respiration, immediate intubation and ventilation will diminish the bulk of the vascular compartment and so lower the intracranial pressure by reducing the arterial carbon dioxide tension, but also at the same time this will ensure adequate oxygenation.

Use of osmotic agents

Mannitol 20% is infused in the dose of 1–2 g/kg over the course of 10 minutes. This will reduce brain oedema which is likely to be present in varying degrees under all the circumstances mentioned. The bladder should be catheterized in order to prevent its sudden distension in the unconscious patients. At the same time dexamethasone 10 mg given intravenously will disperse oedema around a tumour or abscess although there appears to be doubt about its efficacy in traumatic oedema. Further management is dependent on neuroradiological investigation and demands early transfer to a neurosurgical department.

Impairment of vision

Papilloedema may be sufficiently severe to result in seriously diminished visual acuity at first evident as transient visual impairment. If permanent damage is to be prevented the intracranial pressure must be reduced by the use of mannitol and dexamethasone.

Under all circumstances of suspected raised intracranial pressure in childhood, valuable confirmatory and sometimes diagnostic evidence may be obtained from good-quality skull radiographs.

Acute hydrocephalus

See page 353.

Subdural effusion

See page 350.

Further reading

BRUCE, D. A. (1984). Delayed deterioration of consciousness after trivial head injury in childhood: leading article. *British Medical Journal* **289:** 715–716

Chapter 26

Raised intracranial pressure

R. A. Minns

Definition

The normal pressure within the cranium is contributed to by a dynamic equilibrium of CSF, blood, and brain, and is less then 15 mm Hg for the normal adult. Values are much lower in the newborn (about 2 mm Hg) and increase slightly throughout childhood, being 5 mm Hg at 1 year of age and between 6 and 13 mm Hg at about 7 years of age. A normal range for intracranial pressure (ICP) in childhood has been calculated, using the mean ±2 standard deviations (Paraicz, 1982). For adults, values greater than 20 mm Hg are unequivocally raised; for older children over 15 mm Hg is high, over 40 mm Hg is very high, and extremes of 60–80 mm Hg have been recorded in intractable oedema, non-communicating hydrocephalus, and in benign intracranial hypertension.

Pathophysiology

When a situation exists which is likely to give rise to raised ICP, i.e. an increase in one of the cranial compartments, compensatory mechanisms come into operation to maintain normal intracranial pressure, the same mechanisms which protect the brain when sneezing or coughing etc. These buffers are:

1. Shunting of CSF into a distensible spinal compartment.
2. Collapse of the cerebral veins and redistribution of cerebral blood to the arteriolar side of the circuit.
3. Increase of the head circumference in the young child.

When such buffers are exhausted, at a critical intracranial volume, the ICP rises. The compliance or pressure–volume response is an attempt to measure the available residual buffering, and values above unity warn of precipitous rises if more intracranial space is not made available. These sudden plateau waves indicate the need for immediate action with hyperventilation, or a cerebral vasoconstrictor drug such as thiopentone. Measurement of the PVI (pressure–volume index) can be carried out by techniques of infusion or extraction of CSF, but the pressure response to a constant stimulus, such as nasopharyngeal suction can be continuous guide to the compliance in the individual in an Intensive Care Unit.

The causes of raised ICP

1. An increase in the *vascular* compartment (cerebral congestion); this may be due to halothane anaesthesia, cyanotic congenital heart disease, elevated CO_2 states, etc.
2. Expansion of the *brain compartment* (cerebral oedema); this may be of several different types:
   (a) *Vasogenic:* increased permeability of the blood–brain barrier results in expansion of the extracellular fluid spaces of the brain, especially in the white matter. This may be either generalized or focal vasogenic oedema. General insults include trauma, lead encephalopathy, and infarction. Focal oedema is seen surrounding space-occupying lesion such as tumour, clot, haemorrhage, cyst, or abscess.
   (b) *Cytotoxic:* intracellular oedema resulting in diminished extracellular fluid spaces and affecting both grey and white matter. This follows anoxic–ischaemic damage (post-cardiac arrest, post hypoxic states in the newborn (*see* Chapter 71), carbon monoxide poisoning), meningitis, and some toxic encephalopathies. It is sometimes seen in combination with vasogenic oedema.
   (c) *Interstitial:* an increase in the periventricular CSF due to the transependymal retrograde movement of CSF in hydrocephalic states.
   (d) *Hydrostatic:* oedema from an increase in the intravascular pressure, without an increase in the cerebral vascular resistance, causing a diffuse white-matter oedema. This results from trauma, systemic hypertension, hypoxaemia, and hypercapnia.
   (e) *Hypo-osmotic:* this is a diffuse intracellular accumulation of water, a consequence of low plasma osmolality. This occurs in situations of inappropriate ADH secretion and infusion of hypotonic solutions (water intoxication, *see* Chapter 11, pages 123–124).

Expansion of the *CSF compartment* (hydrocephalus) may be thought of as communicating (Arnold–Chiari malformation, intrauterine encephalopathy), or internal, which involves the lateral and third ventricles when there is aqueduct stenosis or mumps aqueductitis etc., or involves all four ventricles when there is outlet obstruction at the fourth ventricle, as in tuberculous meningitis, other forms of adhesive meningitis, post-haemorrhagic or post-meningitic states.

Recognition of raised ICP

Clinical evidence of raised ICP

The clinical signs and symptoms of acutely raised ICP depend on which intracranial compartment is being expanded, so that if the expansion is the CSF compartment, i.e. acute hydrocephalus, the signs and symptoms are expansion of the occipito-frontal circumference, scalp and retinal venous distension, obvious separation of the sutures, a tense non-pulsatile fontanelle, a cranial bruit, pupil changes, and neck retraction. Headache, vomiting, drowsiness, lethargy, and fits are the commonest initial symptoms.

As the hydrocephalus continues to expand, the effects, and signs that result, are due to brain compression and internal herniations. The signs therefore at this stage are similar to those of brain oedema; fits, coma, decerebration, and loss of homeostasis. Ordinarily coma is an infrequent accompaniment of pure hydrocephalus, unless it is severe, when internal herniations are responsible. Where particular parts of the brain have undergone herniation, specific clinical syndromes result, e.g. post-tentorial herniation with the classical coma, ipsilateral hemiparesis and pupillary dilatation; but other cones (foramen magnum, anterior temporal lobe, cingular gyrus herniation etc.) give rise to different combinations of symptoms and signs (*Table 26.1*).

Table 26.1 Clinical features of herniation syndromes

Tentorial herniation	*Foramen magnum cone*	*Cingulate gyrus herniation*
Sunsetting (eyes)	Sudden cardiorespiratory arrest	Diplegia or hemiplegia
Dilated pupil	Bulbar palsy (lower cranial nerve palsies)	Visual symptoms
Sixth nerve palsy	Neck stiffness	
Cortical blindness	Hypotonia	
Hemiplegia	Stridor	
Decerebrate posture*	Spinal flexion	
Coma	Hypotension	
Respiratory irregularities (Cheyne–Stokes respiration, central neurogenic, hyperventilation	Hypothermia	
Systemic hypertension		
Tonic seizures		

* Decerebrate posture: extension and pronation of forearms and extension of legs with equinus position of the feet.

There is no one reliable sign of raised ICP and the only way of knowing what the pressure is, is to measure it. The signs may be unusual (rashes, sweating, hippus, etc.) or unreliable, and in 60 per cent of cases although there are symptoms there will be no signs. The signs of chronic raised pressure are not relevant here.

Radiological recognition of raised ICP

1. *Skull X-ray:* there may be separation of the cranial sutures, flattening of the pituitary fossa and erosion of the posterior clinoid process, 'copper-beaten' appearance, and thinning of the cortical bone.
2. *CT scan:* there may be periventricular lucent zones (hypodense areas), an absent cortical subarachnoid space, slit or shifted ventricles, space occupation, or ventricular dilatation. The ventricular dilatation may be seen as mild, moderate, or severe by simply looking at the scan, or it may be measured by means of a bifrontal ventricular ratio, which is the distance between the lateral edges of both frontal horns divided by the inner diameter of the skull at this level (%). Previously, on pneumoencephalography the cortical mantle was assessed at the vertex, and a similar mantle thickness may be obtained from the ventricle to the inner surface of the skull on CT scan.
3. *Ultrasound scan:* pressure may be seen by reduced or asymmetrical cerebral vascular pulsations, slit or shifted ventricles, ventricular dilatation, space occupation, attenuation of the cerebral parenchyma (it is more echogenic) and ventricular enlargement, which affects the posterior horns first, and thinning of

the cortical mantle which often occurs asymmetrically. The lateral ventricular ratio of Rumack and Johnson (1982) is the ratio between the lateral ventricular width and the hemisphere width; for a normal preterm infant this is 31 per cent, for a normal older child 34 per cent maximum, with mild hydrocephalus having values between 35 and 40 per cent, moderate hydrocephalus 41–50 per cent and severe hydrocephalus over 50 per cent.

Poland *et al.* (1985) have suggested transventricular to transcalvarial diameter ratios as being constant in the 28–48 week post-conceptual age group. Ratios are obtained at two levels in the coronal plane (at the head of the caudate nucleus and at the level of the mid-glomus of the choroid plexus in the atria of the lateral ventricles). Another ratio is constant; this is the thickness of the occipital mantle, divided by the thickness of the frontal mantle in the parasagittal plane.

Direct ICP measurements

Without direct ICP measurements it is impossible to manage raised ICP adequately, both from the point of view of measurement of the degree of elevation, and the ability to monitor normalizing measures.

Ventricular measurements

These provide the most accurate recordings. In the infant short records may be obtained by percutaneous ventricular cannulation via the anterior fontanelle. Prolonged records may be obtained by leaving a fine non-compliant catheter in the ventricle, placed there by a percutaneous puncture through the fontanelle or by using the bedside technique with a bone-marrow needle puncture of the cranial bones (McWilliam and Stephenson, 1984) provided that attention is paid to strict asepsis. The older child with fused cranial bones and acutely ill with raised pressure will require an emergency craniotomy and insertion of a Rickham or Omaya ventriculostomy reservoir (Minns, 1984), as in acute tuberculous meningitis.

Brain surface measurements

This is the only way to measure ICP when there is brain oedema, although the rapid bedside technique described above is used with the slow advancement of the needle and removing the guide wire every 2 mm and looking for a return of CSF. If this is unsuccessful the ventricle may be located manometrically by coupling the catheter to a pressure transducer and looking for a pressure wave on an oscilloscope. Surface measurements in the infant include the insertion of subdural and subarachnoid catheters at the bedside through the anterior fontanelle (Goitein and Amit, 1982; Levene and Evans, 1983).

Alternatively, for the older child a subarachnoid screw can be threaded into a twist-drill hole at the site of the coronal suture (Vries, Becker and Young, 1973). After opening the dura the screw is left *in situ*, primed and an external transducer records the ICP signal which is put through a pre-amplifier and written out on a chart recording or video-display unit. Current research suggests that subarachnoid or epidural screws for measuring ICP are probably less accurate than was originally thought, and that catheter tip epidural transducers inserted via a burrhole correlate better with ventricular pressure recordings.

Principles of management of acute raised ICP

Management depends on which intracranial compartment is expanded, and appropriate measures are taken to reduce this compartment, for example:

1. Reduction of the CSF compartment (in hydrocephalus): by ventricular taps, directly or from a ventriculostomy reservoir, open or closed ventricular drainage, early CSF shunting (ventriculo-peritoneal preferably), or isosorbide (for dosage, *see* page 298) to reduce production of CSF.
2. Reduction of brain compartment (in cerebral oedema): by restricting fluid intake, controlled hyperosmolar dehydration with mannitol, sorbitol, urea, glycerol etc., and also by steroid administration where there is localized peri-tumour oedema.
3. Reduction of cerebral vascular compartment (blood compartment) by hyperventilation, increasing central venous return by elevating the head, positive end-expiratory pressure etc.

There is clearly some overlap in the above measures; thus oedema of the white matter (interstitial oedema) accompanies hydrocephalus. Not infrequently cerebral changes occur in anoxic–ischaemic injury where the pressure initially may be the result of oedema of intracellular type, and after a time, cell membrane function becomes totally deranged with the subsequent loss of response to osmotic diuretics, despite measured elevation of pressure.

In addition to the above measures for reduction of the intracranial contents, other *supportive* measures are aimed at the preservation of the regional cerebral metabolism and avoidance of situations likely to increase existing raised pressure. These are common to all cases of raised pressure, for example:

1. Supportive measures include giving oxygen, glucose, maintenance of systemic arterial pressure, possibly barbiturate administration, cooling etc. (*see* below).
2. Situations known to aggravate raised pressure and therefore worth avoiding include seizures (major fits may induce raised pressure because of compensatory increase in the cerebral blood flow, which may last for 20 minutes (Minns and Brown, 1978)), inhalational cerebral vasodilator anaesthetic agents such as halothane, the intravenous dissociative anaesthetic agent ketamine, insertion of an endotracheal tube without previous mask hyperventilation, and hypoxic or hypercapnic states.

Specific paediatric neurological emergencies with raised ICP

Head injury (see also Chapter 25)

Immediate supportive care is given by providing an airway, inserting an intravenous line, giving a bolus of mannitol, and performing an urgent CT scan.

If the CT scan shows a mass lesion further preoperative mannitol is given and a craniotomy performed for clot evacuation; at the same operation a subarachnoid screw or an epidural catheter transducer is inserted, but if the ventricles are easily cannulated despite the cerebral contusion and oedema, a ventricular drain is preferable. If the CT scan shows no mass lesion but only diffuse oedema, a screw is inserted.

If elevation of the ICP occurs, it is important first to check that there is no jugular compression, that the airway is clear, that the arterial blood gases are satisfactory, that the systemic blood pressure is normal, and to recalibrate the transducer.

If elevations of ICP persist, the patient is hyperventilated, which results in a decrease in the $PaCO_2$. This causes cerebrovascular constriction and decreases the cerebral blood volume. The hyperventilation is continued to a level of 20–25 mm Hg (2.6–3.3 kPa). This is done slowly because rapid lowering of the PCO_2 during recovery from CO_2 narcosis causes a severe alkalosis with a raised arterial blood pH, and multifocal myoclonus and seizures may occur; that is, rapid induction of hypocapnia induces cerebrovascular constriction accompanied by cerebral ischaemia, which offsets the useful effect of raising the PaO_2. Slow reduction of the PCO_2 allows renal compensation to take place (Plum and Posner, 1980). The effect of hyperventilation, however, is rather transient, and mannitol should be given at the same time, to extract water from the normal part of the brain (remote from the lesion) and thus to lower the ICP. The dosage is 5–7 ml/kg of a 20% solution (1.0–1.4 g/kg). The effect of this is rapid and lasts several hours.

If the raised pressure persists, closed ventricular drainage is begun (if a ventricular catheter was previously inserted) or the mannitol is repeated every 4–6 hours.

If the raised pressure still continues hypothermia should be considered. This is induced with chlorpromazine (0.5–1.0 mg/kg IV) and maintained at 30–32°C (86–90°F) by a servo-controlled cooling blanket. Alternatively barbiturates may be useful in the form of thiopentone (1–2 mg/kg IV), phenobarbitone, or pentobarbitone (Nembutal) (3–5 mg/kg initially then 2 mg/kg/hour as an IV infusion for 3 days, with measurement of blood barbiturate levels). Constant infusions or bolus doses have both been used and the effect on the ICP is dramatic. However, there is also a marked reduction in systemic arterial pressure and with disrupted autoregulation of cerebral blood flow these patients frequently depend passively on systemic arterial pressure to provide movement across the cerebrovascular bed. Therefore careful monitoring of the systemic arterial pressure is necessary and barbiturates should not be given if the cerebral perfusion pressure is under 50 mm Hg. The aim in treating raised ICP is to keep the ICP at under 15 mm Hg and the CPP at over 50 mm Hg. Steroids are only useful in head injury patients where there is local oedema from a haematoma, but they also improve compliance of brain tissue and are usually given intravenously at first, although it may be 6 hours before they take full effect. Dexamethasone (0.3 mg/kg/24 hours divided into 4–6 doses; this dose may be halved every 12 hours as soon as the ICP is controlled) is the steroid of choice, sometimes in combination with frusemide or acetazolamide. Other measures include nursing with the head slightly elevated and moving the patient from side to side hourly, an indwelling urinary catheter, and recording the urine output. Measurement of electrolytes and osmolality is also important.

The ICP in children with head injury is of prognostic value, using the outcome categories of Jennett and Bond (1975). Children with an ICP under 20 mm Hg had a significantly better outcome in terms of morbidity and mortality than those with ICP levels between 20 and 40 mm Hg and greater than 40 mm Hg (Minns *et al.*, 1985).

Reye's syndrome (for further details on recognition and management see Chapter 47, pages 415–418)

The first stage in management of this mitochondrial toxic encephalopathy is to stage it according to the Lovejoy system, from stage I to V (*Table 26.2*) (Lovejoy, Smith and Bresnan, 1974).

Table 26.2 Reye's syndrome: Lovejoy staging (Lovejoy *et al.* 1974)

	Stage 1	*Stage 2*	*Stage 3*	*Stage 4*	*Stage 5*
Mental state	Lethargy Sleepiness	Delirium Disorientation	Obtunded (blunting of faculties)	Coma	
Respiration		Hyperventilation	Hyperventilation		Arrest
Other symptoms	Vomiting				Fits
Posture and tone			Decorticate rigidity*	Decerebrate rigidity†	Hypotonia
Reflexes or responses		Exaggerated peripheral reflexes		Loss of 'doll's eye' response	Loss of peripheral reflexes
Ocular movements				Dysconjugate eye movements on caloric testing	
Pupils				Non-reacting dilated pupils; hippus	
Liver function tests	Abnormal	Abnormal	Abnormal	Slightly abnormal	Normal
ECG	Slow (theta waves)	Further slowing (delta waves)	As in Stage 2	Disorganized	Isoelectric

* Decorticate rigidity: flexion of the forearms and extension of the legs.
† Decerebrate rigidity: extension and pronation of the forearms, and the extension of the legs with equinus position of the feet.

ICP is monitored with a subarachnoid bolt or screw or direct brain puncture using the bedside technique with a bone marrow needle or an epidural catheter transducer. This is begun in stage II when the patient is delirious, hyperventilating with brisk reflexes, dominant delta rhythm on ECG and abnormal liver function tests. The ICP is monitored continuously for about 6 days.

Control of raised ICP is by hyperventilation to a $paco_2$ of 25 mm Hg (3.3 kPa). Mannitol is given initially at the same time. This may be repeated when the measured pressure exceeds 20 mm Hg for more than 2 minutes. Sedation is usually by morphine sulphate 0.1 mg/kg every 4 hours or phenobarbitone. Where these measures are unsuccessful in controlling the raised pressure deep hypothermia as outlined before or thiopentone 5 mg/kg with or without the use of dopamine may be necessary to manage acute pressure elevations (*see* Shock, Chapter 10, pages 106–107).

Continuous monitoring of the mean arterial pressure is required to estimate the cerebral perfusion pressure. Continuous display of the EEG is also advisable and arterial and central venous pressure lines aid the intensive care management; patient observations, namely conscious state, pupillary reactions, oculo-cephalic and oculo-vestibular reflexes, tendon reflexes, and postures, are routinely noted.

Hydrocephalus

Acute infantile hydrocephalus (see also Chapter 37)

After the ultrasound and CT scan are obtained and the degree of ventricular dilatation estimated, it is usual to allow ventricular dilatation to occur, hoping for spontaneous arrest by the opening up of alternative CSF absorbtive pathways, until the cortical mantle at the vertex is between 15 and 20 mm or until the lateral ventricular ratio is 45–50 per cent. If no such arrest occurs the raised ICP may need to be relieved, before definitive CSF shunting (to relieve symptoms), by percutaneous ventricular tapping, once or twice a day, or up to 4 hourly if necessary, with strict attention to asepsis. If shunting is delayed, closed ventricular drainage or the use of isosorbide 8 g/kg/24 hours orally, with a daily check on the urea, electrolytes, osmolality, and weight, may be necessary.

Post-haemorrhagic hydrocephalus (post-intraventricular haemorrhage) in the newborn

See Chapter 72, pages 628–629

Post-infection hydrocephalus

In fatal meningitis perivascular inflammatory cells enter the subarachnoid space, traverse the pia and penetrate the cortex along the surface veins. The result is diminished absorption by the arachnoid villi with a resultant *ex-vacuo* hydrocephalus (a defect of CSF absorption, or obstruction involving the villi on the surface of the brain, with consequent ventricular dilatation), and a cortical cerebritis. This occurs particularly with haemophilus influenzae and pneumococcal meningitis, so that the appearances are of surface oedema. In the acute illness, therefore, preventive measures such as fluid restriction (75 per cent of the normal maintenance requirement), steroid administration, or single bolus mannitol administration may be all that is required; however, if the natural course of treated meningitis is not occurring a CT scan will reveal any ventricular enlargement and the need for an interim ventriculostomy reservoir, by which pressure can be controlled.

Acute tuberculous meningitis

This is a special case which frequently presents with hydrocephalus in the acute phase of the illness. There will be alterations of the conscious state and there may be signs of tentorial herniation (hemiparesis, pupillary abnormalities and coma). Ventricular dilatation is more often seen in childhood acute tuberculous meningitis than in adults; Bhargava, Gupta and Tandon (1982) found hydrocephalus in 87 per cent of children, compared with 12 per cent of adults, using CT scan. It is imperative that a CT scan is done immediately, and after confirmation of the hydrocephalus, a ventriculostomy reservoir is inserted immediately. This allows control of the ICP, which is the *priority* in treating tuberculous meningitis. The child is unlikely to die or become blind as a result of the infection in the 24 hours after admission, but may well do so from uncontrolled ICP. Frequent taps of the reservoir or closed ventricular drainage against a pressure head of 10 mm Hg will ensure the controlled relief of CSF pressure. The insertion of a reservoir may avoid the use of a definitive shunt at a later date. Repeated daily pressure readings will show a progressive decline to normal limits. Routine antituberculous chemotherapy should be started (*see* Chapter 36, page 344), as should steroids, always systemically; and, where adhesive arachnoiditis has developed, intrathecally.

Post-hypoxic states in the newborn

See Chapter 71.

Benign intracranial hypertension

Non-specific signs of raised ICP develop, such as intermittent headaches, vomiting, blurring of vision, diplopia, and papilloedema, while the conscious state and higher cortical functions remain normal.

This condition is ill-understood. There may be a defect in the absorption of CSF due to increased vascular resistance at the level of the arachnoid villi. CT scan appearances may show smallish ventricles; Reid, Matheson and Teasdale (1980) measured with a CT scan the volumes of the ventricles and found values significantly lower than in age and sex-matched controls. This probably reflects brain swelling due to engorgement or oedema and not a defect of absorption, but the alternative is an increase of CSF volume accommodated entirely within a distensible subarachnoid space.

Diagnosis is made first by excluding other causes of ICP by the CT scan, in particular excluding midline or 'silent area' neoplasms. One space-occupying lesion which may be missed on CT scan, is the bilateral isodense subdural haematoma with no midline shift.

CSF should be obtained, and at the time of lumbar puncture, a pressure transducer is connected to the lumbar puncture needle, so that with minimal displacement of the CSF, and the patient in a lateral recumbent position, a recording can be made of the ICP. In most cases the pressure is raised initially and returns to normal after gradual removal of CSF. The CSF is usually clear or has a slight pleocytosis.

The EEG usually shows paroxysmal slowing, and a technetium brain scan and a CT scan are the most important investigations. The haemoglobin, haematocrit, calcium, phosphate, electrolytes, 17 keto-steroids, blood gases, and visual field testing for enlarged blind spots etc. are also important.

Treatment is aimed at maintaining a normal ICP, by giving osmotic diuretics, acetazolamide, corticosteroids, or oral glycerol. If more effective measures are necessary, daily or even twice daily lumbar punctures may be required and if this method of treatment needs to be continued, continuous drainage by a theco-peritoneal shunt without laminectomy may be used. The prognosis is usually excellent and most cases resolve within 2–3 months. If obesity is a problem, or withdrawal of steroids has precipitated the episode, steroids should be restarted, with weight reduction and salt restriction.

Coma states (see also Chapter 29)

Management of comatose children has been summarized by Gordon *et al.* (1983). The management of the comatose child involves both diagnosis and support and monitoring of the coma state. There is often overlap between those investigations aimed at discovering an obscure cause, and the supportive investigations which are independent of the cause of the coma.

Diagnostic investigations include, first a CT scan, followed by an examination of CSF either by the lumbar route or from the ventricles. An EEG, metabolic screen, virology, technetium scan, toxicology etc. should follow.

The supportive investigations are aimed at treating the treatable i.e. pressure, fits, infection, and homeostatic disorders, regardless of the cause of the coma; raised ICP should be thought of in all coma states.

The management of the comatose child may present a dilemma: whether or not to measure the ICP invasively. The signs may be inconclusive and radiological investigations unhelpful. Of children in coma due to cranio-cerebral trauma, 54 per cent have raised ICP. Following anoxic–ischaemic injury, such as post-cardiac arrest, only 22 per cent have raised ICP, in the infective encephalopathies such as meningitis or encephalitis, the incidence of raised ICP varies from 50 to 86 per cent. In intracranial neoplasms, apart from pontine gliomas, the ICP is almost always raised and in hydrocephalic states, where there is coma, the pressure is raised in almost 80 per cent of cases.

References

BHARGAVA, S., GUPTA, A. K. and TANDON, P. N. (1982) Tuberculous meningitis; a CT study. *British Journal of Radiology* **55,** 189–196

GOITEIN, K. J. and AMIT, Y. (1982) Percutaneous placement of subdural catheter for measurement of intracranial pressure in small children. *Critical Care Medicine* **10,** 46–48

GORDON, N. S., FOIS, A., JACOBI, G., MINNS, R. A. and SESHIA, S. S. (1983) The management of the comatose child. *Neuropediatrics* **14,** 3–5

JENNETT, B. and BOND, M. R. (1975) Assessment of outcome after severe brain damage. *Lancet,* **i,** 480–484

LEVENE, M. I. and EVANS, D. H. (1983) Continuous measurement of subarachnoid pressure in the severely asphyxiated newborn. *Archives of Disease in Childhood* **58,** 1013–1015

LOVEJOY, F. H., SMITH, A. L. and BRESNAN, N. J. (1974) Clinical staging in Reye's Syndrome. *American Journal of Diseases of Children* **128,** 36–41

McWILLIAM, R. C. and STEPHENSON, J. B. P. (1984) Rapid bedside technique for intracranial pressure monitoring. *Lancet* **ii,** 73–75

MINNS, R. A. (1984) Intracranial pressure monitoring: personal practice. *Archives of Disease in Childhood* **59,** 486–488

MINNS, R. A. and BROWN, J. K. (1978) Intracranial pressure changes associated with childhood seizures. *Developmental Medicine and Child Neurology* **20,** 561–569

MINNS, R. A., MILLER, J. D., WARD, J. D. and STEER, C. R. (1985) The prognostic value of intracranial pressure monitoring in comatose children. In preparation

PARAICZ, E. (1982) *ICP in Infancy and Childhood.* Monographs in Paediatrics. Vol. 15, pp. 1–7. Basel, S. Karger

PLUM, F. and POSNER, J. B. (1980) *The Diagnosis of Stupor and Coma* (3rd edn.) Philadelphia: F. A. Davis Company

POLAND, R. L., SLOVIS, T. L. and SHANKARAN, S. (1985) Normal values for ventricular size as determined by real time sonographic techniques. *Pediatric Radiology* **15,** 12–14

REID, A. C., MATHESON, M. S. and TEASDALE, G. (1980) Volume of the ventricles in benign intracranial hypertension. *Lancet* **ii,** 7–8

RUMACK, C. M. and JOHNSON, M. L. (1982) Real-time ultrasound evaluation of the neonatal brain. *Clinical Ultrasound* **10,** 179–202

VRIES, J. K., BECKER, D. P. and YOUNG, H. F. (1973) A subarachnoid screw for monitoring intracranial pressure. *Journal of Neurosurgery* **39,** 416–419

Chapter 27

Brain death

R. A. Minns

Death has been defined in the Sydney declaration as an irreversible process of cells dying, following functional or somatic death. The majority of deaths occur with the cessation of pulse and respiration, but the concept of brain death has arisen unnaturally and as a result of technological advances in resuscitation where a comatose and apnoeic patient, who would in the ordinary course of events have become anoxic and asystolic, has heart and lung function taken over mechanically by ventilation. Where there is irreversible brain damage this has meant ventilating a dead brain.

It is now medically and legally accepted that death is synonymous with 'brain death', or more precisely, 'brainstem death'. Since the main functions of the brain stem are the capacity of the reticular activating system to generate consciousness by alerting the hemispheres, and at the opposite end of the stem, the control of respiration, the signs of brainstem death are apnoeic coma and absent brainstem reflexes.

Brainstem death may result from two mechanisms: primary stem damage due to haemorrhage or infarct (which rarely causes total loss of stem function) or trauma; or as a secondary stem lesion from raised intracranial pressure. The effects of acutely raised intracranial pressure are internal herniations and cones which result in ischaemic infarction of the stem by kinking the pontine branches of the basilar artery, or stem compression and damage from uncal herniation or foramen magnum cone. While hypoxia selectively affects the cortex more than the stem the ensuing brain oedema from hypoxic encephalopathy may result in coning. Ventilation of a non-functioning brainstem will result in the well-recognized necropsy picture of liquefaction and cerebellotonsillar detachments.

Whilst most brainstem deaths result from head injury and intracranial haemorrhage (particularly subarachnoid haemorrhage from a ruptured aneurysm) 20 per cent are due to other causes of brain oedema, namely cerebral abscess, meningitis, encephalitis, cardiorespiratory arrest, strangulation and drowning etc.

The diagnosis of brainstem death

The diagnosis of brainstem death rests on:

1. Fulfilment of certain preconditions.
2. Exclusion of reversible causes of apnoeic coma.
3. Clinical tests of brain-stem areflexia and apnoea.

Preconditions

Apnoeic coma

The patient is unresponsive and requires ventilation. This excludes patients who are fully conscious, who are drowsy or disorientated, and those showing arousal to light or deep motor stimulation, verbally or by eye opening, grimacing or hand movements. It also excludes those showing arousal to verbal commands, by obeying, showing comprehension, eye-opening, changing pulse rate, or by grimacing. It also excludes those who have sleep–wake cycles.

Irreversible structural brain damage

This is obtained from the history, examination and investigations. If no diagnosis can be made for the cause of the structural brain damage the preconditions have not been met. After 'successful' cardiopulmonary resuscitation, if there is presumed post-anoxic oedema, it is assumed that the preconditions are met. Treatment or the passage of time should not have altered the clinical picture; seizures indicate some intact stem connections, and negate the preconditions.

One can apply the tests for brainstem death only after some time on the ventilator; that is, however long it takes to satisfy the preconditions. The tests should be applied after a minimum of 6 hours, even in the presence of massive brain damage. For most ischaemic events, it should be more than 24 hours; and if there are additional drug effects, it should be 3–4 days before the tests are applied.

Exclusion of reversible causes of apnoeic coma

In considering the differential diagnosis of brainstem death, reversible causes and disorders which simulate apnoeic coma are grouped as drugs effects and other pathological states.

Drugs

The commonest drug effect is from alcohol. This can usually be discounted in paediatric intensive care units. However, barbiturate effects need to be excluded, as they have a temporary depressant effect on both the EEG and brainstem reflexes. If there is any suspicion of intoxication with barbiturates or meprobromate, or if they have been used in the course of management in the intensive care unit, remembering that the blood concentration lags behind the brain concentration, testing of brainstem function cannot be undertaken until the blood level is almost undetectable. Similarly with benzodiazepines, which also have a long half-life.

The effects of neuromuscular blocking drugs (e.g. pancuronium) must be excluded, and if there is no certainty about the timing of the last dose, the peripheral nervous system should be examined. If the knee and ankle jerks are present there is no significant neuromuscular blocking; or nerve stimulation may be performed and if positive, negates any neuromuscular blocking effect.

Other pathological states

These include the following:

1. Electrocution, where severe limb spasm and absent pulses may simulate apnoeic coma.

2. If there is a history of hypothermia the patient needs to be warmed first before clinical testing; certainly the temperature needs to be recorded at the time of testing. Homeostatic derangements from stem damage may result in poikilothermia.
3. Hypothyroid crisis or coma is a possible reversible cause of apnoeic coma but does not occur in childhood.
4. It is important to exclude hypoglycaemia and other *metabolic* abnormalities associated with hepatic, renal, or respiratory failure following cardiac arrest, hypoxia, or hypotension.
5. A history of drowning will be obvious.
6. Rare inherited enzyme deficiencies causing prolonged neuromuscular blockade may be reversed by neostigmine or excluded by peripheral nerve stimulation.

Bilateral paramedian, tegmental area lesions of the brainstem

These may cause coma, but other tests of brainstem function will not all be negative.

Ventral pontine infarction ('locked-in' syndrome)

This usually results from basilar artery occlusion and causes tetraplegia and aphonia, with other stem functions intact, namely conjugate vertical gaze, blink, hearing, pain perception, and breathing.

Brainstem encephalitis

This usually causes external ophthalmoplegia, bulbar paresis, facial diplegia, ataxia and sometimes respiratory difficulties. However, these patients are not in deep coma, and will show movements of the limbs spontaneously, or in response to stimuli.

The Guillain–Barré syndrome

This consists of variable cranial nerve involvement, respiratory paralysis and rarely ophthalmoplegia.

Persistent vegetative state

In the persistent vegetative state (cognitive death) stem function is satisfactory, but cerebral activity above the tentorium is deficient. This usually results from hypoxic states such as cardiorespiratory arrest or from shearing of the subcortical white matter after impact head injury. Such patients breathe normally, swallow, open their eyes, and have conjugate roving eye movements with active reflexes, and primitive postures and movements of the limbs.

In practical terms the clinical findings of most of the above will differentiate them from brainstem death. However, drug effects must be looked for, and hypothermia, hypoglycaemia and other biochemical disorders *must* be excluded by investigation.

Table 27.1 Tests of brainstem function

	Brainstem death	Not brainstem death
Brainstem areflexia (*all* must be absent)	1. Pupils: no response to bright light; may be cadaveric (mid-paralysis).	May be dilated, equal or unequal. Pupils react. Pin-point. Exclude mydriatics.
	2. Blinking and corneal reflex: no response using sterile throat swab.	Present.
	3. Vestibulo-ocular reflexes (calorics): irrigation with 20 ml ice-cold water in wax free canals, right and left; no movement of either eye.	Nystagmus. Tonic deviation to ipsilateral side – contralateral internuclear ophthalmoplegia. Tonic deviation to contralateral side – VI nerve lesion. False negatives: gentamicin – end organ failure. Vestibular suppressants – sedatives, anticholinergic, anticonvulsant, or tricyclic drugs.
	4. Oculocephalic reflex (doll's eye): Negative (not in UK code). Stand at top of patient, hold head, and raise eyelids; head rotated to one side for 3–4 seconds, then through 180° to other side. Not done if cervical trauma.	Normal alert – eyes move in coordination with head. Cadaver – head and eyes move together. Newborn <2 weeks – present. Damaged hemispheres – present, i.e. eyes deviate to opposite side for 1–2 seconds then prompt realignment with head.
	5. Motor response (a) No grimacing to painful stimuli (in V nerve distribution), e.g. supraorbital pressure. (b) No grimacing to painful stimuli of limbs (pencil pressed hard against patient's finger and toe nail). If heart beat continues tendon reflexes may recover or show pathological limb reflexes e.g. flexor withdrawal. (c) No gag or cough reflex or diaphragmatic movement in response to bronchial stimulation by suction catheter passed down trachea.	Abnormal postures such as decorticate (flexion of forearms and extension of legs), or decerebrate (extension and pronation forearms and extension of legs): trismus.
Testing apnoea (most critical)	1. Preoxygenate with 100% oxygen for 10 minutes. 2. If hypocapnic on ventilator – either slow ventilation rate or 5% CO_2 in 95% oxygen for 5 minutes to ensure starting $PaCO_2$ of 5.3 kPa (40 mm Hg). 3. Disconnect. Maintain oxygen diffusion with 100% oxygen at 6 ℓ/min (in well-grown school-age child) via catheter down trachea. 4. Maintain disconnection for 10 minutes (should raise $PaCO_2$ by 2.7 kPa (20 mm Hg)); UK code states $PaCO_2$ should rise to at least 6.65 kPa (50 mm Hg) before documenting incapacity to breathe.	Spontaneous respiration. Gasping.

Tests of brainstem function (Table 27.1)

Retesting

The testing is carried out by two doctors, usually consultants or a consultant and senior registrar. Their findings are recorded in writing and a note is made of the time, the nature of the brain damage, and the duration of the coma. A second test is done after a variable interval which is usually the time that is necessary to establish the diagnosis beyond any doubt. It may be 3 hours, but if delayed for 24 hours asystole frequently occurs before the second test.

If the test for brainstem death is positive and organ donation is envisaged the 'beating heart cadaver' is reconnected to the ventilator until operation. The disconnection should be done by the medical staff and after the diagnosis of brainstem death; if disconnection is not done immediately, asystole will develop some time from 12 hours to 5 days later, but only rarely should artificial ventilation be continued more than 12 hours after declaration of brainstem death.

Additional investigations done in some centres

EEG

This is not essential, according to the UK code. The isoelectric tracing ('electrocerebral silence') has been defined as no electrical activity over 2 mV when recording from the scalp or referential electrode pairs 10 or more cm apart with an interelectrode resistance under 10 000 ohms (or impedances under 6000 ohms) but over 100 ohms. Many depressant drugs produce an isoelectric EEG (barbiturates, meprobromate) as do anoxia, hypothermia, encephalitis and trauma. The EEG may only become isoelectric some time after diagnosis of brain-stem death. A flat EEG, even if due to structural brain damage, is still compatible with survival. It is not expected that the EEG from surface scalp electrodes will pick up activity within the brain stem, but if some activity is found, this suggests that the reticular activating system of the stem is alerting the hemispheres and thus causing cortical activity.

Apart from pathological flattening of the EEG trace, many artefactual effects are possible and this prompted the American EEG Society's 'ad hoc' committee to produce EEG criteria for the determination of cerebral deaths. Recommendations about the minimal technical standards include:

1. Eight scalp electrodes and ear lobe reference electrodes.
2. Interelectrode resistance under 10 000 ohms but over 100 ohms.
3. Deliberate creation of artefact potential at each electrode of the montage.
4. Interelectrode distance of at least 10 cm.
5. Sensitivity increased from 75 mV/mm to 3.5 and 2.5 mV/mm or better during part of the recording.
6. The use of time constants of 0.3–0.4 seconds during part of recording.
7. The use of monitoring devices such as the ECG, and if necessary a chest strain gauge transducer to determine the component due to external interference.
8. Tests for clinical and electrical reactivity to intense stimuli such as pain, loud sound and strong light.
9. A recording time of at least 30 minutes.
10. This to be repeated within 24 hours.

One cannot envisage a situation where an EEG would not be performed in most paediatric intensive care units before disconnection of the ventilator, even if this had to be done to elucidate the cause, or help in management of the case. However, it is not deemed essential; but in situations where organ transplant is contemplated, it would be advisable.

OTHER HOMEOSTATIC DERANGEMENTS

Abnormalities of salt, water, and glucose metabolism may occur with stem death and are estimated by measuring serum electrolytes, osmolality and glucose. Temperature irregularities and an unstable blood pressure are also often confirmatory. A fixed pulse rate suggests absent vagal transmission. If there is no change in the pulse while sucking out the patient, applying eyeball or carotid pressure, giving verbal commands or painful rubbing of the sternum (ciliospinal reflex) vagal afferents are not traversing the stem.

Although the cortex is selectively vulnerable in the young infant and older child, which should mean existing tests of brain-stem death are still applicable, in the newborn period total cessation of conduction in the brain stem auditory pathway has been found to be compatible with a normal outcome. The preterm infant has a brain stem which is particularly susceptible to anoxia, and further studies are necessary in this group of children to validate criteria for brain-stem death.

Further reading

Conference of Medical Royal Colleges and Faculties in the United Kingdom (1976) Diagnosis of brain death. *British Medical Journal* **ii,** 1187–1188

DEAR, P. R. F. and GODFREY, D. J. (1985) Neonatal auditory brainstem response cannot reliably diagnose brainstem death. *Archives of Disease in Childhood* **60,** 17–19

JENNETT, B., GLEAVE, J. and WILSON, P. (1981) Brain death in three neurosurgical units. *British Medical Journal* **282,** 533–539

PALLIS, C. ABC of Brain Stem Death. (a) *British Medical Journal* (1982) **285,** 1409–1412; 1487–149; 1558–1560; 1641–1644; 1720–1722. (b) *Ibid* **286,** 39; 123–124; 209–210; 284–287. Also complete series of above articles published by British Medical Association, London

ROBINSON, R. O. (1981) Brain death in children (Annotation). *Archives of Disease in Childhood* **56,** 657–658

SILVERMAN, D., MASLAND, R. L., SAUNDERS, M. G. and SCHWAB, R. S. (1969) *Minimal Technical Standards for EEG Recording in Suspected Cerebral Death.* American EEG Society's ad hoc committee on EEG criteria for the determination of cerebral death. The Proceedings of the Electro-Physiological Technologists' Association. Published by the Electro-Physiological Technologist's Association

Chapter 28

Convulsions and status epilepticus

(For Convulsions in the Newborn see Chapter 89)

M. J. Noronha

A convulsion or seizure is a symptom: it denotes a sudden, excessive and disorderly discharge of neurones that may be induced by a variety of pathological processes of genetic or acquired origin. The abnormal discharge in the brain may result in a variety of manifestations which include disturbance of movement, sensation, behaviour or consciousness, depending upon the region of the central nervous system involved.

Pathophysiology

During an epileptic seizure, cerebral metabolism increases by 50–100 per cent. In a brief seizure the accompanying increase in cerebral blood flow is sufficient to meet the increased cerebral metabolic needs. However, a prolonged convulsive seizure lasting more than 20–30 minutes is usually accompanied by apnoea and in addition an enormous increase in oxygen and energy demand from the contracting skeletal muscles. This results in:

1. Hypoxaemia.
2. Hypercapnia.
3. Lactic acidosis secondary to anaerobic metabolism.
4. Arterial hypotension and cardiac irregularities.
5. Rise in body temperature secondary to the muscular activity, itself further increasing cerebral metabolic needs.

This chain of events is probably the most important factor in the production of cerebral damage during prolonged convulsive seizures and underlies the importance of their management as acute medical emergencies.

Recognition

A patient is said to be in status epilepticus when seizures occur in succession without intervening periods of recovery. Only the generalized convulsive (tonic–clonic) form presents an immediate threat to life or cerebral damage. Other forms of status epilepticus, such as 'absence' (petit mal or minor seizures), myoclonic, psychomotor and partial-continuous varieties, do not usually require urgent life-saving measures, and there is time for investigation before treatment is commenced.

Management

The single convulsion

This is usually self-limiting and, unless prolonged for more than 5 or 10 minutes, does not require immediate anticonvulsant medication, but the patient must have an adequate airway and be protected from self-injury.

Status epilepticus

The prolonged convulsion is a true medical emergency and the principles of treatment are:

1. An adequate airway must be maintained and oxygen should be given.
2. The patient should be placed in a semi-prone position and protected against self-injury or too zealous therapeutic restraint.
3. The seizures should be controlled by drugs (*see* below).
4. Fluid and electrolyte balance must be maintained.
5. Obvious causes such as infection, tumour, encephalitis, or recent withdrawal of anticonvulsant drugs, should be treated.
6. Laboratory investigations should include (but not on an emergency basis) complete blood count and urinalysis, blood glucose, urea and electrolytes, plasma calcium and phosphorus, radiographs of the skull (for intracranial calcification or evidence of raised intracranial pressure (ICP)); lumbar puncture *except when the ICP is raised.*

Controlling the seizure

1. Diazepam (valium), without dilution, should be given by slow intravenous injection over 2–3 minutes.
   (a) Recommended dose:
      1 year: 0.025 mg/kg.
      1–6 years: 2.5 mg.
      7–12 years: 5 mg.
      12 years: 10 mg.
   (b) Apnoea may occur if the drug is given too quickly.
   (c) The effect is rapid but usually lasts for only 30–60 minutes and it may have to be repeated.
2. Alternatively diazepam (IV solution), without dilution, can be given rectally by a 2.0 ml syringe; the nozzle being lubricated with vaseline to facilitate its passage through the anal canal. The dose is 0.25–0.5 mg/kg body weight up to a maximum of 10 mg in a single dose. The effect is seen usually within 5–10 minutes and this dose can be repeated in a few hours time. If the child is still convulsing 10 minutes after the rectal administration of diazepam, other routes of administration of diazepam or another drug should be tried.
3. A slow intravenous infusion of diazepam can be given instead of repeated bolus injections.
   (a) Diazepam 30 mg in 500 ml of sodium chloride injection (BP) at a rate of 0.05–0.2 mg per minute.
   (b) The total amount of drug given depends on the response, the effect being assessed after each 5 mg is given.

(c) As soon as the seizures subside the infusion can be stopped, to be started again if they recur.
(d) A careful watch must be kept for signs of respiratory depression and hypotension: these complications are only likely to occur to a significant degree when other drugs such as barbiturates have been given parenterally.

4. Alternatively clonazepam (Rivotril, another benzodiazepine derivative) may be given as it is claimed by some to be more effective than diazepam. Clonazepam may be used as a slow intravenous injection of 0.5 mg active substance freshly mixed with 0.5 ml diluent (water for injection) over a period of a minute, and the injection can be repeated in a few minutes if necessary. Alternatively, clonazepam can be given as a slow intravenous infusion (like diazepam); 3 mg are dissolved in 250 ml of either sodium chloride injection (BP) or 5–10% glucose, the rate of infusion depending upon the clinical response.
5. Paraldehyde may be given intramuscularly if there is difficulty in giving an intravenous injection of other drugs. A glass syringe should be used, although an opaque plastic syringe (but not the clear translucent variety) can also be used.
   Dose:
   1 year of age: 1.0–1.5 ml.
   1–5 years: 3 ml.
   6–10 years: 8 ml.
   Over 10 years: 10 ml.
6. The importance of stopping the seizures as quickly as possible in order to minimize the risk of brain damage cannot be overemphasized. If this cannot be achieved with the use of the above-mentioned drugs in generous dosage, the aid of an anaesthetist should be sought without delay so that the patient can be anaesthetized with thiopentone sodium. This should only be done in an intensive treatment unit and maintained until seizures no longer recur as the level of anaesthesia is lightened.

Further reading

DELGADO-ESCUETA, A. V., WASTERLAIN, G., TREIMAN, D. M. and PORTER, R. J. (eds) (1983) Status Epilepticus. In *Advances in Neurology*. Vol 34. pp. 352–358. New York: Raven Press

GORDON, N. (1972) The consequences of major status epilepticus. *Developmental Medicine and Child Neurology* **14,** 228–230

PARSONAGE, M. (1975) Treatment of status epilepticus. *Prescribers Journal* **15,** 81–85

Chapter 29

Coma

M. J. Noronha

Definition

Coma is a state of unconsciousness from which the patient cannot be roused. There is absence of the normal sleep–wake cycles and an inability to arouse spontaneously and in response to stimuli. Consciousness requires intact functioning of the cerebral hemispheres and the reticular activating formation in the upper brainstem.

Recognition

The initial questions are:

1. Where does the lesion(s) lie?
2. In what direction is the process evolving?
3. What is the pathological process and what can be done about it and its effects on the brain?
4. Is there a patent airway with sufficient respiratory exchange?
5. Is the circulation adequate?
6. Is intracranial pressure raised; and, if so, is the increase great enough to be life threatening?
7. Is there a focal neurological deficit which might indicate a localized, surgically remediable lesion?
8. Is the coma likely to be due to remediable metabolic disease, e.g. hypoglycaemia?

Clinical diagnosis

1. A detailed history often provides clues to diagnosis, e.g. trauma, accidental poisoning, infection. Unfortunately a reliable history is often unobtainable and the immediate cause is obscure, so that great reliance is placed on the clinical examination.
2. The major difficulty is to differentiate between primary CNS disease and systemic diseases or poisoning which produce secondary CNS depression.

3. General examination:
   (a) Evidence of external and internal injuries.
   (b) Pulse (bradycardia), temperature and blood pressure.
   (c) Inspection of the skin, e.g. petechiae suggesting meningococcaemia, haemophilus influenzae meningitis, bleeding disorder, or bruising from non-accidental injury.
   (d) Neck stiffness and Brudzinski's sign (may be absent in the critically ill).
   (e) Examination of the head: head circumference, palpation of anterior fontanelle for tension, detection of suture separation and distension of scalp veins, checking for facial oedema and intracranial bruits, transillumination in those under 1 year of age.
   (f) Examination of the eyes: proptosis, lid swelling, unilateral exophthalmos, tension of bulbs on palpation (e.g. low tension in diabetic coma, high tension in hypoglycaemia coma), auscultation over bulbs (intracranial arteriovenous shunt).
   (g) Examination of ear drums and mastoids.
   (h) Examination of mouth and nose (glue odour, blood, CSF).
   (i) Examination of heart, lungs, and abdomen, and auscultation and palpation of major vessels especially in the neck.
4. Evidence of increased intracranial pressure:
   (a) In infants: full, bulging fontanelle, increased head size, separation of sutures, prominent scalp veins, papilloedema.
   (b) Older children: headache, vomiting and papilloedema.
5. Serial evaluation of five physiological functions (level of consciousness, pupillary reactions, eye movements, motor functions, respirations) gives important information about the *level* of the brain involved, the *nature* of the involvement, and the *direction* the disease process is taking.

Level of consciousness

The level of consciousness is best assessed by using the 'Glasgow Coma Scale':

I. *Best motor response*	II. *Verbal response*	III. *Eye opening*
Obeys, 6	Orientated, 5	Spontaneous, 4
Localizes, 5	Confused conversation, 4	To speech, 3
Withdraws (flexion), 4	Inappropriate words, 3	To pain, 2
Abnormal flexion, 3	Incomprehensible sound, 2	Nil, 1
Extensor response, 2	Nil, 1	
Nil, 1		

Coma score = score I + II + III

This scale has been adapted for infants under 24 months of age, as follows;

V_5 – Fixes on, follows and recognizes objects and persons, laughs.
V_4 – Fixes on and follows objects inconstantly, recognition of persons uncertain.
V_3 – Arousable only at times; does not drink.
V_2 – Motor restlessness; unrousable.
V_1 – Complete unresponsiveness; no motor response to visual, acoustic or sensory stimuli.

Pupillary reactions

1. Normally reacting pupils are an encouraging sign.
2. An unequal, widely dilated and non-reacting pupil usually indicates 3rd nerve damage by tentorial herniation of the brain and is an indication for emergency medical or surgical measures to reduce intracranial pressure.
3. A dilated pupil may also be due to eye trauma, a transient postconvulsive finding, and is occasionally congenital.
4. Bilateral fixed dilated pupils often, but not always, imply irreversible brain-stem damage when the condition persists for more than 5 minutes.
5. Pupils may be unreactive in reversible coma from poisoning by sedative or atropine-like drugs, hypothermia, and from previous local instillation of mydriatics.
6. Pinpoint pupils are seen in poisoning with opiates and with pontine lesions.

Eye movements

1. Roving, non-conjugate eye movements suggest a light plane of anaesthesia.
2. Conjugate deviation of eyes suggests a destructive process on the same side or an irritative process on the opposite side of the cerebral hemisphere.
3. Sixth nerve palsy is usually due to increased intracranial pressure; it does not carry as ominous a prognosis as does 3rd nerve dysfunction.
4. 'Doll's eye' phenomenon: with the eyelids open, the head is briskly rotated from side to side. A positive response is a contraversive conjugate eye movement (turn the head to the right, the eyes move conjugately to the left, then the eyes slowly return to the new head position). Absence of this response in a comatose patient implies disturbance of the brainstem or of the oculomotor nerves.
5. 'Caloric stimulation test'; this can be done as a less urgent test to investigate brainstem function.

Motor functions

These can be observed by applying painful stimuli and observing the responses.

1. Cranial nerves:
   (a) Motor reaction to trigeminal stimulation (supraorbital pressure).
   (b) Pharyngeal/gag reflex.
2. Extension spasms (may be unilateral or bilateral, spontaneous or after stimulation over upper sternum):
   (a) Decorticate posturing with arms flexed and legs extended is produced by severe diffuse disturbance of the cerebral cortex and its thalamic connections.
   (b) Decerebrate posturing is characterized by rigid extension and pronation of arms and extension of legs. It indicates midbrain involvement. When decerebrate posturing is unilateral, it is often caused by tentorial herniation, in which case it may be associated with a contralateral 3rd nerve palsy.
   (c) Flaccid limbs appear when the lower pons and medulla are involved.

3. Focal weakness:
   (a) Unilateral eversion of one foot may indicate hemiplegia.
   (b) Unilateral hypotonia, hyporeflexia and unilateral loss of abdominal reflexes.
4. Muscle tone; spastic or rigid, hypotonic.
   Tendon reflexes; increased, decreased, absent.
   Extrapyramidal signs; dystonia, dyskinesia.

Respirations

1. Cheyne–Stokes respiration is periodic breathing in which hyperpnoea regularly alternates with apnoea. It implies bilateral disturbance of deep cerebral and diencephalic structures.
2. Central neurogenic hyperventilation; deep, rapid, regular respirations occur with involvement of midbrain and pontine structures.
3. Ataxic breathing is irregular in rate and depth and indicates involvement of the medulla and the respiratory centre. It is a feature of impending respiratory arrest.

The recognition of the signs of decerebrate rigidity and the accompanying respiratory patterns associated with 'coning' (brain herniation) are most important in any condition in which there is raised intracranial pressure from any cause. This is considered further in the section on lumbar puncture (*see* page 745) and meningitis (*see* page 346).

Epileptic phenomena

Fits – generalized, focal, myoclonic, vegetative signs of possible epileptic origin (ocular bobbing and agitation, and increased rate and length of respiration may also be epileptic phenomena).

Investigations

1. Determination of blood glucose, serum electrolytes, blood gases and pH, blood urea, liver function tests, and blood ammonia. Toxicological analysis on blood and urine (e.g. toluene, barbiturates, salicylates, iron, anticonvulsants, heavy metals, such as lead).
2. Lumbar puncture is usually necessary to rule out bacterial meningitis, but this carries the risk of tentorial herniation in the patient with increased intracranial pressure, especially with a focal brain lesion, e.g. cerebral abscess. *In any comatose child, who has raised intracranial pressure, lumbar puncture is therefore contraindicated.*
2. Computerized axial tomography (CT brain scan) is indicated if a focal lesion is suspected, to assess ventricular size, and to detect other structural changes in the brain. If a CT brain scan is not available cerebral angiography will be required. Real-time ultrasound is indicated if the fontanelle is still open.

Differential diagnosis

Information obtained during the examination will usually enable the child to be placed into one of four categories depending on whether intracranial pressure is raised and on whether focal neurologial signs are present (*Table 29.1*).

Table 29.1 The differential diagnosis of coma

Without focal signs		*With focal signs*	
Normal pressure	*Increased pressure*	*Normal pressure*	*Increased pressure*
Most metabolic encephalopathies; diabetes, hypoglycaemia, hepatic, uraemia	Some metabolic encephalopathies; water intoxication, Reye's syndrome, severe hypoxia	Vascular disease (cerebral artery occlusion)	Trauma; subdural extradural or intracerebral haemorrhage, cerebral contusion
Intoxication. Solvent abuse	Acute lead poisoning		Brain tumour; usually supratentorial
CNS infection; meningitis, encephalitis, cerebral malaria	CNS infection; meningitis, encephalitis	CNS infection; encephalitis	CNS infection; brain abscess, subdural empyema, encephalitis especially herpes simplex
Trauma (concussion)	Trauma; subdural haemorrhage in infants, subarachnoid haemorrhage	Trauma; cerebral contusion	
Epilepsy (postconvulsive state)	Brain tumour; midline, posterior fossa	Epilepsy; postconvulsive state with Todd's paralysis	Vascular disease; arteriovenous malformation
	Hypertensive encephalopathy. Hydrocephalus		

Management

1. The airway and oxygenation must be maintained; the child is nursed on the side to minimize the danger of aspiration. Frequent suction of secretions is required. The comatose patient should never be left unattended.
2. Shock should be treated (*see* Chapter 10).
3. An intravenous line should be set up; fluid intake should be carefully monitored as overhydration is common and results in water intoxication (*see* page 124) because patients often have inappropriate secretion of antidiuretic hormone.
4. Prompt therapeutic intervention may be life saving in the comatose child with a marked increase in intracranial pressure (ICP) (*see also* Chapter 26).
   (a) Obstructive hydrocephalus; this is relieved most quickly and effectively by ventricular tap.

(b) Cerebral oedema (*see also* page 296); several medical measures may be effective – IV mannitol 20% (1–2 g/kg) rapidly over 20–30 minutes or oral glycerol (1 g/kg) repeated 6 hourly. A urinary catheter should be in place to prevent overdistension of the bladder. The effect of these agents is quick but transient and rarely lasts longer than 6 hours. Dexamethasone 0.2–0.4 mg/kg, IV initially, followed by 0.1–0.2 mg/kg i.m. every 6 hours is commonly employed but the therapeutic response is not seen for 3 or 4 hours. These measures are non-specific and should not replace or delay definitive therapy of the underlying disease.

5. Specific treatment is indicated by assessment of the patient, the history, physical examination, laboratory and special investigations.
6. The child should be repeatedly reassessed with a view to altering treatment or seeking further advice, e.g. focal neurological signs and raised intracranial pressure will usually require neurosurgical assistance.

Further reading

BATES, D. (1983) Predicting recovery from coma. *British Journal of Hospital Medicine,* **25**, 276–282

PLUM, F. and POSNER, J. B. (1980) *The Diagnosis of Stupor and Coma,* 3rd edn. Philadelphia: F. A. Davis

TEASDALE, G. and JENNETT, B. (1974) Assessment of coma and impaired consciousness – a practical scale. *Lancet,* **ii,** 81–83

Chapter 30

Acute paraplegia

Ian A. McKinlay

Recognition

Acute paraplegia is sudden loss of power in the legs.

Basic principles

1. Spinal compression requires urgent investigation and relief.
2. Investigation, particularly *lumbar puncture, can induce marked deterioration if acute paraplegia is due to compression, so it should only be performed in collaboration with a neurosurgeon.*
3. Surgical relief of the compression is more important than precise preoperative pathological diagnosis.
4. Commonly acute paraplegia occurs after acute infection, or as post-immunization myelopathy or transverse myelitis. Surgery in such cases is potentially harmful.
5. Patients suspected of having spinal compression should only be moved with extreme care, with support above and below the suspected lesion to avoid increasing the effects of the lesion.

History

1. A history of recent viral infection or immunization should be sought.
2. Evidence of systemic upset suggests continuing viral infection, spinal tuberculosis, osteomyelitis, or leukaemia.
3. Only severe spinal injury causes acute paraplegia. A history of minor injury is commonly obtained from patients with spinal compression. Sudden movement can disturb the blood supply of the compressed cord or the compressing lesion.
4. There may be a history of recent clumsiness of gait and increased tendency to fall as the result of compression.
5. Local aching or girdle pain is commonly associated with spinal tumours or local infection and helps to localize the lesion.
6. Retention of urine is usual in transverse myelitis but a history of bowel or bladder habit change is absent twice as commonly as it is present in spinal compression. Frequency of micturition and constipation are the commonest symptoms.

7. A history of sudden, painful and often transient loss of vision in the preceding weeks or months strongly favours a demyelinating disorder (Devic's disease (neuromyelitis optica)).
8. The more sudden, severe, and painless is the onset of weakness the more likely is the cause to be intrinsic inflammation of the cord.

Examination

1. The patient may have generalized superficial skin lesions in neurofibromatosis or a local superficial abnormality overlying a congenital lesion.
2. Scoliosis may be present below a lesion of long standing.
3. Spinal tenderness elicited by pressure is of great localizing value. It is more marked in the presence of infection.
4. The legs are weak and usually hypotonic and hyporeflexic in acute paraplegia though, with acute deterioration of unrecognized compression, the legs may be spastic and hyperreflexic. Plantar reflexes are difficult to elicit or are extensor.
5. Paralysis may ascend progressively (Landry syndrome) with a poor prognosis.
6. It is difficult to delineate sensory loss precisely. The apparent level may be several segments below the lesion. It is to be distinguished from the glove and stocking sensory loss of the Guillain–Barré syndrome, where weakness and hyporeflexia in the arms will usually be found.
7. Spinal angulation (gibbus) is a very late feature of spinal tuberculosis.

Diagnosis

1. Full blood count, ESR, blood culture, and viral studies on blood, urine, faeces and nasopharyngeal secretions should be done.
2. Plain X-rays of the spine should be taken, including intervertebral foramina (dumb-bell lesions such as neuroblastoma or neurofibroma may widen them). There may be spina bifida occulta or hemivertebrae associated with a congenital lesion. The spinal canal may show widening, sometimes with narrowing of the anteroposterior diameter of a vertebra, or scoliosis in the presence of a slow-growing lesion. The pedicles may be eroded by an infiltrative lesion, or the disc spaces narrowed by tuberculous infection; a paraspinal soft-tissue mass usually indicates a neuroblastoma though tuberculosis also causes this. Nearly 50 per cent of spinal tumours are in the narrow thoracic canal.
3. Lumbar puncture should be performed, preferably by a radiologist, only after discussion with a neurosurgeon. It requires great caution and a fine needle should be used. Only a very small volume of CSF should be removed, and replaced by contrast medium to delineate any compression. Cisternal myelography may be necessary also to show the upper limit of a big lesion. The CSF below the level of compression is often yellow, with very high protein content and few cells, though leukaemic cells may be seen in a freshly prepared specimen. If the fluid is clear there is greater likelihood of myelitis or myelopathy. There may be slight increase in protein, especially the globulin fraction, and in the lymphocyte count. Heavy blood-staining from an atraumatic tap suggests rupture of an angioma. Very frequent reassessment after lumbar puncture will detect deterioration early.

4. Urine collection for vanillylmandelic acid (VMA) and homovanillic acid (HVA) base-line values is often indicated as neuroblastoma is the commonest tumour causing compression. However, surgery may be necessary before the collection is complete.

Management

1. Nurse in a firm bed, immobilizing as far as is possible and as is consistent with skin care.
2. Treat pain with analgesics.
3. Arrange urgent surgical decompression when indicated. Discuss with radiotherapist in addition, when appropriate.
4. Dexamethasone 4 mg i.m. immediately and 2–4 mg i.m. 4 hourly is indicated pending surgery when a compressive lesion is present, especially if lumbar puncture is followed by deterioration. Its advantage in acute myelitis or myelopathy is dubious.
5. Antibiotics (with drainage of a compressing abscess) are indicated in tuberculosis or osteomyelitis.
6. Attention to bowel and bladder function. Catheterization may be necessary temporarily.

Prognosis

Children recover from spinal compression better than do adults so surgery is indicated even when severe disability is present. Recovery is variable after inflammatory disorders but many patients make a good recovery with symptomatic treatment.

Chapter 31

Acute polyneuropathies

M. J. Noronha

The acute polyneuropathies include a group of clinical syndromes of uncertain aetiology characterized by the acute or subacute paralysis of the limbs, at times of the trunk, or of muscles innervated by the cranial nerves. A variable degree of sensory disturbance is present with sphincter disturbances and autonomic dysfunction in severe cases.

Recognition

Most of the acute and subacute neuropathies do not progress and become life-threatening, but serious respiratory, cardiac and central nervous system complications can occur, and deaths have resulted. Although the rate at which symptoms have developed may provide a guide, it is often difficult to predict how rapidly progression will occur.

A thorough general neurological examination should be done to establish a base-line from which the subsequent course may be judged:

1. The degree of weakness in the extremities should be assessed; also the presence or absence of the tendon reflexes.
2. The degree of bulbar and respiratory muscle involvement:
   (a) Dysphagia, dysphonia, and respiratory effort.
   (b) Ability to cough and the presence of infection in the upper or lower respiratory tract.
   (c) Optic fundi, blood pressure and respiratory rate should be checked regularly. In older children tidal volume should be measured with Wright's respirometer.
   (d) Chest X-ray and ECG monitoring are indicated if there is evidence of respiratory or cardiac involvement.

Features of failing respiratory function

1. Restless and anxiety.
2. Increasing pulse rate and respiratory rate.
3. Cyanosis (if oxygen is not being given).

4. Signs of CO_2 retention, warm extremities, high pulse pressure, tremor.
5. If in doubt a blood-gas analysis should be done.
6. If swallowing mechanisms and/or respiratory function fail ($PCO_2 > 6.6$ kPa (> 50 mm Hg) of if $PO_2 < 9$ kPa (< 70 mm Hg) provided the patient is not receiving oxygen), expert advice should be sought from the specialist in charge of the intensive treatment unit as the patient may require to be intubated and ventilated (*see* Acute Respiratory Failure, pages 226–230).

Chapter 32

Poliomyelitis

B. Heyworth

Since the introduction of immunization, particularly with oral polio vaccine, poliomyelitis has become rare in developed countries, though imported cases occur. In developing countries poliomyelitis is widespread, mainly in children under 5 years of age. A common presentation is 'morning paralysis', a flaccid paralysis of a limb in an infant who seems otherwise well, without preceding illness. With improvements in urban sanitation in developing countries, older children may develop respiratory and bulbar paralysis; these are paediatric emergencies.

Recognition

In paralytic poliomyelitis the following respiratory complications may occur:

1. Increasing weakness of the respiratory muscles progressing to respiratory failure.
2. Upper airways obstruction from retained secretions, progressing to respiratory failure.
3. A combination of the above.
4. Superadded pneumonia or atelectasis.
5. Coma with bulbar or bulbospinal poliomyelitis.

Management

1. Ensure an adequate airway by a combination of postural drainage, mechanical suction and perhaps tracheostomy, or endotracheal intubation (ETT).
2. Adequate mechanical respiratory assistance and ventilation by intermittent positive pressure via endotracheal or tracheostomy tube, or by a tank respirator.

Tracheostomy/ETT

This is indicated when posture and suction fail to relieve airways obstruction.

1. In comatose or stuporose patients (usually due to polioencephalitis) when restlessness, diminished reflexes, reduced ventilation and increased secretions make drainage and suction impracticable.
2. In bulbospinal cases where the airway cannot be kept open.
3. In patients with hypoventilation where a respirator is not available.

Intubation may help where persistent atelectasis is a problem.

Intubation should be done early, before the onset of hypercapnia and hypoxia. Adequate humidification and repeated suction are necessary to avoid repeated changes of the tube. It can be removed when swallowing is normal and the patient can cough. Mechanical ventilation will depend on the type of respiratory paralysis.

Respiratory paralysis

This may occur with or without limb or bulbar paralysis, and may occur suddenly. It can be caused by a combination of:

1. *Paralysis of intercostal muscles;* asymmetrical, complete or incomplete.
2. *Paralysis of the diaphragm;* asymmetrical, complete or incomplete.
3. *Paralysis of the respiratory centre;* (*see under* Bulbar poliomyelitis below).

Recognition

Symptoms of the respiratory insufficiency due to (1) and (2) above are:

1. Breathlessness.
2. Restlessness and foreboding of suffocation.
3. Difficulty in coughing and talking.

Signs of respiratory insufficiency are:

1. Tachypnoea.
2. Use of accessory respiratory muscles (alae nasi, sternomastoids, etc.).
3. Inability to take and hold a deep breath.
4. Inability to count 30 after one inspiration.
5. Reduction of the vital capacity (difficult to determine in young children).
6. Reduction of the arterial PO_2 below 10.5 kPa (80 mm Hg) and if severe, a reduction of O_2 saturation below 93 per cent, and/or respiratory acidosis, with a rising PCO_2.

Assessment of the muscles involved must be done frequently.

Intercostal muscles

Inspection may reveal paradoxical enlargement of the thorax during inspiration, with movement of the thorax towards the abdomen. As the patient tires, or towards the end of the examination, there may be increasing use of the accessory muscles. Palpation and measurement of the thorax at several levels and on each side are necessary, so that progress of the paralysis can be assessed.

Diaphragm

Unilateral or incomplete involvement may be revealed only by fluoroscopic screening. Unless associated with intercostal paralysis it does not usually cause trouble. Bilateral paralysis results in paradoxical 'see-saw' movements of the thoraco-abdominal muscles, seen as depression of the epigastrium during inspiration.

Paralysis of the abdominal muscles will produce reduced movement of the umbilicus on coughing. It will contribute little to the overall respiratory embarrassment, except indirectly by failing to clear secretions. Obstruction of the upper airways by secretions, atelectasis and pneumonia can all cause respiratory insufficiency (or increase mortality) in an otherwise mild case.

Prognosis – Without ventilation, respiratory failure is said to carry a 90 per cent mortality. Although ventilation can reduce mortality below 50 per cent only half of those surviving return to a normal life.

Bulbar paralysis (paralysis of the respiratory centre)

Bulbar involvement occurs in 10–20 per cent of cases of paralytic poliomyelitis. Ninety per cent of those with bulbar palsy have spinal paralysis, often of the upper limb girdle and sometimes with diaphragmatic paralysis. Major bulbar poliomyelitis can be very rapid in onset and progression.

Polioencephalitis

This may involve the medulla and can only be diagnosed with certainty when hypoxia and hypercapnia are proved absent. Children seem particularly susceptible. Associated upper cranial nerve palsies, especially of the facial nerve, lethargy, coma, and muscular hypotonia simulate respiratory paresis. There is often peripheral paralysis.

When bulbar or medullary centres are also involved, respirations are constantly irregular and the 'circulation centre' may be affected (*see* below).

Lower cranial nerves

Laryngeal nerve involvement occurs frequently, causing suffocation before difficulty with swallowing is observed. As it is often associated with dysphagia it is difficult to diagnose. Children may present with coughing and choking especially after eating and drinking. Occasionally, regurgitation of fluids through the nose occurs on swallowing, causing refusal to eat or drink. Refusal to eat or drink must be regarded as serious and not put down to temper tantrums. Respiration is difficult because of obstruction and aspiration of fluids into the respiratory tract. Suffocation and salivation, sometimes with frothing, may lead to cyanosis, noisy breathing, and pulmonary atelectasis. But, even when the child has been deeply unconscious, recovery is often complete.

Respiratory centre

Involvement is shown by irregular respiration or apnoea for several seconds. Older children may show inability to change the rate and/or depth of respiration. Retention of secretions with increasing cyanosis indicates obstruction and asphyxia. Auscultation may reveal extensive rales and signs of atelectasis.

Circulation centre

In the absence of asphyxia, tachycardia is significant. The blood pressure is usually unstable. As in tetanus, hypertensive episodes without hypercapnia are grave, indicating extensive involvement of the brainstem. Just before death, multiple ventricular extrasystoles may appear. Vasomotor and secretory disturbances, with flushing of the face, sweating, and excessive salivation may alternate with pallor. Rarely, convulsions, with drowsiness and hallucinations, may occur terminally.

Other cranial nerves can be involved without causing immediate danger.

Management

The management of emergencies in poliomyelitis should start promptly with the major illness, for emergencies can develop with little warning. Pain and paraesthesiae in limbs, trunk or neck are preparalytic symptoms. General management preceding and during an emergency includes:

1. Rest.
2. Measurement of the respiratory rate (4 hourly during waking and sleeping); assessment of the ability to cough and clear secretions; and of respiratory effort, especially the use of accessory muscles.
3. Measurement of temperature and pulse rate, rhythm and volume. Assessment of colour, speech, eating and drinking, bladder and bowel function, weakness, pain, spasm, and tenderness of muscles.
4. Assessment of motor function of limbs, abdomen and chest.

Bulbar poliomyelitis

Most cases do not need tracheostomy, but a clear airway is essential. Nursing the patient head down by raising the foot of the bed about 45 cm (18 in) and using a simple shoulder harness to restrict sliding help in this. If this is not well tolerated, the mattress can be made into an inverted 'V' so that both head and feet are dependent, probably a better position for treatment. A 'baby alarm' system or microphone should be positioned to monitor breathing and possible vomiting.

Respiratory paralysis only

Treatment can be carried out with a tank respirator without the need for tracheostomy. Waiting for severe hypoxia to develop before resorting to artificial respiration is harmful because it increases atelectasis. If a tank respirator is not available, tracheostomy with intermittent positive pressure respiration can be used. Measurement of tidal flow, full blood-gas analysis, and clinical and radiological examination for lung pathology should be done periodically.

Other complications

These tend to occur later in the course of the disease and rarely as presenting complications. In decreasing order of frequency these are:

1. *Shock*. In polioencephalitis and bulbar poliomyelitis shock may be due to affected centres and myocardial damage. It is precipitated by hypoxia and hypercapnia. Respirators operating at too high a pressure can impede the venous return and so reduce the cardiac output causing peripheral circulatory failure.

2. *Paralytic ileus and acute gastric dilatation.* These can be due to central damage in bulbar poliomyelitis, but also caused by shock or hypokalaemia. Increased secretions, vomiting and impaired diaphragmatic movement make postural drainage difficult. Aspiration via a nasogastric tube may help to prevent this complication. Continuous suction should be used and a normal fluid and electrolyte balance should be maintained.
3. *Azotaemia.* This is caused by renal failure secondary to shock and will be associated with metabolic acidosis; it is also aggravated by increased catabolism.
4. *Hyperpyrexia.* This may occur early in polioencephalitis, or may be the result of secondary infection. Tepid sponging should always be used; β-adrenergic blockers may be tried in polioencephalitis.
5. *Hypertension and cardiac arrhythmias.* These are also seen, like hyperpyrexia, in tetanus, and are usually transient and due to hypercapnia. If they are central in origin, β-adrenergic blockade may be successful.
6. *Pulmonary oedema.* This may be secondary to vasomotor centre involvement, hypoxia or ill-judged IV therapy.

One of these complications occurs in 10–40 per cent of cases of poliomyelitis with bulbar palsy or respiratory insufficiency. All are associated with a high mortality.

Further reading (including details of tracheostomy and respirators)

BOWER, A. G. (ed.) (1954) *Poliomyelitis and its Complications.* Baltimore: Williams and Wilkins

CHRISTIE, A. B. (1980) *Infectious Diseases.* (3rd edn) p. 572. Edinburgh: Churchill Livingstone

FOURTH INTERNATIONAL POLIO CONFERENCE (1958) *Poliomyelitis. Paper and Discussions.* Philadelphia: J. B. Lippincott

WORLD HEALTH ORGANISATION (1955) Poliomyelitis. *WHO Monogr Series No. 26.* Geneva: World Health Organisation

Chapter 33

Tetanus in childhood

A. G. Wesley

Tetanus in the child follows a course similar to that in the adult. In only about 50 per cent of cases can the site of injury and invasion of the organism be identified.

Where a recognized injury occurs those with some retained foreign body are most predisposed to tetanus. Otitis media or a burn can be the site of the infection.

Recognition

The minimum incubation period is 5 days. The longer the period of incubation and the longer the invasive period between the first signs of trismus and generalized spasms, the milder the disease.

1. Trismus is the earliest and most constant physical sign.
2. The risus sardonicus is diagnostic.
3. Mild forms of the disease show only muscular hypertonicity.
4. Moderate cases have generalized spasms but these are not prolonged or frequent and do not interfere with respiration or swallowing.
5. Severe cases have spasms which impair pulmonary ventilation in one or more of the following ways:
   (a) Prolonged or frequent spasms which fix the chest wall and diaphragm.
   (b) Laryngospasm with complete obstruction of respiration.
   (c) Pharyngospasm which prevents the swallowing of saliva which lies pooled in the pharynx and is inhaled into the trachea.

Impaired pulmonary ventilation is shown by anxiety, restlessness, a rising pulse and blood pressure, sweating, and cyanosis.

Severe forms of tetanus

Very severe forms show signs of impending failure of the vital centres, with circulatory collapse, respiratory failure, hyperpyrexia, ileus and sometimes, terminally, diminished spasms with muscular flaccidity.

1. Any spasm severe enough to cause apnoea which requires artificial respiration to re-establish breathing is an absolute indication for tracheostomy as a second attack of this type is almost invariably fatal.
2. Very occasionally, severe forms are associated with only focal spasms of the larynx and pharynx.

3. Generalized spasms and trismus due to infections of the central nervous system have to be distinguished from tetanus, but in tetanus the state of consciousness is characteristically clear.
4. Neck stiffness can be confused with meningitis, and abdominal rigidity with peritonitis.

Management

1. If human tetanus immunoglobulin (HTIG) is available, 500 units should be given intramuscularly; otherwise, give 20 000 units of anti-tetanus horse serum (ATS) (10 000 IV and 10 000 i.m.) after testing for sensitivity.
2. Wounds are treated solely on their surgical merits; any wound must be examined carefully for the presence of a foreign body.
3. Procaine-penicillin is given i.m. for 10 days, or cloxacillin if the wound is heavily infected, possibly with a penicillinase-producing staphylococcus.
4. The sedatives used are diazepam 5–10 mg 4 hourly, chlorpromazine 25 mg 4 hourly, or phenobarbitone 100 mg 8 hourly, separately or in combination.
5. Tracheostomy:
   (a) All severe and many moderate cases require tracheostomy. This is best done under general anaesthesia but can be done under local. A high tracheostomy at the level of the third, fourth and fifth rings is essential. If the disease is expected to run a severe course requiring IPPV, a cuffed tracheostomy tube should be inserted in children of 6 years and older. The tube must lie in alignment with the trachea so that the tip does not cause pressure erosion of the tracheal wall or kink the trachea. The position of the head and neck can determine whether pressure effects occur.
   (b) The patient should be placed in a humidified atmosphere after the tracheostomy or a heat moisture exchanger should be attached to the tracheostomy tube.
   (c) Secretions must be kept fluid so that physiotherapy and suctioning are efficient, otherwise bronchial obstruction and infection of the lung are inevitable.
   (d) Change of posture from back to side is required every 4 hours to encourage bronchial drainage and prevent pressure sores.
   (e) Hypersalivation, which is a feature of severe tetanus, requires the mouth and pharynx to be suctioned frequently.
   (f) A rising pulse rate, sweating, fever and increased spasms are more likely to be due to some obstruction of the airway than pulmonary infection or tetanus intoxication. In the older child tracheostomy alone is often enough to break the vicious circle of spasms–asphyxia–increasing spasm.
6. IPPV: very severe forms of tetanus cannot be controlled only with tracheostomy and sedation. They require total muscle paralysis and IPPV. Such cases are recognized:
   (a) By spasms of such severity as to interfere with respiration and which cannot be controlled by sedation, or which require such heavy sedation as to depress respiration.
   (b) By increasing cardiorespiratory distress with rising pulse, especially over 160.
   (c) By hyperpyrexia with a temperature of over 40°C (104°F).

The patient is paralysed with alcuronium and put on a mechanical ventilator. Sedation with chlorpromazine or diazepam by nasogastric tube should be continued. Management thereafter is as for any intensive care patient. There are two special points:

1. A generous amount of daily fluids is required to prevent dehydration since there is increased insensible loss due to sweating and excess salivation (Kerr, 1981). Fluids are given by nasogastric tube supplemented if necessary by the intravenous route in an amount sufficient to exceed the urine output and keep the urine SG at 1010–1015.
2. Sympathetic nervous system overactivity may occur due to the effect of toxin on the autonomic nervous system. The signs are hypertension, tachycardia, sweating and cool to cold limb peripheries (Kerr *et al.*, 1968). To control this alpha- and beta-adrenergic blocking drugs have been used, but central narcosis with morphine is safer and simpler to use. Morphine 1 mg/kg body weight can be given as an infusion over 30 minutes and reduces blood pressure, pulse rate and sweating. The drug is repeated as necessary, usually 8–12 hourly, and is needed until tachycardia and hypertension cease to recur.

IPPV and total muscle paralysis are usually required for 10–15 days, after which the patient is weaned off alcuronium. This is facilitated by the re-introduction of heavy sedation with phenobarbitone 100 mg i.m. 8 hourly being added to the maintenance diazepam or chlorpromazine, and should control residual spasms. This sedation is later lightened and when the patient is breathing spontaneously he is weaned from the ventilator:

1. The tracheostomy tube should be removed only after the patient has recovered sufficiently to swallow feeds without difficulty.
2. Since the disease confers no immunity, active immunization with toxoid should be started before discharge.

Prevention

1. When an injury occurs in which tetanus could be a complication, previously fully immunized individuals need wound care only, providing the last immunizing dose of tetanus toxoid was given not more than a year previously.
2. If the last immunizing dose was longer than a year ago a booster dose of 0.5 ml of tetanus toxoid should be given intramuscularly.
3. If the patient was not fully immunized previously, prophylactic HTIG 250 units i.m. should be given.
4. If HTIG is not available, ATS should be given; but it is essential that skin tests for hypersensitivity be done, and it is safer if the injection is given starting with a small dosage and increasing the volume every half-hour until the full amount is given.
5. Although *Clostridium tetani* is sensitive to penicillin, penicillin alone will not prevent tetanus developing.

References

KERR, J. H. (1981) Insensible fluid loss in severe tetanus. *Intensive Care Medicine,* **7,** 209–212

KERR, J. H., CORBETT, J. L., PRYS-ROBERTS, C., CRAMPTON-SMITH, A. and SPALDING, J. M. K. (1968) Involvement of the sympathetic nervous system in tetanus. *Lancet,* **ii,** 236–241

Chapter 34

Neonatal tetanus: treatment with IPPV

A. G. Wesley

Neonatal tetanus is due to infection of the umbilical cord by unsterile dressings or ligature.

Recognition

The disease manifests seldom less than 5 days and never less than 3 days after birth; in general the prognosis is worse the earlier the onset.

1. Presenting symptoms are: refusal to feed, due to trismus; muscular rigidity or spasms without loss of consciousness.
2. Other features are:
   Risus sardonicus.
   Salivation due to pharyngospasm.
   Rigidity, especially of the abdominal muscles and spasms causing head retraction or arching of the back.
   Respiratory impairment due to spasm of intercostals and diaphragm.
   Nearly always there is some evidence of umbilical infection.
3. The differential diagnosis includes:
   (a) Intracranial haemorrhage or hypoxia.
   (b) Fits from any cause (such as meningitis).
   (c) Tetany from hypocalcaemia or hypomagnesaemia: in these conditions there is 'jitteriness' or convulsions.
   (d) Kernicterus.

Management

In areas where neonatal tetanus is common, facilities for treatment with muscle relaxants and IPPV are not always available. Conservative treatment of severe disease has a mortality of over 90 per cent, and units without facilities for IPPV but with the possibility of transport of cases to a specialized centre must decide early in the course of the disease which cases require transfer. To wait for apnoeic attacks or pulmonary infection or atelectasis before transfer to an IPPV unit is to impair seriously the chance of survival. In general an infant with onset of symptoms at 8 days of age or less is likely to have severe disease and be in need of IPPV.

Procedure

1. On admission all infants receive chlorpromazine 12.5 mg and phenobarbitone 66 mg i.m. Oxygen is given as required.
2. Human tetanus immunoglobulin (HTIG) 500 IU is given i.m. or if not available, horse antitetanus serum (ATS) 20 000 IU half IV and half i.m.
3. Penicillin IV or i.m. is given for 7 days. Gentamicin is added if necessary for umbilical infection with other organisms or for pulmonary infection.
4. Vitamin K_1 1 mg i.m. is given since these children are born at home and would not have received it at birth.
5. Indications for IPPV:
   (a) Severe spasms.
   (b) A severe cyanotic or apnoeic episode.

Management with IPPV

Tracheostomy or nasotracheal intubation

IPPV can be applied through a tracheostomy, which is done under local or general anaesthesia. A high vertical incision through the third and fourth tracheal rings avoids pneumothorax. Polyvinyl chloride (PVC) uncuffed tracheostomy tubes FG 15 or 18 can be used. These usually need distal trimming to avoid impinging on the carina. The attachment to the ventilator circuit should be by a pliable tube, e.g. latex, and the tapes around the neck should not be tied too tightly. This will reduce erosion of the trachea by malalignment of the tracheostomy tube.

Because of the problems encountered in extubating a tracheostomized neonate (granulomata, tracheomalacia and tracheal stenosis) nasotracheal intubation with an uncuffed PVC tube 3.0 mm is an alternative to tracheostomy. Here the tube is passed to within 1–1½ cm of the carina (check by radiograph) and fixed by a stitch to a tape passing across the upper lip and tied around the head. The tape is fixed to the cheeks with non-irritant adhesive. The tube proximal to the stitch is not trimmed but left to attach to the ventilator circuit.

Extubation problems have been less with nasotracheal tube than with a tracheostomy, but accidental dislodgement is a hazard.

Ventilation

The infant will be on mechanical ventilation for 3 or more weeks so the facilities required of the respirator are a warm humidifier, an air–oxygen blender, PEEP, IMV and CPAP.

The initial ventilator settings are inspired oxygen concentration of 30%, rate of 28 per minute, 2 cm H_2O PEEP with inspiratory pressure limited to 15 cm H_2O.

Blood gas analysis once a day during the period of muscle relaxation is usually sufficient for modification of the respiratory controls to keep the child normally ventilated and oxygenated.

Muscle relaxation

Alcuronium chloride 1.25 mg IV or i.m. is repeated whenever spasms recur.

General care

1. Changes in body position allow drainage of upper and lower lung lobes.
2. Chest physiotherapy should be done every 4 hours. Saliva should be sucked out of the mouth before commencing the procedure. Strict sterile precautions are imperative during suction of the endotracheal tube. This is best done with a PVC FG 6 feeding tube. Airway suction may need to be performed more frequently if mucus partially obstructs the endotracheal tube.
3. Feeds: milk feeds, preferably freshly expressed breast milk, are given down a nasogastric tube 3 hourly, aspirating the stomach before each feed; any residue indicates some degree of ileus. If more than one-third of the daily total volume is not absorbed, the milk feeds are temporarily stopped and IV fluids are given.

Weaning from ventilation

After 10 days of muscle paralysis heavy sedation is added, e.g. phenobarbitone 33–66 mg i.m. 8 hourly in addition to chlorpromazine 12.5 mg 6 hourly or diazepam 2 mg 6 hourly which are given via the nasogastric tube.

Alcuronium chloride can usually be stopped after 2 days, along with the phenobarbitone. The oral sedation is continued to minimize residual spasms. IPPV is maintained until this sedation has been stopped. The child is then weaned onto IMV, which is gradually reduced, and finally onto CPAP.

When he is alert and making sucking movements (nasotracheal intubation) or sucking feeds through a small teat (tracheostomy) he is extubated.

Failure to tolerate removal of the tracheostomy tube indicates tracheal granulation tissue or tracheal stenosis, and these complications need expert advice (Smythe, 1964, 1967).

When removing a nasotracheal tube care is needed to prevent laryngeal spasm. This can be achieved by light sedation e.g. 2 diazepam IV or rectally. If recession and stridor occur, the infant is re-intubated and extubation repeated 1 week later.

Active immunization

Both infant and mother should be immunized with toxoid. The maternal immunity produced will protect future infants during the neonatal period. The infant who has had tetanus does *not* have any resultant immunity.

References

SMYTHE, P. M. (1964) The problem of detubating an infant with a tracheostomy. *Journal of Pediatrics,* **65,** 446–453

SMYTHE, P. M. (1967) Treatment of tetanus in neonates. *Lancet,* **i,** 335

Chapter 35

Neonatal tetanus: treatment without IPPV

Elizabeth Lund

It was felt essential to include a section for the many units in various parts of the world without facilities for IPPV and without any possibility of transferring their cases to an IPPV centre. (Editor)

Management

Note: Antitetanus serum and antibiotics should of course be given as in the previous chapter on IPPV treatment.

Good nursing and continuous supervision are essential:

1. On admission: start IV drip with a maintenance electrolyte solution containing 4–5% glucose. When spasms have ceased the child can be weighed, and the fluid requirement for the 24 hours can be calculated on the basis of 160 ml/kg plus an additional 50–60 ml/kg if dehydration is present. Since all cases are acidotic 20 ml of a 4% solution of sodium bicarbonate (10.0 mmol) should be put in the first bottle of IV fluid, preceded by an initial 'bolus' of 6 ml/kg of the sodium bicarbonate solution (3 mmol/kg) given over 5–10 minutes.
2. As soon as the drip is running satisfactorily, give diazepam 2.5 mg into the rubber bulb at the end of the tubing and run in at least 30 drops of fluid to ensure that the diazepam has entered the circulation; this dose can be repeated at 5- to 10-minute intervals, giving up to 10 doses over a period of 4 hours: occasionally very large amounts up to 120 mg over 4 hours will be required. Respiratory arrest from the diazepam is rare, but facilities for intubation should be at the bedside.
3. When muscle relaxation and regular breathing have been produced a nasogastric tube should be passed and chlorpromazine 12.5 mg in the form of a syrup given down the tube, followed by 2–3 ml of sterile water to make certain that the whole dose is in the stomach.
4. Continued treatment:
   (a) Chlorpromazine 12.5 mg every 6 hours through the nasogastric tube; alternating with (b).
   (b) Diazepam syrup 2.5–5.0 mg orally every 6 hours (2.5 mg for infants of 2.5–3.5 kg and 5.0 mg if over 3.5 kg). Additional doses of chlorpromazine or diazepam can be given IV between the 6-hourly doses if the spasms are severe.

5. At the end of 24 hours:
   (a) Slow down the drip to give half the maintenance requirement IV and half by nasogastric tube. The IV drip should be kept going for 3 days in case extra doses of IV diazepam are required.
   (b) Give diazepam syrup orally in the previous dose and increasing or decreasing the dose according to the degree of sedation achieved, as assessed by graded stimuli (*see* below). The diazepam should be given at 6-hourly intervals and should be continued for 1–2 days after the spasms have ceased.

   Assessment of diazepam dosage by stimulation:

Stimulus	
I Lifting the sheet II Touching the abdomen lightly	(A spasm in response to I or II requires an additional dose or an increased dose, as does a spontaneous spasm.)
III Poking the abdomen gently IV Poking the abdomen harder	(Absence of spontaneous spasms or spasms after III or IV stimulus indicates a satisfactory degree of sedation. Spasms after III or IV require continuation of diazepam in the previous dose.)

   (c) Chlorpromazine should be continued for 3–5 weeks but the dose can generally be decreased from the 12th day onwards.

Note: Arrangements should be made for active immunization of the mother, the rest of the family if possible, and the infant, before discharge. *The disease of tetanus confers no immunity.*

Chapter 36

Acute meningitis and encephalitis

Imogen Morgan

Acute bacterial meningitis is a medical emergency. Delay, failure in recognition, or inadequate therapy may result in death, or survival with neurological sequelae such as spasticity, epilepsy, hydrocephalus, deafness, or mental retardation. A diagnostic lumbar puncture is indicated early whenever meningitis is a possibility except in a few rare circumstances (*see* below).

Occasionally the initial cerebrospinal fluid examination may be normal, but if clinical signs persist or evolve a 'second look' lumbar puncture after a few hours may confirm the diagnosis.

The pathogens involved vary with the age of the child (*Table 36.1*). In the neonatal period, maternal perineal flora are usually involved because infection has been acquired before or during birth. *Haemophilus influenzae* affects infants from 20 days old to 5 years, after which it much less common. After the newborn period, *N. meningitidis, H. influenzae*, and *S. pneumoniae* are the most frequent pathogens.

Unusual organisms or recurrent infections may reflect deficient or defective immunity (e.g. patients being treated for leukaemia or malignancy) or an abnormal anatomical connection to the subarachnoid space (e.g. dermal sinus, myelomeningocele, skull fracture). In these cases, normal skin or respiratory tract flora may be involved.

Neonatal meningitis

Recognition

Meningitis is present in 30 per cent of septicaemic neonates. Specific signs of meningitis occur late and carry a poor prognosis and a high index of suspicion is essential. Mortality is high, particularly in Gram negative infections (15–35 per cent) with long-term sequelae demonstrable in at least 30 per cent of survivors.

Predisposing history

1. Maternal illness or fever at delivery.
2. Membranes ruptured for over 24 hours.
3. Maternal colonization (e.g. with group B streptococcus).
4. Risk factors in the infant (birth asphyxia, prematurity, admission to special care unit, respiratory distress, presence of indwelling arterial catheter).

Table 36.1 Organisms found in bacterial meningitis according to infant age

Under 1 month	*Over 1 month*
Common infections	*Common infections*
*Escherichia coli**	*Neisseria meningitidis*
Group B streptococcus*	*Haemophilus influenzae*
Klebsiella sp.	*Streptococcus pneumoniae*
Enterobacter sp.	Group B streptococcus†
Group D streptococcus (enterococcus)	
Staphylococcus aureus	
Listeria monocytogenes	
Less common infections	*Less common infections*
Haemophilus influenzae	Group A streptococcus
Streptococcus pneumoniae	Staphylococcus sp.
N. meningitidis	*Mycobacterium tuberculosis*
Salmonella sp.	Gram negative bacilli
Citrobacter sp.‡	
Serratia sp.	
Proteus mirabilis	
Acinetobacter calcoaceticus	
Pseudomonas aeruginosa	
Bacteroides fragilis (anaerobe)	
Fusobacterium (anaerobe)	
Streptococcus viridans	
Staphylococcus epidermidis	
Pasteurella sp.	

* Together cause 65 per cent of neonatal meningitis.
† At 1–2 months of age.
‡ Very frequent association with cerebral abscess.

Non-specific early symptoms and signs

1. Temperature instability; low or high.
2. 'Not doing well'; poor feeding, lethargy, or irritability.
3. Apnoeic episodes or respiratory irregularity.
4. Vomiting (may contain bile) or abdominal distension.
5. Increasing jaundice.
6. Convulsions; colour changes, abnormal repeated eye or mouth movements, sudden alterations in tone, or jerking limb movements.

Later signs

1. Circulatory failure, shock.
2. Full fontanelle, head retraction, or opisthotonus.
3. Purulent CSF.

Diagnosis

If the diagnosis is suspected, a full septic screen should be performed and the infant commenced on treatment for meningitis. Therapy can be altered or stopped when culture results become available. Delay in initiating treatment, even for a few hours, may adversely affect the outcome.

1. The following specimens should be obtained from the infant: aerobic and anaerobic blood cultures; urine culture; CSF for cell count, Gram stain, glucose, protein, counterimmunoelectrophoresis (CIE), and culture. Swabs from throat, ear, umbilicus, rectum and any septic sites. Pharyngeal aspirate.
2. The following other investigations should be performed: chest X-ray, full blood count with platelet count, coagulation screen, urea and electrolytes, blood glucose, blood gases, viral cultures of CSF, urine, and stool may be indicated.
3. The following specimens should be obtained from the mother: high vaginal swab. Blood and urine cultures if indicated.
4. Examination of the placenta may be informative in early infection.

Note: If the infant is severely shocked, convulsing, or has evidence of brain herniation, diagnostic lumbar puncture must be postponed. A blood culture should be obtained and empirical antibiotic treatment given while the acute problem is managed.

Interpretation of results

1. Indirect evidence of neonatal septicaemia is provided by a peripheral blood film with an absolute neutrophil count of less than 1500/mm^3 or more than 10 000/mm^3 after 24 hours of age. A platelet count of less than 100 000/mm^3, an elevated 'band count', or toxic granulation of neutrophils are also suggestive.
2. If the CSF is thick or under low pressure, it may be difficult to obtain. *Gentle* aspiration by syringe is permissible, or a repeat attempt with the infant supported in a seated position, in a higher interspace, or using a wider bore (20 gauge) needle. The laboratory should be reminded that the samples are from a neonate.

Gram film and culture

These should invariably be performed even if the cell count is not abnormal. Some pathogens are difficult to grow on culture; others may show misleading staining characteristics and morphology due to previous treatment, their true identity being revealed on culture.

Cell count and biochemistry

In the term newborn, the normal CSF cell count is less than 20 cells/mm^3 (30 cells/mm^3 in the first 3 days) with less than 5 neutrophils/mm^3. Protein is less than 2 g/ℓ, and glucose is 50 per cent or more of blood glucose (unless there has been intracranial haemorrhage when persisting hypoglycorrhachia is the rule). Viral meningitis is uncommon in the newborn. Any abnormal CSF cell count or biochemistry usually indicates bacterial meningitis.

Blood-stained CSF

Blood staining may be due to traumatic tap, intracranial haemorrhage, or intracranial haemorrhage with meningitis. The normal ratio of white to red cells

(1:600) will be increased in meningitis. Gram film and culture should be done even if an accurate cell count is not possible.

Other CSF tests

While elevated serum C-reactive protein correlates well with the presence of neonatal sepsis, CSF C-reactive protein and lactate are unreliable tests in neonatal meningitis. Antigen detection by counterimmunoelectrophoresis may be useful.

Management. Antibiotic treatment (Figure 36.1)

Conventional first-line treatment for suspected neonatal septicaemia includes parenteral penicillin or ampicillin with an aminoglycoside (gentamicin or netilmicin).

When Gram negative meningitis complicates septicaemia, however, the therapeutic success of this combination is limited, and is not improved by adding intrathecal or intraventricular aminoglycoside.

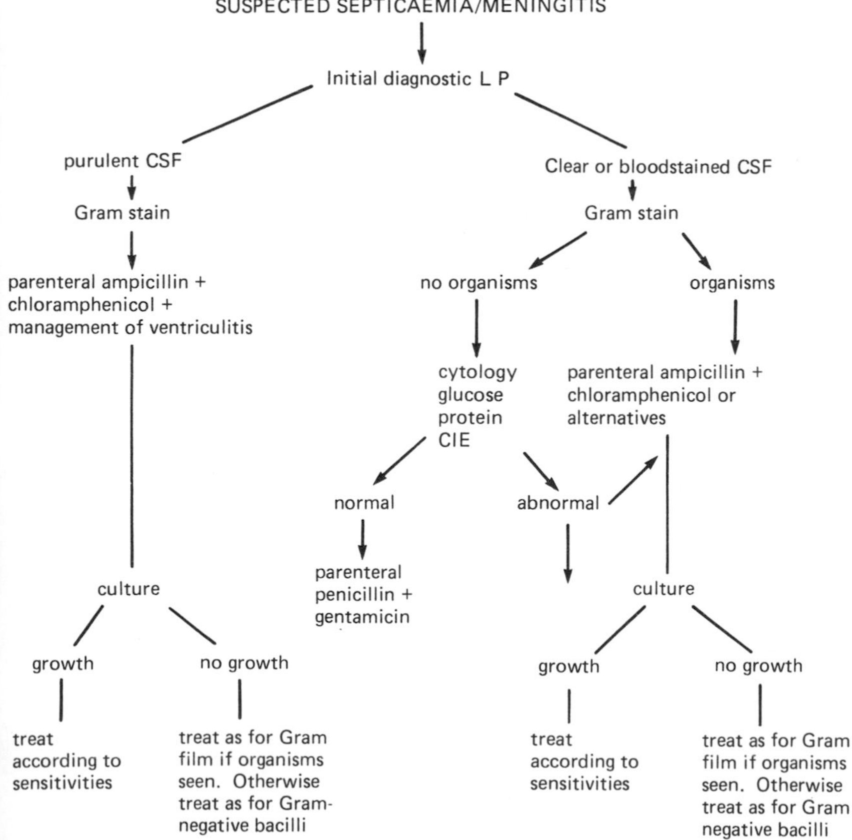

Figure 36.1 Initial management in neonatal meningitis. LP = Lumbar puncture; CIE = counterimmunoelectrophoresis

The initial antibiotic therapy must be active against the usual groups of pathogens (group B streptococci and Gram negative bacilli) and must cross into the cerebrospinal fluid in effective concentration. Where the pathogen is unknown the usual first-line therapy in suspected neonatal meningitis is parenteral ampicillin and chloramphenicol, which fulfils these criteria.

Recently, the newly available antibiotics have been used with some success in place of this combination. Latamoxef (Moxalactam) is particularly active against Gram negative bacilli, but should be used in combination with penicillin where Gram positive infection is a possibility. Cefotaxime and ceftriaxone, newer third-generation cephalosporins with good CSF penetration, when used as monotherapy, appear to offer as effective treatment as the older combinations, with less hazard. Cefuroxime crosses non-inflamed meninges poorly and has limited activity against *E. coli*, suggesting limited usefulness in the neonate.

In all cases, antibiotic treatment is modified when the results of bacterial culture and sensitivities become available, and a second CSF has been examined 1–2 days after starting treatment.

All antibiotics should be given parenterally, preferably intravenously, for a minimum of 10 days after the CSF is sterile.

1. Initial therapy depends on Gram film or antigen detection results. *Two* antibiotics should be used.
   (a) *No organisms seen:* If CSF cytology or biochemistry, or the clinical picture supports the diagnosis of meningitis, parenteral ampicillin 200 mg/kg/day with chloramphenicol 25 mg/kg/day (50 mg/kg/day in term babies after 14 days old) should be given.
   Alternatively, ampicillin with latamoxef (Moxalactam) 100 mg/kg/day, or cefotaxime 200 mg/kg/day alone or ceftriaxone 100 mg/kg/day alone may be used.
   (b) *Gram positive cocci:* Group B streptococci are the commonest cause of neonatal meningitis. One per cent of infants colonized with these organisms develops symptomatic infection. This can be a severe early septicaemia with or without meningitis, or a later meningeal presentation at 10 days to 8 weeks old. Benzylpenicillin 250 000 u/kg/24 hours (150 mg/kg/24 hours) is the treatment of choice, but a second drug should be used initially as group D organisms are less sensitive to penicillin.
   When staphylococcal disease is suspected, methicillin 100 mg/kg/day with gentamicin or vancomycin should be used.
   (c) *Gram negative bacilli:* Initial treatment as in (a) should be given. Ventriculitis complicates over 70 per cent of these infections; a poor outcome correlates with development of ventriculitis, persistence of positive CSF culture, CSF cell count above 10 000 cells/mm^3, or CSF protein higher than 5 g/ℓ.
   (d) *Gram positive bacilli: Listeria monocytogenes* is a short bacillus producing a non-specific maternal infection. The infant inhaling contaminated liquor develops a severe early septicaemia with pneumonia and multiple microabscesses. A late acquired form of this infection presents as meningitis or slowly developing hydrocephalus after 5 days of age in infants of healthy mothers. Parenteral ampicillin is the treatment of choice (*Lancet,* 1980).
2. The final combination of antibiotics is based on results of culture and sensitivities.

No organism may be identified in spite of a polymorph pleocytosis or clinical evidence of meningitis. This may be due to antibiotic treatment before the diagnostic lumbar puncture, anaerobic infection, or a generalized infection mimicking bacterial meningitis. Treatment should be given as for infection with Gram negative bacilli.

3. *Repeat CSF examination and culture should always be performed at 24–36 hours* after antibiotic treatment is commenced. If stained smears demonstrate bacteria, ventriculitis must be sought, and modification of antimicrobial treatment considered.
4. *Minimum duration of treatment.* Treatment should be continued for 14 days in most uncomplicated Gram positive infections and for 21 days in Gram-negative or staphylococcal infections. Where CSF has been purulent or where ventriculitis has developed, daily intraventricular drug treatment should continue until the CSF is sterile on 4 successive days.

Other forms of meningitis

1. *Pseudomonas aeruginosa.* Treatment is difficult since antibiotics to which the organism is usually sensitive do not adequately penetrate the CSF. Daily intrathecal treatment in addition to systemic therapy must be given (gentamicin 1–2 mg daily, kanamycin 2 mg daily, colistin 0.2 mg daily or carbenicillin 10 mg daily). Carbenicillin should not be given alone because of the ready development of resistance.
   Ceftazidime, a third-generation cephalosporin with good CSF penetration, is highly active against pseudomonas and may provide effective treatment when given parenterally, without the need for additional intrathecal treatment.
2. *Anaerobic infections (bacteroides, fusobacterium).* These Gram negative bacilli produce clinical meningitis but do not grow in aerobic culture. Chloramphenicol has been the drug of choice in treatment, but is often unsuccessful in clearing the organisms from the CSF. Recently, the early use of parenteral metronidazole (30 mg/kg/day) has led to recovery without sequelae in newborn infants with bacteroides meningitis (Law and Marks, 1980).
3. *Citrobacter diversus.* Brain abscess develops in 70 per cent of infections. Surgery may be required.

Supportive management

Endotoxic/septic shock

Plasma protein fraction or fresh frozen plasma 10 ml/kg over 30 minutes should be given. Dopamine infusion (initially 5 μg/kg/minute; *see* page 109) may be necessary to improve cardiac output. Blood pressure and urine output should be monitored. The use of irradiated granulocyte transfusion has been advocated in neutropenic septic infants (Christensen *et al.*, 1982).

Convulsions

Fits should be treated with phenobarbitone 10 mg/kg twice at 12 hours apart, then 5 mg/kg/day during the acute illness. Blood levels should be monitored.

If chloramphenicol is being given, serum levels should be monitored, as phenobarbitone will reduce the duration of action of chloramphenicol by induction of hepatic enzymes.

Ventilatory support

Ventilatory support may be required.

Acute complications of neonatal meningitis

Acute ventriculitis

This is very common in neonatal meningitis, particularly in Gram negative infections, and is the commonest cause of therapeutic failure. It is defined as ventricular fluid with greater than 200 cells/mm^3 and containing bacteria. The following features are suspicious:

1. Initially purulent lumbar CSF.
2. Positive culture of lumbar CSF after 24–48 hours of appropriate therapy.
3. Deterioration in general condition after 48 hours.
4. Acute deterioration at any time, with fits, bulging fontanelle, or rapid increase in head circumference.

In these circumstances, cerebral ultrasound or computed tomography should be performed to determine whether ventricular size permits intraventricular drug administration. Diagnostic bilateral ventricular taps should be performed. Usually an aminoglycoside is given daily by the intraventricular route and systemically until the ventricular CSF has been sterile for several days.

Increasing intracranial pressure

This may be due to cerebral necrosis, or acute loculated or generalized hydrocephalus due to obstructed CSF drainage.

See Chapter 26, Raised intracranial pressure.

Meningitis in the older child

Recognition

Classic signs of meningeal irritation are not always demonstrable in infancy, or may be masked by non-specific antibiotic or steroid treatment.

The immediate diagnostic investigation is a lumbar puncture. Additionally, blood cultures, nasal swabs, and needle aspirate cultures of any skin lesions should be taken at the same time.

Suggestive symptoms and signs: under 2 years:

1. Irritability, altered sleep pattern.
2. Lethargy, drowsiness, coma.
3. A convulsion in an ill or febrile child or in any infant under 6 months.
4. Vomiting or respiratory illness where the child appears more ill than expected.
5. Severe shock without obvious cause.
6. Haemorrhagic skin lesions in a febrile child (usually meningococcal).
7. Bulging fontanelle or neck retraction (late).

Over 2 years: (1) to (5) as above with:

1. Fever associated with lethargy or irritability.
2. Headache, neck stiffness.
3. Positive Kernig or Brudzinski sign.

If signs of meningeal irritation are present but lumbar puncture fails to confirm meningitis, an alternative explanation should be sought such as retropharyngeal abscess, cervical adenitis, arthritis or osteomyelitis of cervical spine, subarachnoid haemorrhage, or upper lobe pneumonia.

Diagnosis

Cytology and chemistry of CSF (Table 36.2)

1. Turbid or purulent fluid always indicates bacterial meningitis.
2. If the fluid is clear or opalescent, results of Gram film, cell count, cell morphology, and glucose should be awaited before starting treatment. Gram film and culture should be done even if the cell count is not increased, as very early infection, or a severe meningococcal infection may be present.

Table 36.2 Cytology and chemistry of CSF

Polymorph excess		*Lymphocyte excess*	
Glucose ↓ *Protein* ↑↑	*Glucose N* *Protein* ↑	*Glucose* ↓ *Protein* ↑↑	*Glucose N* *Protein N or* ↑
Bacterial meningitis Mumps meningoencephalitis TB meningitis (rarely)	Early viral infection Poliomyelitis Cerebral abscess	TB meningitis Mumps meningoencephalitis	Viral infection Cerebral abscess Septic thrombophlebitis TB meningitis

Rarer causes of increased cell count with low glucose are:
Lymphocytic choriomeningitis, cryptococcal meningitis, herpes simplex encephalitis, meningeal spread of malignancy, or mycoplasma meningoencephalitis

N = Normal values.

In a *clinically well child*, if a mixed polymorph/lymphocyte pleocytosis is present with negative Gram film and normal glucose, antibiotic therapy may be withheld until a repeat lumbar puncture is performed after 6–12 hours of *close clinical observation*. In early viral meningitis, a predominantly polymorphonuclear picture may change to a predominantly mononuclear one within this time.

3. Where there is bacteraemia, CSF changes may develop at a later stage. For this reason a blood culture should always be taken. If it is positive, lumbar puncture should be repeated after 24 hours.
4. CSF glucose depends on blood glucose. A CSF/blood glucose ratio below 0.4 or a CSF glucose below 2.2 mmol/ℓ is highly specific for bacterial meningitis (Donald, Malan and van der Walt, 1983).

Other CSF tests

1. The 'Phadebact' test (Phadebact CSF test; Pharmacia Diagnostics, New Jersey, USA) uses co-agglutination to detect the antigenic components of common pathogens (*H. influenzae, N. meningitidis, S. pneumoniae,* group B streptococcus). It can be positive even if growth of the organism on culture is inhibited by previous antibiotic treatment (Drow *et al.*, 1983).
2. Counterimmunoelectrophoresis can also detect bacterial antigens rapidly, but requires specialized equipment.
3. CSF lactate is elevated in bacterial but not in viral meningitis. False-negative results occur.
4. CSF C-reactive protein is usually raised in bacterial meningitis, and rarely raised in non-bacterial meningitis. Its rise and fall may be useful when monitoring therapy.

Other tests

A full blood count, platelet count, urea and electrolyte screen, blood glucose determination, and blood culture are also indicated.

Management

Bacterial meningitis is a clinical emergency requiring early diagnosis and immediate treatment. Parenteral antibiotics should be commenced immediately after the diagnostic lumbar puncture. If CSF cannot be obtained, therapy should not be delayed (antigen detection techniques can be used later). *The treatment of shock, seizures, or cerebral oedema should have priority over attempted lumbar puncture.*

Antibiotic treatment

The most common pathogens after 30 days of age are *Haemophilus influenzae*, followed by *Streptococcus pneumoniae,* and *Neisseria meningitidis*. The frequency of *H. influenzae* infection diminishes with advancing age but it remains an important cause of meningitis throughout life.

Intrathecal antibiotics

If the CSF is purulent, intrathecal benzylpenicillin 10 000 units (6 mg) (of specific intrathecal preparation) may be given at the time of diagnostic lumbar puncture. Permanent neurological damage or death may result if the incorrect preparation or excessive dose is administered.

Initial therapy

Initial intravenous antibiotic therapy depends on the results of the Gram stain or antigen detection.

NO ORGANISMS SEEN, OR DETECTED

If the CSF suggests bacterial infection, give ampicillin 300 mg/kg/day plus chloramphenicol 100 mg/kg/day.

GRAM NEGATIVE COCCI (MENINGOCOCCI)

Benzylpenicillin in 250 000 u/kg/day (150 mg/kg/24 hours) in six divided doses for 5–7 days produces adequate CSF drug concentrations in most cases. Penicillin-resistant organisms have been described, but are uncommon.

GRAM POSITIVE COCCI (S. PNEUMONIAE, STREPTOCOCCI OR, RARELY, STAPHYLOCOCCI)

Initial treatment is benzylpenicillin 250 000 u/kg/day (150 mg/kg/24 hr). Some strains of pneumococci are now resistant to penicillin, therefore sensitivity testing should always be performed. Chloramphenicol, cefotaxime 200 mg/kg/day, or ceftriaxone 100 mg/kg/day provide effective alternative treatment (Steele and Bradsher, 1983). In suspected staphylococcal infection, cloxacillin 100 mg/kg/day should be given in addition until sensitivities are known. For recognition and management of raised intracranial pressure in pneumococcal meningitis *see* Chapter 26, page 298.

GRAM NEGATIVE BACILLI OR COCCOBACILLI (H. INFLUENZAE)

Initially, both ampicillin and chloramphenicol should be given, for at least 10 days. Up to 20 per cent of organisms are resistant to ampicillin, while chloramphenicol-resistant organisms are emerging. Organisms resistant to both drugs have now been reported. Latamoxef (Moxalactam) (150 mg/kg/day), ceftriaxone (100 mg/kg/day), and cefotaxime (200 mg/kg/day) have each been successfully used as an alternative treatment in *H. influenzae* meningitis in children (Kaplan *et al.*, 1984). For management of raised intracranial pressure and obstructive hydrocephalus *see* Chapter 26, page 298.

Definitive combination

The definitive combination of antibiotics must be based upon the results of bacterial culture and sensitivities.

Second lumbar puncture

If clinical improvement has not occurred after 48 hours of treatment, a second lumbar puncture should be done. There is no benefit from a lumbar puncture at the end of the course of antibiotics.

Fever

Fever developing after 10 days' treatment is likely to be a drug reaction. Therapy should be stopped and clinical observation carried on while the possibility of septic complications is borne in mind.

Antibiotic prophylaxis

Antibiotic prophylaxis (rifampicin 20 mg/kg/day in two doses for 4 days) should be given to children who are household contacts of cases with meningococcal or *H. influenzae* infections.

Other forms of meningitis

Tuberculous meningitis

The onset is usually more gradual than that of acute bacterial meningitis, but occasionally the history is short. CSF findings may mimic acute bacterial or viral infection (*Table 36.2*). If TB meningitis is considered a possibility acid-fast bacilli should be sought on microscopy though they may not be visible despite prolonged search. Other signs of tuberculous infection may be present, such as choroidal tubercles, splenomegaly, chest X-ray changes, or a history of contact with a case. The Mantoux test should be performed but is sometimes negative in anergic states. Raised intracranial pressure is commonly present with hydrocephalus and signs of tentorial coning at diagnosis; its detection and relief is a matter of urgency (*see* Chapter 26). Initial treatment, which should be started on presumption of infection, is isoniazid 20 mg/kg/day, ethambutol 15 mg/kg/day, rifampicin 20 mg/kg/day, and intramuscular streptomycin 20 mg/kg/day.

Pyridoxine 25 mg/day is given with therapy. Treatment with two drugs is continued after the sensitivities are known (Naughten *et al.*, 1981).

Cryptococcal meningitis

This mycotic meningitis particularly affects immunosuppressed children. Indian ink staining of CSF shows budding yeasts. Treatment is with flucytosine 150 mg/kg/day and amphotericin 0.3 mg/kg/day.

Amoebic meningoencephalitis (Naegleria sp.)

This is a fulminant, usually fatal infection. There may be a history of recent swimming in a freshwater lake. Treatment is with amphotericin, rifampicin, and miconazole (Seidel *et al.*, 1982).

Viral meningitis

Sixty per cent of 'aseptic meningitis' is caused by mumps, Coxsackie, or ECHO viruses. Treatment is symptomatic.

Supportive management in meningitis

Convulsions

Prophylactic anticonvulsants may be indicated for irritable children. Phenytoin or phenobarbitone are suitable, but phenobarbitone will reduce the duration of action of chloramphenicol. Diazepam may induce respiratory depression and increase cerebral oedema.

Shock

Plasma or isotonic crystalloid should be given to maintain blood pressure and urine output while avoiding fluid overload which might increase cerebral oedema. Central venous pressure should be monitored. Dopamine or inotropic agents may be required to improve cardiac output (*see* page 109). Close monitoring to avoid hypoxaemia or hypoglycaemia is required. The use of steroids is controversial since they interfere with antibiotic penetration into CSF (Brady, Kaplan and Taber, 1981).

Disseminated coagulopathy (DIC) (see Chapter 54)

This should be suspected in meningococcal infection with necrotic skin lesions, oozing from puncture sites, leucopenia or thrombocytopenia.

Hyponatraemia and inappropriate ADH secretion

Hyponatraemia is common in bacterial meningitis, correlating with infectious complications and with poor neurological outcome. The effects of inappropriate ADH secretion added to inflammatory cell swelling in the brain may produce water intoxication. If shock is not present, administered fluids should be isotonic and should be restricted initially to 50–60 per cent of maintenance requirements. Serum electrolytes, osmolality, urine volume and osmolality should be monitored daily (Kaplan and Feigin, 1978).

Acute complications of meningitis in the older infant

Subdural empyema

Asymptomatic subdural effusions commonly complicate bacterial meningitis, particularly *H. influenzae* infection. They are caused by increased vascular permeability and eventually resolve spontaneously.

Empyema within the subdural space complicates *H. influenzae, S. pneumoniae*, or coliform meningitis in infants, or sinus infections in older children.

Suspicious signs include:

1. Sudden or progressive increase in head circumference in infants.
2. Separation of sutures on skull X-ray.
3. Sudden increase in fontanelle tension.
4. Persistent illness despite improvement in lumbar CSF.
5. Ophthalmic signs, ophthalmoplegia or papilloedema.
6. Hemisphere signs; convulsions followed by confusion, hemiparesis, hemianopia, or dysphasia.

Immediate computed tomography will confirm the diagnosis. Bilateral subdural taps through the anterior fontanelle or burrholes will be required.

Cerebral abscess

This may result from bloodstream infection, penetrating skull injury, or extension from adjacent sites. Symptoms such as headache and vomiting, with signs including lethargy and fever, may mimic meningitis. Papilloedema and focal neurological signs are common and are indications for immediate computed tomography. Treatment is primarily surgical, along with prolonged intravenous antibiotic treatment (*see* page 350).

Acutely raised intracranial pressure

1. Cerebral oedema increases the mortality and post-infectious morbidity of bacterial meningitis. Inflammatory parenchymal swelling, inappropriate ADH secretion, respiratory depression and water overload contribute to its development. Cerebral perfusion pressure is reduced which, together with the effects of vasculitis, produces cerebral ischaemia, or infarction (Goitein and Tamir, 1983) (for further consideration of diagnosis and management of raised intracranial pressure in bacterial meningitis, *see* Chapter 26, page 298).
2. Brain herniation may be precipitated by lumbar puncture (Horwitz, Boxerbaum and O'Bell, 1980).
3. Similar complications occur from obstructive hydrocephalus, especially in *H. influenzae* infections (*see also* Chapter 26, page 298).

Recognition

1. It is not possible to predict which patients will sustain brain herniation, which is probably the *commonest cause of death in bacterial meningitis.*
2. Classic signs of incipient herniation include:
   (a) Reduction in level of consciousness.
   (b) Loss of pupillary reaction to light.
   (c) Development of hemiparesis, decorticate or decerebrate posturing.
   (d) Abnormal respiration pattern and bradycardia.
   (e) Oculomotor deviation or loss of oculocephalic response.

Management

(*See also* related Chapter 26.)

1. *Suspected brain herniation is an absolute contraindication to lumbar puncture.*
2. *Emergency management of herniation reduces mortality.*
3. *Immediate management includes intubation, hyperventilation, and intravenous mannitol. Intracranial pressure should be monitored if possible.*
4. *In these circumstances, parenteral antibiotics should be started, and lumbar puncture delayed until evidence of brain herniation has disappeared.*

Indications for early computed tomography in bacterial meningitis

In some circumstances, early computed tomography is indicated to permit early diagnosis of complications.

1. Persistent or focal seizures.
2. Prolonged fever.
3. Persistently full fontanelle or signs of raised intracranial pressure.
4. Altered mental status after 48 hours of treatment.
5. Focal neurological signs.
6. Tuberculous meningitis.

Acute viral encephalitis

Acute encephalitis may be caused by direct virus invasion or by post-infectious encephalomyelitis following infections such as measles or vaccinia. Differential diagnosis is from tuberculous meningitis, cerebral abscess, fungal meningitis, or occasionally, cerebral tumour.

Recognition

1. Onset is usually sudden with fever, headache, neck stiffness, and vomiting.
2. An altered level of consciousness follows.
3. Focal or generalized convulsions may occur.
4. In herpes simplex infection there may be bizarre behaviour, memory loss, or hallucinations of taste or smell.
5. Focal signs such as cranial nerve palsies, hemiplegia, speech disturbance, or asymmetrical neurological signs may develop.
6. In herpes infection, herpes labialis may be present.
7. There may be an accompanying exanthem.

Diagnosis

Aetiological diagnosis can be established by isolating the virus from brain or by demonstrating antibody rise in convalescent serum or CSF. Specific therapy is at present available only in herpes simplex virus infection and in true (post-inferior) varicella encephalitis as seen in treated leukaemia (*see* page 492).

1. CSF is clear or opalescent with a lymphocytic cell count of 5–1500 cells/mm^3. Protein is increased and glucose is normal. Red cells may be present in the CSF in herpes virus infections.
2. Electroencephalography usually shows generalized slowing. Localized complexes over the temporal areas are suggestive of herpes simplex infection.
3. Computed tomography scan in herpes simplex encephalitis shows areas of decreased attenuation over the temporal lobes at 3–11 days of illness in 50 per cent of cases.

Management

1. Supportive treatment is the mainstay of management, following the same principles as in bacterial meningitis. Fluid or water overload should be avoided, the development of raised intracranial pressure managed actively, adequate glucose provided, and hypoxaemia avoided.
2. Specific antiviral treatment is available for herpes simplex encephalitis. The state of consciousness is an important prognostic factor, the outcome being uniformly bad once coma has developed. If the diagnosis is likely, early intravenous treatment with acyclovir 5 mg/kg 8 hourly for 10 days should be given. Few adverse effects have been reported from this drug, however resistant virus strains have already been identified.
   Vidarabine, an alternative treatment, requires the administration of an undesirably large fluid volume, and has been associated with adverse gastrointestinal and neurological side-effects (Hirsch and Schooley, 1983).
   Double-blind trials comparing vidarabine and acyclovir are at present being conducted.

References

BRADY, M. T., KAPLAN, S. L. and TABER, L. H. (1981) Association between persistence of pneumococcal meningitis and dexamethasone administration. *Journal of Pediatrics,* **99,** 924–926

CHRISTENSEN, R. D., ROTHSTEIN, G., ANSTALL, H. B. and BYBEE, B. (1982) Granulocyte transfusions in neonates with bacterial infection, neutropenia and depletion of mature marrow neutrophils. *Pediatrics,* **70,** 1–6

DONALD, P. R., MALAN, C. and VAN DER WALT, A. (1983) Simultaneous determination of CSF glucose and blood glucose concentrations in the diagnosis of bacterial meningitis. *Journal of Pediatrics,* **103,** 413–415

DROW, D. L., WELCH, D. F., HENSEL, D., EISENACH, K., LONG, E. and SLIFKIN, M. (1983) Evaluation of the Phadebact CSF test for detection of the four most common causes of bacterial meningitis. *Journal of Clinical Microbiology,* **18,** 1358–1361

GOITEIN, K. J. and TAMIR, I. (1983) Cerebral perfusion pressure in CNS infections of infancy and childhood. *Journal of Pediatrics,* **103,** 40–43

HIRSCH, M. S. and SCHOOLEY, R. T. (1983) Treatment of herpesvirus infections. Part I. *New England Journal of Medicine,* **309,** 963–970

HORWITZ, S. J., BOXERBAUM, B. and O'BELL, J. (1980) Cerebral herniation in bacterial meningitis in childhood. *Annals of Neurology,* **7,** 524–528

KAPLAN, S. L. and FEIGIN, R. D. (1978) The syndrome of inappropriate secretion of antidiuretic hormone in children with bacterial meningitis. *Journal of Pediatrics,* **92,** 758–761

KAPLAN, S. L., MASON, E. O. and MASON, S. K. *et al.* (1984) Prospective comparative trial of moxalactam versus ampicillin or chloramphenicol for treatment of *Haemophilus influenzae* type b meningitis in children. *Journal of Pediatrics,* **104,** 447–453

Lancet (1980). Perinatal listeriosis. *Lancet,* **i,** 911

LAW, B. J. and MARKS, M. I. (1980) Excellent outcome of Bacteroides meningitis in a newborn treated with metronidazole. *Pediatrics,* **66,** 463–465

NAUGHTEN, E., WEINDLING, A. M., NEWTON, R. and BOWER, B. D. (1981) Tuberculous meningitis in children. *Lancet,* **ii,** 973–975

SEIDEL, J. S., HARMATZ, P., VISVESVARA, G. S., COHEN, A., EDWARDS, J. and TURNER, J. (1982) Successful treatment of primary ameobic meningoencephalitis. *New England Journal of Medicine,* **306,** 346–348

STEELE, R. W. and BRADSHER, R. W. (1983) Comparison of ceftriazone with standard therapy for bacterial meningitis. *Journal of Pediatrics,* **103,** 138–141

Further reading

BELL, W. E. and McGUINNESS, G. A. (1982) Suppurative central nervous system infections in the neonate. *Seminars in Perinatology,* **6,** 1–24

DE LOUVOIS, J. (1983) Use of some new antibiotics in the newborn. *Hospital Update,* **9,** 1291–1299

KAPLAN, S. L. and FEIGIN, R. D. (1983) Treatment of meningitis in children. *Pediatric Clinics of North America, 30,* 259–269

McCRACKEN, G. H. and NELSON, J. D. (1983) *Antimicrobial Therapy for Newborns* (2nd edn.). New York: Grune and Stratton

WOOD, M. J. (1984) Antiviral chemotherapy. *Medicine International.* Vol. 2, part 3, pp. 102–110

Chapter 37

Expanding lesions in the head

Ian A. McKinlay

Most expanding lesions in the head do not require emergency treatment on diagnosis. Exceptions are those in patients with signs of raised intracranial pressure, status epilepticus, cerebral abscess or empyema, subdural or large intracerebral haematomas, and those with bulbar palsy.

Recognition

Signs of raised intracranial pressure:

1. Rising pulse rate, respiratory rate and blood pressure.
2. Deteriorating consciousness level; initially loss of highest mental functions.
3. Stiffness of the neck, stridor, and dysphagia.
4. Tense fontanelle or intracranial bruit.
5. Papilloedema (only found in 50 per cent of patients).
6. Dilatation or constriction and sluggish reaction of pupils.
7. Bradycardia and Cheyne–Stokes respiration.

Management

Hazards of lumbar puncture in raised intracranial pressure (see also page 292)

Patients suspected of having expanding lesions in the head should be transferred to a centre where neurosurgical help is available. Lumbar puncture is not an appropriate investigation for tumours, haematomas or abscesses except in discussion with a neurosurgeon and in special circumstances, e.g. if meningitis is thought to coexist with an abscess. If a lumbar puncture is performed a fine needle should be used and the pressure directly measured (rate of drip of fluid is unreliable). Queckenstedt's test should NEVER be attempted and the patient should be frequently monitored for evidence of deterioration for 24 hours as 'coning' can occur many hours after the lumbar puncture. As little CSF as possible should be withdrawn (*see also* page 745). The CSF is usually normal in patients with gliomas and is often unhelpful in patients with cerebral abscess, when it may be normal or show a slight lymphocytosis if the abscess is near the meninges.

Computerized tomography (CT) and electroencephalography are much safer and more reliable investigations. If not available, transfer of the patient should be arranged.

Cerebral abscess

Recognition

This should be suspected in the following circumstances:

1. Unexplained raised intracranial pressure with a short history.
2. Patients whose conscious level or neurological state does not seem consistent with an obvious infection, e.g. meningitis, sinusitis, acute or chronic otitis media (abscess is now more common in acute than chronic otitis media). Forty per cent have fits. The site of the known infection may give a clue to the site of the abscess.
3. After compound head injury with neurological deterioration.
4. In vague short illness with malaise, vomiting, failure to thrive, fits, and often drowsiness or irritability. There may be focal neurological signs. Thirty per cent of cases have no fever, leucocytosis, or raised ESR. Toddlers and older children with cyanotic congenital heart disease are especially susceptible.

Investigations

1. Skull X-ray (sutures, sinuses, mastoids, fractures, osteomyelitis).
2. EEG; focal slow wave activity is helpful evidence.
3. CT scan.
4. Blood culture.
5. Full blood count and ESR.
6. Angiography (blush round avascular area and associated oedema; multiple abscesses may be demonstrated). Often not suitable in polycythaemic patients.

Management

1. Empirical antibiotics (e.g. intravenous cloxacillin and ampicillin or gentamicin) are often indicated before drainage which, if performed prematurely, may be unsuccessful and even harmful.
2. Drainage by a neurosurgeon is indicated if the patient is deteriorating or when the situation is more stable.

Subdural empyema

Presentation and primary source of infection are similar to cerebral abscess. It is commoner in later childhood and in boys more than girls. Early neurosurgical drainage by burrhole is indicated; bilateral collections are common.

Subdural effusion or haematoma (see Chapter 25, page 287, for Acute subdural haematoma)

The commonest causes are trauma (often non-accidental) and meningitis. Effusions may also result from the effects of CSF shunts.

Recognition

1. More than half the patients show vomiting, tense anterior fontanelle and/or suture separation, fits, retinal haemorrhages, and irritability. About 40 per cent are anaemic, 30 per cent have big heads and 10 per cent have skull fractures. If no explanation is forthcoming a full social history should be obtained, skeletal survey X-rays requested and the child carefully inspected for bruises, state of hygiene, and nutrition.
2. The only certain diagnostic test is a subdural tap performed by an experienced person. *See under* Practical procedures, Chapter 93, page 748.
3. CT scan and angiography are commonly positive but often unnecessary. Echo-encephalogram can be misleading with bilateral collections (i.e. no shift) and the EEG is usually normal unless there is coexisting brain injury.

Intracerebral haematoma

Sudden bleeding from a vascular malformation may cause raised intracranial pressure with an intracerebral haematoma. Urgent neurosurgical opinion is required as to the advisability of removing the clot.

Gliomas

Gliomas may cause raised intracranial pressure (*see* above and below), convulsions (*see* Chapter 28 on epilepsy), or bulbar palsy (usually brainstem lesions). The latter may produce acute problems by causing aspiration or respiratory failure. Tube feeding or intravenous fluid, and sometimes assisted ventilation may be needed pending full investigation. Ataxia, hemiplegia, or squint are usually present.

Other causes of raised intracranial pressure and differential diagnosis

Benign intracranial hypertension is diagnosed after investigation, e.g. CT scan. Hypertensive encephalopathy, acute encephalitis and toxic encephalopathy, especially lead encephalopathy, need to be considered. Occasionally migraine with focal signs may cause difficulty in diagnosis, especially from cerebral haemorrhage. Sagittal sinus thrombosis can be diagnosed by CT with contrast or by angiography. Sudden, often painful, visual failure with a central scotoma, especially for red objects, occurs with optic neuritis (cf. peripheral field loss in papilloedema). Though the optic nerve head is oedematous there are no haemorrhages and usually no other neurological signs unless a myelitis coexists. Optic nerve drüsen, a congenital malformation, can be mistaken for papilloedema in patients presenting with headache.

Management of raised intracranial pressure

See Chapter 26.

Chapter 38

Spina bifida and hydrocephalus

Ian A. McKinlay

Spina bifida: examination of newborn

1. Inspect the lesion and record the extent.
2. Cover with a non-adherent dressing, e.g. a single layer of tulle or Mellolin and swabs. It may be useful to mark the lesion, e.g. with a sterile pipe-cleaner for X-ray purposes.
3. Lie the patient prone or on one side to avoid pressure on the lesion.
4. Examine the patient for generalized abnormalities or other congenital lesion (lesions may be multiple).
5. Examine the head for evidence of obvious hydrocephalus or encephalocele. Record the occipitofrontal circumference (OFC) with paper tape and plot on a standard chart.
6. Assess voluntary movement below the lesion by observation and by stimulation above the site of the lesion.
7. Assess the state of sphincters and bladder function.

Investigations

1. X-ray the skull, whole spine, chest and hips for evidence of splayed sutures, lacunar skull, hemivertebrae, other occult spina bifida lesions, rib anomalies, cardiac abnormality, sacral abnormalities, and hip dislocation.
2. Computerized tomography (CT) is helpful in assessing the cause and degree of hydrocephalus. Ultrasonography is an alternative technique. Lacunar skull or silver-beaten appearance on X-ray need not mean severe hydrocephalus. A cortical thickness of less than 22 mm is unlikely to be associated with normal intelligence when present in the newborn.
3. Assess the family situation and parental attitudes to the baby's problem. Most will rely on the informed opinion of the doctor with regard to the prognosis.

Early operation is less important than careful assessment and, in selected patients, repair by an experienced surgeon. Factors often considered to make repair inadvisable, unless parents wish it to be done, include marked hydrocephalus, hemivertebrae, congenital scoliosis, lack of voluntary leg movement other than hip flexion, and other major congenital abnormalities.

The patient not selected for operation should be kept comfortable, with attention to warmth, feeding on request, adequate relief of pain, and regular sedation. This may need to be discussed with parents and colleagues. Parents may be offered a second opinion when there is any doubt about treatment. Both during the first week when decisions about treatment are being made and following such decisions social work involvement can be very helpful.

Acute hydrocephalus

Ninety per cent of patients with spina bifida have an associated Arnold–Chiari malformation, though only 10 per cent have frank clinical hydrocephalus at birth. The clinical features of acute hydrocephalus are irritability, drowsiness, vomiting, stridor, raised blood pressure, tachycardia or bradycardia, tachypnoea or Cheyne–Stokes ventilation, tense fontanelle, distended scalp veins, pupillary abnormalities, ophthalmoplegia, papilloedema, 'setting sun' sign (not diagnostic of raised pressure, however) and neck stiffness. Apart from risks to vital functions the main hazard is rapid visual failure.

Acute hydrocephalus can occur at any time in infancy and childhood, though it is commonest in the first few weeks after birth. The OFC should be measured daily in the newborn period and regularly thereafter with a paper tape and charted to gain early evidence of unduly rapid head growth, which is more important than large head size but normal growth rate. Compensated or arrested hydrocephalus may deteriorate acutely often in the course of an infection (usually upper respiratory tract infection) or after a head injury. Ventricular tapping of CSF through the anterior fontanelle or a burrhole may be life saving (*see* Chapter 93, page 749).

Valve problems

Every opportunity should be taken to assess the feel of valves in different circumstances. Many children with apparently blocked valves are asymptomatic and require no treatment unless there is acute deterioration. In an emergency with a distal catheter block CSF can be obtained by direct puncture of the shunt chamber.

Infection of the valve

Bacteraemic spread of *Staphylococcus albus* or coliforms leads to ventriculitis (and septicaemia with ventriculo-atrial shunts). This is a very rapidly destructive condition and removal of the shunt is urgently required as well as intravenous and intraventricular antibiotic treatment. After valve removal regular removal of CSF and ventricular instillation of antibiotics may be achieved either by ventricular punctures or through a reservoir inserted half an hour after removal of the contaminated shunt and an intravenous high dose of antibiotics (e.g. gentamicin and cloxacillin). The intrathecal dose of gentamicin in the presence of hydrocephalus is 2–3 mg and the intravenous dose 6 mg/kg. The intrathecal dose of cloxacillin is 5 mg.

Catheter disconnection

This can occur proximally or distally. The radio-opaque markers can be found by X-ray if not palpable or visible. There may be swelling due to accumulation of CSF at the site of distal disconnection. The disconnected part usually has to be replaced, but seldom as an urgency.

Overactivity of the valve

This can cause an alarming state of 'upward coning' with shock, very depressed fontanelle, abnormal pulse rate, blood pressure, respiratory pattern, ophthalmoplegia, disturbed consciousness level, or some of these. This is commonest following insertion of the valve and also can lead to an acute subdural haematoma. The patient should be nursed head-down with liberal oral or intravenous fluids. It is commonly transient, but if persistent a valve draining at higher pressure may be needed to replace the existing valve.

Septicaemia

This is relatively common in children with spina bifida, and blood cultures should be taken in any significant infective illness. Urinary tract infection, related to disturbed bladder function and sometimes associated hydronephrosis, or infected valves are common sources. A chronically infected valve is sometimes associated with splenomegaly, anaemia, haematuria, cor pulmonale, or nephrotic syndrome.

Fractures

These are common in the legs of paraplegic patients and are usually painless. The presentation is an audible crack or crepitus, swelling and bruising of the limb, or abnormal mobility. Immobilization in a functional position should be achieved in the least cumbersome way and only until the callus is stable.

Urinary tract

The state of the bladder and urinary tract should be assessed by intravenous pyelography or ultrasound examination of the urinary tract, urine culture from suprapubic aspiration, and cystometrogram. A high-pressure bladder which does not empty effectively is likely to lead to hydronephrosis and urinary tract infection.

Abandonment of treatment

It is as well to take stock of the general state of the child if this is known, before launching into vigorous resuscitative measures for their own sake.

Chapter 39

Acute lead poisoning

Ian Shellshear

The following factors are present in most children with lead poisoning.

Exposure to lead based paints

This is possible in most housing built before 1950, as it was not until then that titanium began to replace lead extensively as a paint base. The paint may be eaten as flakes, or painted material may be chewed or sucked. Occasionally children eat putty containing red lead.

Pica

This behavioural disturbance, often associated with anaemia, is so common as to be regarded as normal from 1–2 years of age. The age of children most affected, 1–5 years, is closely related to mobility and exploration of the environment. Inadequate supervision and poor social circumstances are also important.

Exposure to lead-containing cosmetics and medicines

In Asia and in Arab countries a black make-up is often put round the eyes and inside the lids of infants and small children. This is done to improve the child's appearance and it is also thought to protect against eye infections. Though originally made from lamp black, vegetable dyes or antimony sulphide, adulterated preparations containing lead sulphide are in common use in Asia, the Middle East and in the UK, even though its importation into this country has been banned. These preparations, known in Asia as Surma, Surama, or Kajil, and as Al Kohl in the Middle East, can be absorbed in sufficient quantities to cause lead poisoning (Green *et al.*, 1979; Warley, Blackledge and O'Gorman, 1968). There are also a number of medicines prescribed by Asian traditional practitioners which contain lead.

Recognition

The onset of symptoms in summer, and especially in association with upper respiratory infections, may be related to lead mobilization within the body.

Lead poisoning may present as:

1. Acute encephalopathy: this is usually preceded by anorexia, lethargy, irritability, loss of co-ordination and occasional vomiting. It is followed by gross ataxia associated with forceful vomiting, stupor, convulsions and finally coma. Papilloedema is usually present. Lead toxicity should always be suspected in any unexplained 'encephalitis'.
2. Vague symptoms such as anorexia, constipation and colicky abdominal pains. Peripheral neuropathy as seen in adults rarely occurs in children.
3. In the course of a screening programme or during the investigation of an iron deficiency anaemia. Treatment with iron may mobilize lead and precipitate encephalopathy.

   Increased lead intake may also be suspected when a plain abdominal X-ray shows radio-opaque flakes in the gut and especially if the X-ray is being taken because of abdominal pain. X-rays of the long bones may show radio-opaque metaphyseal lead lines. These are best recognized at the knee, wrist or costochondral junction. Less frequently lead poisoning may be found on investigation of unexplained glycosuria or aminoaciduria. Any of the following investigations may be used for rapid confirmation of a diagnosis of lead poisoning.

Confirmation of the diagnosis

1. The US Public Health Service regards a blood-lead level of greater than 80 μg/100 ml as unequivocal evidence of lead poisoning and recommends that such a case be treated as a medical emergency.
2. Children with a blood lead level between 40 and 80 μg/100 ml should be tested by a sodium calcium edetate mobilization test. If more than 0.5 mg lead are excreted in 24 hours after an i.m. test dose of 25 mg/kg sodium calcium edetate, the child has a potentially dangerous lead burden and treatment should be started.
3. The definitive test is to measure the blood lead, preferably by the dithizone method. For this method 10 ml heparinized blood are required. The atomic absorption micromethod is less reliable unless the laboratory is routinely carrying out lead estimations; 1–5 ml of whole blood (lithium heparin) are required.

In any unexplained encephalopathy the urine should be tested for coproporphyrin, and X-rays of the abdomen and long bones should be taken.

Management

Acute encephalopathy

Lumbar puncture carries a high risk of death by 'coning' (*see* page 745) if lead encephalopathy is present and is contraindicated. If CSF was obtained before the disease was considered, it is usually found to have a raised protein level.

Treatment is aimed at:

1. Reduction of cerebral oedema (*see* Chapter 26).
2. Control of convulsions (*see* page 308).
3. Reduction of the blood-lead level; initially dimercaprol (BAL) should be used in a dose of 4 mg/kg i.m. 4-hourly on the first day reducing to 2.5 mg/kg by the fourth day and then stopping. Four hours after starting dimercaprol, sodium calcium edetate is started in a dose of 50 mg/kg/24 h IV as divided 'push' doses, or i.m. 4-hourly, for 5–7 days. The gut is emptied with an enema to remove the remaining ingested lead.

Acute poisoning without encephalopathy

1. Chelation therapy as above (dimercaprol, sodium calcium edetate).
2. The gut should be emptied as above but using oral laxatives.
3. The home environment must be checked for a source of lead which should include:
   (a) Chewed window sills or cot sides.
   (b) Putty containing 'red lead'.
   (c) Lead soldiers, crayons, coloured newsprint.
   (d) Batteries burned for heat, soft water in lead pipes.
   (e) Stoneware storage of drinking fluids (especially if slightly acid, as lemon juice or cider).
   (f) Housedust, soil around the house
   (g) Proximity to motorways and lead-processing industries.
   (h) The father's occupation both past and present should be investigated.
4. Whatever the presentation, the affected child MUST NOT be returned to the environment where there is still a source of lead. Prevention may involve stripping paint from walls and removing the paint chips, or covering walls with board.
5. It may be necessary to move the family to other accommodation.
6. A long-term plan should be considered which might involve cyclical chelation therapy as described, every 3–4 weeks, while the blood lead remains grossly elevated. The use of oral D-penicillamine 40 mg/kg/24 h, once the blood lead is reduced below the dangerous level, would then be appropriate. D-penicillamine should not be used if there is any possibility of continuing exposure, as it will increase the absorption of ingested lead. Treatment of the anaemia with iron therapy should be delayed until the blood lead is reduced to safe levels since iron can mobilize lead from red cells.
7. The management of associated social difficulties and the education of parents should be considered.
8. Siblings with a history of pica should have their blood lead checked and anaemia (if present) treated.

Further reading

BETTS, P. R., ASTLEY, R. and RAINE, D. N. (1973) Lead intoxication in children in Birmingham. *British Medical Journal,* **i,** 402–406

CHISHOLM, J. J. (1968) The use of chelating agents in the treatment of acute and chronic lead intoxication in childhood. *Journal of Pediatrics,* **73,** 1–38

CHISHOLM, J. J. (1973) Screening for lead poisoning in children. *Pediatrics,* **51,** 280–287

COMMITTEE ON ENVIRONMENT HAZARDS (1971) Lead content of paint applied to surfaces accessible to young children. *Pediatrics,* **49,** 918–921

GREEN, S. D. R., LEALMAN, G. T., ASLAM, M. and DAVIS, S. S. (1979) Surma and blood lead concentrations. *Public Health, London,* **93,** 371–376

HARDY, H. L., CHAMBERLIN, R. I., MALOOF, C. C., BOYLEN, G. W. and HOWELL, M. C. (1971) Lead as an environmental poison. *Clinical Pharmacology and Therapeutics,* **12,** 982–1002

WARLEY, M. A., BLACKLEDGE, P. and O'GORMAN, P. (1968) Lead poisoning and cosmetics. *British Medical Journal,* **i,** 117

Part VIII

Gastrointestinal emergencies

Chapter 40

Acute abdominal emergencies

L. Spitz

Examination of the infant and child with acute abdominal pain

History

Accurate and detailed history taking is essential in arriving at the correct diagnosis. In most cases the history will be obtained from the parents, but, when feasible, the child should be consulted on the finer details.

Pain

ONSET

The sudden onset of acute abdominal pain in a previously well child usually signifies a surgical condition unless there is a clear history of dietary indiscretion.

SITUATION

Localization is inaccurate in the young child, who, irrespective of the site of the disease, invariably points to the umbilical region. Vague periumbilical pain in the older child, except in early appendicitis, is usually of little significance, whereas pain localized to one or other abdominal quadrant is suggestive of local organic disease. For instance, epigastric pain may indicate oesophagitis, peptic ulceration, liver or gallbladder disease, while in colonic disease the pain is referred to the hypogastrium. Pain in the flanks (hypochondrium, loin or lumbar regions) is characteristic of renal pathology (hydronephrosis or pyelonephritis) and a history of frequency of micturition, dysuria, or haematuria should be sought.

NATURE

It is often difficult for a child to describe pain, though he may do so by analogy (e.g. 'It pricks'; 'It feels like squeezing'). The pain may be intermittent and colicky in intestinal obstruction; continuous, intense and sharply defined as in acute appendicitis with localized peritonitis; or a vague dull ache.

PERSISTENCE

Persistence of the pain means persistence of the cause. An attack of abdominal pain lasting more than 3 hours should be regarded as an abdominal emergency until proved otherwise. It is helpful to ascertain whether the pain is persisting, subsiding, or getting worse. Are there any factors which relieve (vomiting, defaecation) or aggravate (movement, micturition) the pain?

RADIATION

Periumbilical pain which radiates and localizes in the right iliac fossa is practically diagnostic of acute appendicitis, but such a history is rarely obtainable from a young child.

ASSOCIATED SYMPTOMS

It is important to establish whether the child feels unwell or is otherwise healthy. The presence of pyrexia, nausea, vomiting, diarrhoea, urinary or respiratory symptoms should be noted. A history of trauma may be extremely important. Alternatively, a minor injury may bring to attention an otherwise asymptomatic mass.

Vomiting

RELATION TO THE ONSET OF PAIN

In surgical conditions vomiting usually occurs *after* the onset of abdominal pain. In gastroenteritis vomiting generally *precedes* colicky abdominal pain and diarrhoea.

TYPE

The presence of bile in the vomitus indicates intestinal obstruction unless proved otherwise. The child requires urgent diagnosis and prompt treatment.

FREQUENCY

In acute appendicitis vomiting may occur on only two or three occasions. It may then cease and not reappear until peritonitis supervenes. In intestinal obstruction the vomiting lasts as long as the obstruction persists, and is usually frequent and copious. Initially, the vomitus contains food only but this is soon replaced by bilious vomiting. Faeculent vomiting is a late feature of intestinal obstruction.

Bowel function

Constipation occurs in the majority of abdominal emergencies. Some parents will have given a laxative to the child before the medical consultation, and diarrhoea from this cause should not be misinterpreted. Diarrhoea may also occur in acute appendicitis when the inflamed organ overlies the sigmoid colon or rectum or where a pelvic abscess has developed.

Micturition

Dysuria, frequency and haematuria are all suggestive of a urinary tract infection. Dysuria and frequency are occasionally seen in acute appendicitis complicated by pelvic peritonitis.

Previous history

A history of previous similar attacks of abdominal pain which resolved spontaneously, especially if vague and periumbilical in location, suggests a functional rather than an organic cause. Nevertheless, acute appendicitis can and does occur in children with so-called recurrent abdominal pain and any change in the nature of the symptoms should alert the clinician to this possibility (*see* below, page 374).

Examination

While obtaining the history, it is essential to gain the confidence of the child. The position and comfort of the child are more important than that of the doctor. The most suitable position may be the mother's lap or curled up in an armchair.

In the older child the examination can be done in the conventional manner, whereas in the tense or unco-operative patient subtle variations are of great value. It is wise to palpate the abdomen before inspecting it.

Gentle palpation with the warm hand under the bedclothes may provide more valuable information than baring the abdomen and upsetting the child. Palpation should start well away from the suspected site of disease while the child's facial expression is observed for signs of pain, such as wincing. Having obtained the maximum information from palpation, the rest of the examination can be conducted, reserving rectal examination and inspection of the ears and throat until the end. Rebound tenderness is a sign with limited value in children, is acutely distressing to the child with peritoneal irritation, and attempts to elicit it should not be made. Inspection and examination of the groin and genitalia should never be omitted. An irreducible inguinal hernia or testicular torsion frequently causes pain which may be referred entirely to the abdomen (*see* page 373).

A general systematic examination should, of course, never be omitted. Particular attention should be directed to the chest for signs of pneumonia, the central nervous system for meningism, and the cardiovascular system for murmurs or congestive cardiac failure. These are particular examples of extra-abdominal conditions which cause abdominal symptoms.

The acute abdomen

The spectrum of disease which may cause abdominal symptoms in the child is so wide and diverse that a complete discussion of all the conditions is beyond the scope of this chapter.

It is intended to present a practical diagnostic approach to some of the more common conditions involved in the differential diagnosis of the acute surgical abdomen encountered in the child, and to outline the principles of management.

Intestinal obstruction in the neonate and infant

Recognition

The classic presenting features of neonatal intestinal obstruction are: (1) vomiting; (2) delay in the passage of meconium; (3) abdominal distension.

A practical diagnostic approach to vomiting in the infant is given in *Figure 40.1*.

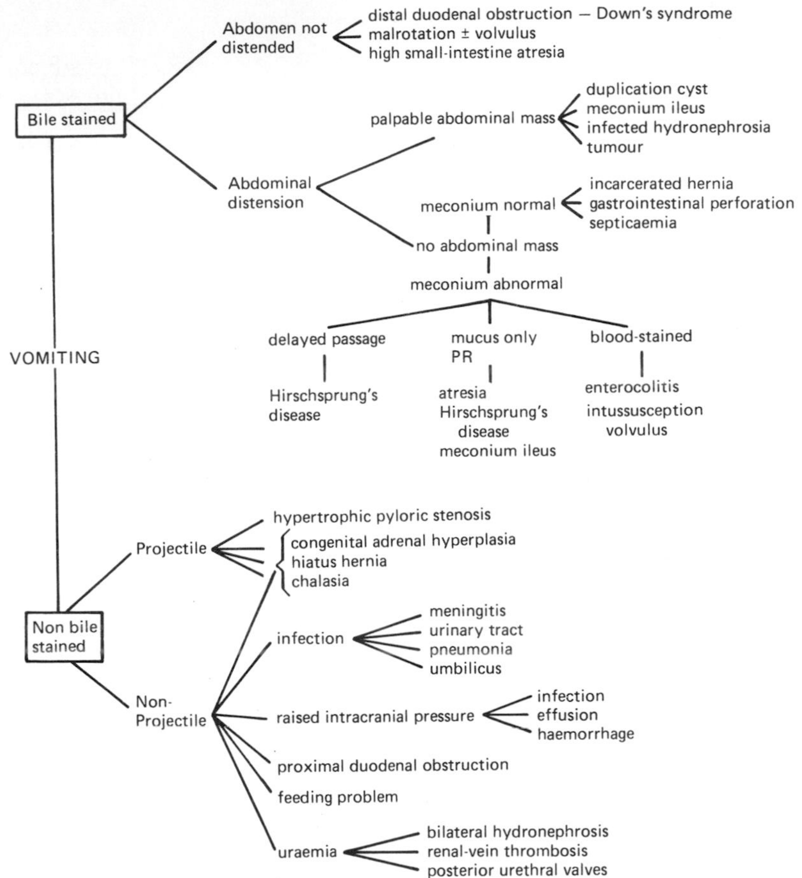

Figure 40.1 Diagnostic approach to vomiting in the newborn. PR = Per rectum

1. Vomiting is the only absolute sign of intestinal obstruction and when the vomitus contains bile-stained material its significance should be obvious. Unless a non-surgical cause for the bile-stained vomiting has been confirmed, a mechanical cause for the intestinal obstruction should be suspected.
2. It is important to recognize that small amounts of meconium may be passed rectally even in the presence of a complete intestinal atresia. Failure to pass meconium within the first 24 hours of life is abnormal. If, in addition to this delay in the passage of meconium, other symptoms of intestinal obstruction are present, which are relieved by the evacuation of a large plug of meconium following either digital examination or a saline rectal wash-out, a presumptive diagnosis of Hirschsprung's disease should be made and only excluded after negative radiological, histopathological, or manometric examination.
3. The degree of abdominal distension is related to the level of the intestinal obstruction. In duodenal obstructions there may be only minimal upper-abdominal fullness, whereas in low colonic lesions massive distension with elevation of the diaphragm, sufficient to produce respiratory embarrassment, may be present.

The presence of periumbilical erythema and/or oedema of the anterior abdominal wall, in addition to the above signs, signifies an intraperitoneal complication such as peritonitis or intestinal gangrene.

Radiography

Radiography of the abdomen is the most useful special investigation. The initial examination should consist of straight erect and supine views of the abdomen, as air is a safe and effective contrast at this age. An upper gastrointestinal study is the most rewarding investigation for suspected proximal intestinal obstructions, particularly malrotation. A contrast enema should be carried out in doubtful cases of distal intestinal obstruction.

The main causes of intestinal obstruction are listed below:

Mechanical:

1. Intraluminal:
   (a) Meconium ileus.
   (b) Meconium plug syndrome.
   (c) 'Inspissated milk' syndrome.
2. Intramural:
   (a) Intestinal atresia and stenosis.
   (b) Hirschsprung's disease.
3. Extraintestinal:
   (a) Malrotation with or without associated volvulus.
   (b) Duplication cysts.
   (c) Obstructed hernia.
   (d) Intussusception.
   (e) Adhesions from previous surgery.

Paralytic (ileus):

1. Gastrointestinal perforation.
2. Necrotizing enterocolitis.
3. Septicaemia, usually with one of the following:
   (a) Pyelonephritis.
   (b) Meningitis.
   (c) Pneumonia.
   (d) Umbilical sepsis.
4. Hypothyroidism; a rare cause of ileus in the newborn (*see* page 478).

Meconium ileus

This occurs as a complication of cystic fibrosis. There may be a family history of the condition. The thick inspissated meconium becomes impacted in the distal small intestine. Symptoms of obstruction occur within the first 24–48 hours of life. The abdomen is distended, and palpable loops of dilated meconium-filled intestine may be felt. The characteristic features on plain X-ray of the abdomen are uneven dilatation of the intestinal loops, a paucity of air-fluid levels and a granular bubbly appearance in the lower abdomen. Calcification denotes an antenatal perforation. A barium enema reveals a narrow, unused microcolon.

Treatment

In uncomplicated cases diatrizoate methyl glucamine (Gastrografin) may be used as a therapeutic enema in an attempt to relieve the obstruction. The procedure which must be performed by an experienced radiologist should be carried out with extreme caution to avoid dehydration as a result of the hypertonicity of the contrast material. Surgical intervention is indicated for complicated meconium ileus such as perforation, atresia or volvulus and in uncomplicated cases which fail to respond to Gastrografin enemas.

Meconium plug syndrome

The infant fails to pass meconium within the first 24 hours of life. The abdomen becomes distended and bilious vomiting may ensue. Rectal examination reveals a 'tight' anus and an empty rectum. A greyish plug of mucoid material followed by a large mass of meconium may be passed on withdrawing the examining finger. In more resistant cases a rectal saline wash-out or Gastrografin enema may be required to relieve the obstruction. Although the condition may be entirely benign and frequently occurs in association with maternal diabetes, respiratory distress syndrome, or prematurity, approximately 20 per cent of cases have Hirschsprung's disease (*see* below).

Intestinal atresia

Duodenal atresia appears to be due to an error in development. It is frequently associated with Down's syndrome, oesophageal atresia, anorectal anomalies, and congenital cardiac deformities. Intestinal atresias are the result of an intrauterine mesenteric vascular catastrophe in which the infarcted intestine is resorbed. The diagnosis is established on plain erect abdominal X-ray. In duodenal atresia there is the typical 'double-bubble' while in atresias further distal in the intestine, dilated bowel loops with multiple air-fluid levels are seen. The treatment is surgical, with restoration of intestinal continuity.

Hirschsprung's disease

This results from an absence of ganglion cells in the wall of the distal intestine. The rectum is always affected, but the disease may extend proximally for a variable distance and may affect the entire colon (5 per cent). The condition may present with complete intestinal obstruction in the neonatal period but the most constant presenting feature is delayed passage of meconium (in excess of 24 hours after birth). Failure to recognize and treat the condition at this stage exposes the infant to the hazard of enterocolitis (profuse watery diarrhoea often containing blood), which has a significant mortality rate. The diagnosis is established by a combination of rectal biopsy (suction technique where experienced histopathological assistance is available), barium enema and anorectal manometry. Treatment is by colostomy in the first instance, followed at a later stage by resection of the aganglionic intestine.

Malrotation

This results from arrest of the normal process of rotation. The ileocaecal region comes to lie in a subhepatic position and the duodenojejunal junction lies to the

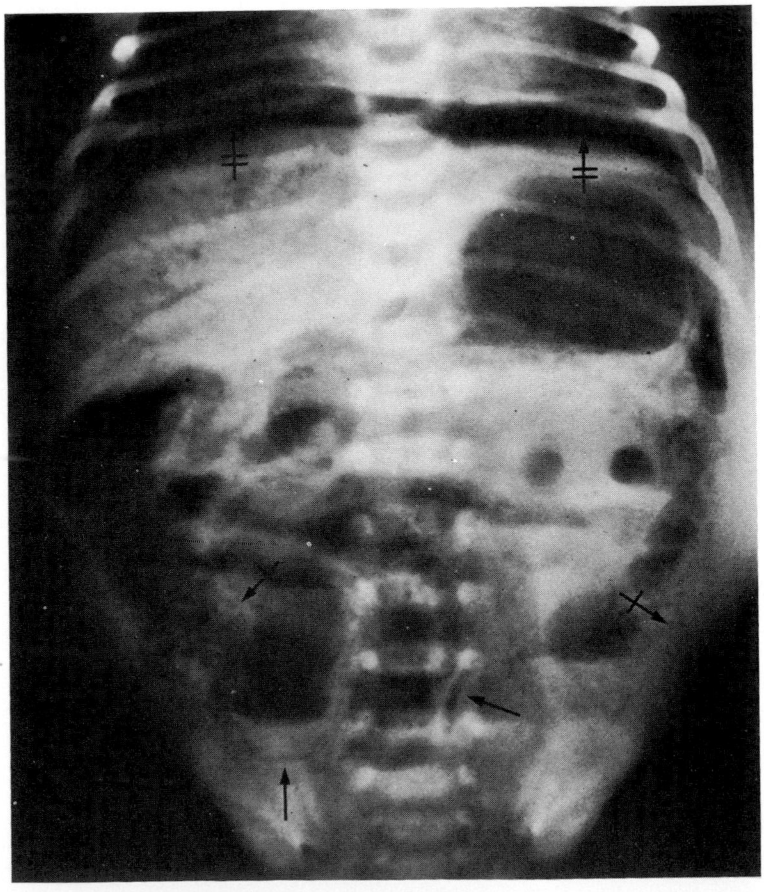

Plate I. *Radiological appearances which may be seen in necrotizing enterocolitis. In addition to gas in the portal venous system in the liver, the following can be seen: Intramural gas producing a halo effect* (*arrows*); *Small gas bubbles in the bowel wall producing an appearance similar to that of faecal contents, which is not a normal finding in this age group* (*single-barred arrows*); *Free air under the diaphragm* (*pneumoperitoneum*) (*double-barred arrows*)

right of the midline. Ladd's bands cross and partially obstruct the descending part of the duodenum causing intermittent bilious vomiting, while the narrow based mesentery of the midgut is prone to undergo volvulus with the danger of ischaemic necrosis of long sections of intestine. The plain abdominal X-ray shows a relatively gasless appearance which may be misleading to the inexperienced, expecting to find air-fluid levels. The diagnosis is best established by upper gastrointestinal contrast examination. The position of the caecum may be defined on barium enema. Treatment consists of urgent surgery, to re-site the intestine.

Septicaemia and intestinal obstruction

The onset of septicaemia is usually acute, with instability of temperature, jaundice, moderate hepatosplenomegaly, and thrombocytopenia, in addition to the usual signs of intestinal obstruction. The poor general condition of the infant, the presence of jaundice, and the diagnostic importance of the thrombocytopenia (jaundice and thrombocytopenia are not invariably present) should alert one to the possibility of septicaemia. The diagnosis is confirmed by positive blood cultures but a full 'infection screen' should be performed, including lumbar puncture, examination of the urine, X-ray of the chest, and swabs from nose, umbilicus, axillae, rectum and any septic skin lesions. In addition to the basic conservative measures for intestinal obstruction, i.e. nasogastric decompression and intravenous infusion, broad-spectrum antibiotic therapy with parenteral gentamicin, and benzylpenicillin or cloxacillin and metronidazole should be started immediately, i.e. before bacteriological culture results are available. *Inadvertent operative intervention should, if possible, be avoided. See also* page 655 for further discussion on septicaemia in the newborn.

Management of intestinal obstruction

Gross fluid and electrolyte imbalances should be corrected by intravenous infusion before the infant is transferred to a hospital equipped to deal with neonatal surgical problems. A large-size nasogastric tube should be passed and the stomach evacuated of its contents before the infant leaves the base hospital, and at regular intervals during transportation, to prevent vomiting and aspiration. The ideal method of transportation for the newborn infant is in a portable incubator, accompanied by an experienced medical attendant. Great care should be paid to maintenance of normal body temperature. It is also important to send a valid consent form for surgery, and a specimen of maternal blood for cross-matching. For a detailed description of the surgical management of the specific lesions, the reader is referred to the standard paediatric surgical texts.

Necrotizing enterocolitis

Recognition

Reluctance to feed, abdominal distension, and bile-stained vomiting with the passage of blood and mucus rectally, are the first symptoms of necrotizing enterocolitis. It is more commonly seen in low birth weight infants, and occurs especially in infants who have undergone some perinatal stress such as hypoxia, hypothermia, hypotension, or have required an exchange transfusion or infusions through the umbilical vein. The diagnosis is confirmed radiologically by the presence of gas within the wall of the intestine (pneumatosis intestinalis). Pneumoperitoneum signifies the presence of an intestinal perforation (*Plate 40.1*).

Management

Early intensive medical therapy, including nasogastric decompression, parenteral nutrition, and parenteral broad-spectrum antibiotics (gentamicin, penicillin and metronidazole) facilitate complete resolution of the pathological process in the majority of cases. It is important to continue with the total parenteral nutrition for 10–14 days and systemic antibiotics for at least 7 days. Oral feeds may then be commenced with extreme caution. Surgical intervention is indicated in the presence of an intestinal perforation, as shown by pneumoperitoneum or signs of local peritonitis, mechanical intestinal obstruction due to stricture formation, or profuse gastrointestinal haemorrhage, and, in those cases which have failed to respond within a reasonable period to vigorous medical therapy. The surgical procedure consists of the resection of obviously gangrenous intestine and the establishment of a proximal and distal enterostomy. The anastomosis between the proximal and distal enterostomies should be delayed until the infant has completely recovered from the acute episode and is thriving.

Intussusception

Intussusception is the most common cause of intestinal obstruction in infants between the ages of 3 months and 2 years. The peak incidence is from 6 to 12 months of age. The ileocaecal region is the site most commonly affected, although any part of the intestine may be involved.

Recognition

Clinical presentation

1. Colicky abdominal pain.
2. Vomiting.
3. Presence of a 'sausage-shaped' abdominal mass.
4. Passage of blood and mucus per rectum.

The onset of an intussusception is usually acute, with classic paroxysms of screaming and drawing up of the knees, accompanied by pallor, but in 10 per cent there is no obvious colic. Attacks usually last between 1 and 2 minutes and occur at intervals of 15–30 minutes. Vomiting is usual, but not invariable, and is initially confined to gastric contents only; but in the neglected case with long-standing intussusception the vomiting becomes faeculent. The 'sausage-shaped' abdominal mass is often difficult to detect, as it may lie beneath the edge of the liver. The mass may be easier to find in a sleeping, relaxed child (sedation may be helpful). The passage of blood and mucus per rectum may be delayed for a number of hours (and in some cases may not occur); its appearance on the examining finger after a rectal examination may lead to a diagnosis, but to wait for its occurrence is not good practice. Early diagnosis is important, for after 24 hours the complications increase significantly.

Confirmation of the diagnosis

The diagnosis of intussusception is usually based on the clinical features. A plain film of the abdomen may show air outlining the head of the intussusception which appears as a soft-tissue mass. It may show evidence of intestinal obstruction or an absence of gas in the right iliac fossa. The barium enema for purely diagnostic purposes is reserved for cases in which the clinical diagnosis is inconclusive.

Management

Nasogastric decompression and correction of fluid and electrolyte imbalance are essential before definitive treatment.

Hydrostatic reduction by barium enema is the treatment of choice for the early uncomplicated case. It is contraindicated in the presence of intestinal obstruction and in the ill, toxic infant who needs resuscitation. Surgical management is the preferred method in cases with prolonged symptoms (over 24 hours), in infants under the age of 3 months, and in the older child where a primary cause for the intussusception, for example polyp, diverticulum duplication, amoebiasis (*see* Chapter 65) or ascariasis (*see* Chapter 42) is more likely to be present. Intussusception may also complicate Henoch–Schöenlein purpura. The recurrence rate following hydrostatic reduction is around 10 per cent while only 2 per cent of intussusceptions recur after operative reduction.

Appendicitis

Acute appendicitis is the condition which most frequently requires emergency abdominal surgery in childhood. It is rare below the age of 2 years, but becomes progressively more common thereafter. *However, this condition must be considered in the differential diagnosis of almost every acute abdominal emergency in children of all ages.*

Recognition

The older child

The clinical features are:

1. Abdominal pain which frequently follows the classic pattern of initial vague colicky periumbilical discomfort, and subsequently radiates to and localizes in the right iliac fossa, where it becomes continuous and more intense. The pain may, however, commence over the appendix area itself. The pain of acute appendicitis may be atypical in presentation, especially in cases with prolonged delay in diagnosis and where the appendix lies in an unusual position, e.g. retrocaecal or retroileal.
2. Vomiting is such a constant feature that in its absence the diagnosis of appendicitis should remain suspect. The vomitus is rarely profuse, and usually contains only stomach contents.
3. Low-grade pyrexia (±38°C (100°F)); a higher fever in the absence of frank perforation or localized abscess is against the diagnosis of acute appendicitis and is more in favour of mesenteric adenitis of viral origin.

4. Bowel habits are generally normal. Mild constipation is common but diarrhoea may occur in the presence of a pelvic abscess.
5. Frequency and pain on micturition are not uncommon and may indicate an inflamed appendix lying in contact with the ureter or bladder.
6. Loss of appetite is characteristic.
7. On examination the child usually lies still and in one fixed position, as movement of the abdomen is painful. It is often obvious that respiratory movement of the lower abdomen is restricted. Localized abdominal tenderness and guarding in the right iliac fossa are the physical signs of an unruptured appendicitis. Rebound tenderness is of no diagnostic value in the child. Involuntary muscle spasm (rigidity) in the right iliac fossa generally indicates a gangrenous or perforated appendicitis with localized peritonitis. A rectal examination, which should be performed as gently as possible, may reveal tenderness or a mass projecting into the anterior wall of the rectum.

The child under 2 years of age

Appendicitis in infancy is usually characterized by a prolonged delay in diagnosis due to the absence of recognizable abdominal signs, a high incidence of perforation (over 80 per cent) and significant mortality (10 per cent) and morbidity (50 per cent) rates. The young infant presents with non-specific symptoms such as lethargy, irritability, vomiting, and pyrexia. Abdominal distension and tenderness are late signs and usually consequent upon rupture and peritonitis. *Diarrhoea is more common than constipation.*

Diagnosis

Appendicitis is generally a clinical diagnosis based on objective signs, but investigations may be helpful. A polymorphonuclear leucocytosis of 12 000–18 000/mm^3 is common but not invariably present. The plain abdominal X-rays may reveal localized ileus in the right iliac fossa. A calcified faecolith is pathognomonic of appendicitis. In early acute pyelonephritis pus cells may not be found in the urine but pain is likely to be felt in the costovertebral angle, i.e. even higher than with a retrocaecal appendicitis. The final diagnosis should be based on objective abdominal findings: *when these are absent or inconclusive the child should be kept under observation in hospital and the physical signs reviewed at regular intervals.*

Management

The acutely ill child with a long-standing perforated appendicitis and peritonitis may present with dehydration and shock. In such cases surgery should be delayed while intensive preoperative resuscitation is carried out. This should include nasogastric decompression, intravenous fluid therapy commencing with 20 ml/kg plasma (or plasma protein fraction) delivered within the first hour followed by 0.9% NaCl with potassium 20 mmol/ℓ added when urine flow is established. Preoperative parenteral antibiotics (gentamicin 6.0 mg/kg/24 h and penicillin and metronidazole 50 mg/kg/24 h) should be started immediately; this will provide protection against Gram positive and negative organisms, as well as the anaerobic bacteroides. The surgical treatment is removal of the inflamed appendix whenever possible. An appendix mass should be treated conservatively and an internal appendicectomy planned 6–8 weeks later. Drainage of an appendix mass is occasionally necessary in children with an abscess that fails to respond to or deteriorates with conservative treatment.

Trauma

Accidental injuries are responsible for over half the deaths in boys between 5 and 14 years of age and for nearly 40 per cent of the total in girls of the same age group. Over 90 per cent of abdominal injuries in childhood are caused by blunt trauma. In order of frequency, the spleen, genitourinary tract, liver, gastrointestinal tract, and pancreas are most commonly involved. A complete physical examination is essential to exclude injuries to other parts of the body, e.g. head injury. Injuries to the abdomen may also result from a blow from the hand (*see* Chapter 58, Non-accidental injury and Child abuse).

Recognition

Persistent abdominal tenderness is the most consistent physical sign of an abdominal visceral injury. When this is accompanied by the signs of hypovolaemic shock the diagnosis of a ruptured liver, spleen, or kidney should be considered. Splenic injury may present less dramatically, with a persistent tachycardia or unexplained pallor. Haematuria, whether macro- or microscopic, demands urgent investigation with ultrasonography and/or intravenous pyelography. Routine erect and supine X-rays of the abdomen and haematological investigations including haematocrit, leucocyte count, and serum amylase should be carried out in all cases with suspected visceral injury.

Management

Laparotomy should be performed only after adequate resuscitation and when sufficient quantities of compatible blood are available for transfusion. *In severe liver trauma continuing rapid loss of blood may preclude attempts at resuscitation and urgent exploration may be life saving.* Conservative management of splenic trauma in an attempt to conserve its immunological properties is now widely practised.

Gastrointestinal bleeding (blood in the stool) (see Chapter 43 for further discussion, including haematemesis)

The main causes of gastrointestinal haemorrhage in infancy and childhood can be divided into conditions occurring in the first year of life and those occurring in the older child (*Table 40.1*). Infectious diarrhoea (especially due to Salmonella and Shigella) may occur at any age and often produces blood and mucus in the stool. *See Figure 40.2* for diagnostic scheme for gastrointestinal haemorrhage.

Investigation of gastrointestinal haemorrhage

1. Particular attention is given to the age of the child, the quantity and colour of the blood passed, the general physical condition of the patient and the presence or absence of associated signs of intestinal obstruction. The anus should be carefully inspected for the presence of a fissure before digital rectal examination.
2. Ancillary investigations include full blood count, platelet count, screening tests for coagulation disorders (*see* page 495), sigmoidoscopy, barium enema and/or meal and follow-through. Technetium scan of the abdomen may reveal ectopic gastric mucosa (Meckel's diverticulum, duplication).

Table 40.1 Causes of gastrointestinal bleeding

<1 year of age	*>1 year of age*
Acute peptic ulceration	Oesophageal varices
Volvulus and gangrene of the intestine	Peptic ulceration
Necrotizing enterocolitis (neonatal period)	Meckel's diverticulum
Meckel's diverticulum	Intussusception
Intussusception	Crohn's disease
Duplications	Ulcerative colitis
Anal fissure	Polyps
	Anal fissure

3. Fibreoptic endoscopy of the upper and/or lower gastrointestinal tract performed within 24–48 hours of the bleeding episode significantly improves the yield of positive diagnoses.

Rectal bleeding associated with bile-stained vomiting and shock in the neonate or in early infancy indicates an intestinal volvulus and requires urgent surgical intervention. Where intestinal obstruction coexists with rectal haemorrhage, surgery is indicated on the assumption that the haemorrhage and the obstruction are due to the same pathological process. In the majority of cases with minor rectal bleeding, no cause is found even after exhaustive investigation. From the practical point of view, therefore, it is safe to ignore minimal rectal bleeding in the young infant. It may be presumed that the bleeding originates from superficial mucosal ulceration. Where the rectal bleeding is severe enough to warrant admission to hospital, or where repeated minor episodes occur, 50 per cent are found to have a

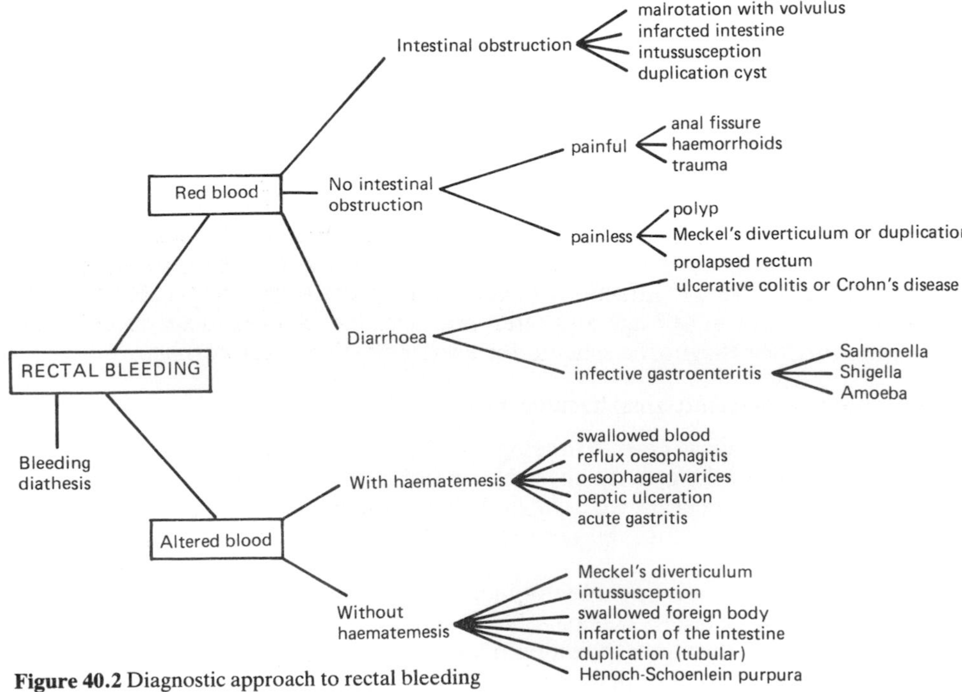

Figure 40.2 Diagnostic approach to rectal bleeding

localized gastrointestinal lesion, 10–20 per cent have a systemic disturbance (e.g. septicaemia, haemorrhagic diathesis) while in approximately one-third of cases no cause can be identified (Spencer, 1964) (*see* fibreoptic endoscopy, above).

Abdominal masses

The finding of an abdominal mass in a child constitutes a surgical emergency requiring urgent and precise elucidation. Hepatomegaly and splenomegaly, which together account for approximately 50 per cent of all abdominal masses, require further investigation but rarely constitute an emergency. Of the masses which are clearly not due to enlargement of the liver or spleen, half are due to cystic lesions of the kidney, and the rest must be considered malignant until proved otherwise. It is impossible to distinguish with any certainty intra-abdominal from retroperitoneal masses in infancy and childhood. Abdominal ultrasonography is the essential initial investigation. Skeletal survey, isotope bone scans, and X-ray of the chest are necessary to detect distant metastases. Other useful investigations are an excretory abdominal urogram and abdominal computerized tomography.

Routine haematological investigations and urinalysis including catecholamine and alpha-fetoprotein estimations are essential ancillary tests. Arteriography may be helpful when the true nature of the lesion remains in doubt. The common malignant conditions encountered in infancy and childhood are neuroblastoma, nephroblastoma (Wilms' tumour), teratoma, and soft-tissue retroperitoneal sarcomas. The best results in the treatment of childhood malignant tumours are achieved by the combined approach of a paediatric surgeon, radiotherapist, oncologist, and radiologist working together and adhering strictly to recognized treatment protocols.

Scrotal pain and swelling (see also page 440 for other causes of acute scrotal swelling)

The two conditions which mimic an acute abdomen are irreducible inguinal hernia and testicular torsion.

Irreducible inguinal hernia

The incidence of irreducibility (incarceration) in inguinal hernia is greatest in the first 3 months of life. For this reason herniotomy is recommended on diagnosis without 'delaying until the child is older'. The early signs and symptoms of incarceration are crying, irritability and vomiting, associated with a swelling in the groin extending for a variable distance into the scrotum. Only later do the features of frank intestinal obstruction and strangulation supervene. Reduction of the hernia by gentle manual pressure may be successful in the early stages. Operation can then be done within 24–48 hours. In the presence of intestinal obstruction or signs of intestinal strangulation, emergency exploration and herniotomy are indicated. Ischaemic damage may also affect the ipsilateral testis.

Testicular torsion

The acute onset of pain and swelling of the testis is an absolute indication for surgical exploration on the provisional diagnosis of testicular torsion. The affected testis should be untwisted and anchored to the scrotum. The testis should generally be retained even in the presence of apparent total gangrene. The other testis should also be anchored to the scrotum at the same time to prevent a similar episode occurring in the future on the opposite side.

Ascaris infestation (see also Chapter 42 for further details)

Parasitic infestation with roundworms (*Ascaris lumbricoides*) may cause bouts of colicky abdominal pain or obstruction.

Recurrent abdominal pain and the acute abdomen

A difficult diagnostic problem is the child who has previously been classified as suffering from recurrent abdominal pain, which implies at least three episodes of pain, severe enough to restrict activity, and extending over a period of more than 3 months. Such a child may at any time develop a true abdominal emergency such as acute appendicitis. Familiarity with the benign course of the previous attacks may delay the realization by the parents or the doctor that the present attack is different from its predecessors, and the actual diagnosis may be greatly delayed. This situation may arise in one of two ways:

1. The previous attacks were caused by an organic condition and were NOT of psychosomatic origin, e.g. malrotation with episodes of incomplete mid-gut volvulus, or hydronephrosis.
2. The previous attacks were genuinely those of recurrent abdominal pain of psychosomatic origin, but the current attack is due to an acute abdominal emergency.

It is important to emphasize the manner in which the clinical presentation of an acute abdominal emergency differs from attacks of psychogenic recurrent abdominal pain.

1. The attack is different from previous attacks.
2. An additional feature not experienced in previous attacks is present, e.g. pyrexia, vomiting (especially if bile-stained), abdominal distension, pain which is sharply localized (especially if lateralized).
3. The attack may last longer than usual.

The child with abdominal pain of organic origin will not sleep, nor will anyone else in the household.

Further reading

FILSTON, H. C. (1982) *Surgical Problems in Children: Recognition and Referral*. St. Louis: C. V. Mosby

HOLDER, T. M. and ASHCRAFT, K. W. (1980) *Pediatric Surgery*. Philadelphia: W. B. Saunders

JONES, P. G. (1976) *Clinical Paediatric Surgery* (2nd edn.). Oxford: Blackwell Scientific Publications

NIXON, H. H. and O'DONNELL, B. (1976) *The Essentials of Paediatric Surgery* (3rd edn.). London: Heinemann

RICKHAM, P. P., LISTER, J. and IRVING, I. M. (1978) *Neonatal Surgery* (2nd edn.). London: Butterworths

SPENCER, R. (1964) Gastrointestinal haemorrhage in infancy and childhood: 476 cases. *Surgery*, **55**, 718–734

Chapter 41

Medical conditions that may mimic acute abdominal emergencies

J. A. Black

The newborn and young infant (Table 41.1)

Table 41.1 Conditions mimicking acute intestinal obstruction in the newborn and young infant

Medical condition	*Clues to diagnosis*	*Diagnostic tests*	*Remarks*
Septicaemia with or without meningitis	Sudden onset of lethargy, pallor, reluctance to feed, abdominal distension, jaundice, bile-stained vomiting.	Lumbar puncture Blood culture Platelet count Full blood count.	*See* page 335.
Hypothyroidism (cretinism) with ileus.	'Physiological' jaundice prolonged beyond 14 days.	Skeletal age at the knee will be delayed in term infants. T_3 or T_4 low. TSH raised.	Occasionally occurs in older infants (*see* page 478)
Cardiac failure with acute hepatic enlargement causing abdominal distension and discomfort.	Large tender liver and tachypnoea; paroxysmal tachycardia the commonest cause in previously healthy infant, with apex beat >250 per minute during paroxysms.	ECG may be abnormal. X-ray of chest may show cardiac enlargement.	*See* page 264.

Older children (Tables 41.2–41.5)

Table 41.2 Conditions mimicking acute appendicitis in older children

Medical condition	*Clues to diagnosis*	*Diagnostic tests*	*Remarks*
Diabetic ketoacidosis.	Known diabetic or previously undetected diabetic; history of thirst and polyuria.	Urine shows ++ of sugar and acetone. Plasma, glucose or Dextrostix >25 mmol/ℓ (>450 mg/100 ml).	Diabetics can also develop acute appendicitis, pyelonephritis, pneumonia etc. (*see* pages 445–446).
Acute pyelonephritis.	Frequency and pain on micturition; high fever and loin tenderness. Sometimes previous attacks.	Urine microscopy shows white cells and organisms.	Pelvic appendicitis may cause similar urinary symptoms (*see* page 370) and slight pyuria but no organisms on microscopy.
Right basal (lobar) pneumonia.	Sudden onset with tachypnoea and high fever.	X-ray of chest shows lobar consolidation.	Pneumonia and acute appendicitis may coexist.
Acute mesenteric adenitis.	High fever, abdominal pain and vomiting, sometimes with constipation or diarrhoea. Acute tonsillitis is commonly present.	If the pain and tenderness are localized in the right iliac fossa, acute appendicitis may only be excluded at laparotomy. White cell counts are generally unhelpful.	*See* page 369.
Acute mesenteric adenitis due to infection with *Yersinia enterocolitica*.	Continuous fever of 38.5–40°C (101–104°F) with abdominal pain; stools may contain mucus and occasionally blood.	Leucocytosis is not common. The organism can be grown from mesenteric glands but is easily confused with Proteus sp.	Infection from contaminated food (*see* pages 396 and 400).
Campylobacter infections.	Diarrhoea with blood and pus in stool.	Isolation of organisms from stool, ileocaecal glands or resected appendix.	Infection from food, often from raw milk (*see* pages 395 and 400).
Acute toxic staphylococcal food poisoning.	Acute past of severe epigastric pain followed by vomiting and diarrhoea. Others in family, school or other close group often simultaneously affected.	Staphylococci may not be isolated from stool or from suspect food if this was cooked after the formation of the heat stable toxin.	*See* page 401.
Pre-icteric hepatitis. Commonly infective hepatitis A in children.	Vomiting and abdominal pain with mild fever and anorexia.	Serum transaminases are raised before clinical jaundice. Bilirubin usually slightly raised.	

Table 41.2 continued

Medical condition	*Clues to diagnosis*	*Diagnostic tests*	*Remarks*
	Liver enlarged and tender. Spleen may be palpable in young children.	Bilirubin present in urine in immediate preicteric phase; increased urobilin less constant.	
Malaria (*see Table 41.4*).			
Sickle-cell crisis (very rarely in children with sickle-cell trait who are not usually anaemic but have positive screening test).	Commonly but not exclusively in children of African race. Anaemia and hepatomegaly; jaundice and splenomegaly are common in young children.	Sickle cells usually visible on direct blood film in sickle-cell anaemia, but in trait only when cells are mixed with reducing agent.	'Sicklers' are as liable as others to develop acute appendicitis, etc. Pneumococcal infections, particularly meningitis and peritonitis are common.
Faecal impaction in cystic fibrosis (*see below*).			

Table 41.3 Conditions mimicking acute intussusception in older children

Medical condition	*Clues to diagnosis*	*Diagnostic tests*	*Remarks*
Acute bacillary dysentery (commonly *Shigella sonnei* in United Kingdom). Similar symptoms may be due to Salmonella infections.	Sudden onset with high fever, severe colicky pain and blood and mucus in stool.	Microscopy of stool showing white cells, may help.	Misdiagnosis may cause admission of a dysentery case to a surgical ward or intussception to an infectious unit, both undesirable (*see* pages 396, 398).
Henoch–Schoenlein (anaphylactoid) purpura.	Severe abdominal pain may precede or accompany one or some of the following: rash, joint swelling, haematuria (often on microscopy only), fresh blood or melaena in the stool.	Careful clinical examination: rash if present, is usually typical; platelet count is *always* normal; ESR and ASO titre are sometimes raised but rarely helpful.	Ileus or intussusception may occur.
Meningococcal septicaemia (with or without meningitis) and attacks of screaming.	Petechiae or skin haemorrhages. Meningitis may be obvious.	Lumbar puncture. Blood culture. Evidence of DIC (*see* page 498).	
Ascaris obstruction (*see below*).			

Table 41.4 Other conditions causing ill-defined acute abdominal pain in older children

Medical condition	*Clues to diagnosis*	*Diagnostic tests*	*Remarks*
Severe constipation.	History of chronic constipation; hard faecal masses in lower abdomen, rectum, and anal canal.	Relief after enema.	Acute retention of urine may also occur causing severe lower abdominal pain.
Faecal impaction in cystic fibrosis.	The diagnosis is generally already known. Obstruction usually occurs in older children. It may mimic acute appendicitis, and intussusception may be a complication.	Sweat test. Sodium level > 70 mmol/ℓ.	
Mumps pancreatitis with or without salivary gland swelling; upper-epigastric pain and vomiting.	Usually other evidence of mumps. Close contact with a known case may help.	Serum amylase is raised in mumps but this may be due to involvement of the salivary glands.	
Ascaris (roundworm) obstruction.	Affects children born or living in a highly infected environment who have heavy infestation. Occasionally a mass of worms may mimic intussusception.	Microscopy of stool for ova. Ill-defined mass may be palpable. Plain film of abdomen may show worms or barium meal may outline them.	Ascariasis is almost universal in some communities, therefore the presence of ova in the stool is difficult to evaluate (*see also* Chapter 42).
Tuberculous adenitis or peritonitis.	Masses of glands in omentum, ± ascites.	Tuberculin test usually positive. Calcified glands sometimes visible in chest X-ray. Diagnostic laparotomy is sometimes necessary.	
Acute lead poisoning with colicky abdominal pain.	History of pica sometimes obtained but often denied.	Opaque flecks in plain film of abdomen; dense lines at the metaphyses. Raised blood level of >50 μg/100 ml. Punctuate basophilia and blue gums quite unreliable.	*See* Chapter 39.

Table 41.4 continued

Medical condition	*Clues to diagnosis*	*Diagnostic tests*	*Remarks*
Haemophilia with haemorrhage into rectus sheath or retroperitoneal tissues.	Diagnosis usually known.	Prolonged partial thromboplastin time (PTT). Whole blood coagulation time too insensitive and *may be normal* in haemophilia. Lowered factor VIII (or IX in Christmas disease).	(*see also* Chapter 54).
Malignant tertian (falciparum) malaria, with acute abdominal pain, with or without diarrhoea or blood in the stool.	Liver may be palpable and tender: splenomegaly variable.	Blood film examination *repeatedly* (thick and thin films)	*See* page 575.
Iliac adenitis	Inguinal glands may also be enlarged. Restriction of movement at the hip sometimes present.	Primary infection on leg or perineum.	
Osteomyelitis of the pelvis (iliac bone).	Onset more acute, with higher fever than in appendicitis. Abdominal rigidity and tenderness on rectal examination may be present. Occasionally fixed flexion of the hip or limitation of medial rotation.	Polymorph leucocytosis, positive blood culture. X-ray only shows changes in late cases (over 10 days).	

Table 41.5 Less common conditions causing acute abdominal pain in older children

Medical condition	*Clues to diagnosis*	*Diagnostic tests*	*Remarks*
Primary peritonitis (pneumococcal or streptococcal).	May complicate nephrotic syndrome. Abdominal distension, with rigidity later unless ascites is present.	Needle aspiration of the peritoneal cavity.	
Polyarteritis nodosa.	Skin rashes, joint pains, proteinuria, haematuria are common.	Skin or muscle biopsy may be diagnostic.	
Familial Mediterranean fever.	History of recurrent pain in joints, chest (pleuritic) or abdomen (peritoneal irritation).	Rectal or renal biopsy may show amyloid.	Inherited as a dominant. Mainly in Sephardic (N. African, Mediterranean) Jews. Occasionally in Armenians, Arabs, or Turks.
Hyperlipidaemia, Type I.	Hepatosplenomegaly, xanthomata.	Marked lipaemia of serum.	Inherited as a recessive.
Acute intermittent porphyria.	Attacks of abdominal pain and constipation. Usually with barbiturates or other precipitating drugs. Urine may be dark, but is not a useful diagnostic point.	Elevated urinary porphobilinogens.	This type of porphyria is inherited as a dominant.
Hereditary angio-oedema.	Previous attacks of localized oedema after trauma, or laryngeal oedema. Abdominal pain due to oedema of intestinal wall.	Low level of complement C 1-esterase inhibitor, or more rarely, normal levels of an inacive molecule.	Inherited as a dominant. History of recurrent abdominal pains or sudden death from laryngeal oedema in parent or close relative (*see also* page 515).

Chapter 42

Abdominal ascariasis

David A. Lloyd

The normal habitat of the roundworm, *Ascaris lumbricoides*, is the human small intestine, where the worms usually live without causing symptoms. Abdominal complications are most likely to occur when there is heavy intestinal infestation, and when worms enter the common bile duct.

Intestinal complications

Intestinal obstruction results when an intertwined mass of worms obstructs the bowel lumen. The impaction is intensified by spasm of the adjacent bowel wall. Serious complications are uncommon, but may be fatal if not recognized early. Prolonged obstruction may lead to necrosis of the intestinal wall, followed by perforation. A loop of bowel impacted with worms may undergo volvulus and will become ischaemic and gangrenous if the volvulus is not urgently relieved. Less common complications are intussusception and appendicitis.

Recognition

The typical features of simple, uncomplicated *Ascaris* obstruction are:

1. A history of vomiting worms or passing worms in the stools.
2. Intermittent abdominal pain, also described as cramp-like or colicky.
3. One or more palpable masses of worms in the abdomen.

The child has often been given a vermifuge 2 or 3 days before the onset of obstructive symptoms. Signs of bowel wall necrosis include fever, apathy, persistent vomiting, constant abdominal pain, abdominal distension, a tender abdominal mass, the passage of blood in the stools, and evidence of generalized peritonitis.

Diagnosis

Plain abdominal radiographs show partial intestinal obstruction in most patients with simple worm impaction, and worm shadows can often be identified. Complete obstruction is less common and may herald bowel wall necrosis. Intestinal volvulus produces the 'whirlpool' or 'target' sign. Stool microscopy confirms *Ascaris* infestation in doubtful cases.

Differential diagnosis

Intussusception causes identical clinical features and may occur in a patient who also has ascariasis. With asciariasis, blood is not found in the stools unless there are ischaemic complications. Ileocolic intussusception can be excluded by barium enema examination.

Management

Most patients with simple worm obstruction recover without an operation, on a regimen consisting of:

1. Resting the gastrointestinal tract by starving the patient, with nasogastric drainage if vomiting is severe or persistent.
2. Intravenous fluids for replacement of losses and maintenance requirements.
3. Parenteral antispasmodics, e.g. hyoscine butylbromide (Buscopan) or avapyrazone with dipyrone Avafortan, Noristan, South Africa.
4. Analgesia, if required.

A vermifuge is given only *after* the acute symptoms have resolved and gastrointestinal function has returned. This is to avoid killing the worms while they are impacted: necrotic worms appear to enhance bowel-wall necrosis.

Indications for operation

Recognition of the patient with compromised bowel is vital, as urgent surgery is essential. Danger signs include:

1. Evidence of intestinal ischaemia, notably:
   (a) A tender abdominal mass.
   (b) Blood in the stools.
   (c) Toxaemia associated with tense abdominal distension and rebound tenderness.
2. Radiological signs of complete intestinal obstruction not responding promptly to conservative management.
3. Failure to respond to adequate conservative management.

Operative management

Preoperative correction of fluid, electrolyte, and acid–base abnormalities is essential. At operation the obstructing worm bolus is disentangled by manipulation and the worms are milked into the colon. Extraction of worms through an enterotomy is occasionally necessary, but should be avoided if possible. Non-viable bowel is resected and primary anastomosis is performed after removing all intestinal worms. An anthelminthic (*see* Appendix A11.7) is prescribed when normal bowel function has returned.

Peritonitis

Worms have been found in the peritoneal cavity of patients with peritonitis. This may follow perforation, for example of a Meckel's diverticulum, but in some patients, usually those with enteritis, an intestinal perforation cannot be identified. Management consists of removing the worms and treating any associated disease.

Biliary and hepatic ascariasis

Not infrequently, worms migrate from the duodenum into the common bile duct, causing biliary colic and cholangitis. With appropriate treatment, the worms usually return to the duodenum. Prolonged or massive biliary infestation is associated with varying degrees of biliary obstruction and secondary bacterial infection. A distended, inflamed common bile duct may perforate. If worms die in the biliary tree, biliary strictures and calculi may result, and may be further complicated by suppurative ascending cholangitis and liver abscesses. Biliary worms may penetrate the liver parenchyma stimulating a granulomatous inflammatory reaction. Secondary infection of the worm nests or liver granulomas results in liver abscesses.

Recognition

Simple biliary ascariasis is characterized by intermittent, colicky abdominal pain and tenderness localized to the right upper quadrant and epigastrium. There is evidence of intestinal ascariasis, notably a history of vomiting worms or passing worms in the stool. The gallbladder may be palpable, but jaundice is rare.

Septic biliary or hepatic complications are associated with pyrexia and toxaemia, and increasing pain, tenderness and guarding in the right upper abdomen progressing to signs of peritonitis. A tender inflammatory mass may become palpable and there may be clinical jaundice.

Diagnosis

Simple biliary ascariasis

1. *Plain abdominal* films confirm the presence of intestinal worms and may show air in the biliary tree.
2. *Ultrasound scanning* demonstrates the distended gallbladder and the worm may be visualized in the dilated common bile duct.
3. *Intravenous cholangiography* confirms the diagnosis in 90 per cent of patients. The worm is seen as a filling defect in the common bile duct.

Complicated biliary and hepatic ascariasis

1. *Plain abdominal X-rays* show intestinal worms and may demonstrate air in the biliary tree or a liver abscess.
2. *Ultrasound scanning* is the most useful investigation. Worms may be identified in the dilated extrahepatic and intrahepatic bile ducts and in the liver parenchyma. Liver abscesses can also be visualized.
3. *Intravenous cholangiography* fails to opacify the biliary tree in 60 per cent of patients with complicated biliary ascariasis, and is of no value in the presence of jaundice.

Other methods of confirming the diagnosis of biliary and hepatic ascariasis include barium meal examination (to show duodenal worms entering the ampulla of Vater), endoscopic retrograde cholangiography and percutaneous transhepatic cholangiography. Haemobilia is an indication for hepatic arteriography.

Management

For simple biliary ascariasis, treatment is identical with that for intestinal ascariasis. The vermifuge may be given early provided there is no evidence of intestinal obstruction, in order to clear worms from the duodenum and encourage withdrawal of the biliary worms from the bile duct. There is a risk of killing worms in the biliary tree, and a non-absorbable vermifuge which is not excreted in the bile (e.g. piperazine; *see* Appendix A11.7) is therefore preferred.

In most patients the worms will spontaneously evacuate the biliary tree and symptoms will resolve in 2 or 3 days. Follow-up ultrasonography or intravenous cholangiography is recommended 10 days after the acute symptoms have subsided, to confirm that the worm has left the biliary tree.

Indications for operation

1. Unremitting severe symptoms not responding to conservative management.
2. Evidence of persistent biliary worms on ultrasound or cholangiography after adequate medical management (usually after 10 days).
3. Evidence of complications, namely: pyrexial illness; jaundice with serum bilirubin greater than 70 mmol/ℓ; increasing tender hepatomegaly; local or generalized peritonitis.

Operative management

Before operation, fluid, electrolyte, and acid–base abnormalities are corrected. Broad-spectrum antimicrobials are given when there is evidence of bacterial infection. A vermifuge is given to clear the intestine of worms. At operation, worms are removed from the biliary tree through a choledochotomy. Worms nests and abscesses in the liver are explored and evacuated. External biliary drainage is established through either a T-tube placed in the common bile duct or a catheter in the gallbladder. Intraoperative cholangiography is performed to confirm complete clearance of the extrahepatic and intrahepatic biliary tree. If large numbers of worms are present in the intestine, they are removed through an enterotomy to prevent reinfestation of the bile ducts.

Fibreoptic endoscopy

In some patients the biliary worm becomes impacted at the ampulla of Vater. These patients have persistent severe pain but no significant septic complications. In this situation the worm may be identified at endoscopy and removed with biopsy forceps, thus avoiding surgery.

Pancreatitis

The pancreatic duct may become obstructed by a worm in the common bile duct, leading to acute pancreatitis. The clinical features resemble those of biliary ascariasis, but the abdominal tenderness and guarding extend towards the left upper quadrant and left lumbar region. The diagnosis is established by ultrasonography, intravenous cholangiography, and serum amylase estimations.

Most patients will respond to non-operative management, as for simple biliary ascariasis. Surgery is indicated when there is failure to respond to treatment or when there are complications such as a pancreatic abscess.

Further reading

LLOYD, D. A. (1982) Hepatic Ascariasis. *South African Journal of Surgery,* **20,** 297–304

LLOYD, D. A. and WHITE, J. A. M. (1982) Biliary disease in the tropics. In Blumgart, L. (ed.) *Clinical Surgery International, Volume 8: The Biliary Tract,* pp. 236–247. Edinburgh: Churchill Livingstone

LOUW, J. H. (1966) Abdominal complications of *Ascaris lumbricoides* infestation in children. *British Journal of Surgery,* **53,** 510–521

Chapter 43

Gastrointestinal bleeding

E. R. Wozniak

Gastrointestinal bleeding may present with haematemesis, fresh rectal bleeding, melaena, abdominal pain, syncope or shock. Having established the necessity and urgency of resuscitation, the following questions must be answered.

1. *Is it blood?* Several substances, including iron and bismuth salts, can mimic melaena and are distinguished with the Haemoccult test.
2. *Is it gastrointestinal?* Blood may be swallowed following epistaxis, dental or oral trauma. The newborn may swallow maternal blood from an antepartum haemorrhage, vaginal bleeding or lesions of the nipple or breast. The Apt test (*see* Appendix 18) distinguishes fetal from materal haemoglobin. The blood may arise from the urogenital tract.
3. *Where is the bleeding site?* Haematemesis is usually due to a lesion above the mid-duodenum. Fresh rectal bleeding is usually due to a low lesion, but the character of blood passed also depends on the length of the gut and the speed of transit. Streaks of blood in the vomitus imply an oesophageal lesion, and over the stool an anorectal lesion.
4. *How much blood has been lost?* The frightened child will have a tachycardia. Blood pressure and haemoglobin may be maintained for some hours following a large bleed. Large volumes of blood may remain in the gut.
5. *Is there underlying disease?* Children with serious diseases such as infection, malignancy or coagulation disorders have the highest mortality.

6. *What is the diagnosis?* This is age dependent, and is discussed below.

Neonates

Haematemesis

1. *Bleeding disorders.* Haemorrhagic disease of the newborn is the commonest and is discussed on page 678. Maternal ingestion of aspirin, anticoagulants or anticonvulsants and maternal immune thrombocytopenia are other causes.
3. *Gastritis*, erosions and ulcers occur in the neonate with perinatal asphyxia or sepsis, and haematemeses may be large.
3. *Anatomical anomalies.* Small bleeds occur in oesophageal atresia, duodenal atresia and stenosis, hiatus hernia or duplications of the bowel.
4. *Oesophagitis* due to gastro-oesophageal reflux is increasingly recognized in neonates.

Rectal bleeding

1. *Intestinal infection,* including enteropathogenic *E. coli* and Campylobacter infection, is one of the commonest causes of colitis in infancy.
2. *Anorectal trauma*, e.g. by rectal thermometers, or anal fissures, cause streaks of blood on the stool.
3. *Necrotizing enterocolitis* occurs usually in sick premature babies. There is abdominal distension and loose stools mixed with blood.
4. *Hirschsprung's disease* may result in an enterocolitis.
5. *Mid-gut volvulus* causes obstruction, gut infarction and sometimes massive rectal bleeding.
6. *Colitis* due to cows' milk allergy is suspected if the neonate has eczema and a family history of atopy. Management is by antigen exclusion.

Infants

Haematemesis

1. *Oesophagitis* is due to gastro-oesophageal reflux and hiatus hernia. Recurrent vomits streaked with blood, pain or dyaphagia occur. Ingestion of corrosives or foreign bodies present in a similar way.
2. *Gastritis* may be due to protracted vomiting especially due to viral infections e.g. measles, or ingestion of corrosives, aspirin, iron, or steroids.
3. *Peptic ulceration* is usually acute and related to burns, serious infection or injury. There is frequent vomiting and bleeds may be large.
4. *Obstruction.* Pyloric stenosis is associated with gastritis and in neglected cases, massive haematemesis may occur. Gastric volvulus, antral or duodenal webs or diaphragms cause intermittent vomiting.

Rectal bleeding

1. *Anal fissure* is the commonest cause. Small streaks of blood are present on the stool. Defaecation is associated with straining or pain.
2. *Intussusception* is commonest under 2 years. There are symptoms suggesting pain, and signs of an abdominal mass or intestinal obstruction. Typical 'redcurrant jelly' stools are not always seen. It may be related to a polyp, Meckel's diverticulum, cystic fibrosis, lymphoid hyperplasia, Henoch–Schoenlein purpura, amoebiasis or ascariasis (*see* Chapter 42). Barium enema may be diagnostic and is often therapeutic; if not, treatment is surgical (*see* Chapter 40, page 368).
3. *Intestinal infection – see* Chapter 45.
4. *Meckel's diverticulum.* The bleed is large, red or tarry, and usually painless. It is most common under 2 years of age. Although usually diagnosed clinically, ^{99}technetium scan may support the diagnosis, but false negatives and positives occur. Management is surgical.
5. *Duplications* of the gut may result in large, painless rectal bleeds, sometimes with signs of intestinal obstruction or a mass. Diagnosis may be made by barium studies or ^{99}technetium scan, but a laparotomy may be necessary.

Children

At all ages, swallowed blood may result in apparent gastrointestinal bleeding.

Haematemesis

1. *Varices.* After, infancy, oesophageal, gastric, or duodenal varices are an important cause of massive haematemesis. The child may have been previously well, and bleeding decompresses the portal system such that splenomegaly may be minimal or absent. A neonatal history of umbilical catheterization or sepsis, exchange transfusion, jaundice or hepatitis may be present. If liver dysfunction is present, cystic fibrosis, α_1-antitrypsin deficiency, Wilson's disease, and chronic active hepatitis should be considered.
2. *Peptic ulceration.* Bleeding may be massive. A past history of abdominal pain, especially at night, and a positive family history is suggestive. Duodenal ulceration is probably more common than gastric ulceration and the frequency increases with age, especially over 8 years. Acute ulceration may occur in serious illness or trauma. Gastritis and oesophagitis occur as in infancy.
3. *Oesophageal tears* may follow prolonged vomiting or retching in adolescents (Mallory–Weiss tear), or ingestion of foreign bodies.
4. *Bleeding disorders* rarely present with haematemesis, but include disseminated intravascular coagulation and thrombocytopenia (*see* pages 493–499).
5. *Tumours.* Gastric or duodenal polyps, or even more rarely, lymphoma, leiomyoma or teratoma may present with bleeding.
6. *Infection.* Candidal oesophagitis in the immunocompromised causes dysphagia, sometimes with haematemesis.

Rectal bleeding

All the causes described in infants may occur.

1. *Polyps* are probably the commonest cause:
   (a) Juvenile polyps are single or multiple, usually colonic and sometimes palpable per rectum. They are non-malignant.
   (b) Peutz–Jeghers syndrome consists of gastrointestinal polyposis and mucocutaneous pigmentation of the lips, mouth and fingers. Polyps cause pain or bleeding.
   (c) Familial polyposis coli usually presents after 10 years with diarrhoea and rectal bleeding. The polyps invariably become malignant.
   (d) Gardner's syndrome is associated with fibromas, epidermoid cysts, and osteomas.
2. *Inflammatory bowel disease* presents most commonly over the age of 10 years. The incidence of Crohn's disease is rising. It may present insidiously with anorexia, abdominal pain or growth failure, and perianal disease or tags may be present. In ulcerative colitis, abdominal pain and tenesmus occur. In both, stools may consist mainly of mucus and blood, and large bleeds may occur. Prednisolone and sulphasalazine are the main therapeutic agents.
3. *Infection.* Viral, Shigella, Salmonella, Campylobacter or Yersinia infection, amoebiasis, schistosomiasis, haemorrhagic fevers (e.g. Dengue, *see* Chapter 66) hookworm and whipworm can cause rectal bleeding, sometimes massive. Clostridia are associated with pseudomembraneous colitis and necrotizing jejunitis.
4. *Vascular malformations.* Cutaneous vascular malformations are present in 50 per cent of patients. Large cavernous haemangiomas are commonest. Other

causes include hereditary haemorrhagic telangiectasia, Klippel–Tremannoy–Weber syndrome, Turner's syndrome, blue-rubber bleb naevus syndrome, and arteriovenous malformations.

5. *Henoch–Schoenlein purpura* occurs in children aged 2–10 years and causes rectal bleeding, abdominal pain and, rarely, haematemesis. It is sometimes associated with intussusception. Purpura, especially of the lower limbs, oedema of the hands or feet and haematuria or hypertension may be present.
6. *Haemolytic uraemic syndrome* may follow gastroenteritis with fresh rectal bleeding and renal failure.
7. *Foreign body* in the rectum causes rectal pain.
8. *Haemorrhoids* occur occasionally in adolescents and are more common in portal hypertension.

Investigation

Blood is taken for grouping, cross-match, haemoglobin, platelets, coagulation studies, liver function tests, electrolytes and urea. A raised urea may be due to a large bleed as well as renal impairment.

Further investigation depends on the likely diagnosis, the amount and rate of bleeding and facilities available.

Haematemesis

Upper gastrointestinal endoscopy is the investigation of choice and should be performed when the patient is stable and preferably within 24 hours. Plain abdominal X-ray is only useful if perforation or obstruction is suspected. Barium studies are performed if endoscopy is not available. Active bleeding of 0.5 ml/minute or more may be localized with arteriography. Selective arterial infusion of drugs or embolization may stop bleeding. Using these techniques, over 80 per cent of patients can be accurately diagnosed.

Rectal bleeding

Many conditions can be diagnosed clinically. The ^{99}technetium scan for Meckel's diverticulum and barium enema for intussusception have been discussed. Proctosigmoidoscopy, colonoscopy or double-contrast barium enema are useful for diagnosing polyps or inflammatory bowel disease. Polypectomy can be performed endoscopically. Active bleeding, including bleeding from vascular malformations, can be localized with ^{99}technetium labelled red cell scans or arteriography.

Management

Most patients require observation and no treatment. The majority of those requiring treatment stop bleeding spontancously and management is supportive.

More aggressive investigation and treatment is required for persistent massive bleeding. Mortality is associated wth the presence of serious underlying disease, coagulation disorders, a haemoglobin less than 7 g/100 ml, a transfusion requirement of more than 85 ml/kg and failure to identify the bleeding site. A joint medical and surgical team approach is essential. Large bleeds require rapid volume replacement using saline or plasma through a large-bore intravenous cannula, with blood transfusion as urgently as possible. Fresh frozen plasma should be given if a coagulation disorder is suspected (*see* page 499).

In suspected upper gastrointestinal bleeding without haematemesis, a nasogastric tube may be passed to determine the presence of blood in the stomach. If positive, some advocate cold saline gastric lavage. Nasogastric intubation can, however, reactivate variceal bleeding.

Peptic ulcer

Bleeding ulcers can be treated with photocoagulation or laser therapy at endoscopy. Cimetidine 2 mg/kg by slow intravenous injection every 4–6 hours is often given, but does not influence acute bleeding. Use of cimetidine and antacids to raise gastric pH above 4 may prevent recurrence of bleeding and is used prophylactically in at-risk patients.

Varices

For Management, *see* Chapter 47, page 418.

Surgery

This is indicated for specific problems such as Meckel's diverticulum. Emergency surgery is required for massive persistent bleeding, more than 85 ml/kg in 1½ hours, since medical management is unlikely to stop bleeding. At laparotomy, the bleeding site is identified in only about 50 per cent of cases. If the site is unknown, preoperative arteriographic localization may greatly assist the surgeon (if time and facilities permit), and endoscopy at the time of laparotomy can be very useful.

Feeding

Oral fluids and soft foods can be given even if bleeding persists, unless investigation or surgery is imminent. Starvation worsens the prognosis.

Further reading

British Medical Journal (1981) Management of gastrointestinal bleeding. *British Medical Journal*, **283**, 456–457

COX, K. and AMENT, M. E. (1979) Upper gastrointestinal bleeding in children and adolescents. *Pediatrics*, **63**, 408–413

LEVINE, M. I. (1979) Rectal bleeding in the first month of life. *Postgraduate Medical Journal*, **55**, 22–23

Chapter 44

Enteritis necroticans: Pigbel

Gregor Lawrence

Pigbel is a necrotizing enteritis caused by *Clostridium welchii* type C (CwC) and its B toxin. There is patchy damage in the upper intestine varying from mucosal to full-thickness gut wall necrosis. Loops of damaged gut are bound together by adhesions and covered with omentum. The mesenteric glands are enlarged and the mesentery thickened. Most of the damage is in the jejunum, in very severe cases the whole small bowel is affected. Haemorrhage into the gut wall often results in a striking striped segmental appearance.

In the Papua New Guinea (PNG) highlands pigbel is second only to pneumonia as a cause of death in children after infancy. It is the most common cause of the acute abdomen. It also occurs in South-East Asia and Africa. *Where the disease is less common clinical diagnosis before operation may be difficult.*

Acute pigbel results from overgrowth and B toxin production by CwC in the gut following a meat-containing meal. The clinical syndrome results from gut damage caused by the toxin: pain with varying degrees of intestinal obstruction, and the effects of fluid loss, electrolyte disturbance and absorbed toxin. In the most severe cases patients die within a short period despite treatment and often without abdominal signs. Severe cases present with pain, intestinal obstruction and shock some days after symptoms begin. Milder cases with pain, less distension and without signs of toxicity are common. Occasional patients are seen with chronic intestinal obstruction from scarring, remote from the acute episode.

Recognition

1. In PNG most pigbel cases follow a meat-containing meal, usually by 1–5 days.
2. Virtually all patients have severe abdominal pain, usually central or epigastric and colicky in nature. In mild cases pain is made worse by eating.
3. Diarrhoea is common, particularly in the first few days. It frequently contains blood and sometimes roundworms (ascaris). Stools often cease as intestinal obstruction supervenes.
4. Vomiting is a common early feature. Vomitus is often dark, like coffee grounds, and may contain ascaris.
5. Intestinal obstruction leads to distension and tenderness, most marked in the upper abdomen. Loops of distended bowel with peristalsis may be seen and tender, thickened, damaged intestine palpated.

Management

Mild pigbel

Treatment is conservative: gut rest by nasogastric aspiration, intravenous replacement of deficits, and fluid maintenance and antibiotics. If the patient does not improve in a day or so, or deteriorates, operation should be considered.

1. Free drainage by nasogastric tube with hourly aspiration.
2. Benzyl penicillin and chloramphenicol intravenously, orally after the drip is removed.
3. With improvement and resolution of obstruction, begin clear fluids. After 24 hours of improvement regrade to stronger fluids and later gradually introduce normal food.
4. If the patient deteriorates, or if obstruction, toxicity, or severe pain persists, surgery is indicated.
5. All patients are given piperazine for ascaris.

Severe pigbel

The treatment of severe pigbel is rescuscitation of the patient in preparation for surgery; they have lost large amounts of blood, body fluids, and protein into the damaged gut and have had a poor intake. Some patients will respond to these measures and not need operation.

1. Nasogastric aspiration and antibiotics as for mild pigbel.
2. *Restoration of circulating blood volume and rehydration is vital:* Transfuse with whole blood; correct fluid deficit with plasma or equivalent; replace continuing losses with normal saline with added potassium chloride (KCl); maintenance fluids with potassium chloride according to weight.
3. Pethidine for pain.

Operate for:

1. Persisting toxicity despite adequate treatment.
2. Persisting obstruction with large amounts of gastric aspirate.
3. Recurrent bleeding or perforation.

Timing of operation

Early operation leads to surgery for some cases that would respond to conservative management. Delay may prolong illness and make nutritional and electrolyte problems worse. Delay such that operation takes place much more than a week after onset makes operation more difficult. The necrotic gut is more fragile and adhesions more dense.

Operation

The aim is to remove severely damaged gut and make end-to-end anastomosis through bowel that is as normal as possible. In most cases a single resection will be possible. Where damage is extensive the surgeon must strike a balance between the amount of gut removed and the patient's future nutritional requirements. More than one join may be needed. Use an upper midline incision. Gently expose and remove involved gut without rupture. Because of the greatly thickened mesentery keep fairly close to the bowel wall when dividing the mesentery. Decompress the remaining gut before anastomosis. Normal serosa is important if making anastomosis in partially damaged gut. Drainage will be necessary if pus is found. Some surgeons drain the area close to the anastomosis. Inspect the entire small bowel. If the distal duodenum is involved, an end-to-side anastomosis may be necessary.

Post operative

Preoperative management is continued until gut function returns. Pigbel patients often develop signs of acute malnutrition due to losses and no intake. Prolonged nasogastric aspiration and IV fluids aggravate this. If facilities are available intravenous nutrition should be used in patients with a prolonged hospital course.

Further reading

LAWRENCE, G., SHANN, F., FREESTONE, D. S. and WALKER, P. D. (1979) Prevention of necrotising enteritis in Papua New Guinea by active immunisation. *Lancet,* **ii,** 227–230

SHANN, F. (1984) The medical management of enteritis necroticans. In (W. M. Davies, ed.) *Pigbel.* Papua New Guinea Institute of Medical Research Monograph Series, 6. pp. 89–94. Goroka.

SHANN, F. and LAWRENCE, G. (1979) The medical management of pigel. *Papua New Guinea Medical Journal,* **22,** 24–29

SHEPHERD, A. (1979) Clinical features and operative treatment of pigbel. *Papua New Guinea Medical Journal,* **22,** 18–23

SMITH, F. (1969) Surgical aspects of enteritis necroticans in the Highlands of New Guinea. *Australian and New Zealand Journal of Surgery,* **38,** 199–205

Chapter 45

Acute gastrointestinal infections

J. A. Walker-Smith

Acute gastroenteritis is an illness with an acute onset of vomiting and diarrhoea, often accompanied by fever and constitutional disturbance.

Illnesses which can cause diarrhoea and vomiting that may be confused with gastroenteritis are listed in *Table 45.1*. The principal causative agents with some important aspects are given in *Table 45.2*.

Table 45.1 Illnesses that can cause diarrhoea and vomiting which may be confused with gastroenteritis

Surgical disorders Acute appendicitis Intussusception Pyloric stenosis Various causes of incomplete intestinal obstruction, including Hirschsprung's disease	*Coeliac disease* *Systemic infections* Septicaemia Pneumonia Meningitis Urinary tract infection Measles (especially if malnourished) Malaria
Inflammatory bowel disease Necrotizing or non-specific enterocolitis Crohn's disease Ulcerative colitis	*Upper respiratory tract infections* Otitis media
Acute food intolerance e.g. cows' milk protein intolerance	*Other disorders* Diabetic pre-coma Haemolytic–uraemic syndrome Haemorrhagic shock and encephalopathy*

* Levin *et al.* (1983).

General points in management of acute gastrointestinal infections

The aim is to maintain or restore adequate hydration and electrolyte balance; usually this is achieved by the oral route. But there are risks in giving soft drinks in a casual manner as their electrolyte content varies greatly (*Table 45.3*), some having a very high potassium content (apple juice and orange juice), and all except Lucozade have a very low sodium content. The methods of oral rehydration are considered in detail in Chapter 46. Only where there is significant dehydration are intravenous fluids required.

In developed countries, if there is 5 per cent dehydration, intravenous fluids are often given; but in developing communities, only if a child is 10 per cent dehydrated and shocked are intravenous fluids recommended (for further details of intravenous rehydration, *see* page 409). For fluid requirements *see* Appendix 3.

Drugs in the treatment of acute gastrointestinal infections

In general there is no place for drug therapy. Antibiotics are ineffective even when there is a bacterial infection and are rarely indicated. In salmonellosis antibiotic therapy prolongs the carriage of salmonellae in the stools. The only exception to this is when there is a salmonella septicaemia. In shigellosis in the more severe cases co-trimoxazole (trimethoprim–sulfamethoxazole; Septrin, Bactrim) is recommended as the organism is often resistant to ampicillin. Antibiotics are only used with enteropathogenic *E. coli* infections when there is an outbreak in a neonatal nursery or when an infant is gravely ill. There is little evidence that this influences the natural history of the infection although it may reduce the number of bacteria in stools and so their infectivity. Oral colistin may be used. Multiple-resistant strains have diminished the effectiveness of neomycin and kanamycin. Erythromycin may be used in the more severe cases of campylobacter infection but antibiotic therapy is not usually required. Only in giardiasis and amoebiasis is drug therapy always indicated (*see* page 396), namely metronidazole or tinidazole. In Yersinia enteritis and enterocolitis antibiotics are only required in severe infections.

The traditional antidiarrhoeal and anti-emetic drugs are not recommended; kaolin and pectin preparations are of no value; opiates and related drugs such as diphenoxylate (Lomotil) are potentially dangerous and should not be prescribed at all; loperamide (Imodium) is also not recommended at present. In the older child when vomiting is the dominant symptom and the diagnosis is clear an anti-emetic such as prochlorperazine (Stemetil) may be used but should never be used as a suppository as absorption is unpredictable, and its use may result in dystonic reactions.

Synopsis of principal infections of the gastrointestinal tract (Table 45.2)

Rotavirus infection

Recognition

Rotavirus infection is the main cause of infantile gastroenteritis throughout the world. It occurs mainly in infants under 3 years of age, in the winter in temperate climates. It begins with vomiting followed by diarrhoea and sometimes mild fever; the vomiting occurs during the first 2 days but the diarrhoea reaches a peak 3–4 days after the onset. The diarrhoea is watery and there may be temporary carbohydrate (glucose or lactose) intolerance. The disease is usually mild but dehydration with a metabolic acidosis may occur. The stools are acid and do not contain blood. The virus in the stool can be identified by electron microscopy. An ELISA (enzyme linked immunoabsorbent assay) test also gives reliable results.

Table 45.2 Some aetiological agents and important features

Condition	*Aetiological agents*	*Clinical features*		*Incubation period*	*Epidemiological features*	*First-line treatment*
		Common	*Others*			
Acute watery diarrhoea	Rotavirus	Vomiting	Fever. Severe dehydration in some.	24–72 hours	Particularly common in infants and young children. World-wide in all socioeconomic groups. Peak in winter in temperate climates.	Oral rehydration therapy.
	Enterotoxigenic *Escherichia coli* (ETEC)	Nausea, vomiting.	Fever, malaise, severe dehydration.	6–72 hours	Infants and young children in developing countries. Travellers' diarrhoea.	Oral rehydration therapy.
	Enteropathogenic *Escherichia coli*	Nausea, vomiting.	Fever	6–72 hours	Nursery outbreaks in developed countries. Children in developed countries. Uncertain in developing countries.	Oral rehydration therapy.
	Non-typhoid Salmonellae	Nausea, vomiting, fever, chills, abdominal pain.	Malaise, blood and mucus in the stools	8–36 hours	Children. Common world-wide. Food-borne outbreaks (animal products e.g. chicken, meat). Warmer seasons.	Oral rehydration therapy.
	Campylobacter	Abdominal pain, fever, malaise.	Chills, blood and pus in the stools.	3–5 days	World-wide distribution. In developed countries may be food-borne (animal products) or transmitted by handling of animals.	Oral rehydration therapy. Erythromycin in severe cases.

	Vibrio cholerae (*see* Chapter 63)	Vomiting, abdominal pain.	Severe dehydration, circulatory collapse, shock.	1–3 days	Children in endemic areas. Adults in newly affected areas. Not found in Latin America.	Oral rehydration therapy. Tetracycline.
	Yersinia enterocolitica	Acute gastrointestinal illness with fever; stools contain pus and occasionally blood. Septicaemia occurs in infants, acute terminal ileitis or mesenteric adenitis in adults and adolescents.		Variable	Infants, children and adults. Usually food-borne (often raw milk).	Oral rehydration therapy. Often self-limiting condition requiring no antibiotics; severe or prolonged illness may require chloramphenicol, gentamicin, colistin or co-trimoxazole according to sensitivities.
Dysentery: Stool is soft and watery with blood and/or pus	Shigellae	Fever, abdominal pain.	Malaise, vomiting, urgency to defaecate. Painful spasm on defaecation.	36–72 hours	Children, poor hygiene, malnutrition, institutions; warmer seasons.	Oral rehydration therapy. Co-trimoxazole.
Prolonged diarrhoea:	*Entamoeba histolytica*	Abdominal discomfort, stools with blood and mucus.	*See* Chapter 65.	2–6 weeks	All age groups. World-wide distribution.	Metronidazole or tinidazole.
For at least 7 days stools have been more frequent than normal	*Giardia lamblia*	Abdominal distension, watery diarrhoea, crampy abdominal pain.	Anorexia, nausea, coeliac-like picture.	1–3 weeks	Young children. Some travellers: common in malnutrition and dysgammaglobulinaemia.	Metronidazole or tinidazole.

Table 45.3 Analysis of popular soft drinks

Brand	*pH*	*Osmolality* (mosmol/kg)	*Electrolytes* (mmol/ℓ)	
			Sodium	*Potassium*
Coca-Cola	2.8	469	3.0	0.1
Pepsi-Cola	2.7	576	1.0	0.1
Seven-up	3.5	388	4.0	0.0
Lucozade	3.0	710	18.0	0.5
Orange juice	4.0	587	1.0	46.0
Apple juice	3.6	694	0.0	27.4
Ribena* diluted 1:3	3.0	1180	4.0	8.0
Ribena diluted 1:4	3.3	862	3.0	6.0
Ribena diluted 1:5	3.4	561	2.0	4.7

* Blackcurrant cordial.
From Head *et al*. (1983).

Management

Usually a glucose–electrolyte solution (*see* Chapter 46) is adequate, but IV fluids are required if there is severe dehydration.

Other stool viruses

Other stool viruses have now been associated with acute gastroenteritis in childhood, especially in early infancy. They include Norwalk agent, adenovirus, astrovirus and calcivirus. All are diagnosed by stool electron microscopy. Management is as for Rotavirus.

Shigellosis

Shigellosis is an acute enterocolitis due to an organism of the shigella group. The term shigellosis is not synonymous with bacillary dysentery, which is infection with *Shigella shiga (Sh. dysenteriae* Type I). Other Shigellae are *S. sonnei, S. flexneri* and *S. boydii*. Shigellosis is highly contagious, requiring a very low infecting dose. Transmission is by person-to-person contact and food/water contamination by human faecal matter, man being the only natural host, although flies may serve as vectors.

Recognition

Approximately 25 per cent of patients will have mild watery diarrhoea. An equal number will have high fever with minor enteric complaints, and the remainder will have diarrhoea accompanied or followed by fever and, in a day or two, cramping abdominal pain, tenderness, and severe diarrhoea containing blood, shed mucosa and/or mucus. Straining to defaecate may be so severe as to cause rectal prolapse, but vomiting is infrequent.

Children under the age of 10 years are particularly severely affected, perhaps due to their poorer sanitation practices or diminished coprantibodies. Furthermore, in younger children, the abrupt rise in body temperature may be accompanied by prostration, meningism or febrile seizures. Acute symptoms may persist for a week or more, with convalescence prolonged over several weeks. Although dehydration and hyponatraemia are common in severe forms, septicaemia and other complications are generally rare.

An Asian pandemic of shigella dysenteriae Type I (*Shigella shiga*) dysentery was first noticed in Bangladesh in 1972 (Rahaman *et al.*, 1974) and has since spread to India and Sri Lanka (Lamabadusuriya, 1986). Bottle-fed malnourished children have been worst effected. Disseminated intravascular coagulation (DIC), prolonged diarrhoea and further deterioration of nutritional status are all characteristic. Haemolytic uraemic syndrome complicating shigella dysentery has also been described (Raghupathy *et al.*, 1978). Personal hygiene such as washing hands with soap and water after defaecation, and before preparation and consumption of food is vital for controlling the spread of the disease.

Diagnosis

The peripheral white cell count is often elevated but regardless of the actual number of cells, there is a predominance of polymorphonuclear cells and their precursors. Examination of the rectum may reveal an oedematous and friable mucosa with ulcers. Stools usually show masses of red and white cells on smear. Laboratory stool culture can be difficult and should be plated out immediately, as a delay of 2 hours decreases recovery by 50 per cent.

Species in the United Kingdom are usually *S. sonnei* or *S. flexneri; S. shiga (S. dysenteriae* Type I, the original *Shiga bacillus*) and *S. boydii* occurring far less commonly. Serotype identification is used in epidemiological control.

Management

The most important consideration is replacement of fluid and electrolyte losses. Antibiotics should be restricted to fulminant infections in debilitated infants. Shigella is sensitive to many antimicrobials, including co-trimoxazole (trimethoprim–sulphamethoxazole) which is the treatment of choice, but the organism is now often resistant to ampicillin. In severe cases other antibiotics are indicated (World Health Organisation, 1978). Furazolidone or nalidixic acid have been recommended in Sri Lanka (Lamabadusuriya, 1986). Antidiarrhoeal drugs are not used because adverse effects have been reported.

The importance of hygiene should be emphasized. In countries where good sanitary facilities exist and where water is available for hand washing, morbidity from Shigella infection is low; but even in developed nations, where personal hygiene is poor, as in day-care centres and custodial institutions, outbreaks of shigellosis have occurred, often involving numerous secondary cases.

Salmonellosis

Salmonellosis or infection with *S. typhimurium* and related organisms is a very variable infection which may produce mild symptoms or a septicaemia.

Recognition

1. Newborn: the infection may be acquired from the mother or from infected feeds. Symptoms may be mild with slight diarrhoea and with occasional flecks of mucus, or a septicaemic illness complicated by meningitis or osteitis.

2. Other age groups:
   (a) Acute gastrointestinal symptoms with fever, headache, vomiting, abdominal pain and watery stools.
   (b) A typhoid-like condition, with a high remittent fever.
   (c) A septicaemia resembling tuberculous meningitis, with lethargy, stiff neck (without meningitis) and splenomegaly.
   (d) Osteitis is a common complication in African children with sickle-cell anaemia.
   (e) Identification is by culture of the blood (or CSF in meningitis) and stools or rectal swab.

Management

1. Oral glucose–electrolyte mixture (*see* Chapter 46).
2. Dehydration requiring IV fluids (*see* Chapter 46).
3. Antibiotics: Amoxycillin should be given parenterally only in a septicaemic illness, or chloramphenicol in meningitis (*see* pages 338 and 343). Otherwise antibiotics are contraindicated as they may lead to a carrier state.

Yersinia enteritis and enterocolitis

Yersinia enterocolitica is a Gram negative rod previously known as *Pasteurella pseudotuberculosis*. It may cause a zoonosis in several animals. It is more common in Belgium and Scandinavia than in Britain.

Recognition

In children, it presents as acute gastroenteritis with diarrhoea containing blood and pus, and fever, but in adolescents and adults as an acute terminal ileitis or mesenteric adrenitis (Vantrappen *et al.*, 1977).

The diagnosis is made by isolating organisms from the stools or by rising titres of Yersinia antibodies. It can also be isolated from ileocaecal lymph nodes and resected appendices. There is no evidence that Yersinia infection can cause Crohn's disease. However, barium studies may show abnormalities of the terminal ileum which could be confused with Crohn's disease. Radiological abnormalities are mainly with changes in mucosal pattern, and the superficial ulcerative skin lesions of Crohn's disease are never seen.

Management

It is often a self-limiting disease like 'gastroenteritis', requiring oral glucose–electrolyte replacement, but no antibiotics. Infants may become severely ill with septicaemia. Severe or prolonged infections may require treatment with chloramphenicol, gentamicin, colistin, or co-trimoxazole (trimethoprim–sulphamethoxazole, Septrin, Bactrim). Family infections are common.

Campylobacter enteritis

Campylobacter is a micro-aerophilic vibrio recently recognized as a cause of acute gastroenteritis (Skirrow, 1977). The highest incidence is in young children most commonly under a year. A healthy carrier state may exist.

The mode of transmission involves ingestion of the organism, carriage to the intestine, and sometimes invasion of the blood. Wild birds and chickens may be an important source of infection.

Recognition

The clinical features vary, but diarrhoea lasting several days with or without fever is most frequent. The diarrhoea may be trivial or severe with watery stools, sometimes containing blood. Aching of limbs may also occur. Vomiting, and severe cramping abdominal pain may be a feature, and the child may be admitted initially as a suspected surgical emergency.

Management

It is often a self-limiting condition requiring only fluid replacement. Severe illness may need treatment with erythromycin.

Food-poisoning organisms

When acute diarrhoea and vomiting rapidly follow the ingestion of bacterially contaminated food, the diagnosis of food poisoning is made. It may result from ingestion of bacteria *per se* or from a preformed toxin, e.g. staphylococcal enterotoxin (*see* below), or the toxin of *Clostridium botulinum* (classic botulism), fortunately rare. *Clostridium perfringens* is an important cause of food-borne diarrhoea and can cause a sometimes fatal enteritis known as 'pigbel' in the highlands of Papua New Guinea and elsewhere (*see* Chapter 44). Infection with salmonella may produce this syndrome (food poisoning) but other organisms such as *Vibrio parahaemolyticus* and *Bacillus cereus* have now been associated with food poisoning.

Vibrio parahaemolyticus is a Gram negative rod associated with the consumption of uncooked seafoods. Its incubation period is 12–48 hours. Acute gastrointestinal symptoms last a few days but are rarely serious.

Bacillus cereus is a Gram negative rod that can produce a toxin. Infection is usually acquired by eating food that has been stored before eating, e.g. Chinese fried rice.

Staphylococcal infections

Staphylococcal toxin enteritis

The toxin has been already formed in infected food, and there is no bacterial infection. Vomiting and diarrhoea develop suddenly, often with acute abdominal pain which initially may suggest acute appendicitis. This is a self-limiting condition, usually of a few hours' duration.

Staphylococcal enterocolitis

This is an acute staphylococcal infection of the gastrointestinal tract, usually resulting from the elimination of the normal flora by a wide-spectrum antibiotic, one of the tetracyclines, clindamycin, or lincomycin. Dehydration may be severe and require urgent IV correction. Antibiotics parenterally, and possibly orally also, should be given, with any of the antibiotics with a high degree of activity against the staphylococcus (e.g. one of the cephalosporins). It is now rare.

References

DUPONT, H. L. and HORNICTZ, R. B. (1973) Adverse effects of Lomotil therapy in Shigellosis. *Journal of the American Medical Association,* **226,** 1525–1528

HEAD, J., HOGARTH, M., PARSLOE, J. and BROOMHALL, J. (1983) *Lancet,* **i,** 1450

LAMABADUSURIYA, S. P. (1985) Shigellosis in Sri Lanka. *Chronic Diarrhoea and Malnutrition* (eds. J. A. Walker-Smith and A. S. McNeish). London: Butterworth (in Press)

LEVIN, M., HJELM, M., KAY, J. D., PINCOTT, J. R., GOULD, J. D. and DINWIDDIE, J. (1983) *Lancet,* **ii,** 64–67

RAGHUPATHY, P., DATE, A., SHASTRY, J. C. M., SUDARASANAM, A. and JADHAR, M. (1978) Haemolytic-uraemic syndrome complicating Shigella dysentery in South Indian children. *British Medical Journal,* **i,** 1518–1521

RAHAMAN, M. M., HUQ, I., DEY, C. R., KIBRIYA, A. K. M. G. and CURLIN, G. (1974) Ampicillin resistant *Shiga bacillus* in Bangladesh. *Lancet,* **i,** 406–407

SKIRROW, M. B. (1977) Campylobacter enteritis: a 'new disease'. *British Medical Journal,* **ii,** 9–11

VANTRAPPEN, G., POUETTE, E., GEBOES, K. *et al.* (1977) Yersinia enterocolitis: Gastroenterological aspects. *Gastroenterology,* **72,** 220–227

WORLD HEALTH ORGANISATION (1978) *Diarrhoeal Diseases Control Programme; Clinical Management of Acute Diarrhoea.* WHO/DDC/79.3

Further reading

CIBA FOUNDATION SYMPOSIUM (1976) *Acute Diarrhoea in Childhood.* 42 (new series). Amsterdam: Elsevier

WALKER-SMITH, J. A. (1979) Gastroenteritis. In *Diseases of the Small Intestine in Childhood* (2nd edn.). Tunbridge Wells: Pitman Medical

WALKER-SMITH, J. A. (1985) Current Opinion in Gastroenterology. I. pp. 119–125

Chapter 46

Rehydration in gastrointestinal infections

D. C. A. Candy

Clinical studies undertaken in diarrhoeal treatment centres in Asia, Africa and Latin America have shown that 80 per cent or more episodes of dehydration can be successfully treated by oral rehydration, without intravenous fluids (Hirschhorn, 1980). Apart from the obvious attractions of oral rehydration therapy, such as cheapness, simplicity, and versatility, oral rehydration may actually be safer than the intravenous route (Santosham *et al.*, 1982).

Physiology

1. The ability to replace electrolyte and water losses from diarrhoea depends on the fact that the jejunum actively absorbs glucose (and other solutes such as galactose, amino acids and peptides) in the presence of sodium. During this process, chloride, potassium and water are also passively absorbed (Dobbins and Binder, 1981).
2. Dehydration may account for one-third of all deaths in areas where diarrhoea is common. These deaths are largely preventable, by exploiting the reserve capacity to absorb sodium and glucose even in the jejunum damaged by rotavirus infection or other organisms. The discovery of coupled sodium and glucose transport in the jejunum is 'potentially the most important medical advance this century' (*Lancet,* 1978).

Oral rehydration regimen (Pizarro *et al.*, 1983)

Assessment of dehydration

This is outlined in *Table 46.1.* Clinical assessment is more difficult in the following groups of patients:

1. Malnourished children, who may have poor tissue turgor and sunken eyes even when well hydrated; thus dehydration may be overestimated.
2. Obese children: dehydration may be underestimated.
3. Children with hyperatraemic dehydration: tissue turgor may be maintained even with severe dehydration.

General examination

In addition to assessment for hydration, signs of extraintestinal infections (e.g. otitis media, meningitis, measles, bronchopneumonia) and possible surgical conditions (e.g. appendicitis, intussusception) should be looked for.

Table 46.1 Clinical assessment of dehydration

Degree of dehydration	*% body weight lost as water*	*Fluid loss* (ml/kg)	*Symptoms and signs*
Mild	less than 5	50	Nil other than mild thirst and oliguria but history of fluid loss (diarrhoea and/or vomiting).
Moderate	5–10	50–100	Thirst, oliguria, dry mouth, decreased tear formation, sunken eyes, decreased tissue turgor, sunken fontanelle.
Severe	Greater than 10	>100	As for moderate dehydration, and also cold extremities, peripheral cyanosis, apathy, acidotic breathing, tachycardia with low BP and impalpable peripheral pulses.

Oral or intravenous rehydration

1. Intravenous rehydration is indicated for patients with greater than 10 per cent dehydration (*Table 46.1*).
2. Oral rehydration is contraindicated in the presence of ileus (gross abdominal distension, decreased bowel sounds and multiple fluid levels on erect abdominal X-ray).
3. *See also* 'Limitations of oral rehydration' (page 407).

Management (Figure 46.1)

Calculation of fluid deficit

1. Weigh the patient.
2. Assess per cent body weight lost as water (from *Table 46.1*).
3. $$\text{Deficit} = \frac{\text{Weight (kg)} \times \text{per cent body weight lost as water}}{100}$$

   Thus: 6 kg child with 5 per cent dehydration (50 ml/kg):

   $$\text{Deficit} = \frac{6 \times 5}{100} = 0.3\,\text{kg} = 300\,\text{ml water } (6 \times 50\,\text{ml/kg})$$

   (1 kg loss of body weight = 1 kg or 1 ℓ of water)

Replacement of deficit (rehydration phase)

1. If shocked (*see Table 46.1:* symptoms and signs indicating greater than 10 per cent body weight lost as water: intravenous plasma (or 0.9 per cent sodium chloride if plasma is unavailable) 20 ml/kg, should be given over 1–2 hours to

restore renal perfusion and urine production. Once shock has been successfully reversed, it may be possible to revert from intravenous to oral rehydration, during the course of treatment.
2. If dehydrated but not shocked, twice the estimated fluid deficit is replaced orally as rehydration solution (assuming 1 ℓ rehydration solution = 1 kg deficit). Giving twice the estimated deficit allows for continuing diarrhoeal losses during the rehydration and nutrition phases (*see* (2) below).

Choice of rehydration solution

1. Commercially available solutions (in the UK) are shown in Appendix 9. The regimen described in this chapter employs the WHO oral rehydration solution (ORS). (For composition *see* foot of *Table 46.2* and Appendix 9 for alternative solutions.) In the UK and many other Western countries solutions with a lower sodium content (35–50 mmol/ℓ) are used. Studies on infants and children throughout the world have shown that this regimen can be used for acute diarrhoea of various aetiologies, in all age groups, regardless of initial serum sodium concentration and without intravenous fluids.
2. Twice the volume of estimated fluid deficit is given as ORS and water, in a ratio of 2:1. If the infant is hyponatraemic (serum sodium less than 130 mmol/ℓ) the entire rehydration volume may be given as ORS.

Table 46.2 Oral rehydration of 6 kg infant with 5 per cent dehydration (50 ml/kg) (Deficit will be 6 × 50 = 200 ml)

	Plasma Na (mmol/ℓ)		
	<130	*130–150*	*>150*
WHO oral rehydration solution*	100 ml/hr for 6 hr	100 ml/hr for 4 hr	50 ml/hr for 8 hr
Water	–	100 ml/hr for 2 hr	50 ml/hr for 4 hr
Half-strength formula feed (or breast milk)	110 ml every 3 hr for 24 hr; then full-strength formula feed		

* Contains per litre: sodium, 90 mmol; potassium, 20 mmol; chloride, 80 mmol; bicarbonate, 30 mmol; glucose, 110 mmol. (3.5 g NaCl, 2.5 g $NaHCO_3$, 1.5 g KCl, 20 g glucose, water 1 litre). (*See also* Appendix 9 for alternative solutions.)

Duration of rehydration phase (Figure 46.1)

1. Twice the estimated fluid deficit is given over 6 hours. During the first 4 hours, ORS is given, followed by water for 2 hours. If the serum sodium level is known to be high (greater than 150 mmol/ℓ) at the start of rehydration, the same volumes of rehydration solution and water is given *over 12 hours*, since rapid rehydration is associated with an increased risk of convulsions.
2. At the end of the rehydration phase the patient is weighed again, and re-examined for signs of dehydration. If dehydration is still present, a further 6-hour course of ORS and water is given, with the volume based on a

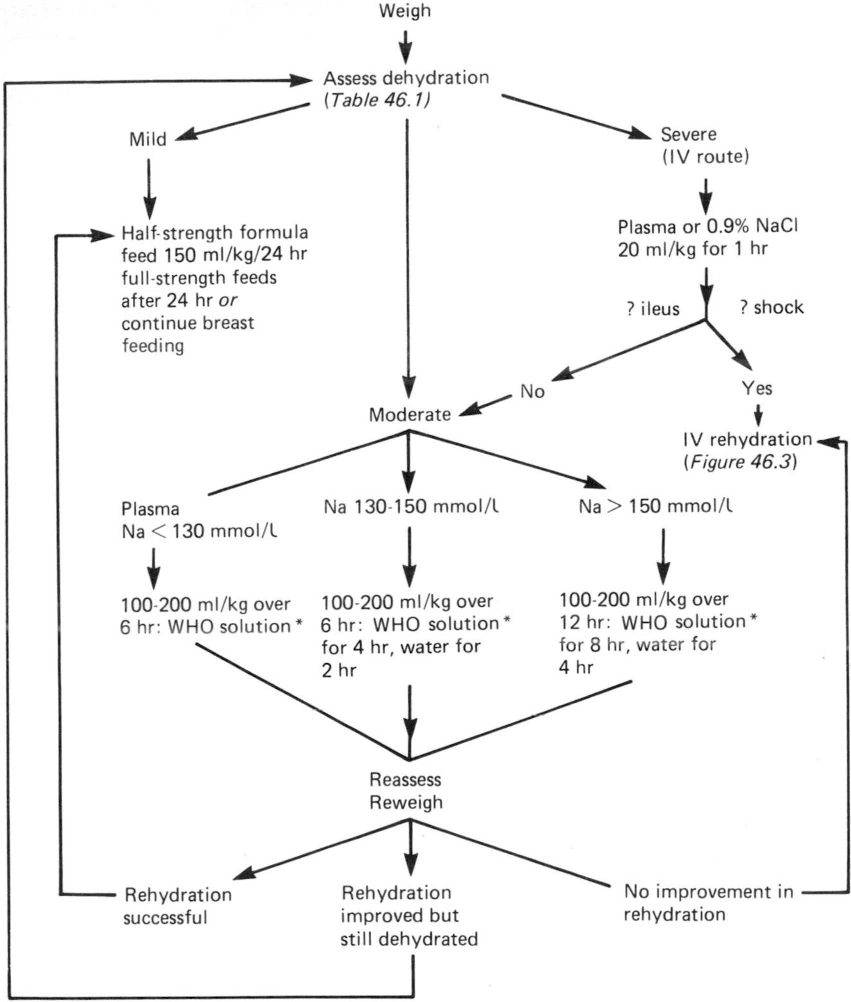

Figure 46.1 Scheme for rehydration according to severity. (**See* foot of *Table 46.2* for composition of WHO solution, and Appendix 9 for alternatives.)

re-estimate of fluid deficit. Those in whom rehydration is judged clinically to be successful enter the nutrition phase of management.

Nutrition phase

1. Breast-fed babies are allowed to breast feed *ad libitum*. Formula-fed babies are given half-strength formula (150 ml/kg/24 hours) as small-volume, frequent feeds, for 24 hours, followed by full-strength formula. No further rehydration solution is given unless signs of dehydration recur.
2. The patient is discharged once the stools become more formed, with instructions to the parents to return if signs of dehydration recur.

Limitations of oral rehydration therapy

Vomiting of ORS fluid

1. This is a common cause of failure of oral rehydration. Even if this is a problem at the outset of oral rehydration, it often improves as fluids and electrolyte deficits are corrected. Oral rehydration solution in frequent small amounts (e.g. by cup and spoon) will diminish the problem, and although loss of ORS occurs, fluid balance is usually positive, as vomiting children can be orally rehydrated. If the fluid is given by the parents, this will increase their confidence in caring for their child, and will emphasize the value of oral rehydration.
2. If parents or nurses are not available to 'cup and spoon', or the patient's intake is poor, rehydration can be given by nasogastric tube (*see* under 'Practical Procedures', page 736). This may also be helpful in vomiting patients.

Carbohydrate intolerance

1. This may be suspected on clinical grounds, when the patient continues to pass large watery stools, and fails to rehydrate with oral fluid.
2. This complication is less likely to be seen with the WHO ORS, which has a lower carbohydrate content, compared with some of the other commercially available solutions (*see* Appendix 9).
3. Carbohydrate malabsorption is a particular feature of viral diarrhoea; for example with rotavirus, up to 30 per cent of administered glucose load may appear in the stool. An adequate clinical response to oral rehydration may still be achieved, as success rates for oral rehydration in rotavirus diarrhoea are as high as in bacterial diarrhoea.

High purging rates

1. Oral therapy fails in patients with very high rates of stool loss (greater than 10 ml/kg/hr).
2. Nasogastric tube infusion of fluid may also assist in this group.
3. The early introduction of nutritious fluids in the nutrition phase of treatment is recommended. Children with acute diarrhoea can absorb from 60–80 per cent of ingested food. If lactose intolerance is suspected, by a considerable increase in large watery stools when milk is introduced, substitution of a low lactose formula (e.g. a soya-based milk) may be required. In practice this is uncommon.

Logistical problems

Since about 500 million attacks of acute diarrhoea occur in children throughout the world every year, it is unlikely that every child can be offered a balanced, physiological electrolyte solution for treatment. Other alternatives must be explored.

1. Simple sugar (domestic sugar, cane or beet sugar = sucrose) and salt solution (*see also* under 'Practical procedures' page 734 for method of preparation at village level and Appendix 24 for alternative methods of measuring salt and sugar). A suitable solution can be prepared under supervision using, for example, a 750 ml beer bottle as a domestic measure, adding ¾ of a level teaspoon of salt (3.7 g) and 8 level (20 g) teaspoons of sugar, filling with water

and shaking well. This will provide a solution of approximately 60 mmol sodium and 80 mmol (3%) sucrose (this has a relatively high sodium content, and therefore water must be given in addition to the ORS, as described on page 405).

2. Problems with this solution include hypokalaemia and acidosis, as would be expected. However, a high success rate is still possible.
3. Potassium can be supplied as bananas. Two to three bananas provide the amount of potassium supplied by oral rehydration with the WHO solution.
4. Plastic, double-ended spoons are available to assist in making up simple sugar salt solutions. (From TALC; Institute of Child Health, 30 Guildford Street, London WC1H 1EH (Tel. 01 242 9789).)
5. When sucrose is unavailable, other sources of carbohydrate can be tried. Heated, ground rice powder (30 g/ℓ) for example has been shown to be as effective as, and possibly more effective than, glucose in oral rehydration fluid (Patra *et al.*, 1982).

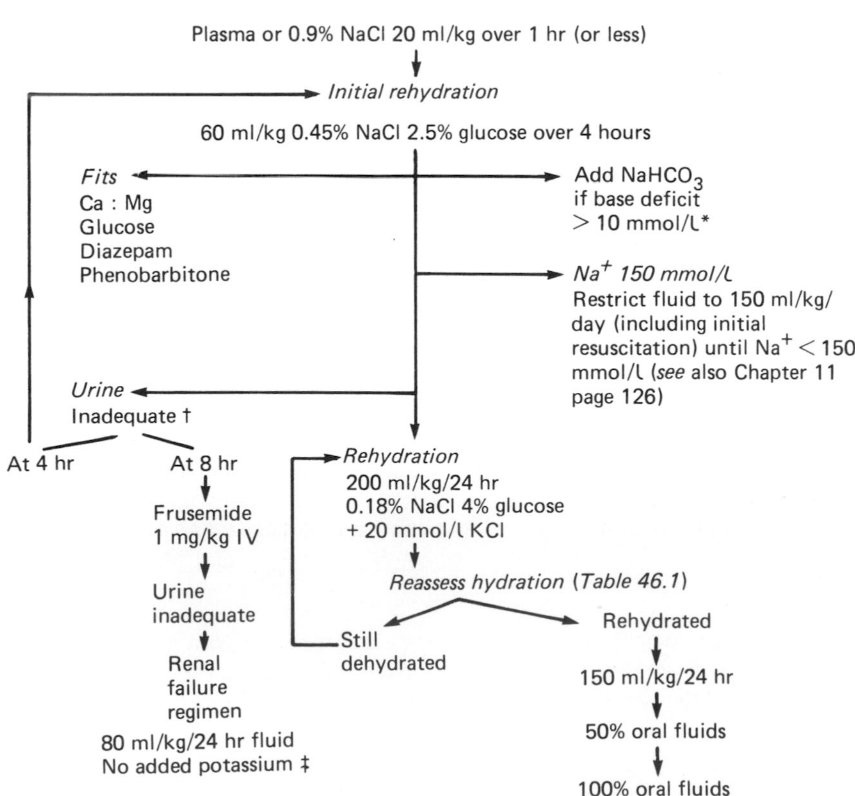

Figure 46.2 Intravenous resuscitation in severe dehydration.
* mmol $NaHCO_3$ = base deficit × weight (kg) × 0.3. Give half over 4 hours, remainder over 12 hours.
† Urine inadequate: <1.0 ml/kg/hr; or urine:plasma creatinine ratio<1; or urine:plasma urea ratio <7.
‡ For management *see* Chapter 48.

Limited impact on morbidity

1. While oral rehydration has a great impact on deaths due to diarrhoeal dehydration, it has, of course, no effect on the incidence of diarrhoea.
2. However oral rehydration can be used as the 'spearhead' of primary health care, in areas of high diarrhoeal morbidity. Once the oral rehydration programme is working, other interventions, such as improved nutrition, and health and hygiene education will be better accepted.

Intravenous rehydration in diarrhoeal diseases (see page 404 for indications and Practical procedures page 739 for method of giving intraperitoneal fluid when IV route is not practicable)

IV plasma (or 0.9% NaCl if unavailable) *is essential in the critically dehydrated child.* Do not delay treatment while blood samples etc. are being obtained. Resuscitation must be commenced in the emergency room in which the child is first seen (*Figure 46.2*).

The IV rehydration scheme in *Figure 46.2* is simple and practical. An example is given in *Figure 46.3*.

Complications

1. Oliguria indicates either continuing dehydration or acute renal failure. Follow the protocol of *Figure 46.2*, using urine volume, or creatinine or urea ratios, and frusemide to distinguish between the two situations. If acute renal failure has occurred, fluid and potassium restriction are required (*see* Chapter 48). The

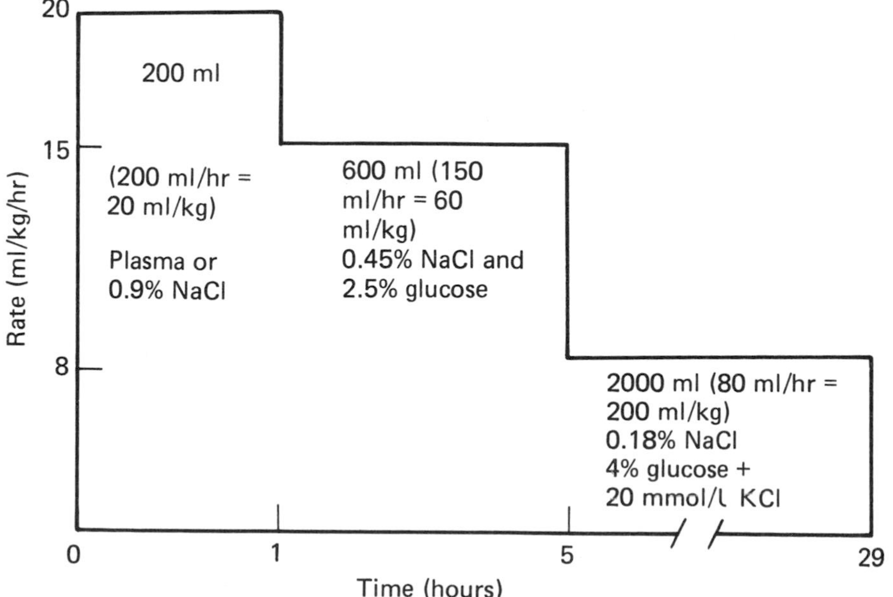

Figure 46.3 An example of IV rehydration of a 10 kg infant (*see also Figure 46.2*)

appearance of polyuria indicates recovery from acute renal tubular necrosis; if this persists, permanent renal damage has occurred. However, complete functional recovery is usual.

2. Convulsions are more likely with IV than with oral rehydration. Restriction of IV fluid to 150 ml/kg for the first 24 hours (*Figure 46.2*) in hypernatraemia will reduce the incidence of convulsions due to cerebral oedema. Management of hypernatraemia should include:
   (a) Prevention: commence phenobarbitone if serum sodium is greater than 150 mmol/ℓ, and rehydrate slowly.
   (b) IV diazepam if convulsions occur.
   (c) Exclude meningitis by lumbar puncture but use extreme care if cerebral oedema is suspected (*see* page 745).
   (d) Febrile convulsions may complicate dysenteric diarrhoea (*see* page 398).
   (e) Correction of hypocalcaemia complicating hypernatraemic dehydration is rarely effective in stopping convulsions.
3. Hypokalaemia is particularly common in malnourished children and may present as hypotension or bradycardia during rehydration. For ECG findings and correction of hypokalaemia *see* page 129.
4. Hyperglycaemia may complicate hypernatraemia. This returns to normal as the hypernatraemia is corrected, and *insulin should be avoided, as affected infants show extreme insulin sensitivity.*

References

DOBBINS, J. W. and BINDER, H. J. (1981) Pathophysiology of diarrhoea: alterations in fluid and electrolyte transport. *Clinics in Gastroenterology,* **10,** 606–625

HIRSCHHORN, N. (1980) The treatment of acute diarrhea in children. An historical and physiological perspective. *American Journal of Clinical Nutrition,* **33,** 637–663

Lancet (1978) Leading article. Water with sugar and salt. *Lancet,* **ii,** 300–301

PATRA, F. C., MAHALANABIS, D., JALAN, K. N., SEN, A. and BANNERJEE, P. (1982) Is oral rice electrolyte solution superior to glucose electrolyte solution in infantile diarrhoea? *Archives of Disease in Childhood,* **57,** 910–912

PIZARRO, D., POSADA, G., VILLAVICENCIO, N., MOHS, E. and LEVINE, M. M. (1983) Oral rehydration in hypernatraemic and hyponatraemic diarrhoeal dehydration. *American Journal of Diseases of Children,* **137,** 730–734

SANTOSHAM, M., DAUM, R. S., DILMAN, L. *et al.* (1982). Oral rehydration therapy of infantile diarrhoea. A controlled study of well-nourished children hospitalized in the United States and Panama. *New England Journal of Medicine,* **306,** 1070–1076

Further reading

SIMMONDS, S., VAUGHAN, P. and GUNN, S. W. (eds) (1983) *Refugee Community Health Care.* Oxford University Press

Chapter 47

Acute liver failure

Alex P. Mowat

Definition

Acute liver failure is a complex, clinical syndrome caused by massive hepatic necrosis producing life-threatening impairment of hepatic function and mental changes. The onset is within 8 weeks of the first symptom of liver disease. There should be no evidence of previous liver disease. The mortality is very high. The hepatic lesion may be completely reversible if the patient can be maintained with intensive care.

Principles of management

1. Early recognition of behaviour disturbance or any neuropsychiatric change in the presence of an acute liver disease.
2. Avoid aggravating factors, e.g. sedation, hypoglycaemia, hypovolaemia, bacterial infections.
3. Maintain homeostasis until hepatic regeneration can occur. Since complications can affect all organs, comprehensive and skilled intensive care is essential.
4. Exclude other causes of coma.
5. Control cerebral oedema.

Specific management for treatable infections or metabolic disorders

Early recognition

Fulminant hepatic failure is suspected when drowsiness or behaviour disturbance occurs in a patient in whom liver disease is recognized because of jaundice and dark bile-containing urine. Less commonly, encephalopathy occurs before jaundice appears.

History

This varies with the age of the patient and the cause of liver damage. In early infancy TORCH (Toxoplasmosis, Rubella, Cytomegalovirus, Herpesvirus) infections, syphilis, varicella or adenoviruses may be responsible. Galactosaemia usually presents between 4 hours and 2 weeks after the first milk-containing feed and fructose intolerance occurs within hours of fructose (or sucrose) ingestion, though this may occur quite late if the infant is exclusively breast fed for some weeks or months. Tyrosinaemia usually presents within 8 weeks of birth. From 2 months of age, the most common infective causes are viral hepatitis types A, B, and non-A, non-B, with leptospirosis, yellow fever, EB virus, and cytomegalovirus occurring in special situations. In viral hepatitis premonitory features include persistent anorexia, progressively deepening jaundice, abdominal pain, fever and vomiting. Following ingestion of the mushroom *Amanita phalloides* ('death cap'), vomiting occurs in 3–6 hours, followed some 6–8 hours later by liver damage. A history of exposure to drugs such as paracetamol, isoniazid (particularly if given with rifampicin), tetracycline, repeated exposure to halothane or to other drugs which may cause liver damage in an idiosyncratic fashion, is essential for establishing a diagnosis of drug-induced liver failure.

Leukaemia, reticulosis, and Wilson's disease are included in differential diagnosis.

Physical examination

There are two cardinal signs, a decrease in liver size, and features of encephalopathy. The liver is likely to be impalpable and the area of hepatic dullness decreased. Encephalopathy usually starts with lethargy but as it deepens there is progressive neurological impairment, decerebrate rigidity, and ultimately brainstem death. In the early stages, uncontrollable, confused, violent combative behaviour with attacks of screaming is frequent. This requires tolerant restraint but *not sedation.* Fetor hepaticus is usually present. There may also be features of the underlying disease and of its complications.

Laboratory assessment

The essential diagnostic investigation is a prothrombin time, prolonged by at least 7 s and uncorrected by parenteral vitamin K. Standard biochemical tests of liver function are abnormal but the severity of the change is no indication of the amount of hepatocellular necrosis or of the prognosis. The serum albumin is low in the late stages. A low albumin early in the disease suggests acute decompensation of chronic liver disease or haemodilution due to excessive intravenous fluids. A blood ammonia, if it can be estimated, may be raised.

Investigations to identify infective, metabolic, or toxic causes of liver damage are essential to assess infectivity and prognosis, and may assist in management. Investigations to monitor management are listed in *Table 47.1.*

Hepatic encephalopathy may be aggravated by a number of factors which must be controlled. These include hypoglycaemia, deficiency of potassium or magnesium, acidosis or alkalosis, sedatives of all sorts, diuretics, excessive nitrogen intake, alimentary bleeding, hypovolaemia, dehydration, bacterial infection, and therapeutic paracentesis.

Specific treatment

This is limited to excluding galactose and fructose from the diet in suspected galactosaemia or fructose intolerance. Leptospirosis may be treated with high doses of penicillin, and toxoplasmosis with pyrimethamine by mouth (1 mg/kg/24 hours in

Table 47.1 Investigations to monitor management

Blood glucose	Nasal swabs
Serum electrolytes including bicarbonate	Urine volume
Urea	Urinary urea, creatinine, sodium, potassium
Creatinine	Urinary osmolality
Serum osmolality	*The following investigations may be appropriate, depending on the severity of the coma*
Standard biochemical tests of liver function	Blood gases
Prothrombin time	Central venous pressure
Full blood count	Brain scan
Blood group	Intracranial pressure monitoring
ECG	EEG
Chest X-ray	Hepatic technetium colloid scan
Urine and blood culture	
Throat swabs	

two equal doses for 72 hours, then half the dose for 14 days), and sulphadimidine by mouth (150 mg/kg/24 hours in four doses for 14 days). Where drugs have caused liver damage, further exposure must be prevented. It is essential to consider and exclude other causes of coma. Aggravating factors must be repeatedly considered and treated if identified, following appropriate investigations.

Intensive care

The patient requires comprehensive care and monitoring for the complications of coma and of fulminant hepatic failure. This requires medical and nursing staff familiar with this disorder. Since the syndrome is variable in severity and complications, different therapeutic measures are applicable in different patients and at different stages in the development of the disorder. Careful clinical assessment should include measurement of pulse rate, blood pressure, central venous pressure, peripheral and core temperature, respiratory rate, and coma grading (*Table 47.2*) and repeated assessment of fluid and electrolyte balance. Biochemical and laboratory investigations necessary for monitoring are given in *Table 47.1.*

Food, fluids and electrolytes

Oral intake of food is stopped and ammonia absorption from the gut minimized by giving neomycin and/or lactulose, and enemas. Intravenous fluids are given at the

Table 47.2 Profile for bedside use in fulminant hepatic failure or Reye's syndrome (*see also* page 297 for Lovejoy staging in Reye's syndrome)

Verbal response	: Normal, confused, incomprehensible, none
Pupillary contraction	: Brisk, sluggish, absent
Eye-opening	: Spontaneous, to verbal stimili, to noxious stimuli
Oculovestibular response	: Normal, partial, or dysconjugate, nil
Absent reflexes	: Conjunctival, corneal, gag
Motor response	: Normal, withdrawal or localized, abnormal flexor, abnormal extensor, none
Respiration	: Normal, rapid, slow, irregular, on respirator

rate of 70% of the normal daily requirements, adjusted for urinary and abnormal losses. Fluids are given as 5, 10 or 20% glucose to minimize endogenous protein catabolism, the concentration given depending on the blood glucose values and urinary sugars. Potassium must be given in a dose of at least 3 mmol/kg/24 hours. No sodium is given initially but abnormal losses must be replaced. When the encephalopathy is of minor severity, calories in the form of carbohydrate may be given orally or by a nasogastric tube.

Respiratory care

Physiotherapy is essential. If mild hypoxia occurs an increase in environmental oxygen may correct this but if it is severe, endotracheal intubation and IPPV using the lowest effective pressures and concentrations of oxygen will be necessary. Hypocapnoea should be maintained by hyperventilation (*see* page 296).

Cardiovascular system

Blood volume depletion decreases tissue perfusion. Therefore, the blood volume must be maintained by infusions of blood, albumin, or fresh frozen plasma, the agent used depending on the haemoglobin and albumin concentration and clotting indices.

Bleeding tendency

Intravenous cimetidine in full doses (IV 10 mg/kg over 2 hours in 5% glucose, repeated 6 hourly) reduces the risk of alimentary bleeding. The only other measure likely to help is the infusion of fresh frozen plasma which contains the missing clotting factors. Fresh frozen plasma is safer than plasma concentrates which may contain infective material. It is better to give fresh frozen plasma if the prothrombin time is prolonged by more than 35 seconds, and to repeat this daily. However, some of the clotting factors have a very short half-life and after 6 hours of completing the infusion the prothrombin time will lengthen. If bleeding has occurred it requires replacement with fresh compatible blood or if this is not available, packed cells and fresh frozen plasma. Thrombocytopenia may require platelet transfusion.

Secondary infection

Respiratory tract infection, urinary tract infection, septicaemia, and peritonitis may all present with few obvious signs. Frequent bacteriological investigation is necessary for early diagnosis. If the patient deteriorates and no other factors have changed, broad-spectrum antibiotics may have to be given parenterally while awaiting the results of bacteriological investigations. Prophylactic antibiotics are not recommended. Fresh frozen plasma by providing complement components may reduce bacterial infection.

Renal failure

This is an important complication which requires effective treatment. In the majority of cases haemodialysis is necessary (*see* Chapter 48).

Cerebral oedema (see also Chapter 26, pages 295–297)

The control of cerebral oedema is a major problem. Mannitol intravenously has a rapid effect in decreasing intracranial pressure but its repeated use, particularly in the presence of renal failure, is hazardous. Dexamethasone or other corticosteroids have no demonstrable effect. The patient should be nursed as upright as possible. Hyperventilation, to achieve a low PCO_2, may help. Intracranial pressure monitoring makes the management of these patients easier, but carries the risk of intracranial haemorrhage.

Encouraging reports of the efficacy of intensive care when combined with haemoperfusion over a charcoal column, combined with prostacycline therapy, has led to a controlled trial of this therapy. Bone marrow depression may require treatment with marrow transplantation.

Reye's syndrome (Encephalopathy with fatty infiltration of the viscera). See also Chapter 26 for further details of management of raised ICP

Definition

Reye's syndrome is a serious, acute disorder of childhood in which vomiting and coma develop within a few days of the onset of what seems to be a mild, unremarkable, viral illness. Death or permanent neurological damage frequently occur although the primary, hepatic lesion, a severe derangement of mitochondrial function, returns to normal within a few days. There are usually no clinical features suggesting hepatic involvement and there is no hepatocellular necrosis.

Principles of management

1. Early recognition and treatment.
2. Intravenous glucose in sufficient quantities to minimize protein catabolism and liberation of fat from tissues.
3. Intensive care to minimize metabolic complications.
4. Control of intracranial pressure by maintaining high serum osmolality, positive pressure ventilation with high doses of sedatives, dexamethasone, and craniectomy.

Early diagnosis

Clinical features

The prodromal illness is usually an unremarkable viral infection without diagnostic clinical features. Influenza B is a frequent prodromal illness in 10–12 year olds, varicella in 5–9 year olds, with diarrhoeal illnesses in toddlers. Over 20 different viruses have been implicated in the prodromal illness. Aspirin may, or may not, have been given. *Profuse and persistent vomiting* is usually the first indication of this disorder. This is associated with or rapidly followed by a *change in the child's mental state*. The diagnosis should be considered in a child who is quiet or withdrawn, rather than waiting for features of more severe neurological involvement such as irrational behaviour, clumsy movements, delirium, convulsions, or deepening coma. Death from medullary coning may occur within 4–60 hours of the onset, or the neurological state may stabilize and improve at any stage short of brain death. In infants, *respiratory difficulties*, tachypnoea, respiratory distress, hyperventilation, apnoea or 'near-miss cot death' are prominent features.

Clinical examination (see Table 47.2)

Abnormalities are those of CNS depression without localizing signs, features of meningeal irritation or increased intracranial pressure. In infants the liver may be enlarged. There are usually *no clinical features of hepatic involvement.* For Lovejoy staging of severity in Reye's syndrome, *see* Chapter 26, page 297.

Investigations of diagnostic importance

A prompt presumptive diagnosis is reached in this clinical setting when hepatic involvement is revealed by a raised aspartate aminotransferase activity or prolonged prothrombin time. The blood ammonia level may be raised and/or the blood glucose value low, but these are not invariable.

The diagnosis is confirmed by percutaneous liver biopsy which shows ultrastructural or histochemical evidence of mitochondrial damage. The first features seen are glycogen depletion followed by a panlobular fat accumulation. In the early stages this can be so fine that it is only demonstrable by electron microscopy or lipid stains. 1–4 days after the onset the lipids coalesce to give microvacuolation of the hepatic parenchyma which is evident on haematoxylin- and eosin-stained sections from paraffin blocks. There is no hepatic necrosis. The fat clears in 2–9 days. Electron microscopy shows bizarre arrangements of mitochondrial structure, glycogen depletion, an increase in perioxisomes, and fat accumulation.

Since increased intracranial pressure is a feature of this disease, *lumbar puncture should be avoided.*

A wide differential diagnosis must be considered. In infants this includes inherited metabolic disorders, particularly urea cycle defects, systemic carnitine deficiency, galactosaemia (newborn) fructose intolerance, and organic acidurias (*see* Chapter 91).

In all age groups other causes of encephalopathy and convulsions, particularly if requiring intramuscular drugs (which raise serum transaminase activity) have to be considered. Shock with hypoxic liver and brain damage accompanying severe bacterial infections, or endotoxaemia, may give a similar picture. Severe viral infections, e.g. varicella, may cause liver damage as well as encephalopathy. Glycogen storage disease, insulin-producing tumours, fulminant hepatic failure before the onset of jaundice, may also cause difficulty. Toxins such as hypoglycin in ackee poisoning (*see* Chapter 70) and some drugs may mimic this disorder.

Treatment

Patients with mild encephalopathy, i.e. drowsiness and slow thought processes, evident for example by difficulty in counting, may stabilize and improve if the blood glucose level is maintained at greater than 8 mmol/ℓ (144 mg/100 ml) by intravenous glucose infusions. The fluid intake should be limited to 70 per cent of the daily requirements. The glucose concentration is adjusted to achieve the necessary blood glucose.

Intensive care

Intensive medical and nursing care are necessary for patients who become unresponsive to verbal stimuli or light pain. The clinical and biochemical monitoring is similar to that in fulminant hepatic failure.

Efforts are concentrated on correcting the metabolic abnormalities and controlling increased intracranial pressure. Renal, pancreatic, and muscular involvement occur, but such organ failure is much less likely than in fulminant hepatic failure.

Aspects of intensive care

1. No food is given by mouth but neomycin and enemas are given, as in fulminant hepatic failure.
2. Intravenous glucose is continued, to give a serum osmolality of between 310 and 330 mosmol/kg with a blood glucose value that is maintained between 11 and 16 mmol/ℓ (200 and 300 mg/100 ml).
3. Acidosis, hypokalaemia, and phosphataemia must be corrected. Dialysis may be required for renal failure.
4. Bleeding is less of a problem than in fulminant hepatic failure. Treatment is similar, although there has been no evaluation of cimetidine therapy.
5. Elective nasotracheal intubation and ventilation with paralysis is undertaken for two reasons:
   (a) To maintain tissue oxygenation by keeping the PO_2 at 150 mm Hg (20 kPa).
   (b) To decrease intracranial pressure by keeping the PCO_2 at between 25 and 30 mm Hg (3.5–4 kPa).
6. Control of intracranial pressure. Physiotherapy, clinical examination, endotracheal suction and coughing frequently increase the intracranial pressure above 20 mm Hg. The aim of treatment is to keep it below this level. Therapy can be adequately monitored only if the intracranial pressure is measured directly using an epidural pressure transducer or by intraventricular catheters (*see also* Chapter 26, page 294).

   High-dose phenobarbitone 30–40 mg/kg intravenously initially followed by 20–30 mg/kg/day maintaining the plasma barbiturate level at 50–60 mg/ℓ; or doses of approximately half that amount combined with morphine 0.1 mg/kg every 1–4 hours, a dose sufficient to keep the pupils small, prevents the increases in intracranial pressure with various stimuli discussed above.

   Dexamethasone 0.1–0.2 mg/kg 6 hourly is thought to minimize intracranial oedema.

   Intravenous mannitol 1–2 g/kg may be used to produce a short-lived decrease in intracranial pressure.

Emergency bi-frontal decompressive craniectomy should be considered for unconscious patients with decorticate rigidity. It must be done before the patient develops signs of medullary compression such as decerebrate rigidity, dilated fixed pupils, or dysconjugate eye movements in response to caloric stimulation of the ocular–vestibular reflex.

Fluid requirements

Patients on ventilators and receiving sedative therapy frequently have a low body temperature. These factors and perhaps inappropriate antidiuretic hormone secretion reduce fluid requirements which may fall to as little as 20–30 per cent of normal maintenance. Close monitoring of all losses is essential.

Gastrointestinal bleeding from oesophageal varices

Bleeding from oesophageal varices is a life-threatening complication of portal hypertension. Whatever the cause, bleeding is unpredictable in its severity and frequency. A single large fatal bleed may be the first indication of portal hypertension. Bleeding causes death in more than 10 per cent of children with extrahepatic portal hypertension and causes even more morbidity and mortality in those with hepatic disease.

Portal hypertension with oesophageal varices in childhood is usually due to extrahepatic portal vein obstruction or intrahepatic disease, but hepatic venous outflow obstruction as in constrictive pericarditis or inferior vena caval obstruction must also be considered. Although the presentation and emergency management are similar irrespective of the cause, the complications, long-term prognosis and management differ according to the underlying disease. All of the diagnostic possibilities cannot be considered here but the following diagnostic points may be helpful:

1. Portal hypertension with normal biochemical tests of liver function is likely to be due to portal vein obstruction or to congenital hepatic fibrosis (the prothrombin time may be prolonged by 4–6 seconds).
2. In congenital hepatic fibrosis it is usual to find an enlarged liver and abnormal renogram.
3. Hepatic outflow obstruction may be detected by careful clinical examination but confirmation requires appropriate cardiovascular studies.
4. The services of an *experienced, critical* ultrasonographer greatly simplifies differential diagnosis.

Principles of management

1. Immediate admission to the nearest hospital with blood transfusion services available.
2. If necessary, replace blood loss and stop further bleeding with cimetidine, antacids, and intravenous glypressin.
3. Treatment to prevent hepatic encephalopathy.
4. Prepare an appropriately sized Sengstaken–Blakemore tube.
5. Transfer to a unit with nursing, medical, and surgical staff experienced in the treatment of bleeding oesophageal varices.
6. Injection sclerotherapy to be started as soon as bleeding has been controlled.

Emergency treatment

General

This is a major emergency. Urgent medical, surgical, and endoscopic consultation at the highest clinical level is necessary to consider the differential diagnosis and management. Careful and repeated observation is necessary. The haemoglobin, white blood count, platelet count, and standard tests of liver function should be determined. Regular monitoring of pulse, blood pressure, urinary output, stool appearance, and the nature of the gastric aspirate obtained via a fine nasogastric tube help in assessing the presence of further bleeding and the patient's response.

Cimetidine is usually given in full doses (*see* page 414). Although there is no evidence that it prevents bleeding from portal hypertension, cimetidine and salt-free antacids may prevent gastric erosions and bleeding from peptic ulceration. Sedatives should be avoided and treatment to prevent hepatic encephalopathy started.

Pharmacological reduction of portal pressure

Vasopressin and its synthetic derivative triglycyl-lysine vasopressin (Glypressin) cause a constriction of the splanchnic arteriolar bed, and a reduction in portal pressure which may allow haemostasis at the bleeding point.

However, they also cause a reduction in hepatic arterial blood flow which in patients with cirrhosis is undesirable. Nevertheless, such drugs may be invaluable in arresting bleeding and in buying time before more effective therapy. The exact dose of the drugs to be used in childhood has not been studied pharmacologically. In adults, vasopressin given intravenously as a bolus of 20 units or by continuous intravenous infusion at a rate of 0.4 units/minute is effective in lowering portal pressure. This dose usually produces marked blanching of the skin, abdominal pain, and defaecation. In children receiving an adult dose multiplied by the child's weight in kilograms divided by 70, a similar response is obtained. Glypressin, which in adults has been shown to be more effective than vasopressin in reducing portal pressure, is given intravenously 6 hourly on the same dose basis, adults receiving 2 mg. Glyceryltrinitrate (nitroglycerine) 0.4 mg sublingually in combination with vasopressin, produces a greater fall in portal pressure than the use of other drugs alone; the use of nitroglycerine has not been studied in children. Somatostatin 250–500 μg/hour by continuous intravenous infusion, in adults, appears to be as effective as vasopressin in preventing bleeding, and there have been no reported side-effects.

Endoscopy

Endoscopy may be essential to ascertain the source of the bleeding. Even if the patient is known to have portal hypertension, bleeding may occur from duodenal ulcers or gastric erosions and not from the varices. In the patient who is bleeding for the first time and who has no history of previous liver disease a particular difficulty arises in that in extrahepatic portal hypertension there may be *no clinical features of portal hypertension* because the spleen contracts with the reduced blood volume following haemorrhage, and is impalpable. A barium meal at this stage is not a sound method of demonstrating varices, and endoscopy may also fail to identify varices, but if done within 24 hours of bleeding it will usually identify the bleeding source.

Hence if bleeding from oesophageal varices is suspected, endoscopy should be delayed until the patient is in the unit where injection sclerotherapy may be used.

Oesophageal tamponade

If bleeding does not stop spontaneously, or with vasopressin or Glypressin, oesophageal tamponade may be life saving. This is done with one or other modification of the Sengstaken–Blakemore tube. This four-lumen tube has a tube which opens in the stomach, a tube leading to a gastric balloon, one leading to an oesophageal balloon, and a fourth lumen for aspirating above the oesophageal balloon. The tamponade is only a temporary measure and must be followed by definitive therapy. The tube should not be left *in situ* for more than 24 hours.

These tubes are very successful in controlling bleeding from varices but they have many complications of which the most important are asphyxia and aspiration. A tube of appropriate size should be selected. The gastric balloon must be large enough to be retained comfortably within the stomach and not be pulled through the gastro-oesophageal sphincter. The volume will vary from 60 to 250 ml. The oesophageal balloon is frequently so long that, the upper end is in the pharynx; if this seems likely, the upper end should be compressed by a tight wrapping of 'Sleek'. The balloon should be tested by inflation, then completely decompressed and lubricated before the tube is passed. These tubes are large and frightening to children. Sedation may be required. A trained anaesthetist with full resuscitation equipment must be in attendance.

The tube is passed into the stomach, which is emptied, the gastric balloon is inflated with a dilute solution of Gastrografin and gently pulled back to the fundus of the stomach so that it is up against the gastro-oesophageal junction. Continuous aspiration via the pharyngeal catheter keeps the pharynx clear of secretion. The oesophageal tube is then inflated with the air to a pressure of 20–30 mm Hg, i.e. slightly greater than that in the portal vein. Gentle traction on the tube is maintained by strapping the tube to the patient's cheek. Skilled nursing observation is essential with this technique.

Obliteration of varices

Sclerosants injected directly into the varix or alongside it causes thrombosis of the varix or thickening of the overlying mucosa and the prevention of subsequent bleeding. The sclerosant is given via a flexible, fibreoptic endoscope. Attention is directed to the area 1–2 cm (¾ in) from the gastro-oesophageal junction where most variceal bleeding originates. A variety of sclerosants are used, ethanolamine oleate being currently the most popular for intravariceal injection, and polidocanol most favoured for those who prefer paravariceal injections. With intravariceal injections at least four sets of injections at intervals of 1–2 weeks are required before the varices are obliterated.

When the varices have been obliterated, repeat endoscopy at intervals of 9–12 months should be undertaken to detect new varices, which can usually be eradicated by one further course of injections.

Oesophageal transection

Oesophageal transection, either transthoracically or with an intra-abdominal technique using a circular stapling gun has a limited place in emergency management. The latter procedure, if combined with gastro-oesophageal devascularization, may give a prolonged period without recurrence of bleeding. Emergency porto-systemic shunts carry a very high operative mortality, and with the long-term risks of porto-systemic encephalopathy; they are rarely done in cirrhotic patients. Shunt procedures in patients with portal vein obstruction are very difficult to perform and have no place in emergency management. The short-term results of shunts in congenital hepatic fibrosis are satisfactory but no long-term studies have been reported.

Bleeding disorders in hepatic disease

Disturbed coagulation in hepatic disease is complex because of the liver's key role in homeostasis. The liver alone manufactures fibrinogen, factor II (prothrombin), and factors V, VII, IX, X, XI and XII; but factor VIII is produced in the reticuloendothelial system within and outside the liver. Factors II, VII, X, and XI are vitamin K dependent. Newborns have negligible vitamin K stores and enteric production is not established until 1 week of age. In sick newborns who are not fed or who are treated with antibiotics vitamin K production is inadequate. Body stores of vitamin K in older children can become depleted over the course of several weeks. Adequate bile production is essential for absorption of this fat-soluble vitamin. The liver is also involved in fibrinolysis and clearing of the activated clotting factors. Plasminogen, a protein produced by the liver, is activated by many factors including hepatocellular necrosis, forming the proteolytic enzyme plasmin which splits the peptide bonds in fibrin and fibrinogen. The fragments produced may have anticoagulant properties, and are normally rapidly cleared by the reticuloendothelial system; this may be inefficient in hepatocellular disease. The following liver-dependent defects in coagulation occur:

1. Congenital defects in carboxylation of vitamin K dependent clotting factors, or in intracellular vitamin K transport.
2. In parenchymal liver disease depression of vitamin K dependent coagulation proteins occurs because of decreased synthesis; vitamin K deficiency due to poor intake, malabsorption, and cholestasis; or increased consumption by fibrinolysis.
3. In all cholestatic disorders, the effects being particularly marked in the first 6 weeks of life, especially in disorders such as galactosaemia and fructose intolerance, in which there is both severe tissue necrosis and cholestasis.

Tests in coagulation disorders:

1. One-stage prothrombin time.
2. Fibrinogen concentration.
3. Fibrin degradation products.
4. Platelet count.

Management

1. Parenteral vitamin K will correct a prolonged one-stage prothrombin time within 3 hours where it has been prolonged owing to cholestasis. Reduction in the prothrombin time by a few seconds may be expected in hepatocellular disease.
2. Stored blood will supply prothrombin, factors VII, VIII, and X, but fresh frozen plasma is required to provide the other clotting factors. It should be noted, however, that factor VII, for example, has a half-life of about 6 hours.
3. Fresh whole blood provides all clotting factors, including platelets. Platelet transfusions are occasionally required.
4. Disseminated intravascular coagulation in hepatic disease is never severe enough to merit heparin therapy.
5. Calcium may be required if large volumes of citrated blood have been given over a short period.

Further reading

CANOSO, R. T., HUTTON, R. A. and DEYKIN, D. (1979) The haemostatic defect of chronic liver disease: kinetic studies using ^{75}Se-Selenomethoinine. *Gastroenterology,* **76,** 450–455

GIMSON, A. E. S. and WILLIAMS, R. (1983) Acute hepatic failure: Aetiological factors, pathogenic mechanisms and treatment. In H. C. Thomas and R. N. M. McSween (eds) *Recent Advances in Hepatology,* 1, pp. 57–69. Edinburgh: Churchill Livingstone

HOWARD, E. R., STAMATAKIS, J. D. and MOWAT, A. P. (1984) Management of oesophageal varices in children by injection sclerotherapy. *Journal of Pediatric Surgery,* **19,** 2–5

LIEBMAN, H. A., FURIE, B. C. and FURIE, B. (1982) Hepatic vitamin K-dependent carboxylation of blood-clotting proteins. *Hepatology,* **2,** 488–494

MOWAT, A. P. (1979) Fulminant hepatic failure. In *Liver Disorders in Childhood,* pp. 126–150. London: Butterworths

MOWAT, A. P. (1979a) *Reye's Syndrome,* pp. 138–146. London: Butterworths

MOWAT, A. P. (1979b) *Treatment of Portal Hypertension,* pp. 308–318. London: Butterworths

NATIONAL INSTITUTE OF HEALTH, BETHESDA, MARYLAND. CONCENSUS CONFERENCE (1981) Diagnosis and treatment of Reye's syndrome. *Journal of The American Association,* **246,** 2441–2444

PSACHAROPOULOS, H. T., MOWAT, A. P., DAVIS, M., PORTMANN, B., SILK, D. P. A. and WILLIAMS, R. (1980) Fulminant hepatic failure in childhood. An analysis of 31 cases. *Archives of Disease in Childhood,* **55,** 252–258

SHAYWITZ, P. A., ROTHSTEIN, P., and VENAS, J. L. (1980) Monitoring and management of increased intracranial pressure in Reye's syndrome: results in 29 children. *Pediatrics,* **66,** 198–204

SHERLOCK, S. (1983) Recent advances in portal hypertension. In H. C. Thomas and R. N. M. MacSween (eds) pp. 237–256. *Recent Advances in Hepatology 1.* Edinburgh: Churchill-Livingstone

Part IX

Genitourinary tract

Chapter 48

Acute renal failure

Richard S. Trompeter

Acute renal failure (ARF) may be defined as a potentially reversible loss or impairment of renal function. Many of the causes of ARF in the adult, such as glomerulonephritis, post-ischaemic and toxic nephropathy and burns also affect children, although the relative importance of different diseases and injuries as causes of the syndrome differs greatly according to age. Of particular importance in this respect is the newborn period, when ARF is relatively common and may be difficult to recognize. The mortality is high and is in part due to the frequent occurrence of ARF with other serious problems, such as severe trauma or congenital heart disease, and to the susceptibility of acutely uraemic patients to severe and frequently fatal secondary complications, such as infection and gastrointestinal haemorrhage.

Successful management requires, firstly, familiarity with the natural history of the specific disorders likely to be involved; and secondly an understanding of the physiology, particularly of the developing infant, and its implications with respect to fluid and electrolyte balance and nutrition.

Fluid and electrolyte balance

The metabolic rate of an individual is approximately proportional to body surface area (SA). The ratio between SA and body mass is inversely related to body size so that the fluid and nutritional requirements are greater in relation to weight in small individuals compared with those in large ones. An adult normally ingests 2–3 per cent of his body weight per day as water, which corresponds to a figure of 15 per cent for an infant in the first 6 months of life. It follows that severe derangements of hydration and biochemistry may occur rapidly in infants in renal failure, and these parameters must be monitored extremely closely if homeostasis is to be maintained.

The resting maintenance water intake* of a child is approximately 1500 ml/24 hours/m^2 SA of which 25% (400 ml/m^2) represents insensible losses and may therefore be taken as the water requirements of the *anuric* patient. An alternative formulation for total water intake, avoiding the necessity for surface area calculations, is given in *Table 48.1*.

* The water required to maintain homeostasis and to replace all losses under hospital conditions, particularly on IV maintenance with glucose electrolyte (low solute load) solution, as opposed to normal physical activity (*see also* Appendix 5).

Table 48.1 Maintenance and energy requirements (under hospital conditions or on IV glucose–electrolyte solutions)

Weight (kg)	*Surface area* (m^2)	*Water/24 hours**		*Energy/24 hours†*	
		ml/kg	ml/m^2	kcal/kg	kcal/m^2
<2.5‡	–	200 or more	Unsuitable in small infants‡	120	Unsuitable in small infants‡
2.5–5.0	0.15–0.25	150	↑	110	↑
5.0–<10.0	>0.25–<0.45	120		100	
10.0	0.45	100		100	
>10.0–<20	>0.45–<0.8	1000 + 50 ml for each kg over 10 kg	1500	1000 + 50 kcal for each kg over 10 kg	1400 (5.8 MJ)
20.0	0.8	1500		1500	
>20	>0.8	1500 + 20 ml for each kg over 20 kg	↓	1500 + 20 kcal for each kg over 20 kg	↓

* *See* Appendix 3 (*Figure A3.1*) for same data in graphic form: figures apply to patients on IV glucose–electrolyte maintenance fluid.
† *See* Appendix 2 for same data in graphic form (*Figure A2.1*) based upon Holliday and Segar (1957). (1 kcal = 4.2 kJ.)
‡ See Appendix 4 for requirements of newborn and low birth weight infants.

Insensible loss (and therefore water requirement in the anuric patient) may be taken as 25 per cent of the resulting total. It is inappropriate to consider managing low birth weight infants anywhere other than in a competent intensive care baby unit, where considerations of water, electrolyte, and energy requirements are part of daily routine. It is important to remember that however the water requirement is arrived at, it increases by approximately 12 per cent for every 1°C (2°F) 'body' temperature above 37°C (98.6°F), and by 30 ml/kg for every 1°C (2°F) 'ambient' temperature above 30°C (86°F), the temperature at which thermal sweating normally begins under resting conditions.

The normal requirement for sodium and potassium is 2–3 mmol/kg/day, with chloride accounting for most of the attendant anion. However, since most of this is replacement of urinary output, in the oliguric patient intake should be based on measured urinary, gastrointestinal, and other losses, and plasma concentrations. Nutritional requirements are directly proportional to surface area, and therefore to normal water requirement, and the provision of an adequate calorie intake is of the utmost importance in patients with ARF. Ensuring an intake of at least 1400 kcal/m^2/day (5800 kJ/m^2/day) to minimize catabolism is one of the most difficult problems the clinician faces in the management of patients with ARF. Children are frequently unable to eat, owing to preceding trauma or surgery, or are anorexic as a consequence of uraemia.

Causes of acute renal failure

Traditionally the oliguric patient with a raised blood urea concentration is allocated to one of three major categories: pre-renal, post-renal, and true renal failure.

Pre-renal failure

This is really a physiological oliguria resulting from poor renal perfusion and represents an attempt by the kidney to conserve salt and water in response to dehydration. *Restoration of adequate circulating volume is promptly followed by the return of urine flow.* Pre-renal failure may be found in association with dehydration, blood loss, hypotension due to trauma, or severe infection, and must be differentiated from true renal failure.

Post-renal failure

This refers to oliguria secondary to obstruction of the lower urinary tract, which in the childhood years is most frequently the result of congenital anomalies. In boys posterior urethral valves may present as oliguric ARF soon after birth. Incomplete obstruction may be missed, only to present as unsuspected and irreversible chronic renal insufficiency in later life.

True renal failure

This is the consequence of intrinsic disease or injury to the kidney itself. In contrast to pre-renal failure, rehydration or restoration of adequate circulation and perfusion will not be followed by a diuresis. The return of normal renal function will only follow resolution or healing of the underlying cause. The principal causes of true ARF are numerous and the more important of these are as follows:

1. Acute tubular necrosis – renal damage due to:
   (a) Anoxia/ischaemia/hypovolaemia/hypotension.
   (b) Septicaemia (especially Gram-negative organisms).
   (c) Nephrotoxins (e.g. mercury, myoglobin).
   (d) Combinations of the above (burns, crush injuries, surgery).
2. Primary glomerular disease (glomerulonephritis):
   (a) Acute post-infective glomerulonephritis.
   (b) The nephritis of Henoch–Schoenlein disease.
   (c) Systemic lupus erythematosus.
   (d) Others.
3. Interstitital nephritis:
   (a) Drug induced (methicillin, diuretics, non-steroidal anti-inflammatory drugs).
   (b) Post-viral.
   (c) Idiopathic.
4. Vascular disorders:
   (a) Haemolytic–uraemic syndrome.
   (b) Renal venous thrombosis.
   (c) Disseminated intravascular coagulation.
5. Crystalluria:
   (a) Uric acid (following anti-tumour or leukaemia therapy), sulphonamides.
   (b) Oxalic acid (ingestion of ethylene glycol or methanol; for further details *see* Chapter 8).

The causes of acute tubular necrosis (ATN) are similar to those for physiological oliguria and this reflects the fact that if severe hypotension, anoxia, or dehydration is allowed to persist untreated, pre-renal failure may progress to ATN. The categories listed are not always clear cut and there is considerable overlap; for example, ATN and renal venous thrombosis may represent the same response to renal injury in the newborn, while glomerulonephritis and interstitial nephritis may coexist in the patient with post-streptococcal disease. Furthermore, the causes of true ARF may be related to the age of the child. In the neonatal period the majority of cases of ARF are secondary to asphyxia or sepsis, and renal venous thrombosis, unilateral or bilateral, is seen in a very ill newborn. Congenital obstructive lesions frequently associated with sepsis or congenital dysplasia may also present in a similar manner in the newborn period. In contrast, after the first year of life the major causes of intrinsic renal failure are glomerulonephritis, the haemolytic uraemic syndrome (HUS), and ATN, ATN often following major surgical procedures.

Recognition

Clinical features

Where renal failure is due to primary renal disease, e.g. glomerulonephritis or the HUS, the oliguria and uraemia are usually associated with oedema and hypertension secondary to salt and water retention. The urine may contain blood, protein, and red cell casts. Fluid retention may lead to congestive cardiac failure, pulmonary oedema or convulsions, which may be the presenting features. A history of a respiratory infection or gastrointestinal disturbance may suggest a specific cause such as glomerulonephritis or the HUS; a rash may be suggestive of Henoch–Schoenlein disease.

Acute tubular necrosis

In ATN the patient's condition will usually reflect the causative disorder. Typical findings are an ill patient, usually dehydrated and possibly shocked. Acidotic respiration, tetany, and other consequences of the complex metabolic disturbance which is likely to present may be seen. Sepsis is common and must be carefully sought in all cases.

The natural history of ATN is distinctive and may be considered in four phases:

1. Aetiology.
2. Oligo-anuric phase.
3. Diuretic or polyuric phase.
4. Recovery.

In a few cases the oliguric phase does not occur and urine output is high from the outset, the so-called polyuric or high-output ATN. This variant may be more common than is generally realized, particularly if milder episodes of ATN are considered, and represents a failure of tubular resorption of filtrate, out of proportion to the fall in GFR.

Diagnosis

Diagnosis involves two stages:

1. Establishing whether the uraemia is of pre-renal, renal or obstructive origin.
2. Identifying the aetiology.

The first step is of the utmost urgency since it dictates the immediate management of the patient. Unless the cause of the ARF is obvious at the outset, obstruction must be excluded without delay. It is therefore useful to perform, as soon as possible after admission, the following:

1. Abdominal ultrasound examination.
2. Plain abdominal X-ray and micturating cystogram.
3. Dynamic renal scan with ^{99m}Tc DTPA.

As a group these investigations will provide the following information:

1. The size and shape of the kidneys.
2. The presence or absence of dilatation of the pelvicalyceal systems, ureters and bladder.
3. The presence or absence of radio-opaque calculi.
4. Whether or not the urethra is obstructed.
5. Some indication of the perfusion and functional state of the kidneys.

By these means obstructive causes may be confidently excluded.

The distinctive functional characteristics of true ARF are a reduced GFR and impaired tubular reabsorption of sodium. In contrast GFR is well maintained and sodium reabsorption is very active in pre-renal failure. Distinction between the two conditions can be made on biochemical grounds without formal demonstration of a low GFR (*Table 48.2*). *In this context the plasma urea concentration has almost no value as simple dehydration alone will produce raised levels similar to those in renal failure, owing to the enhanced reabsorption of urea at a low urine flow rate.* The plasma creatinine concentration, on the other hand, is a reliable guide to GFR and if grossly elevated is diagnostic of the presence of intrinsic renal insufficiency.

Table 48.2 Biochemical differentiation of pre-renal and renal failure

Variable	*Pre-renal failure*	*Renal failure*
Plasma urea	Raised	Raised
Plasma creatinine	Raised	Raised
Urine urea	High	Low
Urine creatinine	High	Low
Urine osmolality	High (>500)	Low (200–400)
Urine specific gravity	High (>1025)	Low (1008–1012)
U:P urea	High (>10)	Low
U:P creatinine	High (>40)	Low
U:P osmolality	High (>2)	Low (1)
FENa	Low (<1%)	High (>3%)
RFI	Low (>1%)	High (>4%)

U:P = urine:plasma ratio, FENa = fractional sodium excretion, RFI = renal failure index.

Investigations early in the course of the disease may reveal a lower level of creatinine which although not diagnostic does not exclude ARF. In this situation examination of the urine is valuable. The urine in ATN has the following characteristics:

1. High sodium and low nitrogen (urea and creatinine) concentration.
2. Approximately isosmolar with plasma (250–400 mosmol/kg water: specific gravity approx: 1010.

The oliguric patient with pre-renal failure produces urine with exactly the opposite composition: high urea, creatinine, and osmolality values and low sodium concentration.

Various permutations of these urinary and plasma values have been used to add precision to the biochemical diagnosis of ARF. The calculated fractional excretion of sodium, i.e. the proportion of filtered sodium excreted in the urine, has been shown to be useful and is calculated by dividing sodium clearance by creatinine clearance, and reduces to the simple formula:

$$\text{FENa}\ (\%) = \frac{U_{Na} \times P_{cr}}{P_{Na} \times U_{Cr}} \times 100$$

where FENa is fractional sodium excretion and the other terms represent urine and plasma concentrations of sodium and creatinine respectively. The value of this calculation has been demonstrated in adults and children and in the neonate. Tests which may be used in the differentiation of ATN from pre-renal failure are listed in *Table 48.2*.

The most difficult diagnostic problem is the child who presents with no recent history of illness or event likely to predispose to ATN. Assuming obstruction has been excluded and an ultrasound examination of the kidneys shows them to be of normal size, the likely diagnoses are:

1. Some form of glomerulonephritis.
2. Acute interstitial nephritis.
3. Haemolytic uraemic syndrome.
4. A drug-induced or toxic form of ATN.

The absence of clinical or serological diagnostic clues indicates the need for urgent renal biopsy, since early specific therapy for some of these conditions may influence the final outcome.

Metabolic complications of ARF

Since the primary function of the kidney is regulation of the volume and composition of the extracellular fluid (ECF), interruption of renal function leads to

Table 48.3 Typical metabolic changes in plasma in ARF

Increased:	Creatinine
	Urea
	Uric acid
	Potassium
	Hydrogen ion (acid)
	Phosphate
	Osmolality
Decreased:	Bicarbonate (metabolic acidosis)
	Calcium
Variable:	Sodium chloride

predictable changes in body chemistry (*Table 48.3*). The alterations in salt and water metabolism are variable and largely reflect intake during the interval between the onset of ARF and the ultimate diagnosis. The patient is frequently oedematous, hypertensive, and hyponatraemic. In addition they are likely to be catabolic as a result of the precipitating cause of the renal failure and any associated infection, and this will lead to the increased production of urea and other products of protein catabolism, such as phosphate, potassium, and hydrogen ion.

Management

Conservative treatment

This consists of adjusting the input of the various dietary components in relation to the damaged kidneys' limited capacity to excrete them. Specific treatments may be indicated for the underlying disease and attention must be given to general care and nutrition.

Shock and dehydration

If depleted, urgent restoration of the circulating blood volume is required, usually with plasma. The status of the circulation should be closely monitored by measurement of central venous pressure and the central–peripheral temperature gap. If peripheral perfusion is poor in the face of a raised venous pressure the careful use of vasodilator drugs is helpful (Chapter 10, page 108). If circulatory failure persists the results may be catastrophic not only to the kidney, but as a consequence of uncontrollable acidosis and hyperkalaemia.

Fluid overload and hypertension

The opposite problem of circulatory overload, if minimal, can be reversed by simply reducing input below normal requirements. Hypertension, cardiac failure,

Table 48.4 Drugs for hypertensive crises in children

Drug	*Onset of action*	*Dose and route*	*Mode of action*	*Comments*
Sodium nitroprusside	Seconds	1 μg/kg/min IV	Vasodilator	Constant infusion, thiocyanate toxicity in renal failure
Hydralazine	Minutes (IV) Hours (IM)	0.15–0.5 mg/kg IV 0.15–0.5 mg/kg IM	Vasodilator	Reflex tachycardia, flushing
Diazoxide	Minutes	1.5–5 mg/kg IV	Vasodilator	Sodium chloride, and water retention, hyperglycaemia with frequent use
Labetalol	Minutes	1–3 mg/kg/hour IV	α- and β-blockade	Constant infusion, caution in congestive cardiac failure, bronchospasm in asthmatics

peripheral, and pulmonary oedema are the clinical features of severe salt and water overload, and may individually, or collectively, be indications for urgent dialysis. Severe pulmonary oedema may require positive pressure ventilation, and occasionally, a venesection may be life saving until effective dialysis or ultrafiltration has been started.

The rapid but controlled lowering of blood pressure is essential in children who present with malignant hypertension or hypertensive encephalopathy. Sudden large reductions in blood pressure have to be avoided if neurological complications are to be prevented. A selection of drugs for use in hypertensive emergencies is shown in *Table 48.4*. Some children with malignant hypertension and ARF are sodium chloride and fluid depleted with intense vasoconstriction. They may be particularly sensitive to vasodilatation and require considerable quantities of saline to maintain and control blood pressure. Thiocyanate toxicity can occur with long-term sodium nitroprusside therapy or with renal insufficiency, and plasma thiocyanate levels should be monitored after 24 hours and treatment stopped if the concentration exceeds 12 mg/100 ml.

When control of the circulation has become stable, balance for water is achieved by restricting input to insensible loss plus a volume equivalent to measured urinary and other losses. Frequent reassessment of fluid balance and daily weighing must be undertaken in order to adjust the rate of fluid intake in the polyuric or diuretic phase.

Sodium

Intake is adjusted according to the plasma concentration and measured output. If output is considerable, estimations ofthe urinary sodium concentration should be undertaken. Insensible losses may be assumed to be sodium free; urine is equivalent to half normal saline (0.45 NaCl; 70–80 mmol sodium/ℓ), and all other losses, e.g. gastrointestinal and wound drainage, are isotonic. When interpreting plasma concentrations of electrolytes as a measure of ECF chemistry, ECF volume can be considered as one third of body weight in infants below 1 year of age and up to one quarter in older children. For example, if a sodium concentration of 135 mmol/ℓ is desirable and the measured value is 125, the deficit is 10 times the body weight (kg) × 0.3 mmol for a 2 year old, assuming the patient is not water overloaded. Hypernatraemia must be avoided, as this will act as an irresistible stimulus to thirst.

Bicarbonate (see also Chapter 11, page 118)

This anion is given in amounts sufficient to correct acidosis, (usually as 8.4% sodium bicarbonate solution), the dose being calculated on the basis of estimated ECF volume as for sodium. If demands exceed that which can be tolerated by the patient's circulation, dialysis should be started.

Potassium (Hyperkalaemia: see also Chapter 11, page 130 for further consideration of management)

As a result of the abrupt loss of renal excretory function hyperkalaemia is inevitable. Potassium accumulates at a rate of 0.2–0.3 mmol/kg/day, resulting in a daily increase in its plasma concentration of between 0.4 and 0.8 mmol/ℓ. The degree of hyperkalaemia is further increased by infection, undernutrition, haemolysis, and acidosis. The most serious consequence of hyperkalaemia is its effect on cardiac conduction, resulting in arrhythmias, heart block, tachycardia, and cardiac arrest. The effects of hyperkalaemia are exacerbated by hyponatraemia and hypocalcaemia, frequently present in ARF. Emergency measures for the treatment of hyperkalaemia are as follows:

1. IV sodium bicarbonate (1 mmol/kg).
2. IV calcium gluconate (0.1–0.2 ml 10% solution/kg).
3. Oral and/or rectal calcium resonium (1 g/kg).
4. IV glucose and insulin (1 ml/kg 50% glucose immediately followed by 0.5 units/kg insulin): 20% glucose should be used for fluid input for 6 hours after this treatment and the blood glucose level monitored every 15 minutes for 2 hours and then hourly.
5. Dialysis.

It should be noted that of the options given, only ion-exchange resin and dialysis achieve the net removal of potassium from the body. It therefore follows that hyperkalaemia in ARF is always an indication for dialysis, even if the conservative measures are successful in temporarily normalizing the plasma potassium concentration. Any manoeuvre which delays dialysis should be regarded as a form of potentially hazardous displacement activity.

Phosphate

Phosphate absorption from the gut is reduced by giving aluminium hydroxide gel by mouth (1–2 ml/kg/24 hours divided into three or four doses), forming insoluble aluminium phosphate in the gut lumen. The dosage can then be titrated against the serum phosphate level. This is worth prescribing in the hyperphosphataemic patient, even if he is not eating, since a significant amount of phosphate is present in the gastrointestinal secretions, particularly saliva.

Calcium (see also Chapter 11, pages 132–136)

Calcium may need to be given in order to correct severe hypocalcaemia, which should not be allowed to persist, particularly in the presence of hyperkalaemia. The combination of hypocalcaemia and hyperphosphataemia will not be corrected by the administration of calcium supplements alone and is an indication for dialysis.

Nutrition

Detailed attention to nutritional requirements is an essential part of the management of the child with renal failure. The objectives of intensive nutritional support in ARF are as follows:

1. To minimize catabolism and limit the rise of urea, potassium, hydrogen ion, and phosphate concentrations in the ECF.
2. To support the child's general condition and prevent malnutrition.

If the child is well enough oral feeding may be possible, otherwise intragastric or jejunal feeding may be necessary. The usual limiting factor in the oliguric patient is volume. It is difficult to concentrate a calorie supplement of 1400 kcal/m^2

(5800 kJ/m^2) into a volume of less than 400 ml/m^2 daily, although using modern highly concentrated energy supplements such as glucose polymers and oil emulsions, adequate calories can be provided. The composition of a typical 'renal feed' is shown in *Table 48.5*, and although there are many ways by which this principle can be achieved the services of a paediatric dietitian are invaluable.

Table 48.5 Composition of a typical 'renal feed'. Suitable for a child with surface area 1.0 m^2, or for a child of normal weight and height for age, weighing 28–30 kg at age of 9 years

Caloreen*	(glucose polymer)	200 g
Prosparol†	(arachis oil emulsion)	130 ml
Water		400 ml (400 ml/m^2)

This provides 1385 kCal (5800 kJ) in a total water content of 465 ml. Protein may be added, e.g. Clinifeed which contains 4 g protein in 100 ml.

* Roussel Laboratories Ltd., Roussel House, North End Road, Wembley Park, Middlesex, HA9 0MF. 01 903 1454.
† Duncan Flockhart & Co. Ltd., 700 Oldfield Lane North, Greenford, Middlesex, UB6 0HD. 01 422 2331

Diuretics

There is no convincing evidence in man that diuretics are of benefit in accelerating the resolution of ATN. A variable protective effect has been demonstrated when the drug is given before renal failure is induced, but not greater than that achieved by saline diuresis. This probably results from a high urine flow rate, preventing occlusion of the lumina of the renal tubules by cell debris. Many diuretics, e.g. frusemide, potentiate the toxic effects of aminoglycosides and other nephrotoxic drugs, and are contraindicated.

Treatment by dialysis

The indications for dialysis are as follows:

1. Hyperkalaemia.
2. Severe acidosis and/or hyponatraemia.
3. Salt and/or water overload (in the presence of hypertension, generalized or pulmonary oedema, and anaemia).
4. Hyperphosphataemia/hypocalcaemia.
5. The very sick patient with involvement of other systems, e.g. uraemic encephalopathy.
6. Failure of early improvement with conservative management.

Often these will be multiple and the need for immediate dialysis will be obvious. Occasionally, however, the choice between conservative management and dialysis may be difficult, but generally the child who is ill, catabolic, and in renal failure should be dialysed early in the course of the illness. This is particularly important in infants and very small children who are less readily controlled conservatively. Factors determining the type of dialysis to use are set out in *Table 48.6*. The choice of methods is between peritoneal dialysis (PD) and haemodialysis (HD), both being highly effective in managing ARF, and local practice determines which is selected in a particular case. Provided that medical and nursing staff are properly

Table 48.6 Dialysis therapy of ARF

Favours haemodialysis	*Favours peritoneal dialysis*
Availability of machinery and experienced personnel	Lack of mechanical and/or technical support
Need for dialysis therapy likely to be of long duration	Need for dialysis likely to be of short duration
Catabolic patient	Non-catabolic patient
Haemodynamically stable, non-hypotensive patient	Haemodynamically unstable patient
Older children	Babies
Undiagnosed intra-abdominal disease	

trained in the techniques, both PD and HD are relatively low-risk procedures, and patients are much more likely to die as a result of failure to begin dialysis early enough.

The basic technique of PD in infants and children is similar to that in adults, although miniaturized equipment is available for paediatric use, notably the cannulae used for insertion into the peritoneal cavity. The conventional sub-umbilical placement of the cannula is not satisfactory in infants and young children, allowing insufficient length of intra-abdominal tubing for efficient dialysis. The preferred sites are in the mid-line above the umbilicus and in either flank above the anterior superior iliac crest. It is essential that 'only' a skilled operator should insert the cannula in order to avoid injury to the liver, spleen and great vessels! 'Priming' the peritoneal cavity by infusion of dialysate, equivalent to the intended cycle volume, through an intravenous needle, will facilitate insertion of the cannula. This manoeuvre separates the viscera and creates a space into which the dialysis cannula can be placed.

The cycle volume of dialysate is reduced according to the size of the patient, effective dialysis requiring 20–50 ml/kg/cycle. Too large a cycle volume may embarrass respiration or compromise venous return from the lower half of the body. The cycle frequency is adjusted according to the clinical and biochemical needs of the patient, rapid exchanges increasing the efficiency of dialysis. The duration and frequency of dialysis on a daily basis will also be reflected by the needs of the individual patient, and if prolonged treatment is envisaged a soft Silastic peritoneal catheter may have to be surgically placed.

HD via arteriovenous shunts or intermittent venous catheterization is the alternative method, but is unsatisfactory in small infants and babies. Not more than 8–10 per cent of the circulating blood volume should be outside the body, i.e. in the extracorporeal circuit, at any one time. Assuming a blood volume of 85 ml/kg, the smallest commercially available equipment requires a priming volume of 70 ml, making the system unsatisfactory for infants weighing less than 8 kg.

Drugs

In ARF no drug should be prescribed unless it is essential and without previous consideration of its safety in the patient with a reduced GFR. As a general rule, if a drug has to be given which is excreted by the kidneys, it is usually safe to give the standard initial therapeutic dose, but to increase the time interval between subsequent doses depending on the drug and the severity of renal failure (*see* Appendix 13); monitoring the plasma level of certain drugs, particularly the aminoglycosides, may be helpful.

The best place for sick children to be treated is a paediatric unit equipped with all the necessary expertise relevant to the child's conditions. In the case of ARF, this means a paediatric unit with more than just occasional experience in the management of renal failure, especially PD and HD. The optimal procedure is therefore to transfer the child to such a centre as soon as ARF is diagnosed, unless his condition or geographical circumstances make this impossible.

Reference

HOLLIDAY, M. A. S. and SEGAR (1957) The maintenance need for water in parenteral fluid therapy. *Pediatrics,* **19,** 823–832

Further reading

BELL, P. R. F. (1984) Haemodialysis in infants. *British Journal of Hospital Medicine,* **32,** 168–174

BENNETT, W. M., SINGER, I. and COGGINS, C. J. (1974) A guide to drug therapy in renal failure. *Journal of the American Medical Association,* **230,** 1544–1533

EDELMANN, C. M. JR. (ed.) (1978) *Pediatric Kidney Disease.* Boston: Little, Brown

McLAREN, D. S. and BURMAN, D. (eds) (1981) *Textbook of Paediatric Nutrition,* 2nd edn. Edinburgh: Churchill Livingstone

RUBIN, M. I. and BARRATT, T. M. (1975) *Pediatric Nephrology.* Baltimore: Williams & Wilkins

SCHRIER, R. W. (1979) Acute renal failure. *Kidney International,* **15,** 205–216

WINTER, R. W. (ed.) (1973). *The Body Fluids in Pediatrics.* Boston: Little, Brown

Chapter 49

Genitourinary emergencies

A. M. K. Rickwood

Acute retention of urine

Inability to void urine from a full bladder may occur as a sudden episode or may represent the end-stage of a previous history of urinary difficulty (acute-on-chronic retention); both events are uncommon in children and are very likely to have some organic cause.

Recognition

Acute retention must be distinguished from the following:

1. Anuria (or severe oliguria). The bladder is not distended. Ultrasound examination will detect or exclude a supra-vesical obstructive uropathy.
2. Extravasation of urine. Outside the neonatal period this is almost always caused by trauma. Urethral injuries are accompanied by bleeding from the urethral meatus (and also from the vagina in females). Urinary retention may occur as a secondary phenomenon. External bleeding is unusual with bladder injuries where extraperitoneal rupture results in extravasation of urine into the pelvic retro-peritoneum and intraperitoneal rupture in urinary ascites. These events may be suspected from the severity of the symptoms and signs; in cases of doubt, ruptured bladder can usually be distinguished from uncomplicated retention by ultrasound examination. In neonates a severe obstructive uropathy (usually posterior urethral valves) can cause spontaneous extravasation (urinary ascites).

Sudden acute retention is extremely uncomfortable. Although spasm of the overlying muscles may prevent palpation of the distended bladder this can be detected by percussion. Relatively painless retention suggests long-standing infravesical obstruction.

Causes of acute retention

1. Intravesical lesions. Acute retention (often with strangury) is the usual presentation of rhabdomyosarcoma, and ureterocoeles occasionally present similarly. Severe haematuria can result in clot retention.
2. Urethral lesions (Stephens, 1983). Impaction of bladder stones in the urethra is still occasionally seen. In boys, urethral strictures may cause acute retention without preceding symptoms; there is sometimes a previous history of trauma (including catheterization) but often there is none.

Pedunculated posterior urethral polyps and ectasia of Cowper's glands tend to cause interrupted micturition rather than retention.

3. Urethral compression or distortion. Retention occasionally results from pelvic tumours or from severe constipation; these are detectable by rectal examination. Hydrocolpos in the neonatal period and haematocolpos at menarche can also cause retention. A feature peculiar to certain female neonates with a urogenital sinus is massive retention of urine within the *vagina* leading to gross lower abdominal distension; inspection of the vulva reveals one orifice only.
4. Neuropathic bladder. This is usually evident from neurological examination but intraspinal tumours can precipitate sudden retention in the absence of abnormal neurological signs or abnormality on plain spinal X-ray.
5. Voluntary suppression of micturition. Children can retain urine by voluntary inhibition of the detrusor or by contracting the external urethral sphincter against a detrusor contraction. This occurs when there is the knowledge, or anticipation, that micturition will be painful and is not uncommon in boys following cystoscopy or circumcision. It can also result from meatal ulceration in the recently circumcised or from ammoniacal ulceration of the prepuce. The same phenomenon occasionally occurs in young children of both sexes for purely emotional or psychological reasons.
6. Miscellaneous. Transient urinary retention (with secondary upper renal tract dilatation) happens in a few neonates for no discernible cause. This condition is self-limiting. The enigmatic 'occult neuropathic bladder' sometimes presents with acute retention. Unconscious and semi-conscious children tend to void at infrequent intervals and may be noted to have an enlarged bladder in consequence. Usually, however, they are capable of complete reflex micturition and true retention is comparatively rare.

Management

Meatal ulceration is treated by sedation, by soaking off any scab with warm water and by topical application of local anaesthetic. Retention secondary to constipation usually responds to an enema.

Acute-on-chronic retention generally requires catheterization. Retention due to voluntary inhibition of micturition and acute retention occurring without obvious cause should be treated initially by a combination of sedation, privacy and a warm bath. If these measures fail some organic cause is likely and catheterization will be necessary.

It is customary to insert a self-retaining balloon catheter and for economy a latex rubber type is advisable in the first instance. The calibre should be kept to a minimum (not exceeding 16 FG in an adolescent) and the balloon size limited to 3–5 ml. With boys, local anaesthetic gel should be instilled into the urethra 5–10 minutes before catheterization. Failure to pass a catheter in a boy suggests the presence of a urethral stricture and in this circumstance suprapubic needle aspiration of the bladder serves as a temporary expedient to relieve discomfort.

Decompression of the renal tract in chronic obstruction

See Appendix 5, page 776.

Haematuria

Recognition

It is essential at the outset to distinguish macroscopic haematuria from other causes of red urine. The latter include beetroot ingestion in susceptible individuals; drugs (e.g. rifampicin, chlorpromazine, danthron (Dorbanex), phenazopyridine (Pyridium)); certain dyes in cold drinks, foods and sweets; and myoglobinuria. Chemical testing for blood excludes these causes while microscopy of a fresh urine specimen distinguishes haematuria from haemoglobinuria.

Infants often present with blood-stained nappies rather than a definite sighting of blood in the urine. In the absence of any obvious external cause (e.g. ammoniacal ulceration of the prepuce), it is safest to regard such cases as having haematuria. Older boys frequently have post-micturition bleeding rather than true haematuria; this is likely to be of urethral origin.

In cases where history and physical examination do not indicate the cause of haematuria, a rapid screening programme comprises testing for proteinuria, microscopy of a fresh urine specimen for casts, pyuria and motile organisms, plain abdominal X-ray to exclude stones, and ultrasound examination to exclude hydronephrosis.

Causes of haematuria

The more common or more important causes of haematuria in children are:

1. Nephritis. Classic post-streptococcal nephritis is now rare in Western countries but still common in the underdeveloped world. Haematuria may occur with Henoch–Schoenlein disease some hours before other manifestations of this condition. In patients with shunted hydrocephalus, haematuria should suggest the possibility of shunt nephritis.
2. Renal vein thrombosis. This follows dehydrating illnesses in small infants; the affected kidney(s) is usually readily palpable.
3. Wilms' tumour. This is rare after the age of 5 years; the involved kidney is always enlarged and usually grossly so.
4. Obstructive uropathies. Painless haematuria is a common presenting symptom, especially of pelviureteric obstruction.
5. Stones. Adolescents sometimes pass small ureteric stones with haematuria and typical ureteric colic. Stone disease otherwise in children usually produces painless haematuria.
6. Renal trauma. Often there is merely contusion of the renal substance. More severe injuries include lacerations into the collecting system, through the cortex or both. Renal pedicle injuries may not produce shock because spasm of the torn vessels prevents massive bleeding. The rare renal pelvis and ureteric injuries may be suspected if there is rapid extravasation of urine.
7. Urinary infection. Bacterial infection is common in girls and in older children is generally accompanied by typical symptoms of cystitis. Bilharzia (*Schistosoma haematobium*) must be considered in children who have been exposed to the infection.
8. Urethral lesions (in boys). These include ectasia of Cowper's and Littré's glands, diverticulum of the fossa navicularis and phimosis due to balanitis xerotica obliterans (Rickwood *et al.,* 1980).

9. Coagulation disorders and thrombocytopenia. Bleeding tends to occur without trauma in haemophilia, Christmas disease and, rarely, in von Willebrand's disease.
10. Homozygous sickle cell disease. This should be considered as a cause of painless haematuria in any child of African descent.
11. Drugs. Phenacetin causes papillary necrosis and cyclophosphamide can induce a severe haemorrhagic cystitis.
12. Factitious haematuria; the simulation of haematuria by the addition of blood to the urine. The blood is usually that of a parent, commonly the mother who may use her menstrual blood. This situation is usually a manifestation of the 'Munchausen by proxy' syndrome in which the parent manufactures illness in the child (*see* Chapter 58).

Management

Most patients require expeditious, rather than emergency, investigation and treatment. If there is good clinical evidence of bacterial urinary infection, antibiotic treatment may be commenced after obtaining a specimen for culture. Emergency action is generally required with:

1. Wilms' tumour.
2. Renal trauma. Emergency IVP is necessary in all cases to assess damage to the affected kidney and to determine the presence and function of the opposite kidney. Ultrasound examination is useful in detecting perirenal collections of blood and urine. Most cases can be managed conservatively with strict bed-rest. Blood transfusion may be required and it is usual to prescribe a broad-spectrum antibiotic. Surgical intervention is limited to patients with severe, persistent bleeding or progressive extravasation of urine.
3. Haematuria sufficient to cause, or threaten, hypovolaemia or clot retention. Treatment depends on cause. A high fluid intake should be given to patients with cyclophosphamide cystitis and bladder wash-outs may be necessary.
4. Factitious haematuria may be confirmed by blood grouping if the parent and child are of different groups, or by observation in hospital.

Acute scrotal conditions

These may present with pain, swelling or both.

Causes

The more usual causes are, in order of incidence (Jones, 1976; Hemalatha and Rickwood, 1981):

1. In neonates and infants:
   (a) Testicular torsion.
   (b) Epididymo-orchitis.
   (c) Acute hydrocoele.

2. In pre-pubertal boys:
   (a) Torson of testicular appendage.
   (b) Idiopathic scrotal oedema.
   (c) Testicular torsion.
   (d) Epididymo-orchitis.
   (e) Trauma.
3. In post-pubertal boys:
   (a) Testicular torsion.
   (b) Epididymo-orchitis.
   (c) Torsion of testicular appendage.
   (d) Trauma.

Recognition

1. Testicular torsion. Hard and apparently painless enlargement of the testis in a neonate is almost certainly due to testicular torsion. In older boys there is characteristically sudden, severe pain, often with abdominal radiation (and which may be mistaken for some abdominal emergency unless the scrotum is examined). Vomiting and loss of sleep are common. In the early stages the testis can be palpated and is exquisitely tender; after 24 hours or so, development of a secondary hydrocoele masks this sign.
2. Torsion of testicular appendage. Pain is not usually more than moderate and abdominal radiation, vomiting and loss of sleep are seldom features of this condition. In the first 24 hours it is often possible to palpate the tender, twisted appendage (usually located posteriorly at the upper pole of the testis) separately from the non-tender testis.
3. Idiopathic scrotal oedema. This condition is virtually painless and often first noticed at bath or bed time. It may be unilateral or bilateral and the characteristic erythema and oedema frequently extend to the perineum, the groin or both. The testes are readily palpable and non-tender.
4. Epididymo-orchitis. Mumps orchitis is uncommon before the age of 12 years and the diagnosis is usually evident from other features of the disease. Epididymo-orchitis in boys is generally secondary to bacterial urinary infection although symptoms of this are often lacking. It is extremely difficult to distinguish from testicular torsion, and the diagnosis can only be made with any confidence in the presence of a known urinary infection.
5. Hydrocoele. Communicating hydrocoeles can appear quite suddenly in infants. The swelling is firm rather than hard and is transilluminable. Scrotal hernias are nearly always readily reducible while incarcerated hernias seldom extend beyond the groin.
6. Trauma. Although this is usually obvious from the history, it is well to remember that a history of trauma does not exclude the possibility of testicular torsion.

Management

Emergency exploration of the scrotum is indicated whenever testicular torsion is suspected or cannot be excluded.

1. Testicular torsion. Torsion rapidly causes infarction, and salvage of the testis is unlikely if the history exceeds 12 hours. For this reason patients with a short history should be explored immediately without regard to the usual period of

pre-anaesthetic starvation. There is evidence that testicular infarction damages the opposite testis and excision of all but unquestionably viable testes is advised. The unaffected testis should always be fixed.

2. Torson of testicular appendage. This can be treated conservatively but, because accurate diagnosis requires considerable experience, it is generally advisable to explore suspected cases and excise the lesion. It is not necessary to explore the opposite hemi-scrotum.
3. Idiopathic scrotal oedema. If there is a confident diagnosis no treatment is required; when there is uncertainty, exploration is advisable.
4. Epididymo-orchitis. Most cases come to exploration. Should urinary infection be documented, it will be necessary to exclude some congenital anomaly predisposing to retrograde spread of infection along the vas deferens (e.g. ectopic ureter).
5. Trauma. Exploration is required only if there is continued bleeding into the scrotum.

Acute penile conditions

Causes

1. Paraphimosis. This occurs when the foreskin has been fully retracted for an extended period and cannot be drawn forward because of the resulting oedema. It is seen in infants whose mothers have been advised at Welfare Clinics to retract the prepuce, but not to draw it forward, and in older boys as the result of a bet or dare, the patient being the victor of this contest.
2. Acute balanoposthitis. In more severe cases oedema and erythema extend along the whole shaft of the penis. If the prepuce is gently retracted pus exudes copiously from beneath it.
3. Zip fastener injuries. The foreskin is trapped in the zip during fastening.

Management

1. Paraphimosis. Reduction under general anaesthetic is kinder in older boys and if oedema is gently squeezed from the prepuce it is usually possible to accomplish reduction without recourse to dorsal slit or circumcision.
2. Balanoposthitis. The foreskin is retracted as far as possible to allow escape of pus. Thereafter the condition resolves rapidly with a combination of sitz baths and a broad-spectrum antibiotic.
3. Zip fastener injuries. Gentle separation of the individual teeth of the zip may free the prepuce. If this fails, separation under general anaesthetic should be attempted; more entangled cases require formal circumcision.

References

HEMALATHA, V. and RICKWOOD, A. M. K. (1981). The diagnosis and management of acute scrotal conditions in boys. *British Journal of Urology,* **53,** 455

JONES, P. G. (ed.) (1976) *Clinical Paediatric Surgery,* 2nd edn., pp. 271–276. Oxford: Blackwell

RICKWOOD, A. M. K., HEMALATHA, V., BATCUP, G. and SPITZ, L. (1980) Phimosis in boys. *British Journal of Urology,* **52,** 147–150

STEPHENS, F. D. (1983) *Congenital Malformations of the Urinary Tract,* pp. 126–149. New York: Praeger

Part X

Metabolic and endocrine emergencies

Chapter 50

Diabetes mellitus

S. A. Greene and J. D. Baum

This chapter gives an outline of the emergency management of: diabetic ketoacidosis; the initiation of treatment in a child newly diagnosed as having diabetes; a surgical operation in a diabetic child; hypoglycaemia; neonatal hyperglycaemia.

Diabetic ketoacidosis

Recognition

This somewhat imprecise title covers conditions ranging from relatively asymptomatic hyperglycaemia with ketonaemia, to severe dehydration with ketoacidosis, hyperglycaemia and coma.

The presenting symptoms of ketoacidosis in diabetes of recent onset are:

1. Vomiting, abdominal pain, headache, thirst, and polyuria.
2. Hyperventilation.
3. Drowsiness or coma.

Preceding symptoms in addition to the above, which may have been present for days or weeks, are frequency of micturition, the recent onset of bed-wetting, loss of weight, and lethargy. An acute infection may precipitate symptoms of ketoacidosis.

In ketoacidosis in a child with established diabetes the symptoms are of shorter duration and may be preceded by a period of unsatisfactory control or be precipitated by an acute infection. The onset may develop over a period of days but can be very rapid, over a few hours.

In prepubertal girls episodes of ketoacidosis may occur at more or less monthly intervals in a cyclical fashion, while after the menarche ketoacidosis may, in rare cases, appear regularly during the 2–3 days before each menstrual period.

In the severely ill child there is evidence of loss of weight and dehydration which may in extreme cases progress to shock, oliguria, or anuria. The main differential diagnosis is between:

1. Acute respiratory disease, particularly lobar pneumonia. The deep pauseless hyperpnoea (Kussmaul respiration) of metabolic acidosis is however quite different from the rather staccato respiration of pneumonia. *Note that diabetes and pneumonia may occur together.*
2. Acute salicylate poisoning, particularly in the pre-school child. Many features of severe salicylate poisoning mimic diabetes; there is a severe metabolic acidosis,

with hyperglycaemia, glycosuria and ketonuria. Plasma glucose level in salicylate poisoning is usually under <14 mmol/ℓ (<250 mg/100 ml) but over 22 mmol/ℓ (>400 mg/100 ml) in diabetic ketoacidosis. A positive test for salicylate in the urine is of little diagnostic value since a diabetic patient may have taken aspirin for symptomatic relief. In severe salicylate poisoning, however, the plasma salicylate level is usually greater than 40 mg/100 ml (in small children acute symptoms of salicylate poisoning may occur with levels as low as 20 mg/100 ml).

3. Acute abdominal conditions. The 'diabetic abdomen' with abdominal pain and rigidity may present diagnostic difficulties: however, the blood glucose level will always be raised and there will usually be associated ketonuria. Even when diabetic ketoacidosis is recognized in a child presenting with abdominal pain care should be taken since *a genuine acute abdominal condition may also be present.* If in doubt a surgical opinion should be obtained.

Management

Initial resuscitation and rehydration

1. The child should be weighed whenever possible. If this is not possible the weight should be assessed from published growth charts (*see* Appendix 1): as an approximation a 1 year old weighs 10 kg; a 6 year old, 20 kg; and a 10 year old, 30 kg.
2. If there is impending circulatory collapse or 'shock' oxygen should be given by face mask.
3. If the child is in coma the duty anaesthetist should be called.
4. An intravenous infusion must be set up, if necessary resorting to a 'cut-down' to secure an adequate infusion line.
5. If there are signs of gastric dilatation, especially if there is a history of persistent vomiting, a stomach tube (narrow gauge) must be passed. Empty the stomach and allow free drainage of stomach contents. The volume of the aspirate should be measured and included in the assessment of fluid balance.
6. *Routine* catheterization of the bladder is not recommended. After rehydration has commenced it is necessary to check for a full bladder if the child is not passing urine. Catheterization at this stage may become necessary. If there is doubt about the child emptying the bladder spontaneously it is better to err on the side of catheterization, since accurate assessment of urine output is essential for safe management.

Clinical observations

A half-hourly record of heart rate and respiratory rate is established and an hourly record of blood pressure and axillary (or rectal) temperature. An ECG monitor should be set up for continuous assessment of heart rate and waveform.

Assessment of the degree of dehydration

1. This involves the assessment and recording of: skin turgor, sunken eyes, dry mouth (this may be dry out of proportion to the degree of dehydation if the child had been mouth breathing), anterior fontanelle tension in infants, heart rate, blood pressure and peripheral skin temperature; ideally this should be measured

and compared with rectal temperature (Aynsley-Green and Pickering, 1974; *see also* Chapter 10, page 98). Children with Kussmaul respiration are usually severely dehydrated, namely 10–15 per cent.

2. As an aid to calculating fluid replacement for a child the degree of dehydration should be classified as:
   Minimal dehydration – 5 per cent dehydrated.
   Moderate dehydration – 10 per cent dehydrated.
   Severe dehydration – 15 per cent dehydrated.

The percentages refer roughly to the percentage of total body weight lost as water and represent the deficit to be made up during rehydration.

Laboratory measurements

It is often difficult to obtain blood samples from a severely dehydrated child. It may be necessary to consider arterial puncture to obtain blood for measurements additional to blood gases.

1. Blood is taken as soon as possible for baseline values of: glucose, urea, Na, K, Cl, HCO_3, haematocrit, and for blood culture.
2. An arterial blood sample is taken (or alternatively a venous sample) for measurement of pH and PCO_2.
3. Cultures for bacteriology from nose, throat and urine should be taken and a portable chest X-ray arranged as soon as possible. The X-ray should include a view of the upper abdomen in the erect position to assess the degree of gastric dilatation.

Intravenous fluids

The first 6 hours: the pattern of rehydration is indicated in *Figure 50.1*.

The total volume to be replaced is the daily maintenance volume together with the calculated fluid deficit:

1. Calculate the daily maintenance fluid requirement:
   Age 1–2 years, 120 ml/kg.
   Age 3–6 years, 100 ml/kg.
   Age 7–9 years, 80 ml/kg.
   Age 10–15 years, 60 ml/kg.
2. The first 60 per cent of the calculated fluid deficit is given in the first 5 hours of therapy: give 20 per cent (1/5) as 0.9% NaCl (without glucose) in the first hour; 10 per cent (1/10) as 0.9% NaCl in the second hour; and 10 per cent (1/10) as 0.9% NaCl in the third hour.
3. This is followed over the next 2 hours by fluid still given at the rate of 10 per cent (1/10) of the calculated fluid deficit per hour. This should be 0.9% NaCl unless the blood glucose falls below 10 mmol/ℓ (180 mg/100 ml) when the change to 0.18% NaCl in 4% glucose should be made.

Example – A 10-year-old child weighing 30 kg and assessed as 10 per cent dehydrated would have a calculated deficit of approximately 3 ℓ (3000 ml), together with a daily maintenance requirement of 1800 ml.

In the first hour give 675 ml fluid replacement (600 ml calculated deficit, 75 ml daily maintenance) as 0.9% saline. For the second, third, fourth and fifth hours

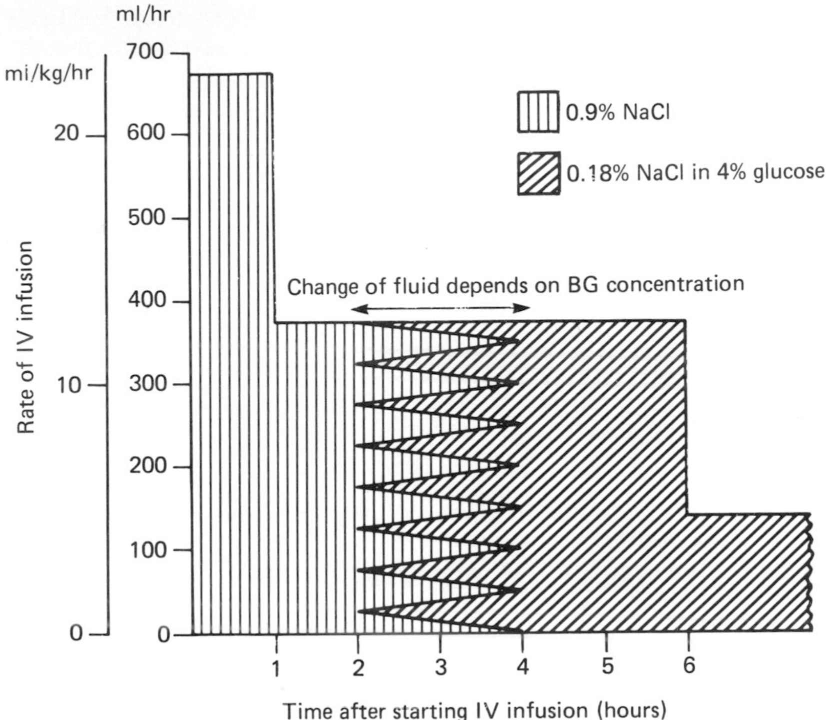

Figure 50.1 The pattern of rehydration for a 10-year-old child weighing 30 kg and assessed as 10 per cent dehydrated. BG = Blood glucose. (For detailed discussion, *see* text)

give 375 ml/hour (300 ml calculated deficit, 75 ml daily maintenance); initially this is as 0.9% saline but should usually change to 0.18% NaCl in 4% glucose between the third to the fifth hour as the blood glucose level falls.

NOTE – Careful recording and continuous calculation of fluid balance (input against output) is required for the safe adjustment of fluid therapy. It is better to avoid large intermittent additions to the fluid input, by constant attention to the fluid balance chart and by reducing the blood glucose below the level of osmotic diuresis as quickly as is reasonably possible. While the blood glucose is raised there will be an inexorable diuresis even in the face of severe dehydration. If the child is not catheterized there is the danger that the fluid balance sums will be seriously misleading unless account is taken of the intermittent passage of large volumes of urine. Once the blood glucose falls below the renal threshold, however, there may be an abrupt reduction in fluid requirement.

Fluid therapy should be reviewed after 5 hours in the light of the clinical and biochemical condition of patient. By this time the blood glucose will often have fallen below the renal threshold and provided that the urinary output has been approximately compensated for, the major proportion of the initial fluid deficit will have been corrected. From 6 hours onwards the rate of infusion should be slowed to correspond with the maintenance requirements for a child of the appropriate age, together with the remaining fluid deficit (i.e. 40 per cent of original calculated deficit). The total calculated fluid deficit should be given within 24 hours of starting intravenous therapy.

If the child is not showing evidence of recovery or has begun to recover and relapses into coma at this stage the possibility of cerebral oedema should be considered (*see* Chapter 26 for further discussion and management of cerebral oedema), or unrecognized hypoglycaemia.

Peripheral circulatory failure (shock) – recognition

Peripheral circulatory failure is indicated by hypotension, tachycardia, vasoconstricted cold white peripheries, and is almost invariably associated with loss of consciousness and Kussmaul respiration. In such a case plasma (or plasma protein fraction) should be given at a rate of 25 ml/kg over the first hour. Thus for a 30 kg child (an average 10 year old) in a state of 'shock' 750 ml of plasma should be run in during the first hour.

Potassium supplements (see also page 127)

1. There is invariably a total body deficit of potassium in patients with ketoacidosis (Soler *et al.*, 1972). The child with newly diagnosed diabetes will frequently have been in a potassium-losing state for many weeks, with polyuria and glycosuria. He is likely to be more severely potassium depleted than the established diabetic with a more acute onset of ketoacidosis.
2. There is no simple guide to total body-potassium depletion but it is important to remember that potassium supplements may be required after the initial resuscitation and rehydration.

   Initially 20 mmol potassium should be added to each 500 ml of fluid (40 mmol/ℓ). It is important that the child should receive the first dose of insulin before potassium is added to the infusion since it is the insulin which drives the potassium out of the extracellular compartment into the cells.
3. It is unnecessary to wait for urine to be passed before adding potassium *unless* there is peripheral circulatory failure, when ischaemic renal damage may have occurred.
4. If a concentration of 40 mmol potassium/ℓ of fluid is maintained throughout the period of rehydration hypokalaemia will usually be avoided. Nevertheless it is advisable to follow the T-wave pattern on the ECG monitor, when hypokalaemia may be indicated by a reduction in the height of the T-wave, a low or absent T-wave and a spread of the QRS complex (*see* page 129).

Insulin

The priorities in the initial management of diabetic ketoacidosis are: first to set up a drip and start intravenous fluids; and secondly to give insulin.

1. INSULIN SHOULD NOT BE GIVEN SUBCUTANEOUSLY SINCE ITS ABSORPTION WILL BE POOR AND IRREGULAR IN A DEHYDRATED CHILD.
2. It is important to avoid large depots of insulin since the insulin may be absorbed irregularly, with the danger of delayed and uncontrolled hypoglycaemia. Short-acting or soluble insulin only should be used, which should now be universally available at a strength of 100 units/ml.
3. Insulin may be given either by continuous intravenous infusion using a reliable infusion pump or by repeated small intramuscular injections.

Intravenous infusion of insulin (Malleson, 1976)

A solution of 1 unit insulin/ml is convenient (50 units soluble insulin in 50 ml of 0.9% NaCl). The solution in the syringe and tubing should be mixed well. The insulin should be connected to the intravenous line by a Y connection or a needle inserted into the rubber connector (do not add insulin to fluid bag or burettes).

The initial starting dose is 0.1 units/kg/hour (e.g. for a 30 kg child give 3 units per hour). This may require frequent adjustment according to the blood glucose response in order to obtain normoglycaemia. The insulin requirement will fall as rehydration proceeds.

Repeated intramuscular insulin (Baum, Jenkins and Aynsley-Green, 1975)

An initial dose of 0.5 units insulin/kg should be given, up to a maximum dose of 10 units. Subsequent doses of 0.1 units insulin/kg are given at two-hourly intervals, to be modified according to hourly blood glucose measurements.

These doses of insulin may need to be modified:

1. If the blood glucose at 2 hours is higher than the initial baseline value, then the second dose of intramuscular insulin should be 0.5 units/kg.
2. If the blood glucose falls below 10 mmol/ℓ (180 mg/100 ml) at any time the dose of insulin should be omitted and the child reassessed after 2 hours.

Insulin resistance

Occasional cases of ketoacidosis which are markedly 'resistant' to insulin have been reported; these require much higher doses of insulin in the initial phase of therapy. Measurement of the blood glucose level after starting insulin will ensure that such cases are recognized and treated with appropriately larger doses of insulin.

Bicarbonate therapy

If there is hyperventilation (Kussmaul respiration) or the initial plasma bicarbonate is less than 12 mmol/ℓ or an arterial pH is less than 7.0, bicarbonate should be added to the infusion. A guide to the approximate dose is as follows:

mmol of bicarbonate = the base deficit × body weight in kilograms × 0.1.

This dose is calculated to correct partially the acidosis since the concurrent rehydration will improve tissue perfusion and reduce further lactic acid production, and the insulin will suppress further lipolysis and ketoacid production (Zimmet *et al.*, 1970). If bicarbonate has been given the pH must be checked within 2 hours. For each millimole of bicarbonate, an extra 1 mmol potassium should be given in the subsequent intravenous fluids, but without exceeding a potassium concentration of 40 mmol/ℓ.

Subsequent management

1. Once the initial resuscitation therapy has been started a flow chart should be constructed to record clinical and biochemical data.
2. A second blood sample is taken 2 hours after the initial baseline biochemical measurements. At the very least, the measurement of blood glucose and

potassium, and bicarbonate, or pH should be repeated if the child is initially acidotic. Preferably blood glucose should be measured hourly if only by reagent strip and finger-prick capillary blood.

3. Additional samples should be sent to the laboratory for the measurement of blood glucose and potassium during the period of clinical recovery, initially at three-hourly intervals.

THE MAIN DANGERS ONCE TREATMENT HAS STARTED ARE HYPOGLYCAEMIA AND HYPOKALAEMIA.

Clinical evidence of recovery

Rehydration should have been achieved and glucose homeostasis restored. Vomiting should have stopped; the peripheral circulation should have been restored; consciousness regained (allowing for an exhausted child being sleepy!); acidosis corrected; and the blood glucose controlled at 4–10 mmol/ℓ (70–180 mg/100 ml). The excretion of ketones in the urine may continue for a day or two: this need not delay subsequent management.

From the onset of resuscitation to the stage of stabilization usually takes from 6 to 24 hours.

Twelve to 24 hours after resuscitation

During the early stage of recovery small sips of fluid are offered. Once oral fluids are tolerated the insulin dose may need to be reduced. For children treated with an intravenous infusion of insulin the transition is made to deep subcutaneous injections of insulin four hourly and finally insulin is given before meals. For children treated with intramuscular insulin the interval between injections is extended to four hourly and then to three times daily before the main meals. The doses of insulin used are gauged by frequent blood glucose measurements timed particularly to occur 2 hours after the main meals. However, in young children some consideration should be given to the distress that may be caused to unnecessarily frequent finger pricking for blood sampling.

Complications

Despite the severity of the dehydration and metabolic disturbance in diabetic ketoacidosis most children respond rapidly to therapy. If the child fails to respond to treatment his clinical condition should be reviewed; hypoglycaemia, previously unrecognized infection (e.g. urinary infection or pneumonia) or the most serious complication, namely the development of acute cerebral oedema, should be considered. Though the cause of this complication is not really understood there is contributory evidence to suggest that rapid changes in the osmolality of the blood may be a factor. This provides an argument in favour of the controlled steady physiological correction of dehydration, hyperglycaemia, and acidaemia. A sudden deterioration of consciousness may indicate the onset of cerebral oedema. This may be confirmed clinically by the finding of papilloedema (although this may be absent) or by ultrasonography or computerized tomography if available. Treatment is empirical including a consideration of the use of mannitol to reduce intracranial pressure, and intermittent positive pressure ventilation to induce hypocapnia (*see also* Chapter 26).

Prevention of ketoacidosis

In children with established diabetes, episodes of ketoacidosis indicate a failure in the education of the parent and the family, and of communication between the family and the hospital. Ketoacidosis may be avoidable if the early signs of loss of control are recognized and acted upon. Reasons for the failure of early identification and communication should be sought after the child has recovered, so that repeat episodes may be prevented.

There will be the occasional established diabetic child who develops an acute intercurrent infection which precipitates ketoacidosis of rapid onset. There are also rare 'brittle' diabetic children, especially teenage girls before the onset of the menarche, who abruptly start vomiting and become ketoacidotic without previous warning.

In new cases of diabetes, ketoacidosis can only be prevented by an awareness of the condition by general practitioners, with a low threshold for testing urine or blood samples for glucose concentrations; this should lead to early diagnosis and referral to hospital.

Stabilization and transfer to maintenance therapy

Diet

After the first 12 hours of intravenous therapy small sips of fluid and then larger drinks can be introduced. After 24 hours the child should begin to tolerate and want a little food.

Insulin

The change from preprandial short acting insulin to intermediate acting insulin should be made relatively early in the stabilization process without waiting for ideal blood glucose control on preprandial insulin therapy.

In the case of the known diabetic patient, unless obviously contraindicated, it is appropriate to return to the normal insulin regimen on the day after satisfactory control has been achieved on preprandial insulin therapy. Extra-short-acting or soluble insulin can be given in addition during the day if indicated by blood glucose results.

The use of frequent capillary blood glucose monitoring has superseded the use of sliding scales of insulin based on urine glucose concentration.

After-care

Following the return to normal hydration and normal diet, stabilization of diabetes is best performed at home. Subsequent management should be supervised at home by the community diabetes nurse supported by telephone contact with other members of the diabetes team and additional visits to the clinic as required.

Discussion should be directed to the prevention of ketoacidosis in the future. The possibility of deliberate manipulation of therapy should be borne in mind, especially for the occasional young teenager presenting with frequent episodes of ketoacidosis, sometimes alternating with hypoglycaemia.

Stabilization of the new diabetic presenting without ketoacidosis

Following diagnosis most children will benefit from starting treatment in hospital although for some children initiation of insulin and dietary therapy at home may be preferred provided there is close supervision from the community diabetes nurse and telephone contact with the clinic medical staff. The majority of children will have had symptoms for several weeks and provided there is no metabolic derangement other than hyperglycaemia (no dehydration, no ketones in the urine) the introduction of insulin can be delayed until the following morning.

If there is polyuria and polydipsia and a markedly raised blood glucose concentration (i.e. greater than 22 mmol/ℓ or 400 mg/100 ml) a small dose of soluble or short-acting insulin may be given at any time during the day of presentation (e.g. 0.3 units/kg body weight).

In cases of dehydration (and if in doubt about the presence of dehydration it is better to err on the side of overestimating the degree of dehydration) and acidosis the therapeutic approach outlined above under ketoacidosis should be started.

Therapy

Insulin

The daily insulin requirement of the new diabetic child can vary considerably. A once daily injection of an intermediate-acting insulin (we prefer human insulin for all new diabetic patients) is usually adequate and a dose of 0.5 units/kg is usually satisfactory to start with. When insulin is given twice daily the same overall total should be used with 2/3 being given in the morning and 1/3 before the main evening meal.

All new patients should be started on 100 strength insulin (100 units/ml) together with plastic disposal syringes. Marks on the syringe equal units of insulin.

Diet

The basic principles of the diet should be introduced to the child and his family by a dietitian in the first day or two. If meals are due before the interview with the dietitian can be arranged, use regular ward food omitting foods obviously high in refined sugar.

The diet is based on normal pre-illness eating patterns as assessed by the dietitian. Average guidelines are:

1. Total daily kilocalories = 1000 + 100 for each year of life until the age of 18.
2. Total energy from carbohydrate = 45–50 per cent of the daily intake (1 g carbohydrate supplies 4 calories).
3. The distribution of daily carbohydrate into three main meals and three snacks is advisable initially, with 20–25 per cent of daily intake at the main meals and 10–15 per cent at the snacks.
4. Encourage whole foods high in dietary fibre and low in animal fats.

Education

Most children and their families are sufficiently distressed at the time of diagnosis to gain little from too much information given in the first few days. Education for the diabetic child is therefore a continuing process taught over subsequent weeks and months in the home and in the clinic.

After-care

Following discharge from the ward newly diagnosed as having diabetes, ensure that the general practitioner has been informed of the diagnosis. In view of the home-care back-up required a telephone call to the general practitioner is preferable to a discharge letter. Where a community diabetes nurse is available it will fall to her to continue instruction on the practical aspects of diabetes, including home visits at the time of daily insulin injections.

Surgery in the diabetic child

It is strongly advised, even for minor surgical procedures such as teeth extraction requiring a general anaesthetic, that the child comes into hospital the day before operation.

Routine minor surgery

On the day before operation insulin and food should be regulated as usual until midnight, and thereafter nothing should be taken by mouth, apart from sips of water.

On the day of operation:

1. Arrange that the child's operation is first on the list (ideally between 8 and 9 am).
2. Set up intravenous infusion 1 hour before operation and give NaCl 0.18% in 4% glucose, at the daily maintenance rate appropriate for the child's weight.
3. Insulin is given 1 hour before the operation by intramuscular injection; in a dose of one sixth of the child's daily requirement in the form of an intermediate-acting insulin, e.g. Monotard (Novo).
4. Follow blood glucose concentration by finger-prick estimations before, during, and hourly after the operation. As recovery proceeds and the situation becomes stable, the frequency of finger-prick testing can be reduced.
5. Additional short-acting insulin should be given during the day at a dose approximating 0.1 unit/kg/body weight if the blood glucose rises above 10 mmol/ℓ (180 mg/100 ml).
6. Most children will be tolerating oral fluids by the late afternoon and possibly eating by early evening, at which stage the intravenous infusion may be stopped.
7. If food is not tolerated as the day goes by, continue intravenous fluids until the following morning, and return to the normal routine with the usual dose of subcutaneous insulin before breakfast.

Emergency or major surgery

Diabetes management during emergency or major surgery is as potentially dangerous as the treatment of ketoacidosis and where possible a senior member of staff with experience in such management should be called to advise from the outset. Management should include intravenous insulin and glucose throughout the operation period.

1. Fluids: provided there is no initial state of dehydration NaCl 0.18% in 4% glucose should be started at a rate corresponding to the normal maintenance requirements for the child's age.
2. Insulin should be given by continuous intravenous infusion at a starting rate of 0.1 unit/kg/hour. This should continue throughout the procedure, the rate being adjusted accordingly to blood glucose levels. The absolute amount of insulin required will depend partly on the child's previous insulin requirements under normal conditions together with the effects of the metabolic response to the surgical stress, which will usually increase the requirement for insulin.
3. With a secure intravenous infusion of glucose–saline together with a controlled infusion of insulin it should be possible to maintain the blood glucose in the range 4–10 mmol/ℓ (70–180 mg/100 ml) throughout the surgery and the post-operative period, provided frequent blood glucose measurements are taken and dealt with appropriately.

Hypoglycaemia

Hypoglycaemia represents a condition of relative insulin excess. It is the single commonest source of anxiety for parents of children with diabetes, particularly so in relation to night-time hypoglycaemia in younger children.

Symptoms

Children usually sense the onset of hypoglycaemia, allowing effective action to be taken. Very young children may not recognize the symptoms themselves and teenagers may either miss early symptoms or ignore them, in which case there may be a rapid progression to more serious symptoms.

Most children show symptoms if their blood glucose falls below 2.5–3 mmol/ℓ (45–55 mg/100 ml). The symptoms of hypoglycaemia differ from child to child and may be inconstant for an individual child, possibly changing over the course of the year. Common symptoms include; faintness, sweating, shivering, nausea, and irritability; vomiting also occurs but rarely.

The child may also complain of abdominal pain, headache or disturbed vision.

The child will usually look pale and feel clammy to the touch. Furthermore, he may appear distant and irritable and may become tearful and difficult to manage.

Uncorrected the symptoms may persist for several hours or may progress over a short period to disturbed or lost consciousness and occasionally to convulsions. In view of the rapidity with which the symptoms of hypoglycaemia may develop urgent intervention is required.

Management at home or at school

The child should be encouraged to eat three or four lumps of table sugar or glucose tablets or to drink a glucose or sucrose sweetened drink. The emergency use of glucose in this way depends of course upon its availability, which in turn depends upon the adequate instruction of the family about the availability of glucose tablets and having glucose- or sucrose-containing drinks available at school. Where possible, if a child has taken glucose for symptoms of hypoglycaemia he should follow this by advancing his next meal or at least having an additional snack, say of biscuits and milk.

Where the hypoglycaemia is more severe attendants may be required to help. For this purpose we have found a 20 ml syringe which contains a concentrated glucose solution invaluable; the glucose solution is injected into the side of the child's mouth (without a needle). Most children, unless they are frankly unconscious, will swallow some of the glucose and enough will be absorbed, allowing recovery. We have had no problems with inhalation of glucose solution at such times.

If these measures fail to revive the child the family may choose to bring the child as an emergency to hospital, or call their family doctor, or try the effect of an intramuscular injection of glucagon. All families with a diabetic child should possess a glucagon kit from which a solution of glucagon can rapidly be prepared and given by intramuscular injection (1 mg for children over 6 years of age; 0.5 mg for children under 6 years of age).

Many children who have experienced severe hypoglycaemic episodes may be sick or have a headache afterwards, which may complicate management or the interpretation of the well-being of the child. Repeated blood glucose measurements at least indicate whether any persisting symptomatology is directly related to extremes of blood glucose concentration.

Hospital management

If a diabetic child presents at the hospital as an emergency certain essential steps should be taken:

1. Establish the diagnosis; an immediate blood glucose measurement should be performed (finger-prick capillary blood or venous blood using an indicator strip with or without a reflectance meter, backed up with a sample sent to clinical biochemistry for measurement). An erroneous result can occur if the child has spilt sugar-containing solutions on his hands during attempts at resuscitation at home.
2. If the admission level of blood glucose is 4 mmol/ℓ (70 mg/100 ml) or greater do not give intravenous glucose. If the child is still unconscious review the diagnosis and consider causes of unconsciousness such as a post-ictal phase following a hypoglycaemic fit. If the child appears well and the blood glucose remains within the normal range it may be appropriate to allow the child to 'sleep it off' under close observation, with frequent blood glucose measurements. If the blood glucose level is less than 2.5 mmol/ℓ (45 mg/100 ml) an intravenous infusion of glucose should be given of around 25–50 g, i.e. 50–100 ml of 50% glucose. This should be followed by an intravenous infusion of 10% glucose at a rate of 100 ml/hour (10 g/hour) until the child regains consciousness and the blood glucose level remains stable within or above the normal range.

Causes of hypoglycaemia

After resuscitation from hypoglycaemia attention should be given to possible causes of hypoglycaemia. These include the incorrect dose of insulin; forgetting to eat snacks or meals; a response to exhausting exercise; a feature of the incubation phase of viral illnesses in some children; or part of the picture of poor and swinging diabetic control as sometimes seen in unstable diabetes.

Treatment is not complete until consideration has been given to the possible cause of the hypoglycaemia and steps taken where possible to prevent its recurrence.

After-care

Children usually recover quickly from hypoglycaemia, particularly if the blood glucose level had been low for a relatively short period of time, e.g. as a reaction to excessive exercise. However, if the blood glucose is low for a long time, as may occur during the night, then after the restoration of blood glucose the child may still have a headache or feel nauseated and may vomit; furthermore if the episode has been nocturnal the child's symptoms may be complicated by fatigue and sleepiness.

Management is not complete until the possible origin of the hypoglycaemia has been discussed with the child and the family and any appropriate changes in management discussed with them. Note that for some families a severe episode of nocturnal hypoglycaemia may very seriously damage their self-confidence about the management of their child's diabetes and an aftermath of anxiety may exist for a long time.

Hyperglycaemia in the newborn

Hyperglycaemia may occur in the newborn in the following situations:

1. The preterm low-birth-weight infant on intravenous glucose; this is the commonest form of neonatal hyperglycaemia, which remits when the concentration or rate of glucose infusion is reduced.
2. The very ill, very low birth-weight preterm infant; it is not uncommon for this biochemical derangement to occur in such infants, frequently in association with an intraventricular haemorrhage. It may represent a disturbance of the hypothalamic regions of the brain.
3. Permanent diabetes mellitus with onset in the newborn period; this is very rare, and the initial management is the same as that for the transient form of neonatal diabetes (*see* below).
4. A post-pancreatectomy diabetes mellitus in the newborn period; children born with hyperinsulinism, particularly due to nesidioblastosis of the pancreas may require total pancreatectomy which inevitably leaves the infant diabetic. The management of such children is no different from that used for the more common form of childhood diabetes, although a relatively smaller dose of insulin may be required (around 0.6–0.7 units/kg/24 hours) and diabetic stability may be rather better than might be anticipated (Greene *et al.*, 1984).

Transient diabetes in the newborn (Ferguson and Milner, 1970)

Recognition

This condition occurs characteristically in low-birth-weight infants especially those born small for dates. More than one such case may present in an individual family. The onset is usually within the first week or two after birth but may present in 24 hours. The infant develops polyuria, loses weight, appears emaciated and dehydrated; however, it is exceptional for the infant to become comatose and often an appearance of wide-eyed alertness is noticed.

The blood glucose is raised, often to levels up to 50 mmol/ℓ (900 mg/100 ml), the blood urea is raised as is the potassium, and the plasma sodium level is often low. There is frequently a metabolic acidosis but characteristically no ketoacidosis nor ketonuria. The condition may be confused with adrenal insufficiency unless glucosuria and hyperglycaemia are identified.

Management

Once recognized the treatment consists of rehydration and the continuous infusion of insulin at a dose of between 1 and 3 units/kg body weight/24 hours. The dose of insulin delivered may require to be modified in accordance with frequent capillary blood glucose measurements.

After initiating treatment the subsequent course is variable. In some infants the condition lasts only a few days while in others it may last for months or blend into permanent diabetes with onset in the newborn period. At the outset it is not possible to be certain with which condition one is dealing. Depending on other aspects of the child it may be simpler to continue with a continuous infusion of insulin daily or, if the child is otherwise well, to transfer to insulin given by subcutaneous injection, perhaps using an intermediate-acting insulin given as two injections a day. Alternatively a continuous subcutaneous infusion of insulin by insulin pump may be appropriate, at least under hospital conditions.

References

AYNSLEY-GREEN, A. and PICKERING, D. (1974) Use of central and peripheral temperature measurements in care of the critically ill child. *Archives of Disease in Childhood,* **49,** 477–481

BAUM, J. D., JENKINS, P. and AYNSLEY-GREEN, A. (1975) Immediate metabolic response to a low dose of insulin in children presenting with diabetes. *Archives of Disease in Childhood,* **50,** 373–378

FERGUSON, A. W. and MILNER, R. D. G. (1970) Transient neonatal diabetes mellitus in sibs. *Archives of Disease in Childhood,* **45,** 80–83

GREENE, S. A., AYNSLEY-GREEN, A., SOLTESZ, G. and BAUM, J. D. (1984) The management of diabetes mellitus following total pancreatectomy in infancy. *Archives of Disease in Childhood,* **59,** 356–359

MALLESON, P. N. (1976) Diabetic ketosis in children treated by adding low-dose insulin to rehydrating fluid. *Archives of Disease in Childhood,* **51,** 373–376

SOLER, N. G., BENNET, M. A., DIXON, K., FITZGERALD, M. G. and MALINS, J. M. (1972) Potassium balance during treatment of diabetic ketoacidosis. *Lancet,* **ii,** 665–667

ZIMMET, P. Z., TAFT, P., ENNIS, G. C. and SHEATH, J. (1970) Acid production in diabetic acidosis: a more rational approach to alkali replacement. *British Medical Journal,* **iii,** 610–612

Further reading

CRAIG, O. (1981) *Childhood Diabetes and its Management.* 2nd edn. London: Butterworths

Chapter 51

Hypoglycaemia

R. D. G. Milner

Hypoglycaemia is encountered commonly in the newborn and less frequently in older infants and children. It is a dangerous condition at any age as the brain is an obligatory consumer of glucose, and hypoglycaemia may result in neuronal damage or death. In neonatal paediatrics so-called 'symptomatic hypoglycaemia' is a misnomer. The term refers to hypoglycaemia associated with abnormal physical signs and contrasts with 'asymptomatic hypoglycaemia' which is purely a laboratory finding. In childhood both symptomatic and asymptomatic hypoglycaemia are found. Hypoglycaemia may be due to too little glucose being delivered to the bloodstream or an accelerated rate of removal. All these points are of importance to the clinician faced with a case of hypoglycaemia since they influence both the pattern of investigation and subsequent management of the patient.

Hypoglycaemia in the newborn (Milner, 1980)

The lower limits of normal blood glucose in the neonate differ from those in later childhood and are shown in *Table 51.1*. The inconsistency of dividing infants into 'term' and 'low birth weight' is not important if precedence is given to the category 'low birth weight' over 'term'. Symptomatic hypoglycaemia is thought to be

Table 51.1 Lower limits of normal blood glucose concentrations (mmol/ℓ; mg/100 ml in parentheses) in newborn infants*

	Before first feed	*After first feed*
Term	1.7 (30)	2.2 (40)
Low birth weight†	1.1 (20)	1.7 (30)

* From Cornblath and Schwartz (1976).
† Less than 2.5 kg birth weight.

followed by a greater prevalence of brain damage than asymptomatic hypoglycaemia and so the neonatologist is always open minded that abnormal clinical signs could be due to hypoglycaemia. The risk of asymptomatic hypoglycaemia becoming symptomatic leads him to be equally vigilant in screening infants known to be at risk (*Table 51.2*).

Table 51.2 Examples of clinical conditions causing neonatal hypoglycaemia

Pathogenesis	*Clinical conditions*
	Excess glucose utilization
Hyperinsulinaemia	
Absolute:	
Fasting	Infant of diabetic mother, erythroblastosis fetalis, nesidioblastosis/insulinoma, Beckwith's syndrome
Post-prandial	Leucine sensitive. Others listed above
Relative:	
Inadequate counter-regulation	Endocrine deficiency, e.g. glucagon, growth hormone
Stress	
(a) Perinatal asphyxia	Cold exposure
(b) Hypermetabolism	
(c) Anoxia	Cardio-respiratory disease
	Inadequate glucose production
Malnutrition	
Prenatal	Light for dates smaller of twins
Postnatal	Iatrogenic
Defective gluconeogenesis	Preterm
	Inborn metabolic errors

Table 51.3 Clinical signs commonly associated with neonatal hypoglycaemia

Central nervous system
Apathy, limpness
Apnoea
Tremors
Irritability, convulsions
Cardiovascular system
Bradycardia
Cyanosis
Respiratory system
Shallow respiration, tachypnoea
Cyanosis

The causal relationship of hypoglycaemia to abnormal neonatal signs is confirmed if the signs disappear on correction of the blood glucose. Clinical signs commonly associated with neonatal hypoglycaemia are listed in *Table 51.3*. None of them is specific; tremor or 'jitteriness' is probably the most characteristic sign, whereas others, such as cyanosis or bradycardia, have other more common causes. The frequency with which asymptomatic hypoglycaemia is diagnosed will depend on how assiduously it is sought. The scheme advocated by Gutberlet and Cornblath

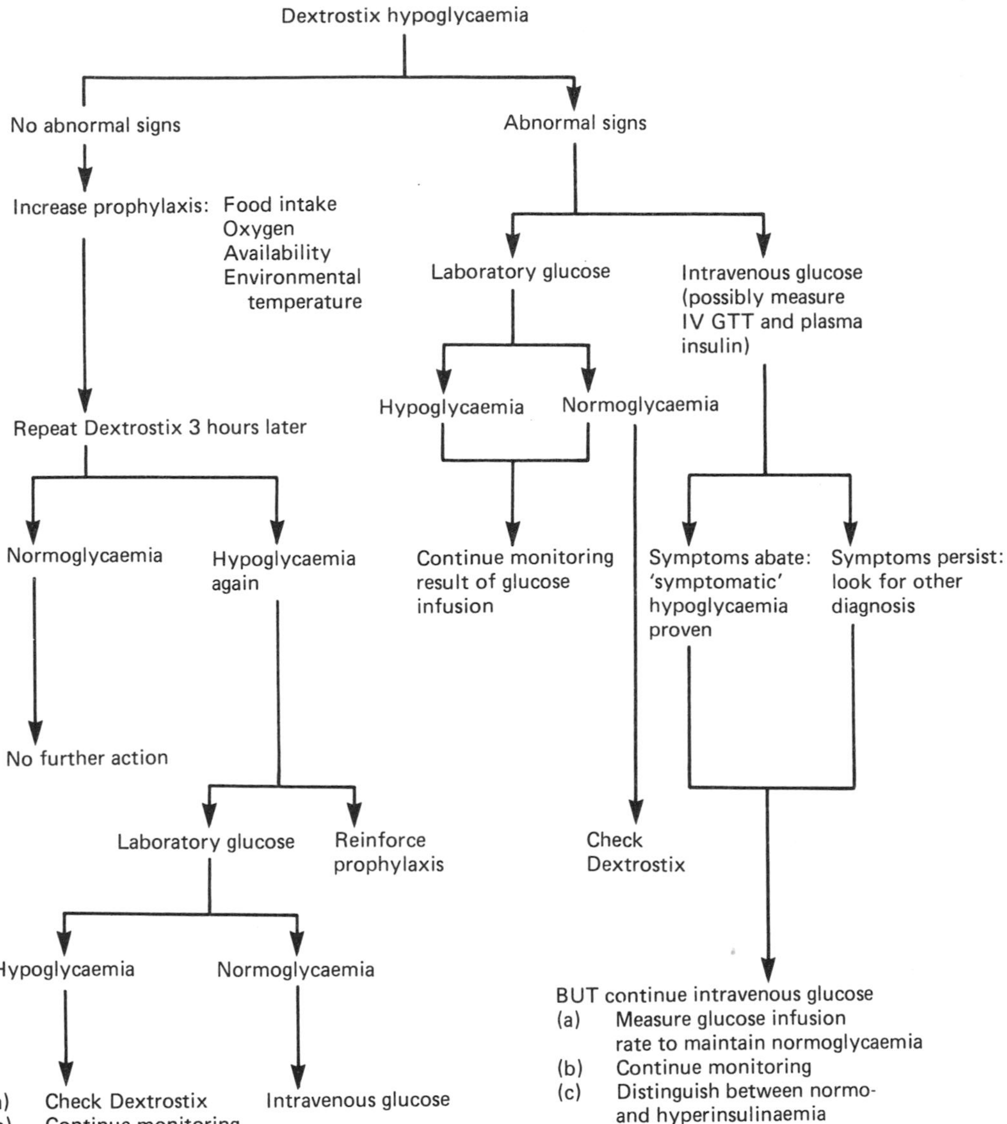

Figure 51.1 Flowchart of the possible actions that may follow the demonstration of neonatal hypoglycaemia. GTT = Glucose tolerance test

(1976) is sensible. They screened (a) all infants born to diabetic mothers or who were light for gestational age (below the 10th centile birth weight); (b) all infants admitted to the intensive care nursery; this included all infants of birth weight below 2.2 kg, all sick infants and all outborn infants; (c) all infants with signs that might be ascribed to hypoglycaemia. In group (a) blood glucose was monitored by Dextrostix at 2, 4, 6, 12, 24 and 48 hours of age; in groups (b) and (c) it was measured at least once. On this basis the frequency of neonatal hypoglycaemia was 4.4 per 1000 inborn infants or 15.5 per 1000 infants of less than 2.5 kg birth weight.

Some neonatal hypoglycaemia is transient (e.g. light-for-dates infants) whereas other cases are persistent (e.g. nesidioblastosis). Although classifications have been made on this basis they are of value mainly in retrospect and the clinician faced with a hypoglycaemic infant is helped if he has a rational scheme for investigation and management (*Figure 51.1*). A system such as this has the merit of maintaining the infant normoglycaemic until the problem has resolved or become manifest as persistent hypoglycaemia. There are a number of practical points that should be noted before the clinical problem is faced.

1. Dextrostix is quoted as a cot-side method of determining blood glucose only as an example. There are several alternative rapid methods available. All stick methods may give false low readings. If this is suspected because the stick and laboratory determination do not agree, the simplest way of checking the remainder of the sticks is for the doctor to perform a Dextrostix blood determination on himself. Alternatively an infant may be oscillating in and out of hypoglycaemia and the Dextrostix may read low but the laboratory glucose may be in the normal range. In such circumstances it is prudent to manage the infant as if he had asymptomatic hypoglycaemia.
2. The tempo of investigation and management depends very much on whether the low Dextrostix result is accompanied by abnormal clinical signs (*Table 51.3*). The majority of cases of asymptomatic hypoglycaemia will respond to appropriate management: early adequate feeding, and nursing at the correct temperature and ambient oxygen concentration.
3. In those cases requiring intravenous glucose (e.g. prolonged proved asymptomatic hypoglycaemia and all cases of symptomatic hypoglycaemia), the infusion should be sited in a peripheral vein if possible and the umbilical vessels used only as a last resort. To deliver adequate glucose without drowning the baby, hypertonic solutions are required and 10% is the preferred strength because the viscosity and acidity of stronger glucose solutions may lead to thrombosis. The rate of infusion and complementary feeding will be adjusted to take account of the infant's overall fluid requirement, but it is worth while remembering that 150 ml 10% glucose/kg/day delivers only 67.5 kcals/kg daily (0.3 MJ/kg daily) which is 60 per cent of the total requirement. Therefore, nutrition should be maintained by a mixture of milk feed and glucose infusion where possible.
4. It is useful to calculate the rate of glucose infusion (mg/kg/min) required to maintain normoglycaemia. In the normal newborn the mean normal glucose production rate is approximately 6 mg/kg/min and if a glucose infusion rate of 10 mg/kg/min or greater is required therapeutically to maintain normoglycaemia this is valuable indirect evidence that the hypoglycaemia is hyperinsulinaemic in origin and not due to a failure of glucose production.
5. In a similar way information about glucose disposal can be obtained if the initial glucose infusion is given in the form of an intravenous glucose tolerance test using a loading dose of 0.5 or 1.0 g glucose/kg body weight. The collection of blood samples at precise times after the glucose bolus permits the calculation of the glucose disappearance rate. If this is abnormally high, hyperinsulinaemic hypoglycaemia is favoured, but proof rests on the measurement of plasma insulin levels. This test will rarely be appropriate for a midnight emergency, but is occasionally of great diagnostic help.

6. An intravenous glucose infusion should never be stopped suddenly because of the likelihood of rebound symptomatic hypoglycaemia. The infusion should be tailed off gradually as oral milk intake is increased and during this time blood glucose levels need regular monitoring.

There remains the problem of what to do with the baby who remains hypoglycaemic despite generous intravenous glucose therapy or the one who cannot be weaned from a glucose infusion because of recurrent rebound hypoglycaemia. The aetiology in such cases is likely to be insulin overproduction, multiple endocrine deficiency, or a rare inborn metabolic error (e.g. galactosaemia, fructose intolerance, or glycogen storage disease). Diazoxide is a rational therapy for hyperinsulinaemia but for some unexplained reason has been found to be largely ineffective when used in the newborn (Crowder *et al.*, 1976). Neither glucagon nor catecholamines have been consistently efficacious in clinical practice and each has undesirable side-effects. In contrast glucocorticoids (e.g. hydrocortisone 5 mg i.m. at 12 hourly intervals) are valuable in weaning an infant from a glucose infusion, despite the mechanism of action not being clearly understood.

Growth hormone deficiency or panhypopituitarism is very rare in the neonatal period but when it does occur hypoglycaemia is the commonest presentation. Such an aetiology should be suspected if hypoglycaemia is refractory to nutritional management, is not associated with excessive glucose consumption, and if a baby boy has microgenitalia (Herber and Milner, 1984). These patients may require glucocorticoids, thyroxine and growth hormone therapy to sustain normoglycaemia.

If hyperinsulinaemia is suspected because of refractory hypoglycaemia and excessive glucose consumption in a patient without a clear diagnosis (e.g. erythroblastosis or infant of a diabetic mother), the plasma insulin should be measured. This may be abnormal in two ways: there may be an inappropriate 'normal' plasma insulin in the face of hypoglycaemia or there may be an exaggerated insulin response to a glucose challenge (Soltesz and Aynsley-Green, 1984). Such patients should be referred without delay to a specialist centre since they are likely to require a laparotomy for the diagnosis/cure of nesidioblastosis or an insulinoma. Delay in making these diagnoses is associated with a high incidence of global retardation in later life (Thomas *et al.*, 1977).

Hypoglycaemia in later infancy and childhood

The lower limit of the normal blood glucose in infancy and childhood is 2.2 mmol/ℓ (40 mg/100 ml). When hypoglycaemia occurs in childhood it is usually genuinely symptomatic, but the explanation of the symptoms is rarely appreciated apart from those occurring in children with diabetes mellitus and those cases where the mother has realized that the symptom may be consistently abated by food. A wide variety of symptoms may be evoked by childhood hypoglycaemia but in an individual patient only one or two are likely to be manifest. Examples of the more common symptoms are given in *Table 51.4*. Unless hypoglycaemia remains in the differential diagnosis entertained by a doctor, symptoms may remain unexplained for a long time, to the serious detriment of the patient. Hypoglycaemia leading to repeated loss of consciousness may cause intellectual impairment or the development of epileptic fits which are triggered initially by hypoglycaemia but later become spontaneous.

Table 51.4 Some symptoms and signs commonly associated with hypoglycaemia in childhood

Excess catechol secretion
Pallor
Sweating
Tachycardia
Central nervous system
Headache
Blurred vision
Irritability, bizarre behaviour
Coma, convulsions
Weakness, wobbly legs
Hunger, tummyache
Vomiting

When fasted the normal child cannot maintain glucose homeostasis for as long as the adult, and hypoglycaemia, which is always associated with ketosis, may be manifest after as little as 20 hours without food (Chaussain *et al.*, 1977). In contrast starved normal adults maintain normoglycaemia for days and the obese for weeks. This is of practical importance because hyperinsulinaemic hypoglycaemia is not associated with ketosis, and testing for ketonuria at the time of hypoglycaemia is a simple, rapid diagnostic step of great precision.

Table 51.5 Examples of causes of hypoglycaemia in childhood

Pathogenesis	*Aetiology*
	Excess glucose utilization
Hyperinsulinaemia	
Absolute:	
Fasting	Insulinoma, nesidioblastosis, insulin overdose, sulphonylurea administration
Post-prandial	Leucine sensitive
Relative	Hypopituitarism
	Inadequate glucose production
Too little glucose intake	Severe malnutrition, clinical diarrhoea
Inadequate glycogenolysis	Glycogen storage disease, glucagon deficiency, fructose intolerance, galactosaemia
Inadequate gluconeogenesis	Normal child, glucose-6-phosphatase deficiency, fructose-1,6-diphosphatase deficiency, Addison's disease, ethanol intoxication

A comprehensive classification is given by Zuppinger (1975).

The principles governing the classification of childhood hypoglycaemia are the same as those in the neonatal period: glucose underproduction and excessive glucose utilization. There is a wide range of uncommon or rare specific causes for each and *Table 51.5* does no more than illustrate some of them. Ackee poisoning (vomiting sickness of Jamaica resulting in severe hypoglycaemia) is discussed in Chapter 70. When faced with the analysis of a particular case the reader will probably need to consult a more detailed text such as Zuppinger (1975) or Soltesz and Aynsley-Green (1984). It is worth remembering that factitious hypoglycaemia may be a manifestation of 'Munchausen syndrome by proxy' and is likely to be missed unless the doctor retains a high index of suspicion. In the same way blood glucose monitoring is necessary on all drunk children or adolescents admitted to hospital if they are not receiving a glucose infusion.

The investigation of suspected hypoglycaemia in childhood starts with measurement of the blood glucose at the time of symptoms. Parents can be taught to use Dextrostix at home but usually the child needs to be admitted to hospital for observation. Advantage can be taken of the admission to undertake planned investigations which are summarized in *Figure 51.2*. The first step involves measuring blood glucose and urinary ketones after an overnight fast (approximately 14 hours) which can be extended to 24 hours if necessary. The establishment of

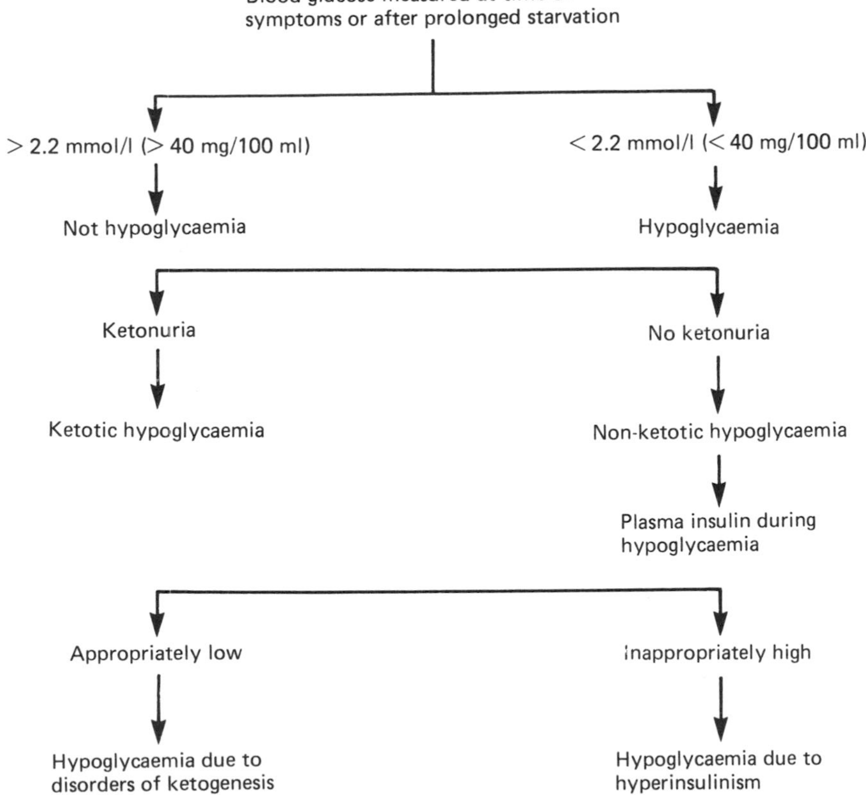

Figure 51.2 Flowchart of the investigations of hypoglycaemia in childhood. (Modified from Soltesz and Aynsley-Green (1984), with kind permission of authors and publishers)

the hypoglycaemia as ketotic or non-ketotic and the measurement of plasma insulin in the latter is crucial to further investigation. When ketonuria is assessed on the ward it should be remembered that Acetest tablets and dipstick methods are very sensitive. If the test is positive on neat urine it should be repeated on urine diluted one drop to ten with tap water; if still positive the ketonuria is clinically important. The words 'inappropriately high plasma insulin' refer to the fact that a plasma insulin in the normal fasting range which does not respond to fluctuations in blood glucose can be sufficient to provoke hypoglycaemia. The plasma insulin during non-hyperinsulinaemic hypoglycaemia is normally under 6 mU/ℓ.

The treatment of hypoglycaemia in childhood divides into the management of the hypoglycaemic episode and the treatment of the underlying cause. The majority of children experiencing hypoglycaemic symptoms are normal, never reach a doctor, and are correctly and empirically managed with extra food. Of those children who present to a doctor a proportion, possibly a majority, will have ketotic hypoglycaemia when fasted. They too should be fed more frequently. Serious hypoglycaemia is likely to be more profound, unequivocal in clinical presentation and to have a specific pathology. The following practical points should be remembered in the management of the acute episode:

1. If the child presents in hypoglycaemic coma, the time to regain consciousness is related both to the degree and to the duration of the hypoglycaemia. The unconsciousness and the hypoglycaemia need not be causally related: other causes of loss of consciousness should be sought. Conversely unconsciousness may be due to hypoglycaemia which is no longer apparent when the blood glucose is determined. In either case a lumbar puncture is helpful because CSF examination will help to elucidate other causes of loss of consciousness such as haemorrhage or infection. In hypoglycaemic unconsciousness the CSF glucose value may remain low (below 1.7 mmol/ℓ (30 mg/100 ml)) when the blood glucose has returned to normal levels.
2. Symptoms of hypoglycaemia are not only related to the absolute blood glucose level but also to the rate of change in blood glucose. A rapid fall in blood glucose from hyperglycaemic to normoglycaemic levels may be associated with symptoms characteristic of hypoglycaemia. This occurs most characteristically in diabetic patients.
3. As in the newborn, strong chemical evidence favouring hypoglycaemia as the cause of symptoms or abnormal signs is their prompt correction by the administration of glucose orally or parenterally.
4. Parenteral glucose is best given as an intravenous bolus of 50% glucose up to a dose of 0.5 g/kg; the viscosity of the solution determines the speed of the injection. If the cause of the hypoglycaemia is unknown, as is most often the case, the bolus injection should be followed by an infusion of 10% glucose. The rate is determined both by the glucose needed to maintain normoglycaemia and by the patient's fluid requirements.

The search for the underlying cause will quickly reveal if the hypoglycaemia is (a) ketotic, (b) non-ketotic with normal insulin secretion, or (c) non-ketotic with inappropriate insulin secretion (*see Figure 51.2*). The plan of investigation of ketotic hypoglycaemia or non-ketotic hypoglycaemia with normal insulin secretion is complicated, since specific tests for a wide variety of rare inborn metabolic errors are involved and the reader must look for these elsewhere (Zuppinger, 1975). If the evidence favours hyperinsulinaemic hypoglycaemia the further management and investigation of the patient become intertwined. This is because the ultimate investigation/treatment may involve a total pancreatectomy and most paediatricians are pragmatic about this procedure (*Figure 51.3*).

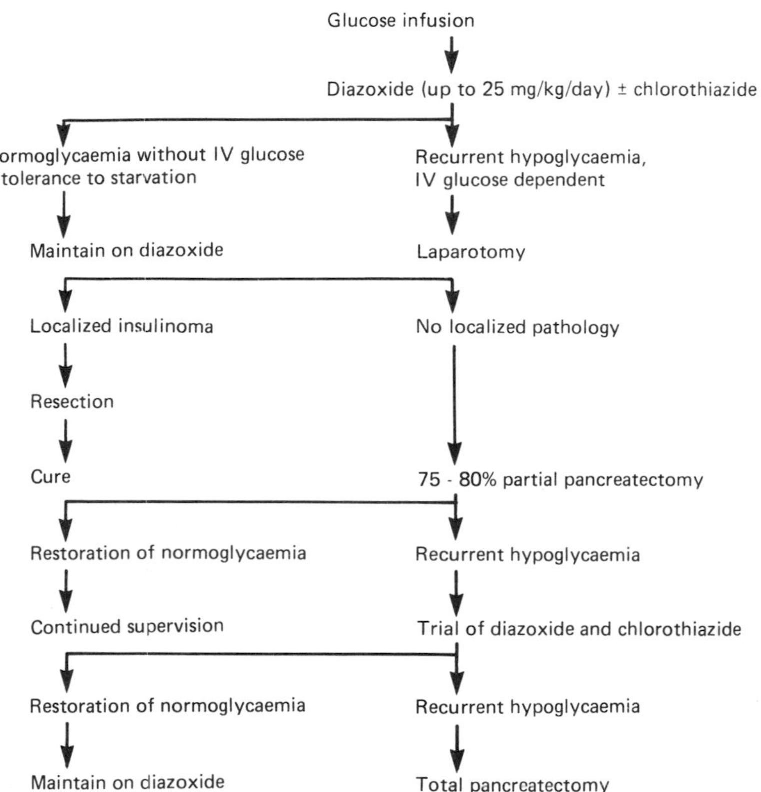

Figure 51.3 Management of hyperinsulinaemic hypoglycaemia in infants and children. (Modified from Soltesz and Aynsley-Green (1984), with kind permission of authors and publishers)

In such cases glucose infusion rates of more than 10 mg/kg/min may be inadequate to maintain normoglycaemia and glucagon (1 mg i.m.) may be needed to produce a transient rise of blood glucose. Diazoxide (up to 25 mg/kg/day) with or without chlorothiazide may provide symptomatic relief. If it does, the child can be maintained on diazoxide, for years if necessary. If diazoxide is not helpful, surgery is indicated, which may culminate in a partial or total pancreatectomy, depending on the pathology found (Soltesz and Aynsley-Green, 1984).

References

CHAUSSAIN, J. L., GEORGES, P., CALZADA, L. and JOB, J. C. (1977) In G. Chinmello and Z. Laron (eds) *Recent Progress in Paediatric Endocrinology,* pp. 113–118. London: Academic Press

CORNBLATH, M. and SCHWARTZ, R. (1976) *Disorders of Carbohydrate Metabolism in Infancy,* 2nd edn., pp. 72–104. Philadelphia: W. B. Saunders

CROWDER, W. L., MacLAREN, N. K., GUTBERLET, R. L., FROST, J. L., MASON, G. R. and CORNBLATH, M. (1976) Neonatal pancreatic β-cell hyperplasia: report of a case with failure of diazoxide and benefit of early subtotal pancreatectomy. *Pediatrics,* **57,** 897–900

GUTBERLET, R. L. and CORNBLATH, M. (1976) Neonatal hypoglycemia revisited, 1975. *Pediatrics,* **58,** 10–17

HERBER, S. M. and MILNER, R. D. G. (1984) Growth hormone deficiency presenting under the age of 2. *Archives of Disease in Childhood,* **59,** 557–560

MILNER, R. D. G. (1980) Neonatal hypoglycaemia. In D. Andreani, P. J. Lefebvre and V. Marks (eds), *Current Views in Hypoglycaemia and Glucagon,* pp. 331–342. London: Academic Press

SOLTESZ, G. and AYNSLEY-GREEN, A. (1984) Hyperinsulinism in infancy and childhood. In P. Frick, G. A. Von Hamack, K. Kochsick, G. A. Martini and A. Prader (eds), *Advances in Internal Medicine and Paediatrics,* Vol 51, pp. 151–202. Berlin: Springer Verlag

THOMAS, C. G. JR., UNDERWOOD, L. E., CARNEY, C. N., DOLCOURT, J. L. and WHITT, J. J. (1977) Neonatal and infantile hypoglycaemia due to insulin excess: new aspects of diagnosis and surgical management. *Annals of Surgery,* **185,** 505–517

ZUPPINGER, K. (1975) Hypoglycaemia in childhood. In F. Falkner, N. Kretchner and E. Rossi (eds), *Monographs in Paediatrics,* Vol. 4. Basel: S. Karger

Chapter 52

Adrenocortical insufficiency and ambiguous genitalia in the newborn

Martin O. Savage

Adrenocortical insufficiency

Adrenocortical insufficiency may be of primary adrenal origin or due to a disorder of the hypothalamic–pituitary system (*Table 52.1*). In primary disorders, there may be congenital hypoplasia or a destructive process involving the cortex or a congenital defect of one of the enzymes responsible for steroidogenesis. The symptoms of adrenocortical insufficiency result from impaired production of the two principal steroid hormones, cortisol and aldosterone.

Table 52.1 Causes of adrenocortical insufficiency

Primary adrenal insufficiency:

- Congenital adrenal hypoplasia
- Congenital adrenal hyperplasia:
  - Deficiency of 21-hydroxylase, 11 β-hydroxylase, 3 β-hydroxysteroid dehydrogenase, 17-α-hydroxylase
- Acute adrenal haemorrhage
- Addison's disease:
  - Autoimmune adrenalitis
  - Tuberculosis
  - Addison–Schilder syndrome

Secondary adrenal insufficiency:

- Hypothalamic–pituitary insufficiency
  - Congenital (idiopathic) panhypopituitarism
  - CNS tumour (e.g. craniopharyngioma)
  - Isolated ACTH deficiency
- Exogenous glucocorticoid therapy

The newborn

The most important symptoms of adrenal insufficiency in newborn infants are those of hypoglycaemia, salt depletion, and circulatory collapse.

Hypoglycaemia

This is a common presenting symptom in both adrenal and pituitary cases, being particularly precipitated by fasting and acute infections. Lack of circulating cortisol results in impaired gluconeogenesis in infants whose glycogen stores become rapidly depleted in the fasting state. The resulting hypoglycaemia usually presents as convulsions, cyanosis, or apnoea. Prolonged jaundice may also indicate cortisol deficiency (*see also* page 471).

Salt depletion

Salt depletion is due to urinary salt-wasting secondary to lack of mineralocorticoid hormone synthesis. The principal mineralocorticoid hormone is aldosterone. This arises in primary adrenal disorders such as congenital adrenal hypoplasia (Black *et al.*, 1977) and in the salt-losing forms of congenital adrenal hyperplasia, i.e. 21-hydroxylase and 3 β-hydroxysteroid dehydrogenase deficiencies.

The clinical features may be acute, such as dehydration and hypovolaemia leading to circulatory collapse, or more insidiously, with vomiting, diarrhoea, poor feeding and failure to thrive. Many salt-depleted infants have been thought to have pyloric stenosis. The biochemical abnormalities are: hyperkalaemia, hyponatraemia, and metabolic acidosis with elevation of plasma renin activity and a low plasma aldosterone value. Urinary sodium excretion is inappropriately high for the state of the sodium balance. Causes of salt depletion in infancy are given in *Table 52.2*. Salt depletion of non-adrenal origin must be considered in all cases.

Table 52.2 Salt-losing conditions in infancy

Name	*External genitalia*		*PRA*	*PAldo*
	46XX	*46XY*		
Congenital adrenal hypoplasia	N	N	↑	↓
Congenital adrenal hyperplasia:				
21-hydroxylase (salt-losing)	Virilized	Usually normal	↑	↓
20-22 desmolase	N	Ambiguous	↑	↓
3β-hydroxysteroid dehydrogenase	Slightly virilized	Ambiguous	↑	↓
Aldosterone biosynthetic defect:				
18-hydroxylase	N	N	↑	↓
Adrenal haemorrhage	N	N	↑	↓
Renal disorders:				
Renal dysplasia	N	N	↑	↑
Tubular defects	N	N	↑	↑
Pseudohypoaldosteronism	N	N	↑	↑ (marked)

PRA, Plasma renin activity; PAldo, plasma aldosterone.

Circulatory collapse

This may be due to more than one cause. It seldom occurs in the absence of salt depletion except when there is acute adrenal haemorrhage when blood loss and cortisol deficiency are probably the main contributing factors.

Principal causes of adrenocortical insufficiency

Congenital adrenal hypoplasia

This developmental defect may be sporadic or familial (X-linked) and the incidence has been estimated to be 1 in 12500 births. The clinical signs are those of complete adrenal insufficiency usually occurring during the first few days of life. Salt depletion and dehydration predominate and the plasma ACTH value is markedly elevated.

Congenital adrenal hyperplasia

This group of disorders inherited as autosomal recessives is characterized by deficiency of one of the enzymes necessary for cortisol synthesis (Hughes, 1982). If the enzyme is also deficient in the mineralocorticoid pathway, salt wasting, which usually presents towards the end of the first week of life, may develop. The commonest form is 21-hydroxylase deficiency, in which the external genitalia are virilized due to excess adrenal androgen secretion. About 60 per cent of affected infants have associated salt loss. Plasma 17-hydroxyprogesterone value, the precursor hormone immediately before the enzyme block, is markedly raised, providing biochemical confirmation of the defect.

Acute adrenal haemorrhage

This condition may occur without warning or as part of a septicaemia. One or both adrenals may be affected (Black and Williams, 1973) and a mass may be palpable in the flank. Adrenal haemorrhage must be distinguished from renal vein thrombosis. Clinically, there is sudden onset of shock and pallor with or without jaundice. An abdominal ultrasound or IVP will show that the kidney on the affected side excretes normally but is displaced downwards and the upper calyces are flattened. Management consists in replacing blood loss, restoring the circulation, and hormone replacement (*see* below). Antibiotics should be given as for a suspected septicaemia: normally benzylpenicillin and gentamicin should be used.

Panhypopituitarism

This is a rare but treatable cause of adrenal insufficiency (Lovinger, Kaplan and Grumbach, 1975). There are multiple anterior pituitary hormone deficiencies, although those that are important neonatally are ACTH and TSH. Hypoglycaemia almost always occurs, responding immediately to hydrocortisone replacement, and thyroxine should be given to treat the hypothyroidism. In male infants the presence of micro-penis from lack of prenatal gonadotrophins is an important pointer to pituitary deficiency. Septo-optic dysplasia, with congenital nystagmus, may also present with multiple pituitary hormone deficiencies. Apnoeic attacks and prolonged conjugated hyperbilirubinaemia are common presenting symptoms of panhypopituitarism in the neonatal period.

Adrenocortical insufficiency in the older child

Addison's disease is an uncommon disorder, the most frequent aetiology being an autoimmune destructive process. The main symptoms are progressive fatigue associated with hyperpigmentation, and postural hypotension. Acute adrenal insufficiency may be precipitated by intercurrent infection. Other autoimmune endocrinopathies, hypoparathyroidism, diabetes mellitus and gonadal failure may coexist.

Recognition of adrenocortical insufficiency

In the newborn period dynamic endocrine studies are difficult and management is aimed at resuscitation and establishment of replacement therapy. The finding of a low plasma cortisol concentration (less than 500 nmol/ℓ) in the presence of stress, i.e. hypoglycaemia or circulatory collapse, is strongly suggestive of adrenal insufficiency. An elevated plasma ACTH level in the same sample will confirm a primary adrenal cause whereas simultaneously low cortisol and ACTH levels are consistent with hypopituitarism. A short synacthen test (0.25 mg i.m. with blood taken for cortisol at 0, 30 and 60 minutes) is usually a sufficient dynamic test of adrenocortical function.

Measurement of plasma sodium and potassium and urinary sodium concentrations may point to mineralocorticoid deficiency which can be confirmed by simultaneous plasma renin activity (high) and plasma aldosterone (low) determinations (Dillon *et al.*, 1976). Plasma 17-hydroxyprogesterone is markedly raised (upper limit of normal range: 15 nmol/ℓ) after the first 24 hours of life in 21-hydroxylase deficiency (Hughes, 1982) and should be measured in all infants with ambiguous genitalia and salt loss.

Management of adrenocortical insufficiency

Salt depletion

1. IV 0.9% NaCl in 5% glucose should be started at the rate of 100–120 ml/kg/24 hours, at an initial rate of 20 ml/kg/hour for 1–2 hours until shock is relieved or improved.
2. In severely shocked infants plasma (or plasma protein fraction) should be substituted for the glucose saline at 20 ml/kg/hour for 1 hour.

Hypoglycaemia

IV 10% glucose should be given to correct hypoglycaemia, followed by hydrocortisone replacement.

Circulatory collapse

1. IV plasma or 0.9% NaCl in 5% glucose should be given at a rate of 20 ml/kg/hour.
2. Hydrocortisone should be given IV in an initial dose of 100 mg followed by a dose of 2 mg/kg/hour i.m. or IV at 4–6 hourly intervals.

Maintenance hormone therapy

1. Hydrocortisone is given in a dose of 20 mg/m^2/24 hours in three divided doses for the first year of life. An example is 5 mg/day for a 4 kg infant given as 2.5, 1.25, 1.25 mg. Larger doses than this physiological replacement may suppress growth. Twice daily replacement is acceptable in older children.

2. 9-α-fludrocortisone is given, 0.1–0.2 mg daily.
3. Deoxycortone pivalate (Percorten M, Ciba) is a depot mineralocorticoid preparation which may be used instead of fludrocortisone. The dose for infants is in the region of 12.5 mg i.m. *monthly*.
4. Salt supplements are given as NaCl solution in a dose of 4–6 mmol sodium/kg/day in divided doses.
5. Steroid cover for surgery:
   (a) *Hydrocortisone* – Intramuscular hydrocortisone 50–100 mg with premedication and six-hourly postoperatively until oral steroids are recommenced. The dose should be gradually reduced to maintenance level over 4–5 days.
   (b) *Fludrocortisone* – This oral steroid will be stopped during surgery. IV NaCl should also be given pre- and postoperatively in a dose of sodium 6 mmol/kg/day.

Ambiguous genitalia

An infant who is born with ambiguity of the external genitalia constitutes a paediatric emergency in two respects (Grant and Savage, 1981). First, the presence of this error of sexual differentiation may indicate an underlying biochemical defect which will in itself have serious consequences for the child. The obvious example is a female infant with salt-losing congenital adrenal hyperplasia. Secondly, urgent investigation is necessary for the infant to be assigned to the correct gender; in the parents' minds this is clearly an emergency.

The aetiology of ambiguous genitalia (Table 52.3)

The three categories of intersex are based on gonadal morphology.

Table 52.3 Classification of ambiguous genitalia

Female pseudohermaphrodite (46 XX)
Congenital adrenal hyperplasia (autosomal recessive, all types). 21-hydroxylase, 11β-hydroxylase, 3β-hydroxysteroid dehydrogenase
Maternal virilizing tumour, maternal progestagen treatment
Male pseudohermaphrodite (46XY)
Impaired testicular function, testosterone biosynthetic defect (usually autosomal recessive)
Impaired peripheral androgen metabolism
Androgen receptor defect (usually X-linked) (complete or incomplete androgen insensitivity)
5-α-reductase deficiency (autosomal recessive)
Abnormal gonadal differentiation
True hermaphrodite, XO/XY gonadal dysgenesis, XX male

Female pseudohermaphroditism

These patients are genetic females (46XX) with normal ovaries, fallopian tubes, and uterus, but virilization of the external genitalia. The virilization occurs from an abnormal production of androgens either by the fetus or mother. The most important cause is virilizing congenital adrenal hyperplasia (*see* above). Other less common causes are virilizing maternal tumours and progestagen therapy during pregnancy. These patients should normally be brought up as girls because, following reconstructive genital surgery and hormone replacement, they have normal female reproductive potential.

Male pseudohermaphroditism

These patients are genetic males (46XY) with normally formed testes but a defect of virilization of the genital structures. Two defects may cause this:

1. Impaired synthesis of testosterone by the fetal testis.
2. An abnormality in peripheral tissue responsiveness to testicular androgens.

The first defect is usually due to an autosomal recessive gene. The second is caused either by a receptor defect (X-linked condition) or to a deficiency of 5-α reductase, which is an autosomal recessive disorder.

One cannot be dogmatic about gender assignment in this group, and each case must be assessed individually from the point of view of the potential of the genitalia and likely pubertal development to fulfill the male role. It is wrong to assign the infant automatically as a male because of the male chromosomes.

Abnormal gonadal formation

This is a heterogeneous group of patients with abnormally formed gonads, in particular testes, which have led to incomplete formation of either a normal male or female fetus. Examples are true hermaphrodites, the XO/XY mosaic patient with asymmetrical development (mixed gonadal dysgenesis) and the XX male. Again, no firm directive can be given for genital assignment which should be based on the structure of the genitalia and the likely pattern of pubertal development.

Table 52.4 Infant with ambiguous genitalia: laboratory investigations

No gonads palpable	Karyotype, plasma 17OH-progesterone, 11-deoxycortisol (urinary 17-oxosteroid excretion)
One gonad palpable	Karyotype, HCG test, gonadal biopsy, laparotomy
Two gonads palpable	Karyotype, HCG test (HCG 1000 u daily × 3) plasma T, DHT, DHEA, $\Delta 4^A$ on days 0 and 3, 'in vitro' androgen binding studies

T, testosterone; DHT, dihydrotestosterone; DHEA, dehydroepiandrosterone; $\Delta 4^A$, androstenedione.

Investigation of ambiguous genitalia (Table 52.4)

The appearance of the external genitalia is of little help in defining the aetiology. A careful family history is important since many of these disorders are genetically determined and a similarly affected sibling may give a firm clue. The most important aspect of the examination is careful palpation for gonads. There are three possibilities:

1. *If no gonads are palpable* – The most likely diagnosis is congenital adrenal hyperplasia which is virtually certain if salt-loss develops. A karyotype is needed

to confirm a 46XX pattern and plasma 17-hydroxyprogesterone level will be elevated in the 21-hydroxylase deficiency.

2. *If two gonads are palpable* – The patient is probably a 46XY male with either an abnormality of testosterone biosynthesis or a peripheral androgen receptor defect. A karyotype is again necessary and measurement of plasma testosterone basally and after HCG stimulation will distinguish a testicular from a peripheral defect.
3. *If one gonad is palpable* – There has been asymmetrical development which may occur in true hermaphroditism or mixed gonadal dysgenesis. Gonadal biopsy or laparotomy to define the internal structures may be necessary.

Choice of gender

Gender assignment will not be covered in detail. The birth of an infant with true ambiguity is rare, and it is unlikely that either the midwife or paediatric resident will have had experience of this difficult situation. Probably the best approach to the family is to explain that there is uncertainty concerning the sex of the child and that investigations and possibly a specialist opinion will be needed. The parents should be reassured that the correct sex will be chosen and that the child will not remain in an intermediate state. If there is genuine doubt, the child's birth should not be registered until the results of investigations have been analysed. The decision concerning gender assignment should be a joint one involving the paediatrician and urologist or plastic surgeon and the child's parents.

References

BLACK, J. and WILLIAMS, D. I. (1973) Natural history of adrenal haemorrhage in the newborn. *Archives of Disease in Childhood,* **48,** 183–190

BLACK, S., BROOK, C. G. D. and COX, P. J. N. (1977) Congenital adrenal hypoplasia and gonadotrophin deficiency. *British Medical Journal,* **ii,** 996

DILLON, M. J., GILLIN, M. E. A., RYNESS, J. M. and DE SWIET, M. (1976) Plasma renin activity and aldosterone concentration in the human newborn. *Archives of Disease in Childhood,* **51,** 537–540

GRANT, D. B. and SAVAGE, M. O. (1981) Clinical aspects of intersex. In C. G. D. Brook (ed.), *Clinical Paediatric Endocrinology,* pp. 40–60. Oxford: Blackwell Scientific Publications

HUGHES, I. A. (1982) Congenital and acquired disorders of the adrenal cortex. In J. Bailey (ed.), *Clinics in Endocrinology and Metabolism,* Vol II(i), pp. 89–125. Philadelphia: W. B. Saunders

LOVINGER, R. D., KAPLAN, S. L. and GRUMBACH, M. M. (1975) Congenital hypopituitarism associated with neonatal hypoglycaemia and microphallus. Four cases secondary to hypothalamic hormone deficiencies. *Journal of Pediatrics,* **87,** 1171–1181

Chapter 53

Disorders of the thyroid gland

N. D. Barnes

Thyroid disease presents acute emergencies only rarely; these may be caused by structural or functional disorders.

Structural disorders

Goitre in the newborn

An enlarged thyroid gland in a newborn infant may compress the trachea and can cause death from asphyxia. The neck of the normal newborn is short and wide so the presence of a goitre may be difficult to detect. Moreover, the size is likely to be underestimated as the gland can almost completely encircle the trachea and may in part be retrosternal.

Recognition

The presence of a goitre should be sought immediately after birth if any predisposing cause is present:

1. Iodine excess, usually due to maternal ingestion of iodide-containing medications for respiratory problems, fortunately now much less widely used; the mother may not have a goitre or hypothyroidism and this fetal risk factor may well have been missed in the antenatal history.
2. Iodine deficiency, in areas of endemic goitre and cretinism; the mother is likely to be goitrous also.
3. Maternal thyrotoxicosis:
   (a) Transplacental passage of thyroid stimulating antibodies from a mother who has had Graves' disease (thyrotoxicosis) whatever her current thyroid status (*see* below).
   (b) Treatment with antithyroid thioamide drugs (carbimazole, methimazole, propylthiouracil), which cross the placenta freely.
4. Familial goitre due to an inherited defect of thyroxine biosynthesis previously detected in a sibling. There are several such disorders; all are recessively inherited, so the risk to each sibling is 1 in 4. Pendred's syndrome, an organification defect, is associated with neural deafness.

Evidence of tracheal compression

1. The infant may have been born by otherwise unexplained face or brow presentation, and will lie with head extended, becoming distressed if the neck is flexed.
2. Stridor on inspiration and expiration may be a prominent feature but is sometimes absent.
3. Severe compression causes fixed upper airway obstruction with dyspnoea, increased respiratory effort, intercostal and subcostal recession. There may be progression to respiratory failure with tachypnoea, tachycardia, cyanosis, exhaustion, and death.

Management

1. All goitrous infants should be observed until it is clear that the danger of tracheal compression is past, and any abnormality of thyroid function is clarified and treated.
2. PA and lateral radiographs of the neck and/or ultrasound examination will confirm tracheal narrowing.
3. The infant should be nursed with head elevated and neck extended over a pillow or sandbag.
4. If the airway is severely obstructed this must be relieved by intubation or tracheostomy with the passage of a tube beyond the narrowed part of the trachea.
5. Definitive relief can then be provided, if necessary, by partial thyroidectomy.

Goitre in childhood

A rapidly enlarging goitre in a child is rare but may be caused by bleeding into a cyst, acute bacterial or subacute viral thyroiditis, or malignant infiltration with lymphomatous tissue. Thyroid cancer in childhood, which often follows external irradiation of the neck, is slow growing. Anaplastic carcinoma is extremely rare.

Acute complications may follow thyroid surgery, especially total thyroidectomy; these include recurrent laryngeal palsies, hypocalcaemic tetany and convulsions from hypoparathyroidism, and tracheal compression from postoperative bleeding.

Functional disorders

Congenital hypothyroidism

The recognition and treatment of congenital hypothyroidism is always urgent because the earlier treatment is started the better the prognosis. In the UK and many other countries all newborn babies are screened for this disease. The incidence is approximately 1 in 4000 live births.

Recognition

Although the maternal and fetal thyroid axes are functionally separate severe symptomatic neonatal hypothyroidism is rare even in athyroidal infants, the typical symptoms and signs usually developing gradually in the early weeks of life. Primary hypothyroidism is confirmed by finding a low serum thyroxine (T_4) for age, a low or normal serum tri-iodothyronine (T_3) and a high serum thyrotropin (TSH). Any anatomical defect can be demonstrated by a thyroid scan with ^{123}I or technetium ^{99m}Tc pertechnetate. If the thyrotropin is low, thyroxine binding globulin deficiency or secondary hypothyroidism due to pituitary or hypothalamic disease must be considered. Acute complications of congenital hypothyroidism include:

1. Respiratory difficulty. In the absence of tracheal compression this may be due to an enlarged tongue, pulmonary immaturity, or neurological depression.
2. Hyperbilirubinaemia. Exaggerated and prolonged 'physiological' jaundice occurs because of immaturity of hepatic glucuronyl transferase activity (*see also* page 682).
3. Functional intestinal obstruction. This may be difficult to distinguish from organic obstruction.
4. Cerebral depression from severe hypothyroidism may mimic neurological disease.
5. In secondary hypothyroidism, hypoglycaemia may occur.

Management

Thyroid hormone replacement should be started as soon as the diagnosis is confirmed. Thyroxine is used for long-term replacement in a dose sufficient to maintain the serum thyroxine (T_4) in the upper part of the normal range for age, approximately 100 μg/m^2/day or 10 μg/kg/day in the newborn.

However, thyroxine has a long plasma half-life, approximately 7 days, and a gradual onset of action mediated by conversion to tri-iodothyronine, so the use of tri-iodothyronine (half-life 2 days) orally or parenterally (IV) in an initial dose of 20 μg/m^2/day may occasionally be indicated when acute complications are present.

Specific measures may be required for the treatment or control of complications until euthyroidism is restored.

Hyperthyroidism

Neonatal thyrotoxicosis (Fisher, 1976)

There are two forms of neonatal thyrotoxicosis. The more common is a transient disorder due to transplacental passage of maternal antibodies to the TSH receptor which causes fetal and neonatal thyroid stimulation. There is also a rare persistent familial form.

Recognition

Neonatal thyrotoxicosis is frequently missed; in severe cases it is a life-threatening disease. Its occurrence is predictable in the presence of active or previously treated maternal Graves' disease (thyrotoxicosis) but the incidence among infants at risk is low, possibly because thyroid stimulating antibody levels fall in pregnancy. However, the higher the antibody level the greater the chance that the baby will be affected.

There is therefore a high change of neonatal thyrotoxicosis if:

1. A previous sibling was affected.
2. The mother has a high level of thyroid stimulating antibodies. At present assays for these antibodies are not widely available.

3. The mother has a history of Graves' disease associated with exophthalmos and pretibial myxoedema. Of particular importance is the occurrence of neonatal thyrotoxicosis when the mother has been previously made euthyroid by thyroidectomy; residual eye signs are usual in such patients.

All such pregnancies should be kept under close observation with special attention to the occurrence of fetal hyperthyroidism, detected by a fetal heart rate consistently greater than 140 beats per minute, and poor intrauterine growth. When this occurs consideration should be given to treatment of the fetus irrespective of the mother's thyroid status. Carbimazole or propylthiouracil will cross the placenta and block the fetal thyroid. The lowest dose sufficient to maintain the fetal heart rate below 140 beats per minute should be given, usually not more than carbimazole 15–20 mg or propylthiouracil 150–200 mg/day. If necessary the mother can be given thyroxine to maintain her euthyroid state since this will not cross the placenta.

All infants at risk should be closely observed clinically and biochemically with total and, if available, free thyroid hormone levels. The onset of symptoms may be delayed in infants whose mothers have received antithyroid agents and sometimes also in those who have not.

The major clinical features are:

1. Low birthweight and skull circumference, small or moderate goitre.
2. Irritability, hyperactivity, restlessness, sweating.
3. Loss of weight or poor gain with normal or excessive intake.
4. Tachycardia, sometimes leading to heart failure, which may develop very suddenly.
5. Thyrotoxic eye signs, proptosis, and lid retraction.

Management

1. Propylthiouracil 10 mg/kg/day or carbimazole or methimazole 1.0 mg/kg/day is given in divided doses by mouth every 4–8 hours. These drugs block iodide binding and thyroid hormone synthesis but have no effect on the secretion of previously synthesized and stored thyroid hormone.
2. Iodide as aqueous iodine (Lugol's) solution (iodine 5%, potassium iodide 10% in water) one drop 8 hourly is therefore used to block thyroid hormone release in severe thyrotoxicosis.
3. Propranolol 2.0 mg/kg/day in divided doses 6–8 hourly may be added to reduce sympathetic stimulation.
4. Complications such as arrhythmias, heart failure, infection, and fever may require specific measures.
5. Antithyroid treatment can generally be withdrawn cautiously after 6–24 weeks. Rapid cessation of treatment has been associated with fatal recurrence.

Thyroid crisis (Mackin, Canary and Pittman, 1974)

Thyrotoxic patients of any age exposed to a precipitating factor such as infection, trauma, surgery, or diabetic ketoacidosis may develop an acute exacerbation of symptoms, so-called thyroid 'crisis' or 'storm'. This complication is often fatal but is increasingly rare, probably because it is more likely to occur in uncontrolled disease which is now seldom seen. The pathogenesis is poorly understood but may be related to dissociation of thyroid hormones from their carrier proteins.

Recognition

There are progressive symptoms of fever, tachycardia, sweating, vomiting and diarrhoea, prostration, and confusion leading to hyperpyrexia and death.

Management

Treatment should aim to control the hypermetabolic state and remove the precipitating cause, and is similar to that for neonatal thyrotoxicosis:

1. Propylthiouracil is the antithyroid drug of choice because in addition to its actions on the thyroid, it inhibits peripheral conversion of thyroxine to tri-iodothyronine. The standard initial dose of 150 mg/m^2/day may be increased up to 600 mg/m^2/day given in divided doses as crushed tablets by nasogastric tube 4–6 hourly. This should be given 1 or 2 hours before iodide to avoid synthesis and storage of a large quantity of hormone in the iodine depleted gland.
2. Intravenous sodium iodide as a continuous infusion giving 1–2 g/day.
3. Intravenous propranolol 0.1 mg/kg up to a maximum of 5 mg 6 hourly giving one quarter of the dose every 10 minutes to four doses. Careful monitoring and the ability to undertake cardiac pacing are necessary. The oral dose is 4 mg/kg/day.
4. Dexamethasone 1–2 mg 6 hourly intravenously.
5. Cooling, O_2, treatment of heart failure and/or dehydration.
6. Measures to control infection, ketoacidosis or other precipitating cause.
7. Plasmapheresis or exchange transfusion have been recommended to remove thyroid hormone.

References

FISHER, D. A. (1976) Pathogenesis and therapy of neonatal Graves' disease. *American Journal of Diseases of Children,* **130,** 133–134

MACKIN, J. F., CANARY, J. J. and PITTMAN, C. S. (1974) Thyroid storm and its management. *New England Journal of Medicine,* **291,** 1396–1398

Further reading

KAPLAN, S. (ed.) (1982) *Clinical Pediatric and Adolescent Endocrinology.* Philadelphia: W. B. Saunders

HERSHMAN, J. A. and BRAY, G. A. (eds) (1979) *The Thyroid: Physiology and Treatment of Disease.* Oxford: Pergamon Press

Part XI

Haematological emergencies

Chapter 54

Haematological emergencies

Judith M. Chessells

Sudden anaemia in childhood (Table 54.1)

(*See* Chapter 84 for Anaemia in the newborn infant)

Recognition

The symptoms depend on the rate of development of the anaemia. If this is rapid, as a result of blood loss or sudden haemolysis, the child may become acutely ill with pallor, tachycardia, and shock. A slower onset over days or weeks may result in

Table 54.1 Sudden anaemia in childhood – clues to the cause

Blood film	*Possible causes*	*Further investigations*
Microspherocytes	Congenital spherocytosis. Autoimmune haemolytic anaemia	Family studies. Osmotic fragility. Direct antiglobulin test. Red cells (in ACD) and serum for investigation
Thalassaemic film	Hb H disease. Other thalassaemias unlikely to cause *acute* anaemia	Reticulocyte preparation (Hb H). Electrophoresis, F and A_2. Family studies
Fragmentation: reduced platelets	Haemolytic uraemic syndrome	Clotting studies. Fibrin degradation products. Urea, creatinine, electrolytes
Shrunken cells (not invariable)	G-6PD deficiency	Enzyme assay
Sickled forms: target cells	Sickle-cell anaemia	Electrophoresis, F and A_2
Reduced platelets, neutropenia ± blast cells	Leukaemia. Aplastic anaemia	Bone marrow
No diagnostic features. WBC and platelets normal. Low reticulocytes	Congenital haemolytic anaemia in aplastic crisis. Pure red-cell aplasia	Assay enzymes, e.g. pyruvate kinase; test for unstable Hb. Bone marrow
Severe hypochromia	Iron deficiency ± thalassaemia trait	Serum iron and total iron-binding capacity. Serum ferritin. Electrophoresis, F and A_2

pallor, lethargy, and anorexia, progressing in extreme instances to congestive cardiac failure. Recognition and assessment of anaemia are notoriously difficult without a haemoglobin estimation, and the diagnosis of chronic anaemia may be made only when a child presents with incidental symptoms, e.g. respiratory infection. Other symptoms such as bruising or limb pains are referable to the cause of the anaemia, e.g. marrow infiltration.

The causes of sudden anaemia

Acute blood loss

1. Obvious: gastrointestinal (*see* Chapter 42, pages 386–389).
2. Not obvious: internal haemorrhage (*see* page 93).

Failure of red cell production

This may occur *de novo* or in patients with a pre-existing haemolytic anaemia. The role of parvovirus has recently been reviewed in this disorder (Davis, 1983). Anaemia usually becomes apparent over days rather than hours. An aplastic crisis may be the presenting feature of hereditary spherocytosis and may complicate most haemolytic anaemias due to enzyme deficiencies. There is a resultant drop in the haemoglobin and reticulocytes; white cells and platelets are not usually affected. Examination of the child shows only pallor and sometimes splenomegaly.

An aplastic crisis may occur in sickle-cell anaemia, and in young children sequestration of cells in the reticuloendothelial system may cause sudden anaemia. The unstable haemoglobins are a rare group of disorders inherited as an autosomal dominant and characterized by congenital non-spherocytic anaemia of variable severity, often associated with splenomegaly. They may be complicated by episodes of red cell aplasia or drug induced haemolysis. Sudden anaemia is uncommon in the thalassaemias except for Hb H disease. Most children with homozygous β-thalassaemia present with chronic anaemia, hepatosplenomegaly, and growth failure after the first few months of life; occasionally the diagnosis is not made until heart failure from anaemia occurs. Children with severe iron deficiency occasionally present as an emergency, usually with an incidental infection. Occasionally a previously normal child may present with anaemia due to *transient* red cell aplasia. This must be distinguished from the true congenital red cell aplasia (Diamond–Blackfan anaemia). Both present with anaemia with reticulocytopenia, the diagnosis being confirmed on bone marrow examination.

Acute leukaemia may present as anaemia alone; there may be no symptoms suggestive of thrombocytopenia or infection but usually some other clinical clue is present, e.g. limb pains. Children with *aplastic* anaemia invariably have bruising, or symptoms referable to neutropenia.

Acute haemolysis

This, especially when intravascular, can be very rapid in onset and cause a shock-like picture resembling haemorrhage or septicaemia. Common causes include:

G6PD deficiency (*see below*)

Oxidant drugs (*see Table 54.3*) may also cause an exacerbation of haemolysis in patients with Hb H disease and unstable haemoglobins. Autoimmune haemolytic anaemia in children often follows an acute infection and may cause intravascular haemolysis and haemoglobinuria. Sudden pallor is often a symptom of the haemolytic uraemic syndrome; the diagnosis should be suggested by the previous history and the finding of fragmentation and thrombocytopenia in the blood film. The possibility of malaria should be considered in patients who have been abroad; thick and thin films should be examined.

Management

1. Blood should be taken for Hb, PCV, film, WBC and differential, platelets, reticulocyte count, direct antiglobulin (Coombs') test, blood grouping, and cross-matching, urea and electrolytes. The results of Hb or PCV and blood film should be available within 30 minutes and may give a clue as to the cause of the anaemia and the further investigations indicated (*see Table 54.1*). If a transfusion is indicated and no diagnosis had been made, blood should be taken into EDTA tubes and a sample of serum saved to facilitate subsequent investigation.
2. Urine must be saved to examine for haemoglobinuria, and stools for evidence of blood loss.
3. Transfusion of blood should be given as necessary. Cross-matching of blood should present no problems but in autoimmune haemolytic anaemia transfusion may be necessary as a life-saving measure despite apparent incompatibility of all cross-matched blood. *If possible seek advice from the regional centre before transfusing* in these circumstances.
4. Further management depends on the cause of the anaemia.
   (a) A bone marrow examination is indicated if there is suspicion of pure red-cell aplasia, leukaemia, or aplastic anaemia.
   (b) A list of drugs to be avoided (*see Table 54.3*) should be given to the parents and family doctor of patients with G6PD deficiency, unstable Hb and Hb H disease.
   (c) Folic acid supplementation is desirable in all chronic haemolytic anaemias.
   (d) In autoimmune haemolytic anaemia arrangements should be made to identify the antibody. In many children haemolysis is complement mediated and no antibody can be detected; such cases recover very rapidly and no specific therapy may be required. In most patients treatment with prednisolone (2 mg/kg/day) is indicated.

Glucose-6-phosphate dehydrogenase deficiency (G6PD)

This is the commonest red-cell enzyme deficiency, affecting many millions of people and present in all ethnic groups, particularly in West Africa, West Indies, the Mediterranean, the Middle East, Thailand and parts of China. The gene is carried on the X chromosome and thus carrier females have intermediate levels of G6PD activity although deficiency, with symptoms, in females is not uncommon. G6PD deficiency is a heterogeneous condition genetically and clinically, and results in varying degrees of enzyme deficiency as assayed in the laboratory, and variable haemolysis in response to oxidant stress. Patients with G6PD deficiency have normal Hb values and slightly reduced red cell survival but, following oxidant stress to the red cell, may become acutely anaemic and jaundiced. The usual source of oxidant stress is a drug (*see Table 54.3*) but haemolysis may also be precipitated by infection and acidosis.

The genetic variant of G6PD found in African patients (A−) is associated with enzyme levels of 5–15 per cent but young red cells and reticulocytes have normal G6PD levels. Hence haemolysis tends to be self-limiting. Patients with the Mediterranean and Far Eastern variants have lower enzyme levels (0–15 per cent) and even young cells have diminished enzyme activity, thus haemolysis is more severe (*Table 54.2*).

Table 54.2 Features of G6PD deficiency

Feature	*African*	*Mediterranean and Far East*
Enzyme levels	5–15%	0–5%
Neonatal haemolysis	? Pre-term infants	Yes
Drug induced haemolysis	Yes	Yes
Favism	No	Sometimes
Severity of haemolysis	Often self-limited	May be fatal

Recognition

Neonatal jaundice (see Chapter 85)

Neonatal jaundice occurring usually after the first day of life is uncommon in Negro (A−) deficiency except in pre-term babies, but common in the Mediterranean and Far Eastern forms. It is often not possible to identify a precipitating factor.

Acute haemolytic anaemia

This usually occurs 3–36 hours after drugs. In Negro patients jaundice haemoglobinuria and haemolysis are self-limited but the more profound haemolysis in Mediterranean patients and in those from the Far East may cause collapse and severe anaemia.

Favism

Rapid intravascular haemolysis may be triggered in some patients with Mediterranean and Far East deficiencies after eating the broad bean (*Vicia faba*) or inhaling its pollen. The offending agent has not been identified and the reason for varying susceptibility to this condition is not clear.

Chronic haemolytic anaemia

This may occur in rare Caucasian variants.

Diagnosis

Deficiency of G6PD should be considered among the causes of acute anaemia in a previously well child. The blood count shows anaemia with normal platelets and possibly a raised white-cell count. The film may show irregular cells in which the haemoglobin appears shrunk away from the cell membrane (diagnostic of a crisis due to G6PD deficiency). Heinz bodies may be seen in the recovery phase.

Drug-induced haemolysis may also occur in Hb H disease and in patients with unstable haemoglobins.

The diagnosis is confirmed by enzyme assay; screening tests may give false negative results, particularly when there is a reticulocytosis in the recovery phase. Blood taken into EDTA will keep at 4°C for several days.

Management

1. Acute haemolysis may necessitate urgent blood transfusion, particularly in Mediterranean and Far Eastern variants.
2. The patients should be given a list of drugs and chemicals to be avoided (*Table 54.3*).

Table 54.3 Agents commonly associated with haemolysis in G6PD deficiency, Hb H disease, and unstable haemoglobins

Anti-malarials:	Chloroquine, primaquine, pamaquine, and quinacrine (Mepacrine).
Analgesics:	Aspirin, phenacetin, acetanilide.
Antibacterial compounds:	Sulphonamides (including co-trimoxazole compounds such as Septrin and Bactrim) and sulphones. Nitrofurantoin, chloramphenicol.
Others:	Vitamin-K analogues, methylene blue, benzene, and naphthalene (moth repellant). Broad beans (*Vicia faba*) in Mediterranean and Far Eastern variants. Acute infections. Diabetic ketoacidosis.*

* Recent evidence suggests that, at least in the Mediterranean variant, diabetic ketoacidosis alone does not precipitate haemolysis (Shaler, Wollver and Menczel. (1984). *British Medical Journal* **288**: 179–180). However, infection as a precipitating cause for haemolysis may also be the reason for the development of the diabetic ketoacidosis.

Sickle-cell disease

Sickle-cell disease is a chronic haemolytic anaemia punctuated by episodes of crisis. The definition includes sickle-cell anaemia, (SS disease), Hb S/β-thalassaemia and Hb S/C disease. Possession of the sickle-cell trait does *not* cause problems except in conditions of severe hypoxia. The diagnosis of sickle-cell disease must be confirmed by haemoglobin electrophoresis and family studies. A blood count and sickling test will not distinguish between sickle-cell trait and conditions with a near normal Hb (e.g. S/C disease).

NOTE: The sickle-cell gene occurs in West Indies, Greece, parts of India and the Middle East as well as in Africa.

Infarctive crises

Intravascular sickling can cause a multiplicity of symptoms. In this type of crisis there is usually *no drop* in the Hb level (6–10 g/100 ml).

Recognition

In infants, pallor, infection, or painful swelling of the dorsum of the hands and feet are common. Older children may have pain in the limbs, chest, back or abdomen often with prostration and fever. The pains may be diffuse and generalized or localized and must be distinguished from osteomyelitis. Prolonged pulmonary episodes resemble pneumonia. Less common problems are priapism, headache, meningisms, cerebrovascular symptoms, haematuria, haemoptysis.

Management

1. Identify and treat any precipitating cause, e.g. infection.
2. Warmth, rest and analgesics (remembering the risk of addiction).
3. Adequate hydration with IV 5% glucose if necessary.
4. There are no specific measures of proved benefit but in a very severe crisis partial exchange transfusion may be indicated.

NOTE: Patients with sickle-cell anaemia are usually unable to concentrate their urine, and may unexpectedly become dehydrated during an acute illness.

Aplastic crisis

Recognition

Sudden increase in pallor may occur in more than one member of a family. A blood count shows a fall in Hb and reticulocyte count.

Management

Transfusion with packed cells.

Sequestration crisis

Recognition

A catastrophic fall in the Hb results from pooling of blood in the reticuloendothelial system. This is particularly common in young children and may be precipitated by pneumococcal infection. Patients may present *in extremis* with enlarged liver and spleen.

Management

Urgent transfusion of packed cells is required. Treatment should be the same as for pneumococcal septicaemia (*see below*).

Haemolytic crisis

True haemolytic crises are uncommon and must be distinguished from hepatitis, gallstones, and coexistent G6PD deficiency. Look for evidence of infection with *Mycoplasma pneumoniae*.

Infections in sickle-cell anaemia

Infection with pneumococcus is particularly common in young children with sickle-cell anaemia who may die rapidly from meningitis or septicaemia. Any acute febrile illness should be promptly treated with benzylpenicillin. The patients are also particularly susceptible to salmonella osteomyelitis which must be distinguished from a painful crisis. Prophylactic penicillin or pneumococcal vaccine should be considered in these patients.

Prevention of crises

It is important to maintain good general health by adequate housing and nutrition, avoidance of chilling, and regular folic acid supplementation. There are no more specific measures available at present.

Acute leukaemia

Recognition

Common presentations of acute leukaemia include sudden or gradual anaemia, limb pains, bruising, acute infection. On examination there is usually enlargement of lymph nodes, liver, and spleen; signs of complications may or may not be present. An uncommon presentation in older children (usually boys) is with a mediastinal mass, sometimes with respiratory obstruction and pleural effusion.

Differential diagnosis

1. Other haematological disorders, e.g. idiopathic thrombocytopenia (ITP), aplastic anaemia.
2. Disseminated malignancy, e.g. neuroblastoma.
3. Musculoskeletal disorders, e.g. Still's disease (juvenile rheumatoid arthritis), osteomyelitis.

Investigation

Except in children with a high white cell count ($>100 \times 10^9/\ell$) who are at risk from intracranial haemorrhage and leucostasis, or those with mediastinal obstruction, treatment of leukaemia itself is not an emergency, but *prevention and treatment of complications should start at once.*

Blood should be taken for Hb, WBC and differential count, film, platelet count and blood group. Serum is saved for cross-matching. Blood should also be saved for uric acid estimation. Chest X-rays, postero-anterior and lateral, should be taken.

Within the next 24–48 hours a bone marrow specimen should be examined *before* starting antileukaemic drugs. If necessary, films can be made and left unfixed and unstained for 2–3 days. Occasionally it is impossible to aspirate marrow, and a trephine biopsy of bone is needed.

Before starting antileukaemic drugs, blood is also taken for urea and electrolytes, plasma proteins, and liver-function tests. If possible a sample of blood and bone marrow should be sent for immunological classification and for cytogenetic analysis.

Management

The management of infection and bleeding is discussed below. Packed cells are given as necessary for anaemia. Allopurinol 50–100 mg should be given by mouth three times daily, and adequate hydration must be ensured to prevent uric acid nephropathy; this is especially important in children with a large leukaemic cell mass. If there is doubt about the type of leukaemia, treat at first as for lymphoblastic leukaemia.

Initial treatment of lymphoblastic leukaemia (Table 54.4)

Patients with acute lymphoblastic leukaemia should preferably be treated in consultation with a special centre. The combination of prednisolone and vincristine, as detailed below, will achieve remission in most patients but more intensive therapy with additional drugs (e.g. anthracyclines and L-asparaginase) is strongly recommended, as improving the chances of prolonged remission.

Prednisolone 40–60 mg/m^2/day orally in 2–3 doses daily.

Vincristine 1.5 mg/m^2 intravenously (to be repeated at weekly intervals for 4 or 5 doses). A laxative is given to avoid the constipating effects of vincristine.

Initial treatment of myeloblastic leukaemia

Children with myeloblastic leukaemia should be referred to a special centre for treatment. If this is impossible the DAT regimen is recommended:

1. Thioguanine 100 mg/m^2 12 hourly by mouth for 5 days (10 doses).
2. Daunorubicin 50 mg/m^2 intravenously on day 1.
3. Cytosine arabinoside 100 mg/m^2 IV 12 hourly for 5 days (10 doses).

This combination is repeated approximately every 1–2 weeks depending on treatment response.

MORE PROBLEMS ARISE FROM PARTIAL TREATMENT OF PATIENTS IN WHOM PROPER DIAGNOSIS AND ASSESSMENT HAVE NOT BEEN MADE, THAN FROM DELAYING ANTILEUKAEMIC TREATMENT FOR A FEW DAYS TO SEEK A SPECIALIST OPINION ABOUT DIAGNOSIS AND MANAGEMENT.

Complications during remission induction

Haemorrhage

This is usually due to thrombocytopenia. Platelet concentrates should be given in a dose of 5 units/m^2 but more liberally in the presence of infection.

Bleeding may also be due to disseminated intravascular coagulation (DIC), particularly in children with the hypergranular promyelocytic variant of myeloid leukaemia. DIC tends to be exacerbated by the start of antileukaemic therapy. Management includes liberal use of platelet concentrates, treatment of any infection present and occasionally heparin therapy.

Leucostasis

Children with a high leucocyte count ($>200 \times 10^9/\ell$) may develop symptoms of cerebral leucostasis, particularly if transfused rapidly with red cells. Give platelets

Table 54.4 Drugs used in acute leukaemia

Drug	*Trade name*	*Route(s) of administration*	*Toxicity*					
			Bone marrow	*Nausea/ vomiting*	*Gastrointestinal*	*CNS*	*Alopecia*	*Other*
Vincristine	Oncovin	IV*	±	–	Constipation ileus	Neuropathy, convulsions	+	–
6-Mercaptopurine (6-MP)	Puri-Nethol	Oral	++†	+	Jaundice	–	–	–
Thioguanine	Lanvis	Oral	++	+	Jaundice	–	–	–
Methotrexate	Methotrexate	Oral, i.m., IV, IT	+	+	Mouth ulcers, diarrhoea hepatitis	Arachnoiditis (IT), encephalopathy	–	Photosensitivity, pneumonitis, osteoporosis
Cyclophosphamide	Endoxana	Oral, IV	++	++	–	–	+	Haemorrhagic cystitis
Daunorubicin	Cerubidin	IV*	+++	++	–	–	+	Cardiotoxic
Doxorubicin	Adriamycin	IV*	+++	++	'Mucositis'	–	+	Cardiotoxic
Cystosine arabinoside (cytarabine)	Cytosar	Oral, s.c., i.m., IV, IT	+++	+++	–	–	–	–
Colaspase (L-asparaginase)	Crasnitin	IV, s.c., i.m.	+	+	Hepatitis, pancreatitis	Confusion	–	Hypofibrinogenaemia, anaphylaxis

* These drugs are sclerosant if they leak outside the vein.
† 6-MP dose should be quartered if given with allopurinol.
± = Infrequent; +++ = marked.

and avoid red cell transfusion if possible until the leucocyte count has dropped. In extreme cases leucophoreses (with continuous flow blood cell separation) or partial exchange transfusion may be indicated.

Bacterial infection

This is particularly serious when children are neutropenic ($<0.5 \times 10^9/\ell$); this is usually at presentation or in relapse. The classic signs of infection are often absent and prompt investigation and treatment are essential. Common organisms include: staphylococci, *E. coli, Pseudomonas aeruginosa.* The neutropenic child with sustained pyrexia should have cultures of blood, nose, throat, urine, rectum, any skin lesions, and a chest X-ray, also lumbar puncture if clinically indicated. Empirical antibiotic therapy should be started, and as no oral combination is effective against the organisms likely to be responsible for infection, broad-spectrum *intravenous* antibiotics should be used. Initially a combination of gentamicin 6–8 mg/kg/day with piperacillin or mezlocillin is a suitable regimen. These antibiotics should be given separately at 8-hourly intervals. The treatment is reviewed as soon as results of cultures become available at 24 and 48 hours. The gentamicin levels at 24 hours should be measured to ensure adequate dosage. Blood creatinine and electrolytes should also be estimated if continued long-term antibiotic treatment is necessary.

Metabolic problems

Patients with a large cell mass are at risk of early metabolic problems (hyperkalaemia, hypocalcaemia) and late urate nephropathy. Ensure adequate urine output with IV glucose saline and monitor for hyperkalaemia.

Problems during remission

Minor infections should be treated in the usual way with antibiotics if indicated; it is not usually necessary to stop antileukaemic drugs.

Live virus vaccines should not be given. Toxoids or killed vaccines may be given if necessary but their efficacy is uncertain. Patients should avoid contact with chickenpox and measles. Zoster immune globulin (dose 250–750 mg) should be given as soon as possible after chickenpox contact. Acyclovir is given IV 1.5 g/m^2/day in three divided doses, i.e. 500 mg/m^2/dose. For oral use, 2.4 g/m^2/day in four divided doses, i.e. 600 mg/m^2 per dose 6-hourly) is effective in patients who develop varicella zoster and should be started promptly in children on cytotoxics who develop severe shingles or chickenpox unmodified by zoster immune globulin. Children who have been in contact with measles should receive immune globulin (0.25 ml/kg i.m. on two consecutive days).

Pneumonia in remission may be due to measles virus, pneumocystis carinii, or especially in marrow transplant recipients, cytomegalovirus. Cytotoxic drugs should be stopped and samples sent for virological and bacteriological investigation. Cough, tachypnoea, silent chest with bilateral X-ray infiltration is suggestive of pneumocystis carinii pneumonia. Treatment should be started with trimethoprim–sulfamethoxazole (co-trimoxazole, Bactrim, Septrin) 20 mg trimethoprim, 100 mg sulfamethoxazole/kg/day in two 12-hourly doses by mouth). If there is no improvement after 48 hours and results of viral immunofluorescence do not establish a diagnosis (e.g. measles) then lung biopsy should be considered.

The CNS in leukaemia

Leukaemic infiltration

This occurs in about 5 per cent *despite* routine prophylaxis. Clinical features include: headache, vomiting, giddiness, papilloedema, and undue weight gain. These findings warrant lumbar puncture with measurement of CSF pressure. The CSF specimen is saved for cytology, and methotrexate (intrathecal preparation) is given in a dose of 10 mg/m^2 (maximum dose 12 mg) intrathecally. This can be repeated at weekly intervals until the CSF is clear. The diagnosis must be confirmed by the presence of *blast cells* in the CSF; if they are not found other causes of CNS disease must be considered or excluded.

Convulsions

These are an uncommon symptom of CNS infiltration. Other causes include haemorrhage (in relapsed patients), vincristine and methotrexate toxicity, and encephalitis. Dystonic reactions from extrapyramidal symptoms due to phenothiazines must be distinguished from a convulsion. Fits should be controlled with anticonvulsants; a lumbar puncture should be done and the CSF specimen saved for cytology.

Progressive neurological deterioration

This may be due to drug encephalopathy, post-infective encephalomyelitis (measles, mumps, herpes simplex), or progressive multifocal leucoencephalopathy. Advice should be sought about further investigation rather than assuming that the symptoms are due to CNS infiltration.

Haematological relapse

Recognition

This may be diagnosed on routine marrow examination or suspected from symptoms like those at presentation, e.g. limb pain.

A fall in the blood count (especially platelets) may be due *either* to relapse or drug toxicity.

Management

If the only feature is a fall in the blood count it is reasonable to do without antileukaemic drugs for a few days and to repeat the count. Other features warrant marrow aspiration as soon as convenient. Complications are treated as at presentation but remembering that the chances of long-term remission are slender in children who relapse on modern combination chemotherapy.

Acute thrombocytopenia

For thrombocytopenia in the newborn infant, *see* page 677.

Recognition

A sudden onset of bruising in a previously well child who has not been traumatized is usually due to idiopathic thrombocytopenic purpura (ITP) (*see Table 54.5* for differential diagnosis). Inquiry should be made about recent viral infections and drug ingestion. Bruising in ITP may be widespread and accompanied by palatal petechiae and mucous membrane haemorrhage. Other signs are uncommon. The absence of anaemia, limb pains, lymphadenopathy and hepatosplenomegaly distinguish ITP from leukaemia. Acute aplastic anaemia usually causes anaemia and infection. The child with DIC is ill from the underlying cause (usually infection). The distribution and type of rash distinguish ITP from anaphylactoid (Henoch–Schoenlein) purpura.

Table 54.5 Thrombocytopenia in childhood

Mechanism	*Bone marrow*	*Examples*
Decreased platelet production	Megakaryocytes, decreased or absent	Aplastic anaemia,* leukaemia,* disseminated malignancy
Excessive destruction of platelets	Megakaryocytes, normal or increased	Postinfective, e.g. rubella, varicella, infectious mononucleosis. Idiopathic,* drug-induced,* Systemic lupus erythematosus
Utilization of platelets	Megakaryocytes, normal or increased	Disseminated or localized intravascular coagulation.*
Splenic pooling of platelets	Megakaryocytes, normal	Portal hypertension, thalassaemia, Gaucher's disease

* Acute onset common.

Investigations

The diagnosis of ITP is confirmed by the following.

Full blood count and film

The results should be made available within the hour. In ITP the only abnormal result usually is a low platelet count (unless substantial blood loss has occurred). Abnormal mononuclear cells may be seen in postviral thrombocytopenia, e.g. infectious mononucleosis.

Bone marrow aspiration

This should be arranged within the next 24–48 hours if there is any doubt about the diagnosis because although leukaemia and marrow failure are unlikely in the presence of a normal Hb and film they cannot be excluded with certainty. NEVER give steroid drugs to a child with ITP without previous bone marrow examination.

Management

ITP in children is a benign condition. If bruising has been sudden in onset, or is severe, admission to hospital for observation and restriction of activity is warranted. A short (2–3 weeks) course of steroids (prednisolone 2 mg/kg/daily) may be indicated in children with extensive mucous membrane bleeding but prolonged steroid therapy should be avoided. Alternatively, in cases with severe bruising a course of IV immunoglobulin (Sandoglobulin) 400 mg/kg/day should be given in three consecutive days. The use of immunoglobulin in ITP has recently been reviewed by Imbach (1985) and Blanchette (1985). Occasionally blood transfusion is needed for epistaxis or gastrointestinal bleeding. Platelet concentrates are ineffective since infused platelets are rapidly destroyed.

Haemophilia and related disorders

Previously undiagnosed patients

Recognition

Haemophilia (factor VIII deficiency) and Christmas disease (factor IX deficiency) are clinically indistinguishable, and one-third of patients have no family history of bleeding. Presenting features of both depend on the levels of factor VIII or IX. Severely affected boys present late in the first year with bleeding from tongue or mouth, lumpy bruises, and muscle bleeds. Haemarthroses are common after age 2–3 years. Mild cases bleed after trauma, surgery, or dental extraction. Neonatal bleeding is uncommon except after circumcision or trauma.

Von Willebrand's disease is inherited as an autosomal dominant; the usual symptoms are epistaxis and mucous membrane bleeding.

Investigations

An atraumatic venepuncture with citrated blood sample filling the bottle is needed. DO NOT puncture femoral or jugular veins or cut down on veins in children with suspected bleeding diathesis. *See Table 54.6* for results of emergency screening tests which should be available within the hour. Plasma that is saved must be deep frozen for further investigations. The partial thromboplastin time with kaolin (PTTK) is

Table 54.6 Screening tests of haemostasis

Condition	*Platelet count*	*Screening test*			
		PT	*PTTK*	*TT*	*BT*
Haemophilia	N	N	ABN	N	N
Christmas disease	N	N	ABN	N	N
Von Willebrand's disease	N	N	ABN	N	ABN
Fibrinogen deficiency	N	ABN	ABN	ABN	ABN
ITP	ABN	N	N	N	*
DIC	ABN	ABN	ABN	ABN	†

N = Normal result; ABN = result usually abnormal; PT = prothrombin time;
PTTK = partial thromboplastin time with kaolin; TT = thrombin time; BT = bleeding time.
* Test not usually indicated in thrombocytopenic patients.
† See text for additional tests.

prolonged in all save mild deficiency of factors VIII and IX but does *not* distinguish between them. For this *assays* are essential. If these cannot be obtained, mixing tests will distinguish between haemophilia and Christmas disease; fresh frozen plasma is the *only* therapeutic material containing both factor VIII and factor IX.

Management of bleeding episodes

Recognition

Haemarthroses are most common in the knee, elbow, and ankle joints; acute bleeds are very painful. Muscle bleeds can occur in limbs (especially the forearm), or abdomen (mimicking appendicitis). Older boys may complain of pain or discomfort in a joint which should be treated as a bleed even in the absence of signs. Haematuria is common in older boys.

Management

Treatment is urgent because delay can result in permanent joint damage or injury to nerves and blood vessels.

IF IN DOUBT TREAT AS A BLEED

Adequate levels of the missing clotting factor must be achieved by prompt intravenous infusion (preferably via 'butterfly' needle) of an adequate amount of the appropriate replacement material. Everything else is of secondary importance.

Haemophilia

Example of dose calculation

A 30 kg boy has a severe haemarthrosis. To raise his factor VIII level to 40 per cent requires 30 × 20 = 600 units of factor VIII. This will have to be given as concentrate *or* cryoprecipitate. One bag of *cryoprecipitate* contains on average about 60 units of factor VIII, so the estimated dose is 10 bags.

Table 54.7 Treatment of haemophilia (factor VIII deficiency)

Type of bleed	*Desirable level after treatment (% normal)*	*Level 24 hours later (% normal)*	*Dose of factor VIII (units/kg body weight)**
Spontaneous bleed Early haemarthrosis	20	5	10–15
Major haemarthrosis	40	10	15–30
Serious accident (major surgery)	100	25	55–70

* 1 unit of factor VIII = amount of factor VIII present in 1 ml fresh normal citrated plasma.
For treatment of Christmas disease *see* text.

Christmas disease

Early bleeds can be treated with fresh frozen plasma 10–15 ml/kg infused as rapidly as possible *or* factor IX concentrate 10–15 units/kg. More severe bleeds require a dose of 40–50 units/kg which must be given as concentrate.

Von Willebrand's disease

Treatment with fresh frozen plasma or cryoprecipitate results in a prolonged rise in factor VIII level.

These instructions for the treatment of haemophilia, Christmas disease and von Willebrand's disease are based on estimations of dose and in any complicated bleed treatment *must* be monitored by factor VIII/IX assay (*see* 'when to seek help' below).

The early complications of treatment

Circulatory overload limits the use of fresh frozen plasma. Allergic reactions to plasma and cryoprecipitate can result in pyrexia, urticarial rash, abdominal pain, and headache. Bronchospasm can occur in severe reactions. These complications should be treated with intravenous antihistamines (e.g. chlorpheniramine 5–10 mg); in severe reactions intravenous hydrocortisone and subcutaneous adrenaline may be necessary. In children who react to cryoprecipitate, the injection should be 'covered' by giving antihistamines beforehand orally or intravenously with the plasma.

Pain

This is relieved by prompt treatment. Severe bleeds may necessitate analgesics but NEVER give aspirin; the risk of addiction must be kept in mind. DO NOT give intramuscular injections.

Admission to hospital

This is not usually needed for early bleeds. Some indications for admission include: established haemarthrosis of knee or ankle, risk to nerve or blood supply (e.g. a large forearm bleed), head and mouth injuries, suspected intra-abdominal bleeding, and wounds requiring suturing.

Rest

Initially the limb must be rested. The arm should be elevated in a forearm bleed.

Further replacement therapy

This is given according to the type and severity of the bleed. One infusion is often enough for early haemarthroses or minor bleeds. The half-life of factor VIII is 12 hours, so treatment twice daily is needed to achieve high enough levels for surgery or following head injury. The half-life of transfused factor IX is about 18 hours so daily treatment is usually adequate.

When to seek help

In any complicated case treatment should be monitored by assay of clotting factors. Advice is available from designated haemophilia centres at all times. Surgical procedures even in the mild haemophiliac should *only* be carried out at such centres.

Disseminated intravascular coagulation

Recognition

Disseminated intravascular coagulation (DIC) occurs as a complication of disease and is not a disease in itself. It should be suspected when bruising, bleeding from venepuncture sites, or, less commonly, thrombosis, occurs in an ill child. The usual underlying cause is septicaemia (e.g. meningococcal infection) but DIC may also occur in acute leukaemia and after cardiopulmonary bypass.

Pathophysiology

Pathological activation of coagulation results in increased utilization of platelets (causing thrombocytopenia) and clotting factors (particularly V and fibrinogen). Secondary fibrinolysis results in formation of fibrin degradation products (FDP) which are in themselves anticoagulant. Fibrin deposition may be generalized or confined to one site or organ (e.g. the kidney in haemolytic–uraemic syndrome or in a cavernous haemangioma). Fragmentation of red cells (micro-angiopathic haemolytic anaemia) can occur as a result of fibrin damage induced in small blood vessels and is more common in localized fibrin deposition.

Tests of haemostasis (*see Table 54.6*) will give variably abnormal results depending on the timing of blood samples, the rate of regeneration of platelets and clotting factors, and whether the stimulus to coagulation is a continuing one.

Management

Recognition and treatment of the underlying cause

The causes and differential diagnosis of DIC in the newborn are discussed elsewhere (*see* page 678 and *Table 83.1*). In older children the diagnosis of DIC is usually apparent clinically and urgent steps to investigate and treat the underlying cause (usually septicaemia) are indicated. All other considerations are of secondary importance.

Assessment of DIC

Blood should be taken for Hb, PCV, film, platelet count and screening tests of haemostasis (results available within 1–2 hours). Estimation of FDP may be available and a sample (EACA is unnecessary except in the newborn; *see* page 676) can be saved for assay of clotting factors. Fragmentation of red cells is an inconstant finding but is always marked in haemolytic–uraemic syndrome; thrombocytopenia is usual and FDPs are present but other clotting tests may be normal in this disorder.

Treatment of DIC

Treatment of DIC itself is often unnecessary since the coagulation status improves as the underlying cause of DIC is removed. If bleeding is severe replacement of platelets and fresh frozen plasma may be necessary: heparin therapy is indicated in cases with overt thrombotic complications. Heparin should be given intravenously at a dose of 25 units/kg body weight/hour as a continuous infusion or 100 units/kg every 4–6 hours as a 'push' dose. Response to therapy is judged by clinical improvement; normalization of clotting tests and platelet count is often delayed for some days and the results are masked by heparin, but the prothrombin time may shorten if previously prolonged. Laboratory control of heparin dosage is also difficult in these circumstances but the thrombin time should be checked at 12–24 hours; if this is markedly prolonged it indicates a heparin effect and protamine neutralization may be used to estimate heparin levels.

Use and availability of blood products

Whole blood

Whole blood should be used only when the patient needs both plasma and red cells, as in severe haemorrhage. It is *not* a useful source of platelets and clotting factors. Blood taken into acid citrate dextrose (ACD) or citrate phosphate dextrose (CPD) can be used for up to 21 days. Blood taken into heparin (e.g. for the neonate) should be used within 24 hours.

Packed cells

Packed cells are preferable to whole blood in treatment of anaemia. The volume in ml of packed cells needed = desired rise in grams Hb × 3 × weight in kg. For example, to raise Hb from 4 g to 8 g/100 ml in a 20 kg child, requires 4 × 3 × 20 = 240 ml packed cells.

Red cells are now usually packed by the transfusion service in a system of plastic bags; if prepared by aspiration of plasma from bottled blood they should be used at once. For patients needing repeated transfusions, washed, filtered, or frozen cells are available from some centres.

Platelet concentrates

Platelet transfusions are of use in treatment of thrombocytopenia due to marrow failure (e.g. leukaemia) but of little value in ITP. They are prepared by transfusion centres as concentrates (usually from 2 to 5 donors) and should be given within 24–48 hours of preparation (where possible give 5 units/m^2). They have a short life after transfusion (half-life: 3–4 days), and more transfusions are needed in the presence of infection. Where a cell separator is available sufficient platelets to achieve haemostasis can be obtained from one donor.

Granulocytes

Granulocytes can be obtained in sufficient numbers from normal donors only by use of a cell separator. Granulocyte transfusions should be considered in management of the febrile neutropenic patient ($<0.5 \times 10^9/\ell$) with a proven serious bacterial infection unresponsive to antibiotics. If indicated, a course of daily transfusions should be given for 4–5 days.

Fresh frozen plasma

Plasma stored at or below −20°C (−4°F) contains all clotting factors. It can be used for minor bleeds in factor VIII and IX deficiency or in bleeding due to liver disease. The dose is up to 15–20 ml/kg given as quickly as possible. Do NOT confuse with freeze–dried plasma stored at room temperature which is used only as a volume expander. Do NOT confuse with the plasma left after removal of cryoprecipitate which no longer contains factor VIII or fibrinogen.

Cryoprecipitate

Cryoprecipitate contains factor VIII and fibrinogen and is available from most transfusion centres. It is used in the treatment of haemophilia (*see* page 496). It must be stored at or below −20°C (−4°F): bags must be aspirated with care to avoid leaving much of the factor VIII activity behind. The content of factor VIII is extremely variable and should be monitored regularly.

Human AHG concentrate

Factor VIII concentrate is used in treatment of haemophilia, is freeze-dried, and of guaranteed potency. Supplies of the NHS concentrate are inadequate at present and commercial concentrate is used to treat many haemophiliacs. Concentrate is the most suitable preparation for home therapy.

Factor IX concentrate

Concentrates rich in factor IX (which also contain II, X, and sometimes VII) are made by the plasma fractionation centres at Oxford and Edinburgh and are available for treatment of Christmas disease.

Plasma protein factor (PPF)

This contains mainly albumin and is used as a volume expander or to replace protein loss. It is of no use in clotting disorders.

References

BLANCHETTE, V. S. (1985) Intravenous gamma-globulin (Sandoglobulin) therapy in the management of four patients with immune thrombocytopenia. *Vox Sanguinis,* **49,** Suppl. 1, 32–41

IMBACH, P. (1985) A Multicentre European trial of intravenous gammaglobulin in immune thrombocytopenia in childhood. *Vox Sanguinis,* **49,** Suppl. 1, 25–31

SHALEV, O., WOLLNER, A. and MENZEL, J. (1984) Diabetic ketoacidosis does not precipitate haemolysis in patients with Mediterranean variants of glucose-6-phosphate dehydrogenase deficiency. *British Medical Journal,* **288,** 179–180

Further reading

CHESSELLS, J. M. (1982) Acute lymphoblastic leukaemia. *Seminars in Hematology,* **19,** 155–171

DAVIS, L. R. (1983) Annotation. Aplastic crises in haemolytic anaemias: the role of a parvovirus-like agent. *British Journal of Haematology,* **55,** 391–393

Lancet (1983) Early infant death in sickle cell disease. *Lancet,* **i,** 1141–1142

LIGHTSEY, A. L. (1980) Thrombocytopenia in children. *Pediatric Clinics of North America,* **27,** 293–308

MONTGOMERY, R. R. and HATHAWAY, W. E. (1980) Acute bleeding emergencies. *Pediatric Clinics of North America,* **27,** 327–344

NINANE, J. and CHESSELLS, J. M. (1981) Serious infections during continuing treatment of acute lymphoblastic leukaemia. *Archives of Disease in Childhood,* **56,** 841–844

PIOMELLI, S. and VORA, S. (1981) G-6PD deficiency and related disorders of the pentose pathway. In G. D. Nathan and F. A. Oski, *Haematology of Infancy and Childhood* (2nd edn.) pp. 608–642. Philadelphia: W. B. Saunders

Part XII

Acute skin conditions

Chapter 55

Dermatological emergencies

David J. Atherton

Genuine dermatological emergencies are relatively few, but paediatricians at all levels rarely feel at ease with children presenting with possibly serious acute skin disorders, particularly when it seems difficult to make a diagnosis.

Fortunately, skin diseases generally cause surprisingly little systemic disturbance. Although the skin is of crucial importance in both fluid and thermal balance, very large areas need to be damaged before problems arise. However, serious physiological derangement can occur without being recognized, a good example being that of the collodion baby, where acute renal failure may complicate massive percutaneous fluid loss. Permanent brain damage may result from hyperpyrexia consequent upon failure of sweating in hypohidrotic ectodermal dysplasia, without anyone ever considering the diagnosis. Occasionally, other medical emergencies have a similarly unsuspected dermatological basis. A good example is cold urticaria, which may be a relatively common cause of unexplained drowning. Massive cutaneous histamine release, induced by immersion in cold water, can in this condition lead to collapse during swimming. If cold urticaria is not recognized, and the parents are not warned of its potential danger, their child may pay the price with its life.

The conditions considered in this chapter are divided into those occurring in the immediate neonatal period, and those occurring thereafter.

Emergencies in the immediate neonatal period

'Harlequin', 'collodion' babies and subsequent ichthyosis (see Table 55.1 for modes of inheritance)

Collodion babies

RECOGNITION

Occasionally babies are born encased in a collodion-like membrane. Such babies will usually go on to manifest one of a variety of ichthyoses, but in a proportion, the skin will become perfectly normal within a few months. However, there is presently no way of knowing the prognosis during the initial days of life, and, for this reason, every effort should be made to save the child.

Table 55.1 Dermatological emergencies: modes of inheritance of genetic disorders

Harlequin and collodion babies	Autosomal recessive (these are genetically distinct conditions)
Epidermolysis bullosa	Severe forms are autosomal recessive
Bullous ichthyosiform erythroderma	Autosomal dominant
Incontinentia pigmenti	X-linked dominant
Acrodermatitis enteropathica (*see under* zinc deficiency)	Autosomal recessive
Hereditary angioedema	Autosomal dominant

MANAGEMENT

The collodion membrane can cause a variety of problems. Fluid loss is particularly important. The skin may not seem wet and the fluid loss may therefore be imperceptible. Apply white soft paraffin liberally to waterproof the skin.

Inability to control heat loss is another potentially serious problem. It is best to nurse such infants in an incubator in high humidity with intravenous fluid replacement.

During the hours after birth, the collodion membrane tends to tighten and may restrict movement. The most serious result of this is interference with respiration, though in practice it is rare for genuine respiratory difficulty to occur.

Harlequin fetus

There is a very rare condition termed 'harlequin' fetus in which the enclosing membrane consists of an armour-like casing rather than the more polythene-like covering in the usual collodion baby. This condition is genetically distinct from the form of ichthyosis causing the collodion baby and is incompatible with survival. The casing tends to break up into large plates separated by raw fissures. Efforts to improve chest movement by cutting the skin are not worthwhile in view of the uniformly poor prognosis.

Bullous, erosive and postular eruptions

The variety of such eruptions can cause diagnostic problems, especially for the inexperienced.

Epidermolysis bullosa

This term covers several disorders, all characterized by mechanical fragility of the skin, from birth. The prognosis varies in the different types. Precise categorization of individual cases should be undertaken by units specializing in this work, and such infants should therefore be transferred to an appropriate unit at the earliest moment.

RECOGNITION

Neonates with epidermolysis bullosa may have an intact skin at birth but, during the next 48 hours, extensive skin loss may occur, particularly at sites of mechanical trauma such as the heels, feet and hands. Bullae developing on the trunk where the baby has been handled are especially characteristic. The mucosae are frequently affected, and oral erosions can result in major feeding problems. In some forms, death during the neonatal period is the rule, but most infants with epidermolysis bullosa will survive, and in a proportion of these the ultimate prognosis is fairly good.

MANAGEMENT

The most important aspect of management is nursing care, the principal aim being to minimize handling and other sources of skin trauma. Topical antibiotics and antiseptics should be avoided because of the dangers of percutaneous absorption. The skin should be kept clean by bathing. The best dressings are Vaseline gauze, covered with Melolin and held in place by light, conforming bandages such as Johnson and Johnson's 'J-form'. Bulky dressings on the arms and legs act as buffers against knocks.

Special soft teats with an enlarged opening are advisable for the bottle-fed infant. Spoon feeding may be necessary. The baby should be offered feeds frequently as pain may limit the volume taken on each occasion.

Since prenatal diagnosis is now available, parents with affected children must receive genetic counselling. This happens in any case if the child reaches a specialized dermatolotical unit; however, it may be overlooked if the infant dies shortly after birth.

Bullous ichthyosiform erythroderma

RECOGNITION AND MANAGEMENT

This is an unusual variety of ichthyosis. The infant is usually red at birth, and shortly afterwards separation of extensive areas of skin may occur at sites of trauma, as in epidermolysis bullosa. In fact, initial differentiation of these conditions can be difficult. Initial treatment is, however, much the same, though the mucous membranes will not be affected.

Neonatal herpes simplex (*see also* ***page 652***)

Transmission of herpes simplex virus to the neonate from the genital tract during delivery may lead to neonatal herpes simplex infection. About 50 per cent of affected infants have skin or mucosal lesions, but only in about 10 per cent will involvement be limited to these sites.

RECOGNITION

Lesions generally appear between the second and twentieth day, unless intrauterine infection has occurred, in which case lesions may be present at birth. The common type of lesion consists of isolated vesicles, but clustered lesions may also be seen. The scalp and the face are the most commonly affected sites. Occasionally, the eruption is generalized and bullous rather than vesicular, and widespread erosions may occur in the absence of obvious vesicles or bullae, leading to an appearance rather similar to epidermolysis bullosa.

Recognition of the virus is by Tzanck smear, by electron microscopy direct immunofluorescence or by tissue culture. To prepare a Tzanck smear, open a fresh vesicle, scrape the base with a sharp scalpel blade, smear the collected material onto a glass slide and dry. Examine by light microscopy after staining with Giemsa's stain, looking for characteristic syncytia of multinucleate epidermal cells.

MANAGEMENT

Treatment is with intravenous or oral acyclovir (*see* pages 653 and 845 for dosage).

Bullous impetigo and staphylococcal scalded skin syndrome (SSSS)

These conditions are not confined to the neonatal period but are particularly common at this time.

BULLOUS IMPETIGO

Bullous impetigo is caused by phage group II strains of *Staphylococcus aureus*, particularly phage type 71. Epidemics of bullous impetigo occur in neonates, due to transmission of infection in the nursery, principally by nursing or medical staff.

Recognition

In the newborn, the condition usually arises during the first week of life. The perineum, periumbilical area, and the neck creases are common sites for the initial lesions. Rapidly enlarging bullae, with thin delicate walls and a narrow red areola, contain clear fluid at first, which may become turbid or frankly purulent later. The condition may remain localized or become disseminated.

Management

Untreated, generalized bullous impetigo in the neonate is associated with a significant mortality, and serious complications include lung abscess, staphylococcal pneumonia, osteomyelitis and septicaemia. Diagnosis is by culture of blister fluid or swabs from the base of the eroded lesions. Treatment is with an appropriate anti-staphylococcal antibiotic such as fusidic acid (Fucidin) or flucloxacillin; this should be started immediately without awaiting the results of cultures.

STAPHYLOCOCCAL SCALDED SKIN SYNDROME (SSSS)

This is often incorrectly called toxic epidermal necrolysis (TEN). The latter is an entirely separate disorder, which rarely, if ever, occurs during the neonatal period. SSSS in neonates has also often been termed 'Ritter's disease', which is inappropriate as 'Ritter' is a German title of nobility, not a name. In any case, the term is best abandoned since SSSS is the same condition whether it occurs in neonates or older children.

SSSS is caused by an epidermolytic toxin elaborated by certain strains of *Staphylococcus aureus*, which reaches the skin via the circulation from a distant focus of infection, usually the middle ear, pharynx, conjunctiva, umbilicus or at the site of circumcision or herniorrhaphy. The very much greater incidence of disseminated disease in neonates is believed to reflect their less efficient metabolism and excretion of the toxin (Elias, Fritsch and Epstein, 1977).

Recognition
The first sign of the disease is a faint macular, orange-red, scarlatiniform eruption, generally occurring in association with purulent conjunctivitis or an upper respiratory tract infection. Usual sites are the central part of the face, axillae and the groins. Tenderness of the skin is an early and striking feature. The presence of impetiginous crusting around the nose and mouth is characteristic. The eruption extends rapidly, and over the next 24–48 hours turns to a more confluent deep erythema with oedema. The child is pyrexial and distressed. The surface then becomes wrinkled before starting to separate, leaving raw red erosions.

The rapid onset with marked cutaneous tenderness distinguishes SSSS from most other causes of erythroderma and skin separation in infancy. The rarity of clinically apparent bullae and the confluent nature of the eruption differentiates it from most other bullous disorders.

Diagnosis can generally be confidently made clinically. It may be extremely difficult to culture the causative *Staphylococcus*, and it must be borne in mind that the organism may not be present on the skin itself even in affected areas. Swabs should be taken from appropriate sites as listed above.

Management
Treatment is as for bullous impetigo. In severe cases, intravenous fluid therapy may be required, and attention to temperature regulation.

Recovery is usually rapid even without antibiotic therapy, though infants occasionally die in spite of such treatment.

Bullous mastocytosis

RECOGNITION

Bullae may occur as a manifestation of mastocytosis during the neonatal period. Occasionally the bullae arise on what appears to be normal skin, and in such cases the diagnosis may not be appreciated before a skin biopsy. In most cases, however, there are other clues to the diagnosis, in the form of urticarial and nodular lesions.

Diagnosis is confirmed by skin biopsy but, even then, it can be missed unless special mast cell stains are employed.

MANAGEMENT

Treatment is rarely necessary, but the child may be made more comfortable by large doses of oral antihistamines. The ultimate prognosis is very good in the majority of cases.

Incontinentia pigmenti

RECOGNITION

This is a rare condition transmitted by an X-linked dominant gene (Carney, 1976). It is presumed to be lethal to the male fetus and occurs almost exclusively in girls. The disease presents during the neonatal period, often at birth, with vesicles or pustules arranged in lines and whorls. The child is generally otherwise well. Other problems may occur in these patients including mental retardation, fits, spastic paralysis, blindness, cataracts, and partial anodontia.

Eosinophilia is a constant feature during the early stages. The skin lesions heal, to leave residual hyperpigmentation, which remains long after the vesicular or pustular phase has passed.

Most important of all in the differential diagnosis is neonatal herpes simplex. The two can be rapidly distinguished by microscopy of a stained smear of pustule contents. This will contain large numbers of eosinophils in incontinentia pigmenti.

MANAGEMENT

There is no specific treatment. The blistering phase usually ceases spontaneously within the first few weeks of life.

Sclerema neonatorum

Sclerema neonatorum is a rare disorder which generally appears during the first week of life, though it can occur at any time up to about 3 months (Warwick, Ruttenberg and Quie, 1963). It is generally considered to be a non-specific sign of grave illness and has a mortality of around 75 per cent. It occurs particularly in the premature and the small-for-dates infant. It does not occur in otherwise healthy infants, always arising during the course of one of a variety of severe illnesses, particularly pneumonia, gastroenteritis, peritonitis, congenital heart disease and other major developmental defects. Cold does not appear to be an important aetiological factor in most cases.

Recognition

The condition presents as a woody induration of the skin, starting on the buttocks, thighs or trunk and spreading rapidly and symmetrically to involve almost the whole body with the exception of the palms, soles and genitalia. The skin is hard and cold to touch, and yellowish white in colour, often with purplish mottling. It does not pit with pressure. Mobility of limbs and thorax is restricted.

The prognosis is poor, but is determined largely by the nature of the underlying disease. In infants who survive, the appearance of the skin returns to normal without long-term complications.

Management

Treatment is that of the underlying disease. Systemic corticosteroids are not effective.

Necrotizing fasciitis

This name is given to a distinctive form of cellulitis which seems to be a special problem in the neonate, though it may occur at any age (Lally *et al.*, 1984).

Recognition

In the neonate it appears to be a complication of physical birth trauma, omphalitis, or surgical procedures such as circumcision. Initially, the child develops what appears to be straightforward cellulitis. However, the child becomes disproportionately toxic and the area affected extends extremely rapidly. Bullae may appear in the centre of the affected areas followed rapidly by necrosis. Gas gangrene is excluded by the absence of tissue crepitus.

Management

A wide variety of bacteria have been associated with necrotizing fasciitis but particularly *Streptococcus pyogenes*. Antibiotic therapy appears to be of limited value in this potentially lethal situation, and the most important aspect of treatment is early surgical excision of necrotic tissue.

Congenital melanocytic naevi

Small moles are not uncommon at birth. However, occasionally babies are born with very extensive moles which are often nodular and/or hairy. These lesions do not generally lead to ill health during the neonatal period and there is usually no feeling of urgency about removing them. However, they are mentioned here because it is now widely believed that they are best treated by superficial removal during the first weeks of life. Such babies should be referred to a paediatric dermatology unit as soon as possible.

Emergencies after the immediate neonatal period

Problems with vascular naevi

There exists a wide variety of developmental vascular malformations, several of which can on occasion cause serious problems, almost always during infancy.

The Kasabach–Merritt syndrome

A better name for this condition would be the haemangioma–haemorrhage syndrome, as it consists of the association of an angiomatous naevus with thrombocytopenia and haemorrhage. The angiomatous naevi which cause this condition are generally large, single subcutaneous lesions which are generally present at birth. These angiomas characteristically occur on the neck, trunk and limbs and are rarely of the common 'strawberry' type. Haemorrhage appears initially to be a consequence of platelet sequestration and consumption of clotting factors within the vascular bed of the angioma. Activation of the fibrinolytic system leads to secondary consumption coagulopathy.

RECOGNITION

The coagulation defect nearly always becomes apparent during the first weeks of life, and is most commonly preceded by bleeding into and around the angioma itself, manifested by an increase in size, induration and by superficial ecchymoses. The resulting rapid expansion in the angioma may cause potentially lethal compression. Internal bleeding may occur at many sites and is associated with a significant mortality.

MANAGEMENT

The choice of treatment depends to a great extent on the severity of the coagulation defect and upon the presence or absence of compression. There is some evidence that systemic corticosteroids can not only reduce the size of the angioma but can also have a direct beneficial effect on the coagulation defect. Initial dosage needs to be about 3 mg/kg daily oral prednisolone. Other treatments include radiotherapy and surgical excision. If systemic corticosteroid treatment is not rapidly effective and the child appears to be in danger, referral to a special centre is advisable. In the medium term, spontaneous improvement should be anticipated (Esterley, 1983).

Diffuse neonatal haemangiomatosis

RECOGNITION

Some infants are born with multiple small angiomatous naevi of 'strawberry' type, or develop these within the first few weeks of life (Esterley *et al.*, 1984). In many such cases, the disorder is associated with analogous systemic angiomata, which may be found at many sites including the liver, gastrointestinal tract, lungs and CNS. Where such systemic lesions occur, mortality is high, death generally occurring during the first few months of life. High output cardiac failure is the commonest cause of death, usually resulting from shunting of blood in the liver. In some cases, the cutaneous component is minimal or absent. Where affected infants have survived, the angiomata have generally regressed spontaneously.

MANAGEMENT

Once high output cardiac failure becomes obvious, treatment is aimed at rapid reduction of the shunt. Oral prednisolone 2–4 mg/kg/day may cause regression of the hepatic angiomata and reversal of cardiac failure. Hepatic artery ligation, partial lobectomy or embolization may be indicated if this approach fails.

Obstruction or compression

RECOGNITION

Angiomatous naevi may cause obstructive symptoms at a variety of sites during their phase of rapid growth. The danger of obstruction must always be borne in mind when infants present with angiomata at critical sites such as the neck.

MANAGEMENT

Systemic corticosteroid treatment needs to be considered in any child in whom respiratory obstruction seems imminent. If obstruction has already occurred, laryngeal intubation or tracheostomy may be urgently required to save life.

Bullous, erosive and pustular eruptions

Pyoderma gangrenosum

RECOGNITION

Pyoderma gangrenosum is a disorder of unknown aetiology which may be the presenting symptom of a number of systemic diseases, for example ulcerative colitis (Holt, 1979). The cutaneous lesions of pyoderma gangrenosum initially take the form of pustules, boil-like lesions, or bullae. These rapidly extend with necrosis and ulceration creating what may be very large ulcers. The condition is usually painful. So much effort may be made to identify the supposed causative infectious agent that the diagnosis of pyoderma gangrenosum may be ignored. The diagnosis is, however, often a difficult one to make initially and exclusion of an infectious cause is undoubtedly important. Skin biopsy tends not be diagnostic, but histology will help to exclude some of the possible infectious causes, and simultaneously provides tissue for culture.

MANAGEMENT

Once the diagnosis is suspected, an early search for a possible underlying cause is important. Treatment of the skin lesions is with high doses of systemic corticosteroids.

Herpes simplex and eczema herpeticum

RECOGNITION (HERPES SIMPLEX)

Herpes simplex infections after the neonatal period are normally acquired from adults with herpes labialis. The most common presentation is with painful gingivo-stomatitis which may be associated with vesicular and pustular lesions around the mouth. Occasionally the site of the primary infection occurs elsewhere; vulvo-vaginitis is the commonest. The lesions initially take the form of clustered vesicles and pustules, which are often umbilicated. The roof of the vesicles or pustules is rapidly shed to produce painful ulcers.

Diagnosis is by microscopic examination of a smear (*see* page 506), by growing the virus *in vitro* in tissue culture, or by direct identification of the virus in vesicle fluid by electron microscopy or by direct immunofluorescence.

MANAGEMENT

If the symptoms warrant systemic treatment, oral or intravenous acyclovir should be given (*see* pages 653 and 845 for dosage). Careful attention should be paid to fluid intake where painful oral lesions are present.

RECOGNITION (ECZEMA HERPETICUM)

Eczema herpeticum is a variety of primary herpes simplex infection and is a specific complication of atopic eczema (Atherton and Marshall, 1982). It is perhaps not widely appreciated how commonly this occurs; although the infection may be severe it is usually mild and often overlooked. Clustered vesicles or pustules are superimposed on atopic eczema, which itself need not be severe. The clinical features are as described for other primary herpes simplex infections of the skin, but the diagnosis may not be appreciated by the inexperienced who may fail to distinguish it from a secondary staphylococcal infection of the underlying atopic eczema. The skin around the eyes is a predilection site for eczema herpeticum and the eyes themselves are at risk of corneal ulceration. In such cases, ophthalmological advice should be sought, and local acyclovir used whether or not this agent is given systemically.

Bullous impetigo and staphylococcal scalded skin syndrome (SSSS)

Bullous impetigo probably remains the commonest cause of bullae throughout childhood. Conversely, SSSS is now relatively uncommon. The clinical features of the two disorders are essentially the same at all ages (*see* page 506).

Chronic acquired bullous dermatoses

Pemphigus and pemphigoid are both exceedingly rare in childhood and are among the least common causes of blistering in children.

Dermatitis herpetiformis (DH) does occasionally occur in children but tends to present as a rather trivial, if itchy, eruption in which intact vesicles may not be a major feature.

RECOGNITION

The least unusual of the chronic acquired blistering disorders in childhood is a condition usually termed chronic bullous dermatosis of childhood (CBDC). This disorder rarely occurs during the first year of life. Thereafter, it may have its onset at any time until about the tenth year. The onset tends to be rather abrupt, with large blisters appearing suddenly and often rapidly becoming extensive. The genitalia, buttocks, and inner thighs are the common sites, as are the scalp and the perioral area of the face. Mucous membrane involvement may occur. The bullae generally arise on otherwise normal skin, and heal with post-inflammatory hyperpigmentation. Clustering of new lesions around a healing blister is rather characteristic. Lesions occur in crops over a period of months or years, but recurrences are rarely as severe as the initial attack, and eventually the disorder 'burns itself out'.

Skin biopsies in DH and CBDC tend to be difficult to distinguish, often showing little more than a rather non-specific subepidermal bulla. Accurate distinction is achieved by direct immunofluorescence which shows granular deposition of IgA in the dermal papillae in perilesional skin in DH, and linear deposition of IgA along the basement membrane zone in CBDC. Whereas gluten enteropathy (coeliac disease) is extremely common in children with DH, it does not occur in CBDC.

MANAGEMENT

Dapsone is very effective in DH; sulphapyridine is an alternative. Either dapsone or sulphapyridine control the majority of cases of CBDC (*see* page 814 (dapsone) and 832 (sulphapyridine) for dosage), but a few require prednisolone in addition.

Erythema multiforme

RECOGNITION

When erythema multiforme is severe, it tends to present with bullae. On the skin, the bullae tend to occur on dusky-red and rather urticarial plaques. Well-developed target lesions may not be obvious but, where present, are highly characteristic.

The eruption is symmetrical, and has a preference for the palms and soles, the backs of the hands and feet and the extensor surfaces of the arms and legs. In children, lesions often also occur on the face. The trunk and neck may be affected where the condition is extensive. Mucosal lesions are frequent in children, and may occur with very little or even no cutaneous involvement at all. The lips tend to become swollen, eroded and studded with haemorrhagic crusts. Erosions within the mouth may make it impossible for the child to eat or drink. The nasal mucosa, conjunctivae, anorectal and urogenital mucosae may all be affected, and constitutional symptoms such as fever, malaise, myalgia and arthralgia are not uncommon when the disorder is severe.

The term Stevens–Johnson syndrome is probably best abandoned as it is not a separate disorder, and merely denotes severe cases of bullous erythema multiforme.

In the majority of cases, the condition, though uncomfortable, is self-limiting, resolving without treatment and without sequelae, though recurrences are not uncommon. In a few patients, severe complications may occur. Eye involvement may lead to corneal ulceration, keratitis and uveitis. Serious pulmonary and renal involvement may also occur on rare occasions.

A clinical diagnosis is all that is required in the great majority of cases. The histological picture in the skin is, however, generally diagnostic.

MANAGEMENT

Treatment is mostly symptomatic. Oral hygiene is important where the mouth is affected. In such cases, intravenous fluid therapy is essential and nasogastric or parenteral nutrition require careful consideration. Ophthalmological advice should be sought where the eyes are involved. Systemic steroids probably do not affect the course of the disease and are best avoided (Rasmussen, 1976).

Many cases of erythema multiforme in childhood are precipitated either by herpes labialis or by streptococcal pharyngitis. Occasionally drugs are responsible. An underlying cause should be sought especially carefully in recurrent cases.

Toxic epidermal necrolysis (TEN)

TEN has frequently been confused in the literature with SSSS (*see* page 506). The two disorders are entirely distinct in terms of aetiology, pathology, and treatment; the only possible confusion is a clinical one. TEN is much less common in childhood than SSSS. There is, on the other hand, a much greater overlap between TEN and bullous erythema multiforme; indeed the two disorders may simply be different clinical presentations of a single pathological entity.

RECOGNITION

TEN presents in its most characteristic form as confluent necrosis of the skin leading to the formation of extensive erosions. From the diagnostic point of view it is important to distinguish TEN from SSSS because of the need to start antibiotic therapy as soon as possible in the latter. Clinical differentiation from SSSS is based firstly on the generally severe involvement of mucous membranes in TEN, whereas they are uninvolved in SSSS, and secondly on the presence of striking cutaneous tenderness in SSSS, which is largely absent in TEN. Histological distinction is very reliable. The level of cleavage in TEN is subepidermal; in SSSS it is intraepidermal. If necessary, this histological distinction can be made using a frozen section of bulla roof, one of the only indications for frozen sections in dermatology.

MANAGEMENT

Treatment with systemic corticosteroids should be avoided and probably increases the significant mortality of TEN. Symptomatic treatment should be undertaken as for bullous erythema multiforme (*see* above).

When a cause for TEN can be identified it generally appears to be a drug.

Thermal, chemical and solar burns

Thermal burns are dealt with in Chapter 4, and solar burns in Chapter 60. Diagnosis of any of these different types of burn is rarely a problem and their management is similar.

Eczematous eruptions

Leiner's syndrome

This is a rather ill-defined entity. The concept is nevertheless helpful to the clinician. Infants with extensive or universal eczema of the 'seborrhoeic' type may fail to thrive and may develop diarrhoea, which frequently appears to result from cows' milk hypersensitivity. The combination of these three features constitutes Leiner's syndrome, and is important because it carries a significant mortality. Infants presenting with this triad, or with the first two components of the triad, are often found to be immunodeficient; careful immunological appraisal is therefore essential in every case. Such infants should be referred to a specialist paediatric dermatology unit if they are well enough to be moved.

Histiocytosis X

RECOGNITION

The diagnosis of histiocytosis X should be considered in any child presenting with a rash having a 'seborrhoeic' distribution, i.e. mainly in the proximal flexures. Clinical features which should make one suspicious include any papular element to the eruption, and, particularly importantly, any petechial component. The diagnosis is frequently overlooked for many months. The child may be unwell, but this is not always so. There may be associated involvement of intraoral structures, bones, hepatosplenomegaly and other signs of systemic involvement. Suspicion of this disease should lead to referral to a specialist paediatric oncology or dermatology unit.

Zinc deficiency

Symptomatic zinc deficiency is not as unusual as frequently supposed, particularly in the first 2 years of life. It may arise as a result of acrodermatitis enteropathica, an inherited disorder of gastrointestinal zinc absorption, or may be acquired, particularly during early infancy, when it seems to be a consequence of prematurity and/or an inadequate supply of zinc in the mother's milk (Aggett *et al.*, 1980). It may also occur in older children particularly, as a consequence of inadequate zinc provision during parenteral nutrition; this is now unusual.

RECOGNITION

The child presents with persistent, gradually extending, eczematous eruption of the anogenital area and the face, where it usually starts around the mouth and nostrils. The eruption is symmetrical and often rather glazed, with marginal peeling. Diarrhoea, alopecia, and malaise tend to be rather late manifestations.

From the diagnostic point of view it is important to be aware that plasma zinc levels are not always low, even in seriously zinc deficient children.

MANAGEMENT

The best diagnostic test is a trial of oral zinc therapy; where the diagnosis is correct, one will be rewarded by a dramatic clinical response. Zinc sulphate should be given, in elixir form, in a dose of approximately 10 mg/kg daily.

Follow-up of children presenting in infancy with zinc deficiency should be undertaken by special centres.

Genetically determined metabolic disorders with skin lesions

The development of unusual skin or mucocutaneous lesions, accompanied by psychomotor retardation or regression, fits or ataxia, or acidotic breathing ('heavy breathing') requires urgent referral for biochemical investigation to the nearest unit with facilities for the investigation of rare metabolic disorders (*see also* Chapter 91).

Three conditions, all inherited as autosomal recessives, may present as follows:

1. Biotinidase deficiency (late-onset multiple carboxylase deficiency, Wolf *et al.*, 1983). The onset is usually between the ages of 3 and 10 months, with a skin rash, followed by loss of hair, fits, ataxia, and developmental delay. Deep breathing may be observed, due to a metabolic acidosis.
2. Oculocutaneous tyrosinaemia (tyrosinaemia type II, tyrosine aminotransferase deficiency) (Ney *et al.*, 1983). The onset may be as early as 2 weeks or as late as 6 months. The first symptom is usually photophobia, due to keratitis, followed by the development of tender, red, scaly lesions of the palms and soles. Psychomotor retardation, either mild or severe, may be obvious in older children.
3. Prolidase deficiency (Powell, Kurovsky and Maniscalco, 1977). Dry scaly lesions develop with ulceration and slow wound healing. Recurrent upper respiratory tract infections are usual; minor seizures may occur and mental retardation is common. The onset is usually from the age of 3–6 months.

Hereditary angioedema

Recognition

This is a very rare but potentially lethal disorder in which subcutaneous oedema may be accompanied by submucosal oedema of the respiratory and gastrointestinal tracts (Frank *et al.*, 1976). The history is generally one of recurrent localized swellings on the trunk, limbs and genitalia which do not itch and which, in contrast to ordinary urticaria, tend to last for several days. Swelling in the mouth or throat may cause difficulty with breathing, and fatal respiratory obstruction is a real danger. There is often a family history of sudden death, for which respiratory obstruction is the usual explanation. Distressing colicky abdominal pain is another characteristic symptom. The disease may start in childhood but sometimes does not become manifest until adult life.

Hereditary angioedema is transmitted by an autosomal dominant gene and affected individuals lack the enzyme C_1 esterase inhibitor, or have normal serum levels of a non-functioning enzyme.

Management

In an acute attack, rest, IV diuretics and fresh plasma may be life saving. Tracheostomy may be necessary. Inject purified C_1 esterase inhibitor if available. Long-term treatment with low dosage non-virilizing androgens such as danazol is effective in reducing the frequency and severity of attacks. As surgical procedures tend to precipitate attacks, prophylactic treatment with ε-aminocaproic acid (EACA), tranexamic acid or fresh frozen plasma should be given.

References

AGGETT, P. J., ATHERTON, D. J., MORE, J., DAVEY, J., DELVES, H. T. and HARRIES, J. T. (1980) Symptomatic zinc deficiency in a breast-fed pre-term infant. *Archives of Disease in Childhood,* **55,** 547–550

ATHERTON, D. J. and MARSHALL, W. C. (1982) Eczema herpeticum. *Practitioner,* **226,** 971–973

CARNEY, R. G. (1976) Incontinentia pigmenti. *Archives of Dermatology,* **112,** 535–542

ELIAS, P. M., FRITISCH, D. and EPSTEIN, E. H. (1977) Staphylococcal scalded skin syndrome. *Archives of Dermatology,* **113,** 207–219

ESTERLEY, N. B. (1983) Kasabach Merritt syndrome in infants. *Journal of the American Academy of Dermatologists,* **8,** 504–513

ESTERLEY, N. B., MARGILETH, A. M., KAHN, G. *et al.* (1984) The management of disseminated eruptive haemangiomata in infants. *Pediatric Dermatology,* **1,** 312–317

FRANK, M. M., GELFAND, J. A. and ATKINSON, J. P. (1976) Hereditary angioedema: the clinical syndrome and its management. *Annals of Internal Medicine,* **84,** 580–593

HOLT, P. J. A. (1979) The current status of pyoderma gangrenosum. *Clinical and Experimental Dermatology,* **4,** 509–516

LALLY, K. P., ATKINSON, J. B., WOOLLEY, M. M. and MAHOUR, G. H. (1984) Necrotizing fasciitis. *Annals of Surgery,* **199,** 101–103

NEY, D., BAY, C., SCHNEIDER, J. A., KELTS, D. and NYHAN, W. L. (1983) Dietary management of oculocutaneous tyrosinaemia in an 11-year-old child. *American Journal of Diseases of Children,* **137,** 995–1000

ORKIN, M., GOOD, R. A., CLAWSON, C. C., FISHER, I. and WINDHORST, D. B. (1970) Bullous mastocytosis. *Archives of Dermatology,* **101,** 547–564

POWELL, G. F., KUROVSKY, A. and MANISCALCO, R. M. (1977) Prolidase deficiency; report of a second case, with quantitation of the excessive excretion of amino-acids. *Journal of Pediatrics,* **91,** 242–246

RASMUSSEN, J. E. (1976) Erythema multiforme in children. *British Journal of Dermatology,* **95,** 181–185

WARWICK, W. J., RUTTENBERG, H. D. and QUIE, P. G . (1963) Sclerema neonatorum – a sign, not a disease. *Journal of American Medical Association,* **184,** 680–683

WOLF, B., GRIER, R. E., ALLEN, R. J. *et al.* (1983) Phenotypic variation in biotinidase deficiency. *Journal of Pediatrics,* **103,** 233–237

Further reading

HURWITZ, S. (1981) *Clinical Pediatric Dermatology.* Philadelphia: W. B. Saunders

ROOK, A. *et al.* (in press) *Textbook of Dermatology* (4th edn.). Oxford: Blackwell Scientific Publications

SOLOMON, L. M. and ESTERLEY, M. B. (1973) *Neonatal Dermatology.* Philadelphia: W. B. Saunders

Part XIII

Psychiatric emergencies

Chapter 56

Acute psychiatric conditions

F. G. Thorpe

Psychiatric emergencies are not common in paediatric practice and apart from anorexia nervosa, non-accidental injury, and some adolescent suicidal attempts, they are seldom life-or-death situations. Nevertheless, prompt action is necessary to prevent further suffering to the child and family, and, in young pre-adolescents, to interrupt behaviour patterns that are adversely affecting personality development. A careful history will usually reveal that the crisis is the culmination of increasingly maladaptive behaviour which has been manifest for some time. Children presenting with phobic anxiety states may have shown similar reactions before, such as the school-phobic child who experienced separation anxiety on starting school, or on returning to school after every holiday, until finally attendance became impossible. The aetiology of psychiatric disorder in childhood is multi-factorial. The initial contact with the parents is of vital importance and many parents may require psychiatric treatment in their own right; those who rationalize their own failure by blaming the school, other children in the neighbourhood, or accept the child's escape into somatic illness as a means of avoiding stress. The real urgency may sometimes be related to the parent's hidden guilt rather than to the presenting problems of the child.

Suicidal attempts

About 20 per cent of acute medical admissions are now for drug overdose and approximately 0.6 per cent of adolescents between the ages of 12 and 16 years make a suicidal attempt in any one year, although for most of these the general practitioner is the central figure.

Recognition

Children and adolescents who make suicidal threats or attempts require urgent help. The clinician is sometimes uncertain whether to request a psychiatric opinion, particularly as there may well be a tendency to cover up suicidal attempts because of the social stigma and the desire by the parents to regard such events as being due to 'irresponsible hysterical behaviour'. It is six times more common in girls than boys, but the boys are often more seriously disturbed. The frequency increases with age and reaches its peak in adolescence. Serious mental illness in the form of schizophrenia or depressive psychosis is rarely the cause of suicidal attempt; the majority are reactively depressed, being faced with an unbearable situation from which they want to escape. In many cases the attempt is staged without the real goal of death, and the clinician must remember that the younger child does not comprehend the finality of death, and imagines himself being able to witness the impact of his act upon his parents and others causing his unhappiness. The younger generation see their parents taking tablets, or hear them expressing suicidal thoughts or making actual suicidal attempts, so it is not surprising that they do likewise. The commonest method is the ingestion of tablets, usually the property of their parents, many of whom are themselves depressed or have personality disorders.

The attempt, which may be caused by anger internalized as guilt and depression, is a way of manipulating another person to gain love, or is designed to punish them. It is a signal of distress and warrants immediate psychiatric help because of the tendency, in both the parent and the child, to suppress information concerning motives and underlying family tensions. When the act is a desire to join a dead relative, usually combined with the withdrawal of love by the remaining depressed parent, the motive is usually obvious. Fortunately, we do not see many successful suicides in children under the age of 12 years but of these, boys succeed five times more frequently than girls.

Management

The paediatrician's role

Direct authoritative approaches which go straight into details of the attempt and its motives are invariably met with denial. It is better to adopt a more gentle non-demanding, unhurried approach and this usually requires the skills of someone with child psychiatric training. The objective should be to set up a meeting of the child, his parents and the psychiatrist within 48 hours. A minimum of questioning by casualty officers and paediatric housemen is indicated, and they should restrict their activities to the management of the immediate medical problem and the child's admission to a place of safety where psychiatric assessment can take place.

Psychiatrist's role

Most of the affected children will reveal severe family and environmental stresses which require urgent attention, and many of their mothers will be suffering from depressive illness. Paternal rejection, desertion, or even death are common. Although the majority settle in hospital some remain depressed and need to be transferred to an appropriate psychiatric inpatient unit where they can be treated with antidepressants and given psychotherapy over a prolonged period. The treatment of acute depression is considered below. The resolution of family tensions requires all the skills of a psychiatric team, casework for the parents, and possibly other members of the household, by a skilled psychiatric social worker. Even so, one in ten young people will make a further attempt within a year, so adequate follow-up is essential.

Anorexia nervosa

Although anorexia nervosa is typically a condition of adolescent girls, it is seen sometimes in pre-adolescent children and also in boys. These young people present in a state of extreme emaciation and a resolute determination not to eat food. Their parents are extremely concerned about their welfare but may have become rejecting and hostile after long periods of tempting with tasty morsels and bribing, leading finally to unsuccessful attempts at force-feeding.

Recognition

The following criteria are essential in making the diagnosis.

Attitude to food

The patient has a characteristic attitude towards food and will avoid carbohydrates, which are regarded as fattening. The subsequent loss of weight is marked and, depending upon parental concern, the weight may well have fallen below the 3rd centile. In addition, other methods may be used to lose weight and get rid of nutrients, such as purging, self-induced vomiting, excessive indulgence in exercise, and the hiding away of food which is claimed to have been eaten.

Amenorrhoea

In pubertal girls there is amenorrhoea, or in younger children, if the condition persists, delayed onset of menstruation when all secondary sexual characteristics are fully developed. The output of pituitary gonadotrophin is reduced but pituitary function is otherwise normal and the long-held view that it resembles Simmonds' disease is now recognized as incorrect.

Fear of obesity

There is a distinctive psychopathology in all cases centred around a morbid fear of becoming obese and an aspiration to an ideal weight far below the mean. Anorexic patients may have a perceptual distortion of body image which accounts for this. Depression superimposed upon an obsessive–compulsive personality is a common feature and may precede the onset of food refusal. Self-mutilation is sometimes observed, and characteristically these patients remain very active and apparently full of energy until the terminal stages of the illness, *which can be fatal.*

Past history

Often the child has had an above-average birth weight, with infant feeding problems, obesity in infancy, and an early menarche.

Anorexia nervosa may be seen psychologically as a subconscious reluctance to reach sexual maturity, and most of these girls have sexual problems which require psychotherapeutic help and even so sometimes persist into adult life. There is invariably conflict with the mother, with problems of identification.

Clinical features

These are secondary to the nutritional deficiency, and include bradycardia, hypotension, acrocyanosis, growth of lanugo hair, dry skin, reduced basal metabolic rate, and avitaminosis.

Management

General approach

Treatment is a matter of extreme urgency as the condition can be fatal, and admission to hospital is required. All cases of anorexia nervosa encountered in paediatric practice require the involvement of a child psychiatrist at the earliest opportunity, and, in addition to the treatment of the patient, the parents will require help to sort out their own attitudes towards their child. Unless the patient is extremely debilitated, requiring intravenous feeding and specialized medical care, treatment is better carried out in a psychiatric unit, as they are extremely manipulative and unreliable. They can become very depressed and possibly suicidal as they begin to gain weight, and sometimes develop an insatiable appetite with eating 'binges' followed by forced vomiting, leading to a condition now recognized as bulimia nervosa. A kind but firm, well-structured approach is required, and will test to the limit the nursing skills of the staff. The younger patient will probably be amenable to psychotherapy but the ability to respond diminishes with age, so that it may be almost impossible to establish a rapport with the older adolescent. Conjoint family therapy can then be helpful.

Diet

In the early stages a 2000 kilocalorie (8.4 MJ) liquid diet containing glucose and protein hydrolysate may be necessary but with skilful nursing the patient can soon commence a 3000 kilocalorie (12.6 MJ) solid diet. The unpleasant taste of the liquid diet appeals to the self-punitive aspects of the anorexic personality, and it is generally taken well.

Drugs

Chlorpromazine is the drug of choice and high doses such as 75–100 mg three times daily may be required in older adolescents. Vitamin deficiencies require treatment and when food intake is reasonable the use of anabolic steroids such as nandrolone (Deca-Durabolin (Organon)) i.m. 12.5–25 mg every 3 weeks may increase food uptake.

School phobia

Recognition

Background

Certain children display abnormal reactions to school of such intensity that they are now commonly termed school phobia, or more appropriately, neurotic school refusal. They must be regarded as emergencies, firstly because of the nature of the impact they make upon the parents, teachers, and various education officers responsible for school attendance; and secondly because the condition may become chronic in the absence of therapeutic intervention. Neurotic school refusal can sometimes be overlooked when the child expresses anxiety predominantly through somatic pathways (e.g. complaints of pain) and the unwary clinician becomes preoccupied with excessive, unnecessary physical investigations. The symptoms may occur during a child's initial school experience, or at the beginning of each new school term, but commonly reach crisis level on commencing secondary education at the age of 11 or 12 years, often following absence for a minor illness. A phobia is an irrational fear and the reaction is one of intense anxiety, amounting in many cases to panic about the school, from which the child protects himself by withdrawal. The psychopathology is usually one of separation anxiety, the child and mother having developed a neurotic bond so that neither can function adequately alone. It is not uncommon to find a mother with agoraphobia, but in every case the attitude towards the child will be one of anxious over-protection, and fathers tend to be passive or sometimes absent. These children function well academically, are frequently of above-average intelligence, and over-achieve because they fear the teacher's reprimand, or escape into work to avoid social contact with other children. They will rationalize their absence from school by finding fault with their teacher or peer group, and the mother is only too willing to accept this.

Physical symptoms

Children who escape into physical illness display less overt anxiety but present with nausea, vomiting, abdominal pain, headache or limb pains, and both they and their parents lose sight of the true nature of the neurotic conflict. Enquiry will usually reveal that the child wants to go to school if only he could understand his problems, in contrast to the truant who wilfully avoids school as part of a delinquent syndrome, and whose parents are unaware of his absence and not particularly interested. Symptoms are at their worst first thing on school mornings, and minimal at week-ends and during school holidays. The child's immaturity may also be shown in aggressive ways, leading to ambivalent feelings about parents, which in older children may find actual verbal expression.

Management

General approach

All cases of school phobia require urgent referral to the Child Psychiatric Services as their treatment is complex, time consuming and aimed at breaking down the neurotic bond between the child and parent. This will involve psychotherapeutic treatment for both, and in severe cases separation may be achieved only by admitting the child to a psychiatric unit. The child should be returned to school at the earliest opportunity and to do this it will be necessary to get the close co-operation of the Education Services. Behaviour modification techniques using progressive desensitization are useful methods of treatment.

Drug treatment

Medication alone will never resolve the problem but may diminish anxiety while the above procedures are carried out. Diazepam 2–5 mg three times daily, according to the age of child, may be used. The mother herself may well need psychiatric treatment for neurotic depression when she finally releases her child.

Psychometric assessment

This should always be done by an educational psychologist to exclude the rare case with a specific learning difficulty, inappropriate school placement, or any other real stress in school.

Resistant cases

These sometimes occur in adolescence, the personality remaining too immature to cope with the complexities of comprehensive education. If there is no 'nurture class' within the comprehensive school a transfer into a day school for maladjusted children is necessary.

Acute depression

Recognition

Background

Depressive states are not as common in children as in adults. When seen they are neurotic depressions in which anxiety is partly or completely replaced by depressive mood. They are sometimes masked, taking the form of behaviour disorders of various types, often with a self-punitive content, or even habit disorders such as encopresis. These conditions are not acute and should be dealt with in the usual way.

Common presenting symptoms

About a quarter of children attending psychiatric clinics present with the symptom of depression. This is significantly associated with anxiety, sleep disturbance, irritability, suicidal thoughts, eating disturbances, school refusal, phobias, alimentary disorders, obsessions, and hypochondriasis. For the diagnosis of depressive disorder, lowered mood should have been present for at least 4 weeks and should be associated with at least two of the above symptoms. In addition the symptoms must be severe enough to interfere with everyday life. Feelings of unworthiness and lowered self-esteem are common and the possibility of an actual suicidal attempt must always be considered. The child with acute depression is usually facing overwhelming environmental stress within the family and loss of love objects is common, including parental separation, desertion, or death. The child with a chronic handicap may also develop severe depressive reactions, especially with the onset of adolescence.

Possible endogenous depression

The depression becomes of psychotic intensity only when there is loss of contact with reality, and this is very rare in the pre-adolescent child. However, depressions do sometimes develop in a secure, stable environment and respond dramatically to appropriate antidepressant medication and so appear to have been endogenous in type. The parents of such children may themselves exhibit a cyclothymic temperament, with alternating depression and exuberance.

Management

General approach

All the patients require urgent psychiatric help and, if the depression seems profound, admission to a paediatric ward pending psychiatric consultation should be considered, particularly if there have been suicidal threats. The only firm contraindication to such an admission is the child still in mourning after bereavement. Reactive depressions in young people respond well to psychotherapeutic help once the nature of the stress has been identified and dealt with. The resolution of conflicts in very disturbed families can be a long-term problem; social-work skills have to be used and inpatient care may be appropriate.

Drug treatment

Tricyclic antidepressant drugs or monoamine oxidase inhibitors may be life saving in adolescents, but should be prescribed only on the recommendations of a psychiatrist and the normal dietary precautions taken with the latter. (Avoidance of Bovril, Oxo or other meat extracts, broad bean pods, cheese, Marmite and other yeast extracts, wines, beers and other alcohol, pickled herrings, flavoured textured vegetable proteins (*Monthly Index of Medical Specialities,* 1983; London, Medical Publications).

Adolescents will require between 50 and 150 mg daily of imipramine, the dose being gradually increased over a period of 2–3 weeks, or phenelzine 30–60 mg daily, in divided doses.

Hysteria

Recognition

Background

It is important not to confuse hysteria with the somatic symptoms produced by anxiety, such as recurrent abdominal pain, headaches, nausea, vomiting, frequency of micturition, and diarrhoea. In hysteria the somatic symptoms are based upon the patient's inability to cope with reality and his attempt to resolve his conflict by 'dissociation', in which the anxiety about his basic conflict is 'converted' into an hysterical symptom. This symptom usually has secondary gain, commonly avoidance of the original situation, and may also have a symbolic meaning or be imitative of a near relative with a similar symptom due to organic causes. Thus a child may develop a disorder of gait because for some reason he is unable to leave his mother; he may also be immature and literally 'unable to stand on his own two feet'. Because the anxiety has been converted into a somatic symptom, patients with hysteria sometimes show a singular lack of concern for their disability, a state known as 'belle indifférence'. Although at one time this was an essential criterion for the diagnosis of hysteria, it is less common in hysterical patients today.

Hysteria is rare in childhood and increases only slightly in frequency during adolescence. The diagnosis must be made with extreme caution as nearly half the cases will eventually be found to have organic illness, especially those with disorders of vision. Although obvious emotional causes for the condition can sometimes be found, this is not always so. In pure hysteria there is often a rapid onset of symptoms and a family history of hysterical symptoms. In pre-adolescence it is equally common in both sexes but in adolescence and adult life females predominate. Epidemic hysteria is also seen in groups of adolescent girls.

Clinical features

Hysteria may present in any of the following ways:

1. Disorders of mobility, including abnormalities of gait, psychogenic paralyses, aphonia.
2. Disorders of perception, including loss of vision, deafness, insensitivity to pain, and other disorders of sensation.
3. Disorders of consciousness, including fits and fugues, which are more common in adolescence.

Signs not compatible with known organic disease are demonstrable in many cases as the condition portrayed is the creation of the patient's own mind. A few cases, however, will be extremely difficult to diagnose with any degree of certainty and prolonged observation will be necessary.

Management

A high proportion of young people with hysterical symptoms find themselves admitted to paediatric wards for further assessment. Whether or not this is the case early psychiatric involvement and a full neurological investigation is a matter of urgency as early intervention improves the prognosis. These cases require the closest cooperation between paediatricians and child psychiatrists, and in some cases prolonged treatment is necessary. A full psychosocial investigation is required to try to uncover the source of stress, either exogenous or endogenous, which if successful will give psychotherapeutic directives to be used to enable the patient to 'reconvert' to normal function. Although environmental manipulation is seldom successful with adults, some success may be achieved with children. Opportunities should be given for the patient to give up symptoms without 'losing face'. Strong suggestion can be used but hypnosis has its dangers and should be attempted only by a psychiatrist with special skills. Drugs have little to offer in treatment unless abreactive techniques are used.

Drug abuse and dependence

Recognition

Background

The possibility of drug abuse must always be considered in patients with toxic confusional states or psychotic-like reactions. At one time this problem was uncommon but in recent years adolescent drug taking has increased in Western countries, and experimentation with drugs may also occur in young teenage children. It usually starts at parties or group meetings in an attempt to produce uninhibited relaxation or excitement, and although sometimes a substitute for the alcoholic habits of previous generations, the two can be mixed for extra 'kicks', with dangerous results. Therefore, many young people presenting for emergency treatment may not be drug addicts, but nevertheless nearly every case warrants further investigation.

Toxic substances

SOLVENT ABUSE (THIS IS DEALT WITH SEPARATELY IN CHAPTER 57)

SOFT DRUGS

The clinician is more likely to meet patients in early adolescence on 'soft drugs' which cause the minimum of physical dependence but considerable psychological dependence because of the enjoyment obtained. If a drug provides a personality need, dependence is more likely to occur and there may be progression to 'hard drugs', but this is by no means the rule. The 'soft drugs' include stimulants, like caffeine, amphetamine (including Drinamyl) and cocaine, and hallucinogens such as cannabis (Marihuana, 'pot') or lysergic acid diethylamide (LSD). Since the medical profession has virtually ceased to prescribed amphetamines and the chemists do not carry stocks which may be stolen, amphetamine dependence is probably not on the increase. It does, however, sometimes produce a psychotic state with delusions and hallucinations not unlike an acute attack of schizophrenia. Methedrine is often self-administered by intravenous injection. Euphoria, flight of ideas, and vivid hallucinatory experiences dominate the picture with LSD, and less so with cannabis. The former can produce states very similar to schizophrenic excitability and may precipitate latent psychosis in vulnerable subjects. It is usually taken on blotting paper or a sugar lump and cannot be reliably detected in the urine.

SEDATIVES

Barbiturates and compound drugs such as glutethimide, and methaqualone and diphenhydramine (Mandrax) and are also used by adolescents and may present varying clinical pictures. They are more readily available on the drug market and are frequently taken with alcohol. When dependence develops, withdrawal should only be attempted in hospital as it can be complicated by convulsions and hyperpyrexia.

HARD DRUGS

It is increasingly likely that the paediatrician will encounter patients on 'hard drugs' like narcotics (opiates, particularly heroin which is now smoked ('chasing the dragon'), pethidine, methadone and others). Should this occur specialist psychiatric services will be urgently required.

DRUNKENNESS IN ADOLESCENCE

Teenagers have become attracted to alcohol. The pub has become the social club and one study showed that 15 per cent of 14-year-old girls frequent pubs regularly. Alcohol is more readily available in the family and parents permit their children a drink on social occasions. Alcoholism is not seen in young children; but in adolescents, in addition to acute alcoholic poisoning, social problems are common, leading sometimes to psychological dependence upon alcohol. The association between intoxication and antisocial behaviour is well known and the resulting violence may bring young patients to casualty departments with a variety of physical injuries. Frequent attenders require further investigation by a social worker, and those who are psychologically dependent should be referred for psychiatric opinion as a matter of urgency.

Management

The clinician must use his knowledge of toxicology in dealing with the immediate medical emergency and identifying the overdose syndrome. Urine and blood samples should be taken where appropriate. When psychotic-like states are encountered psychiatric opinion may be needed to exclude acute schizophrenia. All cases of suspected drug abuse ultimately require thorough medical, psychological, and sociological investigation, particularly to determine the source of the offending drugs and warn the appropriate authorities. When drug dependence is present skilled psychiatric treatment is a matter of urgency and referral to a drug addiction unit may be necessary.

Further reading

CRISP, A. H. (1967) Anorexia nervosa. *British Journal of Hospital Medicine,* **1,** 713–718

HAWTON, K. (1982) Attempted suicide in children and adolescents. *Journal of Child Psychology and Psychiatry,* **23** (4), 497–503

HERSOV, L. (1976) Hysteria. In M. Rutter and L. Hersov (eds) *Child Psychiatry: Modern Approaches,* pp. 437–441. Oxford: Blackwell

KAHN, J. H. and NURSTEN, J. P. (1968) *Unwillingly to School.* Oxford: Pergamon Press

PEARCE, J. (1977) Depressive disorder in childhood. *Journal of Child Psychology and Psychiatry,* **18,** 79–82

Chapter 57

Abuse of solvents and other volatile substances

Martyn Gay

Since the 1970s solvent abuse has become an increasing problem in the United Kingdom, affecting mainly adolescent boys and young male adults, although primary school children, older adults, and girls may also be involved. The practice is usually a group activity, but in about 10 per cent it is a solitary one. The substance used is usually a volatile glue, but may be any substance which is both volatile and capable of giving a mood-altering effect, including dry-cleaning fluid, petrol, butane gas, paint stripper, etc. Fumes are inhaled from the container direct or from a bag into which the substance has been poured. To enhance the effect the substance may be heated. Occasionally, and more dangerously, aerosols are sprayed directly into the mouth or nose.

As a group, the volatile organic solvents are lipophilic, are easily absorbed, and are cerebral depressants. The effects are primarily those of altered levels of consciousness and in many ways parallel those of alcohol ingestion; but due to the rapid absorption from the lungs, their action on the central nervous system occurs much faster. They are rapidly eliminated from the body, leaving few tell-tale signs, within an hour or so of inhalation.

Recognition

Within a few minutes after experiencing an initial euphoria, the person becomes uncoordinated, losing fine control and judgement. This may progress to disinhibition, disorientation, dysphasia, ataxia, and alteration in perception, the user describing dream-like states and 'the buzz' with visual and auditory hallucinations which may be frightening, but which are frequently described as pleasant. Delusions may occur, for example the person may think he can fly or have some strange physical powers. As a consequence of these effects the person may engage in risk-taking behaviour or totally fail to appreciate danger, and present to the Casualty Department because of an accident; for example, a fall, road accident, drowning, or fights. The person may become violent, either as a direct result of cerebral depression or secondary to his delusions or hallucinations, and may present to the Casualty Department via the Police.

The substances themselves are not without danger. Unconsciousness can result from a high blood level, which is easily obtained owing to the rapid absorption. The evidence with regard to morbidity affecting kidneys, liver, central nervous system and bone marrow, is related mainly to studies on individuals who have been exposed to chronic high levels of industrial solvents, principally as an occupational hazard. Early reports on glue sniffing suggest that such complications are probably rare, are not necessarily dose related and are dependent on the chemical abused. Toluene, the active ingredient in many common glues, is reported to have caused acute, sub-acute, and chronic encephalopathy which may present as coma, dysarthria, convulsions, and visual disturbances, including diplopia and persistent hallucinations. In addition, dementia and cerebellar ataxia occur. Renal damage includes transient haematuria and proteinuria as well as reversible renal shut-down.

Psychological sequelae include listlessness, apathy, impaired concentration, and temporary memory loss. There is often an associated deterioration in school or work performance. Secretive behaviour, theft to obtain the solvents, or solitary abuse of them as well as using other drugs all suggest psychological dependence. Physical addiction is probably rare, but tolerance does occur. Death, where it occurs, relates not only to the substance used but its method of use, and accidents occurring while intoxicated. Suicidal behaviour, drowning, falls, road accidents, burns and suffocation from inhalation asphyxia, and from inhaling within the plastic bag have occurred. Sudden 'sniffer's death' occurs occasionally where solvent abuse, particularly aerosol solvent, is associated with strenuous exercise resulting in raised carbon dioxide and catecholamines levels which appear to cause a fatal arrythmia. Half of all solvent abuse deaths appear to be due to a direct toxic effect of the substance used.

The diagnosis in most cases presents no difficulty. The patient often smells of glue or other solvents; there are frequently glue stains on the clothes and there may be a rash around the mouth or nose, a chemical dermatitis from the substance abused. It is important to consider the possibility in unconscious or apparently drunk adolescents and young adults. Toluene can be detected in the blood for some hours after inhalation.

Management

For those aged over 16, after the effect of the substance has worn off, there is usually no need for treatment, although if they appear psychologically dependent or request help, a referral to a psychiatrist would be appropriate. If the patient is under 16, the parents or other responsible adult need to be informed. The majority of abusers, probably about 90 per cent, carry out the practice for a short time as a peer group activity, before giving it up. Their parents may, however, need guidance. Those who participate alone, are abusing other drugs including alcohol, have been involved for over 6 months, or who are suffering side effects, may require further help and should be referred to the relevant local agencies such as child psychiatrist or paediatrician, social worker, voluntary agency or self-help group.

Further reading

ANDERSON, H. R., MACNAIR, R. S. and RAMSEY, J. R. (1985) Deaths from abuse of volatile substances: a national epidemiological study. *British Medical Journal,* **290,** 304–307

CHANNER, K. S. and STANLEY, S. (1983) Persistent visual hallucinations secondary to chronic solvent encephalopathy: Case report and review of literature. *Journal of Neurology, Neurosurgery and Psychiatry,* **46,** 83–86

Human Toxicology (1982) Proceedings of Symposium on Solvent Abuse. *Human Toxicology,* **1,** 201–349

Part XIV

Medicosocial and medicolegal emergencies

Chapter 58

Non-accidental injury and child abuse (Battered Baby syndrome, Silverman's syndrome, non-organic failure to thrive)

N. J. Spencer

Child abuse, though now widely recognized, was not formally described until 1962. Exact statistics are difficult to obtain; Ellerstein (1981) estimates that 1–3 per cent of American children are abused or neglected; physical injury occurs in 0.9/1000 children aged under 5 in Sheffield (Gordon, 1983; unpublished observations).

Actual physical injury is only one aspect of child abuse; others include nutritional deprivation, 'imprisonment' within the home, 'scapegoating', emotional abuse, sexual abuse, deliberate poisoning, withholding essential medical care, and fabricating signs and symptoms to provoke medical intervention, ('Munchhausen by proxy'; Meadow, 1977).

Recognition

'At risk' families

'At risk' families should be recognized if possible in the antenatal period. Predisposing factors are one or more of the following:

1. Absence of normal 'nesting' behaviour.
2. Young, single, unsupported mother.
3. Previous history of child abuse in the family.
4. Maternal depression (often unrecognized).
5. Deprivation during childhood of one or both parents.
6. Parental violent criminal record.
7. Alcoholism or drug abuse.
8. Overcrowding with or without poor economic circumstances.
9. Prolonged parent–child separation from birth.

Early warning signs

Serious physical injury may be prevented if early signs of breakdown in the parent–child relationships are recognized. Common early warning signs are:

1. Feeding difficulties in infancy: persistent crying or vomiting, failure to gain weight.
2. Severe chronic napkin eruptions.

3. Frequent attendances at casualty departments, or hospital admission for complaints inconsistent with clinical findings. Parents may fail to visit or enquire after the child's progress.
4. In the pre-school child, repeated accidental ingestion of household remedies or drugs.
5. In the school child, poor school attendance, sudden inexplicable deterioration of school work, neglected appearance, apathetic or withdrawn behaviour, poor weight gain or growth.
6. Bizarre or disturbed behaviour in the pre-school or school child.

Physical injury

Types of injury

1. Bruises: often of varying ages and in a recognizable pattern (e.g. fingers or belt buckle). The site of bruising can help to distinguish accidental from non-accidental; lumbar bruises are suspicious in under 5's, head and facial injuries common in normal children between 18 months and 3 years but not at other ages (Robertson *et al.*, 1982).
2. Skin lesions: bite marks, scratches, cigarette burns, excoriations, scalds (particularly 'glove', 'stocking' or 'grid' distributions).
3. Oral lesions: frenal tears and lip injuries particularly in non-mobile infants; luxated, intruded, avulsed, or fractured teeth.
4. Limb injuries: swelling of elbow joint or femur in infants, spiral fractures caused by twisting. Old unexplained fractures on skeletal survey.
5. Viscus rupture or haematoma: presenting as abdominal distension, bile-stained vomiting or shock.
6. Subdural haematoma: due to shaking, and presenting in infants as vomiting, or bulging fontanelle.
7. Fabricated symptoms, such as haematuria produced by addition of adult blood (often menstrual blood); effects of drugs given to the child to provoke symptoms ('Munchausen by proxy').

Incompatible story

When physical injury has occurred the story may be incompatible with the clinical findings, frequently changing, inconsistent with the child's motor development, or improbably complex. The interval between the time of injury and presentation at hospital may be inexplicably long. The parents' attitude may be inappropriate; unduly aggressive, apparently unconcerned or over-anxious.

Other forms of abuse

1. Emotional abuse: this can be defined as the deliberate withholding by parent or guardian of the love and affection necessary to the proper development of the child's personality and self-esteem. Its significance has been recognized only recently. Recognition is difficult; the infant may be withdrawn, listless, immobile, failing to thrive or showing 'frozen watchfulness'. The mother–child relationship may be 'cold' with lack of eye contact and playful interaction. Older children may be aggressive, unduly fearful, withdrawn and depressed, or show

bizarre behaviour. They may form immediate attachments to any (or all) adults but show no apparent regret at parental absence. 'Scapegoating' should be suspected when one child in contrast to its siblings shows the above features.

2. Non-organic failure to thrive (psychosocial dwarfism): food deprivation should be considered as a cause of failure to thrive when clinical and laboratory investigation fail to reveal a pathology. These children often have a voracious appetite and gain weight rapidly on admission to hospital. Associated physical and emotional neglect may be obvious but more careful investigation of the family dynamics is often necessary to establish the diagnosis.
3. Sexual abuse (covered more fully in Chapter 59): Kempe (1978) defines sexual abuse as, 'The involvement of dependent, developmentally immature children and adolescents in sexual activities that they do not fully comprehend, to which they are unable to give informed consent or that violate the social taboos of family rules'. Sexual abuse ranges from child rape to occasional genital fondling by an adult known to the child. Most sexual child abuse occurs within the child's family and it is often concealed by all family members (including the child). Recognition is difficult in the absence of genital or perineal trauma and a high index of suspicion is necessary, particularly when young girls present with ill-defined, non-specific abdominal or urinary symptoms.

Management of suspected child abuse

Hospital admission and urgent legal procedures

The child is admitted at once to hospital for observation and investigation. Admission is often welcomed by parents as a relief of emotional tension. If the parents refuse admission or attempt to remove the child against medical advice, a Place of Safety Order can be obtained at any hour through a magistrate on application by a social worker, an NSPCC officer or, in exceptional cases, a police officer. A Place of Safety Order, which is enforceable by the police, expires after 28 days (8 days if on police application) but can be renewed for a further 28 days (an Interim Order) through another application to a Juvenile Court.

Initial history and examination

Whenever possible the child and parents should be seen on admission by a senior member of the paediatric medical staff. Complete, dated, and legibly signed notes should be made containing as much of the following as possible:

1. The parents' own account of the injuries (conflicting and/or changing accounts should be recorded).
2. Details of social history, family composition, and adults present at the time the injuries were said to have occurred.
3. Full medical history of child and siblings.
4. Accurate descriptions of all injuries with sketches and an estimate of the age of each injury.
5. An objective description of the state of cleanliness of the child's hair, skin, nails and clothing.
6. Child's height, weight and head circumference entered on appropriate charts.
7. Details of full physical examination including fundoscopy following dilation of the pupils.

8. An assessment of the child's approximate level of psychomotor achievement, the child's response to adults, and general behaviour. This is particularly important if emotional abuse is suspected.
9. Colour photographs of the injuries should be taken as soon as possible.

Investigations and differential diagnosis

Investigations should include platelet count, prothrombin time, partial thromboplastin time, a cuff (Hess's) test for capillary fragility and a full radiographic examination of the whole skeleton (skeletal survey) which may show multiple fractures of different ages, spiral fractures of the long bones, chip fractures of the metaphyses, displaced epiphyses, calcified subperiosteal haematoma, and new bone formation in the mandible. These, with the clinical examination, will help to exclude bleeding disorders, coagulation defects, capillary fragility, scurvy, and various causes (infantile cortical hyperostosis, osteogenesis imperfecta, syphilis, cystinosis) with similar radiographic changes.

When non-organic failure to thrive is suspected, the child should be observed for a period on an adequate diet; these children often gain weight rapidly on admission to hospital. Non-invasive investigation of urine and stool for infection, infestation, or evidence of malabsorption can be made during the observation period. Jejunal biopsy and other invasive investigations should be reserved for those children who fail to gain weight despite an adequate diet.

'Mongolian blue spots' and lesions made by 'coin-rubbing' (Golden and Duster, 1977) and 'cupping' (Sandler and Haynes, 1978) must be remembered in the differential diagnosis of physical abuse.

Talking to and assessing the parents

Every effort must be made by all hospital staff to gain the confidence of the parents as well as the child. Accusations, explicit or implicit, must be avoided. The consultant paediatrician should see the parents as soon as possible after admission (definitely before a case conference is held) and work with them towards an understanding of what has happened. If a case conference is to be held, its purpose should be explained to the parents. The parents should be seen by the hospital social worker who will also gather information from other sources about the family.

A psychiatric assessment of the parents is helpful: unrecognized depression may be discovered, treatment of which may make it possible to return the child safely to the home; a prognosis can usually be given for response to treatment or case work.

Use of Child Abuse Registers

Registers of abused children and those considered 'at risk' are kept in most areas in the UK. Information should be sought as soon as possible if diagnostic doubt exists or important urgently required background details are unavailable to the admitting hospital.

Case conference

If possible this should be called within 48 hours of admitting the child to hospital and should involve the paediatrician, psychiatrist, any other specialist involved (e.g. orthopaedic surgeon), hospital and local authority social workers, the worker originally involved in bringing the child to hospital, and any others with recent or relevant knowledge of the family. The conference may include the very important family doctor, health visitor, probation officer, NSPCC representative, school teacher, education welfare officer, school nurse and the police.

A doctor is considered to be within his rights in relation to confidentiality in giving all necessary information to safeguard the child without the permission of the parents (*Annual Report of the Medical Defence Union*, 1972).

Even though many helpers may be called in, a small group reaches a decision more quickly. An experienced worker (preferably not directly involved in the case) should chair the conference and guide the discussion.

The objects of a case conference are:

1. To correlate all relevant information.
2. To agree on a plan of action.
3. To nominate one person to work with the parents, to prevent a multiplicity of visits, to avoid contradictory statements, and to establish a good relationship.
4. To decide whether the child's name should be entered in the Child Abuse Register and, if so, in which category (overt, suspected, or at risk).

Long-term planning

This is outside the scope of this chapter but should involve an attempt to improve the attitudes of parents in order that the child can, at some time, return safely to the family.

References

Annual Report of Medical Defence Union (1972) p. 21

ELLERSTEIN, M. S. (1981) *Child Abuse and Neglect – A Medical Reference.* New York: Wiley Medical Publications

GOLDEN, S. M. and DUSTER, M. C. (1977) Hazards of misdiagnosis due to Vietnamese folk medicine. *Clinical Pediatrics,* **16,** 949–950

KEMPE, C. H. (1978) Sexual abuse, another hidden pediatric problem. *Pediatrics,* **62,** 382–389

MEADOW, R. (1977) Munchausen syndrome by proxy – the hinterland of child abuse. *Lancet,* **ii,** 343–345

ROBERTSON, D. M., BARBOR, P. and HULL, D. (1982) Unusual injury? Recent injury in normal children and children with suspected non-accidental injury. *British Medical Journal,* **285,** 1399–1401

SANDLER, A. P. and HAYNES, V. (1978) Non-accidental trauma and medical folk belief: a case of cupping. *Pediatrics,* **61,** 921–922

Further reading

ELLERSTEIN, N. S. (1981) *Child Abuse and Neglect: a Medical Reference.* New York: Wiley Medical Publications

HELFER, R. E. and KEMPE, C. H. (1973) *The Battered Child* (2nd edn.) University of Chicago

KEMPE, C. H. and HELFER, P. E. (1972) *Helping the Battered Child and his Family.* Philadelphia: J. B. Lippincott

SCHMITT, B. D. and KEMPE, C. H. (1975) *Management and Prevention of The Battered Child Syndrome. Folia Traumatologica.* Basle: Ciba-Geigy

Chapter 59

Sexual interference with children

Alan Usher

In recent years, initially in the USA but more recently in the UK, publication from a variety of descriptions – medical, sociological and psychiatric – have drawn attention to the widespread sexual abuse of children, even infants, which had not been fully recognized or appreciated. This abuse is nearly always perpetrated by men, often within the family and its circle of acquaintances; and only occasionally by strangers, when it may be associated with child abduction. Such abuse can be divided into two categories – major sexual interference where the assailant makes a serious attempt to insert his penis into either the child's vagina or its anus and thus enjoy a form of coitus, and minor sexual interference where he contents himself with some lesser degree of molestation.

Minor sexual interference

This form shades almost imperceptibly from hugging and caressing children through 'bottom patting' to touching and fondling the child's private parts outside and inside the clothing, digital penetration of the vulva or anus and frank masturbation. Sometimes the adult will persuade the child to handle him indecently (which constitutes a separate offence under the 1967 Sexual Offences Act) or will attempt to have oral sex with it or more frequently will indulge in intercrural intercourse either from behind or in front. These practices rarely result in physical harm, except that in very young girls the hymen, being small and usually membranous, may be ruptured by even the passage of a finger through its hiatus and occasionally there can be small tears of the vagina inflicted accidentally by jagged finger nails. The only physical traces of such acts apart from those noted above are likely to be some evanescent reddening of the labia (a not uncommon finding in young girls anyway from a variety of causes) and the inner aspects of the thighs together with the deposition of semen on thighs, buttocks, clothing and in the oral cavity according to where (and if) ejaculation has taken place. Such cases are generally classed as 'indecent assault' or 'indecency with children' by the police.

Major sexual interference

The first penetration of the vulva by the erect adult penis in an older co-operative girl (unlawful sexual intercourse if the girl is not yet aged 16) usually results in stretching and eventual rupture of the hymen in its posterior segment with transient pain and bleeding; the tear takes some 10 days to heal. In a proportion of girls, those with a crenated distensible hymen, there is no tear even after several penetrations; the vaginal introitus merely distends and the hymen stretches. Eventually, however, with repeated penetrations, the hymen becomes deficient and largely disappears. In a younger child, forcible penetration may result in serious injury with tearing of the hymen, the fourchette and even the perineum and rectum. The only real proof that penetration was due to a penis is the finding of semen in the vagina or the rectum. Where the act has been accomplished by force (rape), evidence of resistance is likely to be found in proportion to the age and size of the child; a 5-year-old girl may well be overcome by the sheer weight of her assailant on top of her and thus show little evidence of resistance, whilst a muscular 15 year old is more likely to show bruises over the sacrum, shoulder blades, wrists and arms as well as between the knees and on the throat. She may also show scratches upon her thighs, neck and vulva in addition to the signs of recent defloration.

Penile penetration of the anus (buggery) especially without the aid of lubricants produces initially a painful, bruised anus often with radial bleeding tears of the mucosa and spasm of the anal sphincter which may last for several days. Swabs taken from inside the rectum as well as from the external anal margin may reveal the presence of semen and/or lubricants, as well as venereal disease. Gross damage to the anus, including complete tearing of the sphincter, may be caused in the small child thus abused.

Repeated acts of buggery produce in the passive partner epithelialization of the anus, often with radial fissures, a lax sphincter with loss of normal sphincteric reflex and very rarely, loss of the ischiorectal pads of fat producing a 'funnel' anus.

Examination

The best person to examine a child thought to have been molested sexually is undoubtedly a trained police surgeon, who, in the UK, can always be contacted by the local police. If, however, this service is not available, the most senior clinician involved should be asked to make the examination. In all cases the examination should not be done unless a third person is present. This doctor should be given all the information available concerning the incident and should see the parents, obtaining their formal consent to examination before interviewing the child, not only about this episode but, where appropriate, about any previous sexual experience. The victim's story and responses to questions should be taken down verbatim; they often include naïve descriptions of abnormal practices which a child of that age could not be expected to be aware of, and these make compelling evidence in court. Descriptions of acts that might be expected to leave physical signs e.g. punching, choking or nipping should be underlined in the doctor's notes, so that he is reminded to search for corroboration on examination.

The examination should be carried out under the best conditions possible, even in the operating theatre, should the child's condition merit this. Clothing worn at the time should be retained, each garment separately, in large (X-ray) envelopes labelled and listed. Swabs from the mouth, anus, vagina, rectum, vulva etc. should be sealed, labelled and listed, as should 'universal bottles' containing nail clippings, head and pubic hair, stain scrapings, etc. Trace evidence such as foreign hairs or fibres seen on the child's skin may be 'lifted' using short (i.e. 5 cm long) strips of wide Sellotape which are then stuck on to numbered microscope slides or pieces of old X-ray film. Some forensic science laboratories provide to the police and hospitals in their areas made-up sexual crime kits, containing the appropriate swabs, containers etc., together with instructions on how to take the samples.

The extent of the examination will vary with the nature of the case, but young children who cannot be relied upon to tell the whole story and cases of rape, where the signs of resistance are of vital importance, should always be examined from head to toe, including the anus and the genitalia. Notes and diagrams must be made at the time or immediately afterwards while the facts are fresh in the mind, and retained personally by the examiner, who should copy a summary into the case notes. Bacteriology specimens must be dealt with by a hospital laboratory. The rest of the labelled, dated and listed specimens should be handed over to and signed for by a police officer who will transmit them to the nearest Government Forensic Laboratory. The child's parents should be re-interviewed and told the results of the examination. They should be encouraged to play the matter down as much as possible unless in fact the child begins to display symptoms suggesting the need for referral to a consultant child psychiatrist.

Report

The police are involved in a high proportion of these cases since parents are generally very keen to bring this type of offender to book. The officer in the case will usually be glad to have an immediate verbal report from the doctor, following his examination, stating whether the findings are consistent with what was alleged or suspected to have taken place. Later, when laboratory examination of the specimens which have been taken is complete, the examiner, using his notes, should write a full report in the form of a statement for use in court. This is in three parts, the first setting out the examiner's name, profession, qualifications, position and experience and stating when, where and how he came to make the examination; the second recounting the factual part of the examination i.e. his observations; and the third his reasonable deductions from these facts.

References

FURNISS, T., BINGLEY-MILLER, L. and BENTOVIM, A. (1984) Therapeutic approach to sexual abuse. *Archives of Disease in Childhood,* **59,** 865–870

KEMPE, C. H. (1978) Sexual abuse, another hidden problem. *Pediatrics,* **62,** 382–389

MRAZEK, P. B. and KEMPE, C. H. (eds) (1981) *Sexually Abused Children and Their Families.* Oxford: Pergamon Press

PORTER, R. (ed.) (1984) *Sexual Abuse Within the Family.* Ciba Foundation; London: Tavistock Publications

RUSSELL, D. E. H. (1983) Incidence and prevalence of intrafamilial and extrafamilial sexual abuse in female children. *Child Abuse and Neglect,* **7,** 147–151

SGROI, S. M. (1975) Sexual molestation of children – the last frontier in child abuse. *Children Today,* **4,** 18–21

SUMMIT, R. C. (1983) The child sexual abuse accommodation syndrome. *Child Abuse and Neglect,* **7,** 177–193

SUMMIT, R. (1985) Sexual assault against children. In *Assault Against Children* (Meur, J. H., ed.), p. 47. London: Taylor & Francis

TILLELI, J. A., TUREK, D. and JAFFER, A. C. (1986) Sexual abuse of children. *New England Journal of Medicine,* **302,** 319–323

Further reading

BURGESS, S. H. and HILTON, J. E. (eds) (1978) Sexual offences. In *The New Police Surgeon,* pp. 221–286. London: Hutchinson

Part XV

Tropical and sub-tropical disorders

Chapter 60

Heat-related illnesses and hyperpyrexia

John C. Vance

The acute clinical states associated with exposure to excessive heat are described separately; but they rarely occur in a pure form and various combinations can be expected. The main diagnostic points are given in *Table 60.1*. *Always look for a predisposing condition.*

Sunburn

Recognition

1. Predisposing factors:
   (a) Naturally occurring ultraviolet light (wavelength 290–330 nm). Maximum sunburn response is produced at 305 nm.
   (b) Climate, geography and environment.
   (c) Fair-skinned individuals (e.g. red haired or albino).
   (d) Infants left outside for prolonged periods (not necessarily in direct sunlight).
2. Nature of burn:
   (a) Erythema alone.
   (b) Partial thickness burn with erythema and blister formation.
   (c) Pain.
3. Pyrexia or hyperpyrexia due to:
   (a) Extensive areas of involvement.
   (b) Impaired sweating.
   (c) Water or salt depletion.

Management

1. General:
   (a) Analgesia: paracetamol 25 mg/kg daily.
   (b) Fluid replacement. Most children with sunburn are not clinically dehydrated (i.e. their fluid loss is less than 5 per cent of their body weight). Oral glucose solution (5% concentration) or sweetened fruit juice given in amounts up to 5 per cent of the child's body weight should suffice.
   (c) Tetanus toxoid or combined diphtheria and tetanus vaccine 0.5 ml.

Table 60.1 Differential diagnosis of heat-related illnesses

Diagnosis	*Predisposing cause(s)*	*Symptoms*	*Rectal temperature*	*Thirst*	*Urine volume*	*Chlorides in urine*	*Plasma sodium*
Heat syncope	Lack of acclimatization	Fainting	N	0	N	+	N
Heat cramps	Muscular work with sodium depletion and drinking water to relieve thirst	Cramps in muscles used	N	0	N	0 or ↓	N or ↓
Heat exhaustion (water depletion)	Infants, ill or retarded children unable to drink freely	Irritability in infants; giddiness or faintness in children; dry mouth	N or ↑	↑ ↑	↓	+	N or ↑
Heat exhaustion (sodium depletion)	Any salt-losing state: sweating, cystic fibrosis, gastroenteritis, adrenogenital syndrome (adrenal hyperplasia)	Apathy in infants. Weakness, lassitude in children	N	0	N	0	N or ↓
Heatstroke	Environmental overheating, sodium depletion, impaired sweating (*Figure 60.1*)	Listlessness and headache, leads to sweating ceasing, leads to hyperpyrexia, leads to coma ± fits	↑ ↑	+	↓	0	N or ↓

N = Normal; 0 = absent; + = present; ↑ = increase; ↑ ↑ = marked increase; ↓ = reduced.

2. Local:
   (a) Dilute Burrow's solution* (diluted 1/10–1/20), or cold water compresses 15 minutes four times a day.
   (b) Emollients to soothe and relieve dryness of skin. *Antihistamine creams should not be used.*
   (c) Prevention of superinfection if burn is severe. There are two alternative methods:
      (i) Elastomeric copolymer film with adhesive backing is applied to the burn for 7 days. This prevents entry of organisms and decreases oral fluid requirements.
      (ii) Silver sulphadiazine cream 1% with chlorhexidine digluconate 0.2% applied daily to the burn after gentle bathing.

Heat syncope

Recognition

1. Predisposing factors:
   (a) Older children unaccustomed to hot climate.
   (b) Prolonged standing.
   (c) Postural change such as stooping.
   (d) Exercise.
   (e) Excessive clothing.
2. Syncopal attack without water or salt depletion.

Management

1. Reassurance.
2. Environmental control:
   (a) Limitation of outdoor activities.
   (b) Reduction of indoor temperature with ventilation, fans and air-conditioning.
   (c) Adequate fluid intake.
   (d) Light airy clothing.

Heat cramps

Recognition

1. Predisposing factors:
   (a) May or may not be acclimatized.
   (b) Vigorous exercise; for example, long distance running for periods longer than 1 hour.
   (c) Climate; high temperature with low humidity or lower temperature with high humidity.

* *Burrow's solution* – Aluminium sulphate 22.5 g, calcium carbonate 10 g, tartaric acid 4.5 g, acetic acid 25 ml, purified water 75 ml. To prepare the solution:

1. Dissolve aluminium sulphate in 60 ml purified water.
2. Add acetic acid and then calcium carbonate, and mix with the remaining 15 ml of water.
3. Allow to stand for not less than 24 hours in a cool place, stirring occasionally.
4. Filter.
5. Add tartaric acid to filtered solution and mix.
6. Store at a temperature of less than 25°C in well-filled containers.
7. The solution should be freshly prepared and should be discarded after 7 days.

   (d) Profuse sweating with total body depletion of sodium.
   (e) Excessive drinking of fluids with low sodium concentration.
2. Painful contractions of skeletal muscles (especially in legs). These can be reproduced by:
   (a) Exposing the muscle to cold.
   (b) Prolonged contraction.
3. No hyperpyrexia.
4. No clinical dehydration (i.e. fluid loss of less than 5 per cent of body weight).
5. Laboratory tests:
   (a) Absence of chloride in urine (Fantus test).
   (b) Serum sodium and chloride may be normal or reduced, depending on severity.

Management

1. Administration of lost sodium chloride. Alternatives:
   (a) Oral sodium chloride 0.9% flavoured with fruit juice to reduce vomiting; 1 ℓ will replace 10 g lost sodium chloride. The maximum volume of replacement fluid which can be given is about 5 per cent of the child's body weight. This is in addition to the usual daily fluid requirements.
   (b) One gram sodium chloride tablet crushed and mixed with each 100 ml (3½ oz) of water.
   (c) One teaspoon of salt mixed with each 400 ml of water (2 cups).
   (d) IV sodium chloride 0.9% if vomiting is a problem.
2. *This should be done carefully as too much salt given may lead to salt poisoning.*
3. *Administration should be followed with serial serum sodium levels (if possible) and serial estimations of chloride in the urine.*
4. *Treat any coexistent condition.*

Heat exhaustion (heat prostration)

This term describes two major syndromes which present with cardiovascular insufficiency due to water-deficiency dehydration, salt (sodium) deficiency or a mixture of both. At rest, infants aged about 12 months in an atmosphere of 30°C (86°F) and low relative humidity lose sweat at approximately 1.0–1.2 ml/kg/hr.

Water-depletion heat exhaustion

Recognition

1. Predisposing factors:
   (a) Water depletion due to inadequate replacement of water lost from sweating.
   (b) Fever due to an intercurrent illness increases fluid requirements by approximately 12 per cent for each 1°C (2°F) rise in body temperature.
   (c) Illnesses which lead to fluid loss, e.g. gastroenteritis.
   (d) Unacclimatized areas. Heat exhaustion is more likely to occur where excessive environmental heat is unusual. Children acclimatize more slowly than adults to changes in heat.
   (e) Infants who are unable to provide themselves with extra fluid.
   (f) Mentally retarded children.

   (g) Other chronic neurological disorders, e.g. cerebral palsy.
   (h) Head injury or recent neurosurgery.
2. Clinical features in infants.
   (a) Irritability.
   (b) Anorexia.
   (c) Thirst.
   (d) Dry mucous membranes.
   (e) Oliguria or anuria.
   (f) Signs of hypernatraemic dehydration.
   (g) Fits.
   (h) Hyperpyrexia.
   (i) Heatstroke in severe cases.
3. Clinical features in older children (as well as above):
   (a) Fatigue.
   (b) Giddiness.
4. Laboratory tests:
   (a) High urinary specific gravity or osmolality.
   (b) Chloride in urine (Fantus test).
   (c) Serum sodium:
      (i) Normal in older children.
      (ii) Elevated (>140 mmol/ℓ) in infants and those with retardation or chronic neurological disease.

Management

1. Infants:
   (a) Serum sodium >150 mmol/ℓ. Treat as for hypernatraemic dehydration from any cause.
   (b) Serum sodium <150 mmol/ℓ:
      (i) Increase oral fluid intake by giving extra water (equivalent to the volume of the child's usual feed) between feeds and diluting the usual feeds to half-strength by the addition of water. This treatment is only likely to be effective if the child is less than 5 per cent dehydrated.
      (ii) If IV fluids are required because of severe dehydration without hypernatraemia, or because of vomiting of refusal of feeds, sodium chloride 0.18% (N/5 saline) in 4% glucose should be used. The volume given will be determined by the degree of clinical dehydration. *Completely salt-free solutions such as 5% or 10% glucose may cause water intoxication and should not be given.*
2. Older children:
   (a) Oral replacement is usually sufficient.
   (b) Children with mental retardation and chronic neurological conditions may require IV therapy (*see* above).
3. *Treat any coexistent condition.*

Salt-depletion (sodium-depletion) heat exhaustion

Recognition

1. Predisposing factors:
   (a) Excessive losses of sodium and water in sweat.
   (b) Fever.

(c) Illnesses which lead to fluid loss.
(d) Unacclimatized individuals.
(e) Infancy.
(f) Mental retardation.
(g) Chronic neurological disorders.
(h) Obesity.
(i) *Cystic fibrosis.*
(j) Diabetes insipidus.
(k) Diabetes mellitus (*see* Chapter 50, pages 445–458).
(l) *Adrenogenital syndrome* (adrenal hyperplasia) (*see* Chapter 52, pages 469–475).
(m) Chronic heart failure.
(n) Malnutrition.
(o) Anorexia nervosa (*see* Chapter 56).
(p) Sweating insufficiency syndromes.

2. Clinical features in infancy:
   (a) Apathy.
   (b) Refusal to feed.
   (c) Signs of dehydration:
      (i) Sunken eyes.
      (ii) Decreased tissue turgor.
      (iii) Depressed fontanelle.
      (iv) Skin; pale and cold.
      (v) Peripheral cyanosis.
      (vi) Hypotension.
      (vii) Tachycardia.
   (d) *Sweating present.*
   (e) *No thirst.*
   (f) *Normal urine output.*
3. Laboratory tests:
   (a) *Chloride absent from urine* (unless renal salt-losing state or adrenal insufficiency).
   (b) Serum and urine sodium levels low.

Management

1. Acutely ill; IV normal saline (sodium chloride 0.9%) initially at 20–30 ml/kg/hr.
2. Less acutely ill with normal periphral circulation; *see* Heat cramps.
3. *Treat any coexistent condition.*

Heatstroke (sunstroke)

Heatstroke implies the presence of hyperpyrexia; that is the rectal temperature above 40.5°C (105°F), with cerebral symptoms. It represents a state of thermoregulatory failure, usually of sudden onset, after exposure to very high ambient temperatures, strenuous exercise or both. It is associated with cellular damage to the central nervous system and generalized anhidrosis. Heatstroke is often fatal despite aggressive therapy. Children are at potentially greater risk from heat stress than adults because of their greater surface area relative to body weight. Also, if they are unable to move away from the external heat source, the risk is increased.

Predisposing factors (Figure 60.1)

More than one of these factors will frequently contribute to heat stroke.

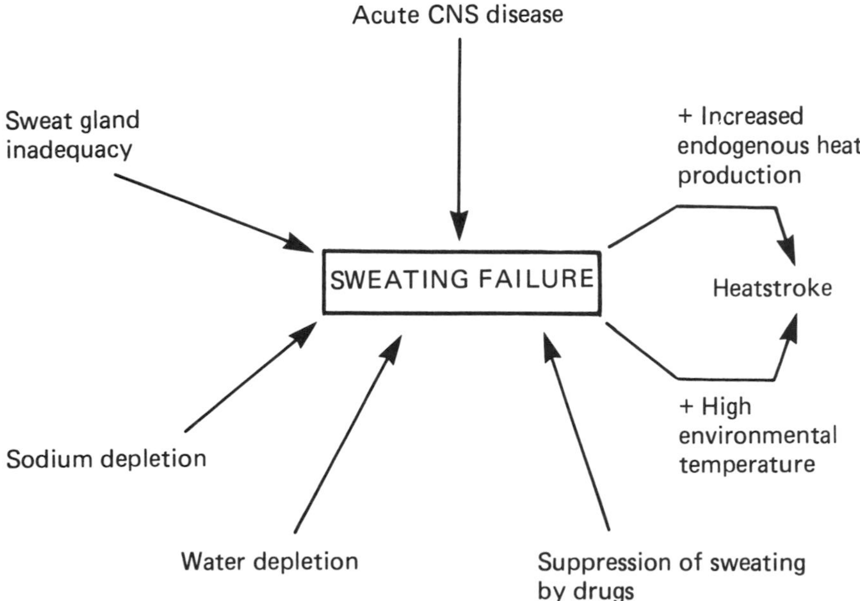

Figure 60.1 Pathogenesis of heatstroke. Heatstroke is caused by a failure of heat loss (lack of sweating) combined with increased heat production (infection; muscular work as in status epilepticus) with or without high environmental temperature

Environmental

1. Children at any age:
   (a) Rapidly rising and high absolute ambient temperature (e.g. heatwaves).
   (b) High humidity.
   (c) Poor ventilation.
   (d) Glass-enclosed areas, such as motor cars or ships' cabins, produce a 'glasshouse effect' thus causing a rapidly rising and high absolute ambient temperature.
   (e) Excessive clothing in hot weather or occlusive dressings in burns patients.
2. Neonates (particularly preterm infants)
   (a) Radiant warmers.
   (b) Phototherapy.
   (c) Faulty incubators.
   (d) Hot water bottles.

Physical exertion

With the increased awareness and interest in physical fitness, children are now participating with their parents in long-distance runs. Parents and race organizers should be aware of potential problems. When the ambient temperature is higher than skin temperature, children have less tolerance to exercise than adults because of:

1. Greater surface area: mass ratio which is used for heat dissipation.
2. Greater metabolic heat production per mass unit.
3. Less sweating capacity.
4. Less capacity to convey heat from body core to skin.

Medical conditions

1. Nutritional:
   (a) Failure to supply extra fluids in hot weather.
   (b) Malnutrition.
   (c) Obesity.
2. Fever:
   Children who are pyrexial due to an infection or disease of any nature will have less ability to dissipate their body's heat if the ambient temperature is high.
3. Diseases which cause excess fluid loss:
   (a) Vomiting from any cause (e.g. infectious disease).
   (b) Gastroenteritis.
   (c) Diabetes mellitus.
   (d) Diabetes insipidus.
4. Diseases that cause excess salt loss:
   (a) *Cystic fibrosis*.
   (b) *Adrenogenital syndrome* (adrenal hyperplasia).
   (c) Children who are currently being treated with corticosteroids or have been in the recent past.
5. Hereditary defects of the sweat glands:
   (a) Anhidrotic ectodermal dysplasia.
   (b) Congenital ichthyosis.
6. Acquired skin conditions with impaired sweating:
   (a) Extensive sunburn or thermal burns.
   (b) Eczema.
   (c) Psoriasis.
7. Anhidrotic heat exhaustion – miliaria (prickly heat). This results from obstruction of the sweat glands with keratinous plugs leading to retention of sweat. There are two major forms, crystallina and rubra. In miliaria crystallina, superficial skin vesicles are present without erythema and rupture readily. Miliaria rubra is less superficial and consists of papulovesicles and intense erythema. Most commonly they are localized to flexural areas.
8. Diseases of the central nervous system:
   (a) Mental retardation (children unable to obtain extra fluids by themselves).
   (b) Cerebral palsy.
   (c) Epilepsy; central effect, increased metabolism during convulsions.
   (d) Paraplegia or quadriplegia (including spina bifida).
   (e) Head injury or after neurosurgery.
9. Psychiatric conditions; anorexia nervosa.
10. Other conditions:
    (a) Asthma.
    (b) Hyperthyroidism.
    (c) Chronic heart disease.
    (d) Hypokalaemia enhances the adverse effects of heat and may predispose to rhabdomyolysis.

Drugs

1. Drugs of addiction.
   (a) Alcohol: inhibits secretion of antidiuretic hormone, producing relative dehydration.
   (b) LSD; increases heat production.
2. Anticholinergic drugs; e.g. atropine or derivatives used in the treatment of eye, bowel disorders or motion sickness; decreased sweat production.
3. Psychotropic drugs:
   (a) Tranquilizers have anticholinergic properties, e.g. chlorpromazine.
   (b) Tricyclic antidepressants have anticholinergic properties, e.g. imipramine, amitriptyline.
   (c) Monoamine oxidase inhibitors, e.g. isocarboxazid, probably act through increased CNS stimulation and heat production.
   (d) Amphetamines probably act through increased CNS stimulation and heat production.
4. Antihistamines, e.g. promethazine hydrochloride, diphenhydramine hydrochloride, chorpheniramine maleate. All these drugs have anticholinergic effect on sweat glands.
5. Inhalational anaesthetics, e.g. ether, halothane, and nitrous oxide contribute to heat stress only:
   (a) In association with atropine-like anaesthetic pre-medication.
   (b) In the presence of malignant hyperpyrexia.
6. Diuretics produce increased fluid loss in urine.
7. Beta-adrenergic blockers, e.g. propranolol, decrease cardiac rate and output.

Recognition

1. Prodromal symptoms. These usually occur from a few minutes to hours (occasionally days) before the onset of heatstroke:
   (a) Gastrointestinal symptoms:
      (i) Anorexia.
      (ii) Nausea.
      (iii) Vomiting.
      (iv) Dysphagia.
      (v) Diarrhoea.
   (b) Central nervous symptoms:
      (i) Headache.
      (ii) Dizziness.
      (iii) Faintness.
      (iv) Confusion.
      (v) Dysarthria.
      (vi) Purposeless movements.
   (c) Musculoskeletal symptoms:
      (i) Cramps.
      (ii) Weakness.
      (iii) Staggering gait.
   (d) *Anhidrosis for up to 48 hours before main symptoms start.*
2. Hyperpyrexia; rectal temprature 40.5°C (105°F) or more.

3. Central nervous system abnormalities:
   (a) Disturbed sensorium:
      (i) Disorientation.
      (ii) Delirium.
      (iii) Hallucinations.
      (iv) Photophobia.
      (v) Stupor.
      (vi) Coma.
   (b) Ataxia.
   (c) Convulsions.
      (i) Focal.
      (ii) General.
   (d) Decerebrate rigidity.
4. Skin abnormalities:
   (a) Red, hot and dry.
   (b) Miliaria crystallina or rubra (prickly heat).
   (c) Blotchy cyanosis of head and face.
   (d) Doughy feel to skin in infants.
5. Cardiovascular abnormalities:
   (a) Tachycardia:
      (i) Initially full volume.
      (ii) Later feeble.
   (b) Blood pressure.
      (i) Initially slightly raised or normal.
      (ii) Later low.
6. Breathing pattern abnormalities:
   (a) Initially rapid or irregular.
   (b) Later Kussmaul type.
   (c) Terminally Cheyne–Stokes type.
7. Renal abnormalities; oliguria leading to anuria.
8. Liver abnormalities; jaundice.
9. Haematological abnormalities; bleeding into skin and elsewhere due to DIC.

Laboratory investigations

1. Confirm diagnosis:
   (a) *Presence of high rectal temperature.*
   (b) Chlorides usually reduced or absent in urine.
   (c) Exclude other diseases:
      (i) *Cerebral malaria in endemic areas.* Thick and thin films for MT (*Plasmodium falciparum*) malaria (*see* Chapter 62).
      (ii) CNS infections, e.g. meningitis, encephalitis. CSF pressure, red cells and protein, normal or slightly elevated.
      (iii) Other infections.
2. Plasma biochemistry:
   (a) Sodium:
      (i) Usually normal or low.
      (ii) Occasionally elevated in infants.
      (iii) Depends on relative amount of salt and water loss.

(b) Potassium:
 (i) Usually low and may aggravate the effects of the heat.
 (ii) If high represents tissue destruction, renal failure and metabolic acidosis.
(c) Creatinine and urea; often elevated due to pre-renal or renal failure.
(d) Uric acid; may be elevated due to tissue destruction.
(e) Acid–base status; usually metabolic acidosis.
(f) Liver function tests:
 (i) Bilirubin may be elevated.
 (ii) Transaminases may be elevated.

3. Haematology:
   (a) White cell count; leucocytosis often present.
   (b) Coagulation profile:
      (i) Prolonged prothrombin time.
      (ii) Prolonged partial thromboplastin time.
      (iii) Thrombocytopenia.
      (iv) Hypofibrinogenaemia.
      (v) Elevated fibrin split products.
      (vi) Decreased concentration of individual clotting factors.
4. Urinalysis:
   (a) Proteinuria.
   (b) Haematuria.
   (c) Myoglobinuria.
   (d) Casts.
   (e) Cells:
      (i) Red.
      (ii) White.

Management

1. *Reduction of body (rectal) temperature* – Body (rectal) temperature should be reduced as quickly as possible, ideally within 1 hour, to prevent permanent sequelae. Measure temperature every 15 minutes to assess progress. Active cooling should be discontinued when temperature reaches 38.9°C (102°F). The method of cooling will depend on the facilities available but the general principles are as follows:
   (a) Environment:
      (i) Cool room (18°C; 65°F).
      (ii) Low humidity.
   (b) Cool patient (four alternatives given):
      (i) Immerse in bath filled with ice chips until temperature drops.
      (ii) Sponge with ice cold water.
      (iii) Wrap in wet sheets and evaporate water from sheets, using fans.
      (iv) Apply rubbing alcohol to skin and evaporate with fans.
   (c) Avoid peripheral vasoconstriction by vigorous massaging of the extremities.
   (d) Control shivering by use of i.m. chlorpromazine (1 mg/kg for age under 12 months; 10 mg at 12 months; 25 mg at 7 years; and up to 50 mg at 14 years).
2. Maintenance of cardiovascular balance. Correct fluid, electrolyte and acid–base imbalance as indicated by the patient's clinical condition, serum biochemistry and renal function.

3. Maintenance of respiration:
   (a) Maintain airway with oropharyngeal or endotracheal intubation as necessary.
   (b) Oxygen.
4. Control convulsions.
   (a) Give IV diazepam initially.
   (b) Follow up with phenobarbitone orally or i.m.
5. *Treat any coexistent condition* – e.g. MT (falciparum) (cerebral) malaria with parenteral chloroquine if there is a strong possibility of this, even if it cannot be proved.
6. Treat DIC.
7. Stop any drugs which may be aggravating heatstroke.

Hyperpyrexia

Hyperpyrexia is a symptom, not a diagnosis, and is defined as a RECTAL TEMPERATURE of 40.5°C (105°F) or more. If cerebral symptoms are present the diagnosis may be heatstroke (under appropriate conditions) or an infection of the CNS such as meningitis, encephalitis, or cerebral malaria.

Hyperpyrexia may occur in severely ill children who have cutaneous vasoconstriction from shock, and does not require suppression of sweating for the body temperature to rise. It may also be a complication of tetanus and polioencephalitis.

Recognition

Rectal temperature of 40.5°C (105°F) or more. Any of the conditions which cause heatstroke may cause hyperpyrexia, but hyperpyrexia does occur in temperate climates. Hyperpyrexia in association with an anaesthetic or operation should suggest *malignant hyperpyrexia*.

Management

1. Treat as for heatstroke (*see* above).
2. When sufficiently improved, investigate for underlying disease.

Further reading

American Academy of Pediatrics, Committee on Sports Medicine (1982) Climatic heat stress and the exercising child. *Pediatrics,* **69,** 808–809

BACON, C. J. (1983) Overheating in infancy. *Archives of Disease in Childhood,* **58,** 673–674

ELLIS, F. P. (1976) Heat illness. II. Pathogenesis. *Transactions of the Royal Society of Tropical Medicine and Hygiene,* **70,** 412–418

GOTTSCHALK, P. G. and THOMAS, J. E. (1967) Heat stroke: recognition and principles of management. *Clinical Pediatrics,* **6,** 576–578

KILBOURNE, E. M., CHOI, D., JONES, T. S. *et al.* (1982) Risk factors for heatstroke – a case–control study. *Journal of the American Medical Association,* **247,** 3332–3336

MITTAL, S. K. (1981) Heat illnesses in children. *Indian Pediatrics,* **18,** 401–404

VANCE, J. C. (1983) Heat stress in cars. In J. Pearn (ed.) *Accidents to Children. Their Incidence, Causes and Effects,* pp. 55–59. Melbourne: Child Accident Prevention Foundation of Australia

Chapter 61

Venomous bites and stings

John Pearn

Introduction

Emergency management of the envenomed child is a problem of tropical and subtropical parts of the world. The event is always dramatic with severe pain; collapse is common and emergency action is often required.

Nothing replaces local knowledge of venomous creatures (*Table 61.1*) and the practical aspects of management. With snakebite, the doctor in Central and Western Africa should know about the viperid snakes, puff-adders and carpet vipers; the puff-adder causes more deaths than all other African snakes. For those in southern Africa, a knowledge of the cobras, adders, boomslangs and mambas is essential; for those in America, knowledge of the *Crotalidae* (rattlesnakes, pit vipers) and *Elapidae* (*Table 61.1*); and in Australia and New Guinea all who work with children should be informed about the *Elapidae* which are some of the world's most poisonous snakes. The main areas of risk are indicated in *Table 61.1.*

History and symptoms (Table 61.2)

A mother may find a toddler playing with the snake, or sometimes the young child will say that he has been bitten, and even older children may not realize the danger of handling snakes (Munro and Pearn, 1978). Snakebite, or other forms of poisoning, must always be suspected in any child in a tropical or sub-tropical environment who presents with bizarre signs. In children presenting in an otherwise inexplicable unconscious state, envenomation must always be considered.

In Africa, Asia, Australia and New Guinea, elapid bites produce a variety of symptoms and signs. In Africa and Asia, viperid snakes may cause the same symptoms, but local pain is usually the predominant feature, rapidly progressing to signs of local tissue damage often with lymphangitis.

The *Crotalidae* (rattlesnakes, pit vipers and bush-master) of the Americas and Asia produce very severe local tissue damage, with pain, weakness, sweating, and nausea in over half the victims who are bitten.

Many older children and adults, who think that they have been bitten, develop snake fright (weakness, faintness, perioral numbness from hyperventilation etc.), but must be given the benefit of the doubt, and must be treated in the field as cases of true potential envenomation.

Table 61.1 Common poisonous snakes causing snakebite in childhood

Family	*Central and West Africa*	*Southern Africa*	*America*	*Asia*	*Australia and New Guinea*	*Europe*
Crotalidae	–	–	Rattlesnakes; pit vipers	–	–	–
Elapidae	Cobras; Mambas	Cobras; Boomslangs; Mambas; Rinkals	Coral snakes	Kraits; Cobras	Tiger snakes; brown snakes; Death adders; Taipans (all poisonous land snakes in this region are Elapids)	–
Viperidae	Puff adders; Carpet vipers	Puff adders; Horned adders; common night adders	–	Adders; Vipers	–	Common adder or viper
Hydrophiidae	–	Only in Indian Ocean, e.g. the Yellow and Black Seasnake	Only on Pacific coast	Various types in coastal waters, e.g. *Enhydrina; hydrophis sp.*	Various types; in coastal waters of the Western Pacific and the Indian Oceans, e.g. *Enhydrina schistosa; Hydrophis elegans*	–

Table 61.2 The main clinical features of snake bites

Family	*Local lesions and symptoms*	*General symptoms and signs*	*Antivenom available*
Crotalidae	Local pain; burning; swelling; with oozing of blood from the bite site	Collapse, sweating, tachycardia, hypotension, shock	Yes
Elapidae	Stinging or burning pain; ache or pain in regional lymph nodes; swelling and ooze at the bite site; (bite may be initially painless); fang marks often with teeth marks; occasionally no visible sign will be present in potentially fatal envenomations	'Tight feeling' in the chest, face, or throat; faintness, collapse, nausea, vomiting, hypotension, weakness, diplopia, bulbar paralysis; paralytic respiratory failure. Onset of neurotoxic symptoms may be delayed for up to 10 hours after the bite	Yes
Viperidae	Local pain, burning; swelling, oozing; necrosis in cases of African puffer and adder bites; teeth and fang marks usually present	Collapse, sweating, tachycardia, hypotension. Abdominal pain and diarrhoea in European adder bites. Non-clotting of blood with oozing and haemorrhages (for most species with the exception of African puff adders)	Yes
Hydrophiidae	Local lesions and symptoms; often little or no signs of fang marks or the snake bite itself. Occasionally lacerations from teeth marks, sometimes faint redness and later swelling	Generalized muscle pains; neurotoxic signs – blurred vision, weakness, diplopia, bulbar paralysis, respiratory paralysis and failure; ± myoglobinuria and acute renal failure	Yes

Signs

The signs of snake envenomation are pleomorphic, and local signs may be absent. The appearance of the bite site varies according to the family of snake (Elapid versus Crotalid, for example), the species (venomous versus non-venomous), the type of venom, the type of strike, and whether multiple strikes were delivered. In most cases two distinct fang marks are present within minutes of the child having been bitten.

Irrespective of the species involved, teeth marks or scratches may be present. Both venomous and non-venomous snakes have four rows of teeth in their upper jaws, and mandibular teeth in the lower jaw. Many bites occur without significant envenomation. The wound may continue to ooze blood, and may swell within several hours after the strike.

Systemic signs include collapse, hypotension, cardiac arrhythmias, fits, and a miscellany of neurological signs of lower motor neuron type. Life threatening signs of bulbar paralysis may occur within 30 minutes of bites by neurotoxic elapid snakes such as Asian Kraits and the Australian Taipans and Brown snakes. Significant bites by adult Elapids generally produce early neurotoxic signs, whereas viper and cobra bites (Africa and Asia) produce prostration, sweating, tachycardia and hypotension.

Species identification

Only in exceptional cases can a victim or onlooker identify snakes accurately in the field (Morrison *et al.*, 1983). Many near-tragedies have occurred because a venomous snake is misidentified by an 'expert' as non-venomous; or because the wrong antivenom is administered because of misidentification as far as genus is concerned. Therefore, only in exceptional circumstances should one be dogmatic about the type of snake involved in a confirmed or suspected snake bite, without formal identification by a zoologist or an expert, or by specific venom identification using an immunoassay detection kit.

First aid (Table 61.3)

A tight compressive bandage will effectively occlude lymph and tissue fluid flow in the envenomed limb, with immobilization using a splint; the compression immobilization technique is also effective and appropriate first aid for bites by Crotalid snakes.

One applies a compressive bandage, immobilizes the limb (over 80 per cent of bites are on limbs), labels the patient, and seeks advice from an expert with local experience. The bandage should be as tight as possible, should cover the bite site, and to prevent painful lymphatic and venous engorgement the bandage should be wound distally to proximally. In remote areas, evacuation by air should not be undertaken before consulting an expert, if there are no symptoms or signs of envenomation. If the compressive bandage is properly applied, an envenomed patient is safe for 1–1½ hours after the bite by an Elapid snake, and possibly for longer. Clothing or other material with venom on it should be sent with the patient for venom identification. One person should stay with the child at all times in case cardiopulmonary resuscitation is required. The correct sequence of first aid measures is listed in *Table 61.3*.

Hospital management (Table 61.4)

An intravenous line should be inserted, blood and urine should be collected for venom estimation, baseline electrolyte and haematological studies, and the patient is nursed in a place where cardiopulmonary resuscitation equipment is available.

Table 61.3 First aid for snakebite

1. Apply immediate hard pressure over the bite site with a finger or hand.
2. Apply a very tight constrictive bandage over the bitten limb, starting over the bite site, and winding from distal to proximal.
3. Apply a splint outside the compressive bandage.
4. Keep the patient at rest, and control the situation firmly.
5. Collect any clothing etc. which may have venom on it, for laboratory diagnosis of the species of snake.
6. One person must stay with the victim at all times, to administer cardiopulmonary resuscitation if required.
7. Label the patient with time and details of the bite or suspected bite, and details of first aid.
8. Summon medical aid, or take the patient to a place of definitive care.
9. Commence cardiopulmonary resuscitation if required.

Table 61.4 General principles of management of envenomed children

1. Dose of antivenom is not age related; children need just as much as do adults; injected venom requires a neutralizing dose of antivenom, irrespective of the size or age of the victim.
2. Antivenom should be given early but it is probably never too late to administer antivenom. Even if the patient is still ill 72 hours after the bite, antivenom may still provide significant venom neutralization.
3. Pain relief is very important, and is often underrated in the management of envenomed children.
4. Allergic reactions to venoms are common.
5. Scrupulous adherence to the principles of cardiopulmonary resuscitation is important.
6. Venoms are always mixtures of different toxic substances, and multiple body systems are usually affected at different times after envenomation.
7. Nothing replaces local knowledge; the best sources of help are local zoos, museums, universities, and poison information centres.
8. An accurate identification of the offending creature is of enormous help; but too specific management of the case where false reliance is placed on a supposed accurate identification of the venomous species has led in the past to fatalities and many near-fatalities.

The hospital management of snakebite has been simplified by enzyme immunoassay methods (Elisa) where this is available, to detect minute quantities of venom and to identify the offending species of snake (Coulter *et al.*, 1980).

Polyvalent antivenom should be assembled near the patient, and only when all these procedures have been undertaken, should the constrictive bandage be *slowly* removed, as this is less likely to cause a sudden bolus surge of venom. In most cases no signs of envenomation will develop, and after a period of observation they can be discharged. However, all children should be admitted for overnight observation. When signs of true envenomation are present *ab initio*, or develop following the removal of the constrictive bandage, antivenom should be infused. Antihistamines and steroids should be given before the infusion of antivenom, and adrenaline tartrate (1 in 1000) should be drawn up in a syringe at the bedside before antivenom is administered. If anaphylaxis occurs either from the venom itself, or from antivenom, adrenaline should be used subcutaneously, into the trachea, or intramuscularly. Anaphylactic collapse following antivenom varies in different parts of the world where different antivenoms are used but does not usually occur in more than 3 per cent of cases.

If antivenom is going to be used it should be given early, but it is never too late to administer it. In most cases one ampule of antivenom will neutralize the bite of an average sized snake; the dose should be repeated up to 24 hours after the initial administration if an inadequate clinical response is observed. The systemic effects of severe envenomation may include acute renal failure, multi-organ damage, and severe local necrosis.

Management of potential local tissue damage at the bite site is controversial; fasciotomy in cases of rattlesnake bites is no longer advocated. With severe and prolonged neurotoxic envenomation, complete recovery can occur even after 16 weeks of mechanical ventilation.

Hymenoptera (bees, wasps, hornets, ants)

Although trivial stings are common, severe envenomation and allergic reactions necessitate emergency treatment. First aid and hospital management are similar for all cases of hymenopteran envenomation.

Bee stings

Bee stings must never be taken lightly. In the United States and in the UK, more deaths occur from anaphylaxis following wasp and bee stings than from all other venomous bites or stings combined. In Australia, more victims die from bee stings than from shark attacks.

The common domestic honey bee (*Apis mellifera*) or feral swarms originating from it, causes problems in all parts of the world. Venom sac and barb become avulsed when she disengages, and remain in the skin. Problems result either from swarm attacks, or from hypersensitivity and anaphylaxis from single stings.

Mass envenomation

Mass envenomation by swarm attacks occurs occasionally, and allergic reactions are not necessarily a component of this syndrome. The victims are usually comatose or semi-comatose, are hot and flushed, and may be shocked. Often several individuals are involved. Pain may be intense, but the victim usually lies still and seems afraid to move. Treatment consists of adrenaline, antihistamines, intravenous infusions, and pain relief with narcotics.

Anaphylaxis

Allergic reactions to single (or several) stings are common, and anaphylaxis is a real and much feared complication. Children at particular risk are those with a history of asthma, and those who have manifested crescendo reactions to more than one bee sting in the past (Pearn, 1982). Hypotension, bronchospasm, low cardiac output and mucoid oversecretion from mucous membranes occur.

First aid

Remove the sting with a fingernail, and apply ammonia or any other basic solution, or a protein-denaturing agent such as aluminium sulphate (20%). The site should be cooled. Cardiopulmonary resuscitation may be required. Adrenaline, salbutamol or terbutaline inhaler, if available, may be life saving in the field.

Hospital management

Hospital management consists of inhalational adrenaline or salbutamol, or intravenous adrenaline tartrate (1 in 1000), intravenous antihistamines and steroids. If sympathomimetics (e.g. adrenaline or salbutamol) and antihistamines cannot be given, permanent brain damage may result from cerebral hypoperfusion.

Prevention

Children who have manifested serious reactions in the past, and children with a known allergic diathesis, especially asthmatic children, are at significantly increased risk from hymenopteran envenomation. All such children should always have an inhalational aerosol of salbutamol or adrenaline available both at home, and when on holiday, and thus should accompany the 'at risk' child to school camps, holidays, scout and youth camps; custodians in charge of such children should be adequately briefed.

Arachnids

Children are particularly vulnerable to arachnid bites. Local knowledge of dangerous species and their clinical effects is important as some lethal species have a very limited habitat. Almost all arachnids possess venoms, and have a world-wide distribution. Scorpion bites are a problem in Africa, Asia, India and the Americas, and tick envenomation in Australia and in North America.

Spiders and scorpions

The symptoms and signs of spider and scorpion envenomation are similar, intense local burning pain which may last for hours and sometimes days, with pain spreading to the local lymph node regions. Signs of envenomation depend on whether the venom has primarily a local dermatonecrotic or histotoxic effect (such as the American fiddleback, *Loxosceles*), or whether its action is largely systemic as in the case of *Latrodectus* (the Red-back or Black Widow spider), or the Sydney funnel-web (*Atrax robustus*).

Latrodectus species (Red Back, Black Widow)

This is a universal spider and is the major cause of serious child arachnid stings. They are called the Red Back spider in Australia and in New Guinea, the Katipo in New Zealand, and the Black Widow in the Americas and in Europe. Its toxin does not cause death in healthy adults but it may cause incapacitation; but children may be at considerable risk. Its colour streak, although usually reddish, may be pink or brown, or even pale cream. Local symptoms include a burning stinging pain, sometimes with a local area of sweating and occasionally local muscle fasciculation. Generalized symptoms include sweating, nausea, vomiting and collapse.

First aid

If the spider or scorpion is seen to bite, and if there is known to be a risk of fatality from local species, a constrictive bandage should be applied with a splint for immobilization. If a known local species is likely to cause a necrotizing lesion a constrictive bandage or ligature is contraindicated, and the limb should be immobilized. The area should be treated with ice packs, standard cardiopulmonary resuscitation techniques applied as appropriate, and specialist advice sought.

Hospital management

If pain is severe, locally injected lignocaine and systemic analgesics should be used. Antivenom should be used to treat *Latrodectus* stings (Red Back or Black Widow spider) if symptoms and signs are significant. Scorpion antivenom should be used only if local species are known to be a problem (not in Australasia). In the case of the Australian funnel-web spider (*Atrax robustus*) children are at grave risk, and sophisticated management in an intensive care unit may be required; and the newly developed antivenom should be injected with all speed, with the usual safeguards against anaphylaxis.

Ticks

There are five essential themes:

1. Allergic reactions.
2. Tick paralysis.
3. Foreign body granuloma.
4. Infections.
5. Zoonoses.

Attached ticks may remain undiscovered for days in young children, and puzzling symptoms and signs may develop. A child may be infested with one or two partly engorged adults, or may experience multiple infestation with several dozen nymph or larval ticks. Allergic reactions, when they occur, can be very serious. Tick paralysis is confined largely to children, and only occurs when an attached tick is overlooked and remains embedded in the child's skin for several days.

Allergic effects

Anaphylaxis with collapse may occur following contact with ticks. To have a tick simply walk over one's hand produces in some people the most intolerable and intense itching, which develops almost instantaneously with sensations unlike any others experienced by the victims. Larvae as well as adults can cause allergic reactions (Pearn, 1977). Severe local erythema and oedema may develop within 2–3 hours of attachment of even a tiny nymph. If the tick is embedded on the head, gross facial and neck swelling may occur within several hours, occasionally progressing to tracheopharyngeal compression within 5–6 hours after the onset of symptoms. Those who experience allergic attacks from ticks describe crescendo-type reactions with a gradual evolution to hypersensitivity with each exposure.

With attachment by an adult female, a lump usually remains at the site of the attachment for many weeks or months after removal of the tick, but it ultimately disappears. The retention of residual mouth parts is the cause of the foreign body granuloma which develops.

Infection

Tick bite may be followed by Rickettsial infection. In the last 5 years Lyme arthritis has been recognized, an epidemic form of brief but clinically severe asymmetrical oligoarticular involvement of larger joints. One to three weeks after the attachment of Ixodid ticks, patients experience skin rashes, malaise, fatigue, chills and fever, headaches and muscle aches, nausea and sometimes prostration. Aseptic meningitis, cranial nerve palsies, and sensory radiculopathies have also been described. The micro-organism responsible, of which ticks are presumably the vectors, remains unknown.

Tick paralysis

Tick paralysis is potentially life threatening, and resembles poliomyelitis or Guillain–Barré syndrome. In Western countries with a high immunization rate against poliomyelitis, one should never diagnose poliomyelitis without first excluding tick paralysis.

Tick paralysis may be localized (Pearn, 1977) or generalized. A feature of children is the progressive ascending flaccid paralysis which may intensify for up to 24 hours after removal of the tick; also there may be marked asymmetry, affecting also the iris dilators. Recovery after acute paralysis may take 4–7 days, and full strength may sometimes not return until 28 days after the removal of the tick.

First aid and medical management

The tick should be removed with one's fingers. In the field, it should be removed with a corkscrewing type of action. If a pair of fine surgical scissors are available, the points should be slightly separated and the tick levered from the skin. In virtually all cases, once the tick is removed recovery is complete, without sequelae. Allergic or anaphylactic reactions should be treated appropriately. In children who are paralysed an effective (canine) antivenom is available, but it is probably better to be conservative in its use and to nurse the child in an intensive care unit, if respiratory effort is still adequate for ventilation.

Marine envenomations

Their camouflage often hides marine creatures until trodden upon. Problems of marine envenomation are not limited to any one zoo-geographic region. Medusans (jelly fish), stonefish and other venomous fish, molluscs, echinoderms, sponges and sea snakes have a world-wide distribution.

Sea snakes

Sea snakes are found throughout the Indian and Pacific Oceans. Although they are common in shallow water, bites are rare. The venom is very toxic but the snakes are not aggressive and clinical toxicity is uncommon. There is a risk to fishermen removing their catch by hand from nets at night (especially in South-East Asian waters). Children become envenomed only from handling snakes, or when a snake is injured (Mercer, McGill and Ibrahim, 1981). Bites by sea snakes tend to be painless, and usually the skin lesion is insignificant, or even absent (Reid, 1961).

First aid

First aid for bites or suspected bites is identical with that for bites by terrestrial snakes. The pressure-bandage–immobilization technique is very effective and has proven very efficient in the case of envenomation by the most common sea snake causing problems, *Enhydrina schistosa* (Sutherland *et al.*, 1981). The clinical syndrome is primary neurotoxic.

Hospital management

Hospital management is identical with that of bites by terrestrial elapid snakes. Sea snake antivenom is available from the Commonwealth Serum Laboratories (Melbourne, Australia) and from the Haffkine Institute, Bombay. These antivenoms offer cross-protection against many sea snake species. The antivenom is given intravenously and is very effective. If sea snake antivenom is not available, Australian Tiger Snake antivenom offers some protection.

Fish stings

Children can be severely envenomed by stone-fish, cat-fish, scorpion-fish, sting-rays and a number of toleost fishes known by various local names. Accidental stings may result from either handling a colourful attractive specimen such as the butterfly cod or scorpion fish (*Pterois volitans*); by inadvertently stepping upon sedentary species such as the common stone-fish; or by removing a specimen from a fishing line. The descending foot presses down on the spine (opening a wound or track), releasing the toxin into the subcutaneous tissues.

Stone-fishes are found throughout the Indo-Pacific and African littorals and are not only the most venomous of the teleost fishes but also the most sessile and sedentary, and are a special danger to children when reefing or wading with bare feet. Stone-fishes inject more venom than do other fish, and their venom appears to be more potent than other fish venom. Victims complain of sudden burning excruciating pain which has a sickening visceral quality. The foot or hand becomes swollen very quickly, and shock may develop. Death is rare from envenomation by teleost fish.

First aid

First aid for all fish envenomations consists of bathing the envenomed limb in as hot water as the victim can comfortably bear. It is important to test the water as the stung foot or hand may be partially anaesthetic. Urgent pain relief is essential. A ligature or compressive bandage is contraindicated. Even a tiny amount of stone-fish venom may cause extreme pain, and gross swelling is usual.

Hospital management

Clinical management consists of injecting lignocaine 1% along the tracks of the spines, and for a stone-fish wound, the use of antivenom. This should be given intramuscularly in a limb not involved in the sting, or intravenously if a patient is shocked and collapsed. Antivenom should not be injected in or around the area of the sting. Intravenous pethidine or morphine is required in most cases of significant envenomation by stone-fishes. Surgical débridement for the lacerations is necessary, and antibiotic and tetanus cover are essential.

Medusans (jellyfish)

Physalia species (Portuguese man-of-war; Blue bottles)

These are found in all temperate and tropical waters of the world. Children may be stung while swimming in the water, or when handling them when they are stranded on the sand. The bubble-like float has beneath it a festoon of small tentacles, and one long fishing tentacle containing the nematocysts which become arranged into stinging buttons when it contracts. Victims who touch these tentacles experience excruciating pain of an intense burning type. Headache and shock may occur. Some children become drowsy and may sleep after being stung. Large specimens deliver an increased dose of venom.

FIRST AID

First aid consists of using vinegar on the stung skin, with subsequent removal of the tentacles. Hot liquids poured onto the stung areas will also help. Other remedies such as aluminium sulphate 20% or meat tenderizer are also effective. Methylated spirits or alcohol actually causes discharge of nematocysts adherent to the skin.

HOSPITAL MANAGEMENT

Medical management consists of the application of 5% lignocaine jelly, oral or parenteral antihistamines, and oral analgesia.

Box jellyfish

In tropical Indo-West Pacific waters exists the world's most dangerous medusan, the box jellyfish *Chironex fleckeri* which is a serious threat to human life in summer months. Victims become entangled in the tentacles of the creature which is very difficult to see in the water. The nematocysts discharge venom which is a mixture of a 'lethal component' having cardiotoxic properties, and a dermatonecrotic factor which causes striated skin lesions. Victims may die within minutes while still in the water. Overwhelming pain occurs following entanglement and causes acute mania or demented behaviour.

FIRST AID

First aid consists in rescuing the patient, and the avoidance of contact with the adhering tentacles oneself. Cardiopulmonary resuscitation (CPR) is thought to be potentially life saving; and if the patient survives, the venom is detoxified or inactivated quickly. Besides administering CPR, the envenomed area should be dealt with as described under Portuguese man-of-war.

HOSPITAL MANAGEMENT

This consists in life support measures, effective pain relief (usually intravenous narcotics) and antivenom if available. The recent advent of a specific antivenom for cubo-medusoid stings is a great advance (Williamson, Callanan and Hartwick, 1980).

Molluscs

Certain cone shells contain very toxic venoms, and are potentially lethal to humans. Children should be warned about collecting cone shells until they are old enough to know the danger of local species which may be venomous. Collectors of any age should always use a scoop or small net for shells of this genus.

Octopus

The blue-ringed octopus of Indo-Pacific waters is potentially deadly. Its electric blue and yellow coloration, which flashes when the creature is disturbed, is appealing to children. A bite results in the injection of tetrodotoxin (which paralyses the cellular sodium pump) and absorption is very rapid.

First aid

First aid is an arterial tourniquet or a very tight compressive bandage with immobilization, with CPR if required. No antivenom is available and hospital management of respiratory and cardiac failure must be supportive.

Envenomation and drowning

A special problem with all marine envenomations is the risk of drowning. So incapacitating is the sting of stone-fish, for example, that the victim may be drowned even in quite shallow water. Similarly, victims of the box jellyfish who are not killed quickly become maniacal from the acute pain, and are at risk from drowning before rescue or extraction from the water can be effected. In hospital care, lung complications of secondary drowning (Pearn, 1980) may be overlooked in the drama of the primary envenomation features, if one is not aware of this potential complication.

Antivenom

SOME CENTRES OFFERING ADVICE, AND POSSIBLE SOURCES OF ANTIVENOM:

Africa
South African Institute for Medical Research, Hospital Street, Johannesburg (P.O. Box 1038, Johannesburg, 2000, South Africa).
Tel: Johannesburg 725-0511.
Institut Pasteur d'Algérie, rue Docteur Laveran, Alger, Algeria.

Australia, New Guinea, and the Pacific
Commonwealth Serum Laboratories, 45 Poplar Avenue, Parkville, Melbourne Victoria, 3052, Australia.
Tel: (03) 389 1911.

India
The Haffkine Institute, Parel, Bombay 12, India.

South America
Instituto Butantan, Caixa Postal 65, Sao Paulo, Brazil.

South-East Asia
Queen Saovabha Memorial Institute, Rama 4 Road, Bangkok, Thailand.

United Kingdom
Main antivenom centres in Britain. A comprehensive stock of antivenoms for bites by foreign snakes is held at the two main antivenom centres:

1. Walton Hospital, Rice Lane, Liverpool L9 1EA. (Tel: 051 525 3611), in conjunction with Liverpool School of Tropical Medicine, Pembroke Place, Liverpool L3 5QA (Tel: 051 708 9393).
2. The National Poisons Information Centre, New Cross Hospital, Avonley Road, London SE14 5ER (Tel: 01-407 7600).

Advice on management of bites by foreign venomous snakes is available from the Liverpool School of Tropical Medicine. (Out of office hours: Walton Hospital: Tel: 051-525 3611.)

United States

Antivenin Index. A catalogue of available antivenoms stored in the United States; number of vials stored at each facility; includes antivenoms to both indigenous snakes of North America, and to exotic species held in the USA. (Published by The American Association of Zoological Parts and Aquariums, with the Oklahoma City Zoo; with the Oklahoma Poison Information Centre.)
Tel: Oklahoma City (405-271-5454).

Denver Poisons Information Centre. Poisindex Central Office.
Tel: Denver (800-332-3073).

Wyeth Laboratories, Box 8299, Philadelphia, Pa 19101, USA.

Western Europe

Institut Pasteur (Annexe de Garches), 91 Hauts-de-Seine, Paris, France, *or* 28 rue du Docteur Roux, Cedex 15, Paris, France.

Behring Institu, Behringwerke AG, Postfach 167, D355 Marburg/Lahn, West Germany.

Institute of Immunology, Rockefellerova 2, Zagreb, Yugoslavia.

Institute for Sera and Vaccines. W. Pieck Street, Prague 2, Czechoslovakia.

References

COULTER, A. R., HARRIS, R. D. and SUTHERLAND, S. K. (1980) Enzyme immunoassay for the rapid clinical identification of snake venom. *Medical Journal of Australia,* **i,** 433–435

MERCER, H. P., McGILL, J. J. and IBRAHIM, R. A. (1981) Envenomation by sea snake in Queensland. *Medical Journal of Australia,* **i,** 130–132

MORRISON, J. J., PEARN, J. H., COVACEVICH, J. and NIXON, J. (1983) Can Australians identify snakes? *Medical Journal of Australia,* **ii,** 66–70

MUNRO, J. G. and PEARN, J. H. (1978) Snakebite in children. *Australian Paediatric Journal,* **14,** 248–253

PEARN, J. (1977) The clinical features of tick bite. *Medical Journal of Australia,* **ii,** 313–318

PEARN, J. H. (1980) Secondary drowning involving children. *British Medical Journal,* **ii,** 1103–1105

PEARN, J. (1982) Acute bee sting reactions: treatment and prevention. *Current Therapeutics,* **23,** 39–43

REID, H. A. (1961) Diagnosis, prognosis and treatment of sea-snake bite. *Lancet,* **ii,** 399–402

SUTHERLAND, S. K., COULTER, A. R. and HARRIS, R. D. (1979) Rationalization of first-aid measures for elapid snakebite. *Lancet,* **i,** 183–186

SUTHERLAND, S. K., COULTER, A. R., HARRIS, R. D., LOVERING, K. E. and ROBERTS, I. D. (1981) A study of the major Australian snake venoms in the monkey (*Macaca fascicularis*). 1. The movement of injected venom, methods which retard this movement, and the response to antivenoms. *Pathology,* **13,** 13–27

WILLIAMSON, J. A., CALLANAN, V. I. and HARTWICK, R. F. (1980) Serious envenomation by the Northern Australian box-jellyfish (*Chironex fleckeri*). *Medical Journal of Australia,* **i,** 13–15

Further reading

CAMERON, A. M. (1981) Venomous fishes hazardous to humans. In J. Pearn (ed.) *Toxins and Man,* Chapter 6, pp. 29–45. Brisbane: Division of Health Education and Information

COOPER, B. J. (1974) Quote in S. K. Sutherland, Venomous Australian creatures: the action of their toxins and the care of the envenomated patient. *Anaesthesia and Intensive Care,* **2,** 316–328

ENDEAN, R. (1981) The Box Jelly-fish or 'Sea wasp'. In J. Pearn (ed.) *Animal Toxins and Man,* Chapter 7, pp. 46–54. Brisbane: Division of Health Education and Information

PEARN, J. and MUNRO, C. (1981) Snakebite in childhood. In J. Pearn (ed.) *Animal Toxins and Man,* Chapter 11, pp. 104–111. Brisbane: Division of Health Education and Information

RUSSELL, F. E. (1983) First Aid. *Snake Venom Poisoning,* pp. 261–280. New York: Scholium International

RUSSELL, F. E., GANS, C. and MINTON, S. (1978) Poisonous snakes. *Clinical Medicine,* **85,** 13–30

SUTHERLAND, S. K. (1983a) Family Hydrophiidae, Sea Snakes. In *Australian Animal Toxins,* Chapter 6, pp. 158–184; and Treatment of snakebite in Australia, Chapter 17, pp. 185–221. Melbourne: Oxford University Press

SUTHERLAND, S. K. (1983b) Genus Synanceia, stonefishes. In *Australian Animal Toxins,* Chapter 28, pp. 400–410. Melbourne: Oxford University Press

SUTHERLAND, S. K. (1983c) *Chironex fleckeri* Southcott, the Box Jellyfish or Sea Wasp. In *Australian Animal Toxins,* pp. 359–373. Melbourne: Oxford University Press

SUTHERLAND, S. K. (1983d) Genus Atrax Cambridge, the Funnel-web spiders. In *Australian Animal Toxins,* Chapter 20, pp. 255–298. Melbourne: Oxford University Press

TURNER, B., SULLIVAN, P. and PENNEFATHER, J. (1980) Disarming the bluebottle, treatment of Physalia envenomation. *Medical Journal of Australia,* **ii,** 394–395

VISSER, J. (1979) *Common Snakes of South Africa.* Cape Town: Purnell

Chapter 62

Malaria

J. Paget Stanfield

Malaria is among the major world-wide causes of mortality and morbidity in children.

With the resurgence of malaria in many areas from which it had been almost eradicated, and children frequently travelling from non-malarious areas into endemic areas, malaria is occurring at all ages and in unlikely places where the index of suspicion is low.

Recognition

Plasmodium (P.) falciparum is the most virulent ('malignant tertian malaria'); *P. vivax, malariae* and *ovale* have much less severe effects, and do not usually produce medical emergencies.

Malaria is particularly lethal during pregnancy for both mother and fetus, especially in primiparae and during the second trimester.

Malarial infection during pregnancy may produce:

1. Severe maternal illness with risk of abortion, premature labour, hypoglycaemia, severe haemorrhage, severe anaemia, a septicaemic-like illness or death.
2. Fetal death.
3. Premature delivery.
4. Small-for-dates infant.
5. A combination of (3) and (4).
6. Congenital malaria from transplacental transmission especially in the absence of antibody (i.e. non-immune mother). This may not manifest itself for up to 3 months after delivery and is not as rare as was previously thought. Transplacentally transmitted malaria is particularly dangerous if the mother and infant move to a non-malarious area with a low index of suspicion.

Emergency treatment is necessary in severe falciparum infections especially in non-immune patients during pregnancy; and in three groups of children:

1. Infection, usually falciparum, in the infant and young child with waning or absent maternally-transferred immunity.
2. Infection, usually falciparum, in the older non-immune child. This may occur in children visiting endemic malarious areas from malaria-free countries who have omitted prophylaxis or are infected with a resistant strain. It is increasingly a risk

in indigenous children who suddenly stop taking prophylaxis after the first 2 or 3 years of life. Falciparum infection in non-immune children should always be regarded as an emergency.
3. Infection in malnourished, anaemic, or otherwise sick or infected children.

The usual acute presentation is with fever, vomiting and convulsions and one or more of the acute 'complications'. These syndromes are (with considerable overlap):

1. The acute neurological syndromes.
2. Hyperpyrexia.
3. Collapse, or 'algid' malaria.
4. Severe haemolytic anaemia.
5. The gastrointestinal syndrome.
6. The acute renal syndrome.

All or any of these could be the result of other acute diseases, but malaria must never be forgotten. The younger the child the less specific will be the symptoms, and the more difficult to distinguish from other possible acute infections.

Uncomplicated acute malaria causes no specific physical signs. The spleen and liver enlarge but such enlargement is not limited to malarial infection.

Attributing the findings in a severely ill infant or child to malaria should be easy, by means of a blood film. However, difficulties may arise:

1. The density of the parasitaemia may not correspond to the severity of the symptoms. The number of parasites in the blood not only indicates severity but also the degree of immunity and the duration and efficacy of any previous antimalarial therapy or chemoprophylaxis.
2. A non-immune child, or one who has received a parenteral dose of antimalarial drug shortly before admission, may be severely ill from malaria and yet have very few parasites in the blood film. On the other hand, a heavy parasitaemia may be present in an immune older child in a hyperendemic area in whom symptoms are slight.
3. Parasitaemia may mask another underlying infection. The presence of parasites in the blood of children from endemic areas is so common that they may well be evident where the primary cause of the symptoms, such as a severe meningococcal septicaemia, is entirely different.
4. A mild attack of malaria may precipitate severe symptoms of an underlying disease, such as a crisis in a child with sickle-cell anaemia.
5. Previous treatment may complicate the diagnosis:
   (a) By reducing the parasitaemia without immediately altering the symptoms, as in cerebral malaria.
   (b) By inducing toxic effects, such as the haemolysis in glucose-6-phosphate dehydrogenase (G6PD) deficiency by the 8-amino-quinoline drugs (primaquine, pamaquine) or the sudden collapse and death produced by too large a dose of parenteral chloroquine or quinine. Toxic effects also result from home or herbal remedies which may produce gastrointestinal or hepatic symptoms unrelated to the malarial infection; bizarre symptoms should raise this suspicion. The association of blackwater fever following repeated inadequate courses of quinine, particularly in the non-immune patient, has never been adequately explained.

The child may be so severely ill that there may seem to be no time to take a blood film and examine it, but it is very important before starting any antimalarial therapy, particularly parenteral therapy, on suspicion, to collect a thick and thin film for examination as soon as possible. In certain situations the diagnosis of the contribution of malaria in an acute illness requiring emergency antimalarial therapy may well have to depend retrospectively on the response.

Management

Initial emergency treatment of malaria aims to suppress the asexual cycle of the parasite within the red cells. Such suppressive schizonticides must be highly active against *P. falciparum* and need to be capable of being given parenterally to obtain an immediate effect. Daily parasite counts are essential to monitor treatment.

Chloroquine (a 4-aminoquinoline) and quinine are the two common drugs in present use, though if the oral route is considered possible amodiaquine can replace chloroquine, with its very similar action. Recent powerful schizonticides, such as mefloquine, are now available to use in combination with or actually to replace quinine in chloroquine-resistant falciparum malaria. Falciparum strains resistant to chloroquine are widespread throughout South East Asia where quinine is now the first-line treatment in most areas. Several foci are also established in South and Central America. In East Africa up to one third of falciparum infections are R2 or R3 resistant*, and resistance is now being reported in West Africa.

1. Chloroquine is available in variously named commercial preparations for use both orally (tablet and syrup) and parenterally. It is important to make certain of the content of chloroquine base in each tablet or ampoule before use. The usual preparations contain 150 mg chloroquine base per tablet and 40 mg chloroquine base/ml injectable solution.
2. Amodiaquine is usually prepared with 200 mg amodiaquine base in each tablet.
3. Quinine is prepared in tablets containing 300 mg salt, equivalent to 250 mg quinine base, or in ampoules for parenteral use containing quinine dihydrochloride 300 or 500 mg (equivalent to 250 mg or 415 mg quinine base) in 1 or 2 ml of water; ampoules of 650 mg quinine dihydrochloride, equivalent to about 500 mg of base, are also available.

All of these preparations have a bitter taste. Chloroquine base 150 mg is equivalent to chloroquine sulphate (Nivaquine) 200 mg and chloroquine phosphate (Avloclor or Malarivon) 250 mg. Quinine anhydrous base 100 mg is equivalent to quinine dihydrochloride (the usual parenteral preparation) 122 mg, quinine hydrochloride 122 mg, quinine bisulphate 169 mg (*British National Formulary* 1986 No. 11).

Chloroquine therapy (doses given as base)

Immediate treatment

In severe infection chloroquine is given intramuscularly in a dose of 5 mg/kg body weight. A second similar dose can be given between 12 and 24 hours after the first

* Definitions of sensitivity and resistance: S – Clearance of asexual parasitaemia within 7 days of the first dose of treatment, without recrudescence. R1 – Clearance of asexual parasitaemia as in sensitivity, followed by recrudescence. R2 – Marked reduction of asexual parasitaemia, but no clearance. R3 – No reduction in asexual parasitaemia.

but the total amount over 24 hours must not exceed these two doses. In very ill, collapsed children chloroquine can be given intravenously; 5 mg/kg is given slowly over 4–6 hours in an appropriate amount of fluid. If a 'bolus' dose is needed this should be no more than one-fifth of the initial dose (1 mg/kg), through as large a syringe as slowly as possible; the remainder can then be given intramuscularly. Parenteral chloroquine in higher doses exposes the child to the risk of sudden death. It is therefore necessary to make careful notes of the amount of parenteral chloroquine administered to any infant or child. These should be attached in some inseparable manner to the patient if transferred to a more central unit.

Oral treatment

As soon as possible oral therapy should be commenced though it may, rarely, be necessary to continue parenteral chloroquine (5 mg/kg daily) for up to the next two 24-hour periods if the child is severely collapsed, comatose or vomiting. Oral therapy is given by nasogastric tube or in crushed tablet or syrup form by spoon depending on the state of consciousness. The dose must be repeated if obviously vomited within the next half hour.

1. *For infants under 1 year* the dose is 75 mg (half a 150 mg tablet) twice in the first day initially (½ tablet as a loading dose followed by a further ½ tablet in 6–8 hours). This is followed by 37–75 mg (¼–½ tablet) daily for the next 2 or 3 days.
2. For children from 1 to 3 years these doses should be doubled (2 tablets in the first 24 hours as a loading dose followed by ½–1 tablet daily).
3. For children over 3 years the loading dose should be 2 tablets followed by 1 tablet daily for 3 days.

The loading oral dose is omitted if parenteral therapy has been given.

Quinine therapy (doses given as base)

In areas of chloroquine resistance quinine replaces chloroquine. Amodiaquine (Camoquin), as a base, in the same dosage as chloroquine, is being used as the second-line drug in Africa. However, it cannot be given parenterally. The initial dose of quinine is 10–15 mg/kg, the higher dose is advocated in Thailand infused intravenously slowly over 4–6 hours in a solution of quinine base through a 100 ml metering chamber. 5–10 mg/kg can be repeated 8–12 hourly until the child has sufficiently improved to start oral therapy. Below 1 year it is safer to commence with doses at the lower limit of the range depending on the gravity of the illness and the likelihood of quinine resistance. The infusion must be given very slowly in children because very high levels in the plasma may cause hypotension, shock, and sudden death. Single intramuscular doses of 10–15 mg/kg should be used if the IV route is not possible. If given 12 hourly for up to four doses, satisfactory plasma levels of quinine of around 10 μg/kg are obtained. Tissue necrosis is avoided by giving the drug deeply and diffusely into the muscles of the thigh. Oral quinine 20–30 mg/kg daily given in three divided doses with a supplementary second-line antimalarial drug should replace parenteral therapy as soon as possible. Like chloroquine the taste is very bitter and it will have to be given determinedly and skilfully, preferably by nasogastric tube.

Complications

The acute neurological syndromes

Recognition

The distinction between 'cerebral malaria', falciparum malaria with febrile convulsions, and encephalitic syndromes with parasites in the blood smear is difficult. Hypoglycaemia may occur in severe falciparum malaria particularly in pregnancy and in undernourished children. Quinine has been found to stimulate insulin production and its use may increase the risk of hypoglycaemia. A blood glucose should always be done to exclude this as the cause of convulsions or coma. Cerebral malaria is never associated with other than *P. falciparum* and so can be ruled out if the parasites are all clearly *P. vivax*.

The infant or child presents with convulsions or coma with initial fever of varying degree. There is a parasitaemia, usually heavy, and the cerebrospinal fluid is clear, with or without pleocytosis and slightly raised protein. Recent work has shown that CSF lactate concentration rises in cerebral malaria, associated with a fall in CSF glucose. Levels of lactate above 6 mmol/ℓ (normal range 1.1–2.2 mmol/ℓ) indicate a poor prognosis (White *et al.*, 1985). The CSF must ALWAYS be examined even when there is a parasitaemia, to exclude a coexisting meningitis.

Diagnosis is not easy and treatment must be directed to the treatable condition, i.e. malaria. *An unconscious or convulsing child with malarial parasites in the blood, especially if they are recognized to be falciparum, ought to be treated as if the diagnosis is cerebral malaria until proved otherwise, by virtue of rapid recovery, or by evidence indicating some other cause for the symptoms.*

Management

1. Specific intravenous schizonticidal antimalarial therapy is started immediately. If the intravenous route is not immediately possible an initial intramuscular dose may be given. The sooner such effective therapy is commenced following loss of consciousness the better the chances of recovery. Recovery is usually complete. If coma persists for longer than 24 hours, IV mannitol may be given on the basis that this may reduce cerebral oedema. Dexamethasone has been advocated for this purpose but a recent carefully conducted double blind trial indicated that its use prolong the period of unconsciousness and increased the likelihood of sequelae such as pneumonia and gastrointestinal bleeding (Warrell *et al.*, 1982). There is no evidence that anticoagulant or fibrinolytic drugs affect the prognosis and they may increase the likelihood of bleeding. Recovery after prolonged coma is often slow even after total elimination of circulating parasites and may never be complete.
2. Convulsions must be controlled by IV diazepam or a combination of i.m. phenobarbitone and i.m. paraldehyde (*see* pages 308–309).
3. In addition to the specific therapy of convulsions and coma, adequate hydration and nutrition must be maintained either by nasogastric tube or, if vomiting is severe, by intravenous infusion. Hypoglycaemia and acidosis should be kept in mind. Intravenous glucose, 20% or 50%, as a bolus will raise the blood glucose immediately but it may be necessary to continue with a 5% or 10% infusion to provide for the increased requirements, until parasitaemia has been controlled. A synthetic somatostatin, SM 201–995, has been found to antagonize quinine-induced insulin release, thus abolishing hypoglycaemia (in adults)

(Phillips *et al.*, 1986). For further details of treatment of hypoglycaemia *see* page 406. Rectal temperature must be taken regularly, 6-hourly, because hyperpyrexia increases the risk of further convulsions or brain damage. In prolonged coma intragastric milk feeding will be necessary.

Acute hyperpyrexia

See page 547 for description.

Management

See page 552 for treatment of hyperpyrexia. A swinging recurrent fever is usually characteristic of malaria and care must be taken not to let the temperature fall below normal, especially in infants. The fever will also tend to fall after convulsions are controlled with diazepam or paraldehyde. Once the antimalarial therapy has begun to reduce the parasitaemia the spiking temperature will fall.

The collapsed child or 'algid' malaria

This may be the terminal phase of severe falciparum malaria, but can appear rapidly, with a short history of fever, diarrhoea and vomiting, or may follow an overdose of parenteral chloroquine or quinine. Occasionally a concomitant Gram-negative septicaemia develops, associated with a pulmonary or urinary tract infection. In such cases the child will fail to recover after antimalarial treatment despite a clearing of parasitaemia, or will suddenly deteriorate for no apparent reason.

Recognition

The child is pale, with cold extremities and a weak rapid pulse. Rectal temperature may be very high, or low. The condition resembles shock, owing to a combination of fluid and electrolyte loss, anaemia, hyperpyrexia, and toxaemia. Bleeding may occur in severe falciparum malaria with nose bleeds, oozing from gums and venepuncture sites, and retinal haemorrhages. Melaena may be a terminal symptom. Blood and urine should be cultured and broad-spectrum antibiotics given if a septicaemia is suspected.

Management

Severely collapsed children will need all the resuscitative measures available. This is the condition 'par excellence' requiring intravenous antimalarial therapy, followed or accompanied by plasma or blood if there is severe anaemia. Not more than 20 ml/kg should be given, 5 ml/kg rapidly and the remainder slowly. The rate and amount of blood given should be monitored by regular pulse, blood pressure, and central venous pressure measurement. Intravenous or intramuscular hydrocortisone (50–100 mg per dose) can also be used.

Severe haemolytic anaemia syndrome

Recognition

Pallor and slight-to-moderate jaundice develop in the course of a febrile illness. Splenomegaly may be considerable. Tachypnoea, cardiac and hepatic enlargement, pulmonary oedema and neck-vein engorgement indicate a 'high-output' cardiac failure. This is a fairly common presentation in infants of non-immune status, and may be superimposed on an already anaemic state such as iron deficiency or sickle-cell anaemia. G6PD deficiency may be present, with haemoglobinaemia and haemoglobinuria.

Management

Control the parasitaemia as rapidly as possible.

A slow blood transfusion, preferably of packed or sedimented red cells, is indicated if the haemoglobin is below 5 g/100 ml (though haemoglobinaemia may mask the full reduction of red cells available), or if there is any indication of cardiac failure not responding to bed rest. Cardiomegaly and moderately increased venous pressure are often indicators of a haemodynamic adaptation to a low haemoglobin, and digoxin and diuretics given in such circumstances can interfere with this adaptation.

During the blood transfusion, which should not exceed 20 ml/kg given over not less than 6 hours, careful watch should be kept for increasing hepatic enlargement or neck-vein engorgement. Diuretics (frusemide 2–5 mg) can be given in the transfusion or separately during transfusion, intramuscularly either as a routine, or in the presence of increasing venous congestion. A limited exchange transfusion has proved life saving. Some workers give 10 ml/kg blood intravenously to restore an immediate quantity of non-parasitized red cells, and give the remaining 10 ml/kg intraperitoneally.

The gastrointestinal syndrome

Recognition

Malaria is often present in the infant with gastrointestinal symptoms. Vomiting is a major feature; the diarrhoea is rarely as copious and watery as in primary gastroenteritis. Occasionally abdominal pain occurs but it is rarely severe. In severe illness gastrointestinal bleeding may occur with haematemesis and melaena.

Management

In any febrile infant with diarrhoea a blood slide should be taken and chloroquine given if in any doubt. Vomiting usually stops dramatically after antimalarial therapy. Intragastric glucose-electrolyte solution (*see* page 730) is usually all that is required for rehydration, with chlorpromazine (1 mg/kg per dose) if vomiting is severe. Intravenous fluid and electrolyte replacement may be necessary initially until the antimalarial therapy becomes effective, and as a vehicle for intravenous antimalarials.

The acute renal syndrome

The kidney may be affected by severe haemolysis, dehydration, electrolyte disturbances, and toxaemia.

Recognition

1. Prerenal azotaemia may occur in infants in whom fever, vomiting and diarrhoea have occurred without adequate rehydration. Adequate rehydration should be accomplished during antimalarial therapy.
2. In algid malaria or during an acute haemolytic episode, oliguria may develop, progressing to anuria; the urine may be red or dark brown due to haemoglobin ('blackwater fever'). Uraemia ensues rapidly with vomiting, acidosis and hyperkalaemia.

Tubular obstruction is probably not the cause of the renal failure: but partial or total cortical necrosis certainly occurs, and DIC probably occurs in some cases. The haemoglobin casts are probably a measure of the acuteness and degree of haemolysis and haemoglobinaemia.

Management *(see also* ***page 431****)*

Antimalarial therapy must be started immediately, and then with care, if anuria supervenes. Management of the renal failure will depend on the glomerular and tubular function, measured most simply by urine flow and level of blood urea. An in-dwelling catheter may be necessary to assess urine output, though some prefer intermittent bladder puncture.

If urine flow is maintained and blood urea and serum potassium are not rising rapidly, the fluid intake orally or intravenously will be adjusted to the urine output. A rapidly rising urea and serum potassium with falling urine output or anuria are indications for peritoneal dialysis or subsequent haemodialysis.

Malaria in pregnancy

Malaria in pregnancy must be regarded seriously and treated immediately. The danger of hypoglycaemia has already been mentioned.

Fortunately, the use of quinine and chloroquine intravenously in therapeutic doses rarely appears to cause fetal damage. The full adult dose of chloroquine is 200–300 mg (base) in 4–5% glucose saline intravenously up to three times in the 24 hours and continued daily until there is marked improvement, when oral therapy can commence. Intramuscular chloroquine has almost as rapid an action and is well tolerated. It should be given in up to three single doses of 300–400 mg (base) (10 ml of a 5% solution) in 24 hours. Quinine should be given if possible intravenously in a dose of 10 mg (base)/kg to a maximum of 500 mg (base) in 10 ml/kg 0.9% sodium chloride to a maximum of 500 ml over 4 hours. This should be repeated every 12–24 hours until considerable improvement has been obtained. More concentrated boluses can be given as 250–500 mg by syringe in 20 ml 'glucose saline' over not less than 10 minutes. If quinine is given any more rapidly intravenously there is a risk of hypotension and cardiac arrhythmia. Quinine is less satisfactorily given deep intramuscularly in single doses of 16 mg/kg base (equivalent to 20 mg/kg quinine dihydrochloride) not exceeding 1000 mg quinine dihydrochloride and a total dosage of 2000 mg in 24 hours.

In severe anaemia blood transfusion will be necessary as a life-saving measure. Caesarean section may be necessary to save the fetus from further hypoxia and to remove a large reservoir of parasitized cells sequestered in the placenta. If blood glucose levels are low, IV glucose should be given in an initial bolus by injection and then as a continuous infusion of a 10% solution.

References

British National Formulary (1986) No. 11, pp. 219–221. London: British Medical Association and the Pharmaceutical Society of Great Britain.

PHILLIPS, R. E., *et al.* (1986) Effectiveness of SMS 201–995 in the treatment of quinine-induced hyperinsulinaemia. *Lancet,* **i,** 713–715

Further reading

CHONGSUPPHAJAISIDDHI, T. Malaria. In *Diseases of The Subtropics and Tropics* (Stanfield, J. P., *et al.,* eds), 4th edn. London: Edward Arnold (In press)

CHONGSUPPHAJAISIDDHI, T., SABHAREON, A. and ATTANATH, P. (1983) Treatment of quinine resistant falciparum malaria. *Southeast Asian Journal of Tropical Medicine and Public Health,* **14,** 357–362

BRUCE-CHWATT, L. J. (ed.) (1981) *Chemotherapy of Malaria* (2nd edn.). Geneva: World Health Organization

GILLES, H. M. (1984) Malaria. *Medicine International,* **2,** 141–145

HALL, A. P. (1976) The treatment of malaria. *British Medical Journal,* **i,** 323–328

McGREGOR, J. A. (ed.) (1982) *British Medical Bulletin,* **38,** 115–125

MIGASENA, S. (1983) Hypoglycaemia in falciparum malaria. *Annals of Tropical Medicine and Parasitology,* **77,** 323–324

PHILLIPS, R. E. *et al.* (1986) Effectiveness of SMS 201–995 in the treatment of quinine induced hyperinsulinaemia. *Lancet,* **i,** 713–715

RANSOME-KUTI, O. (1972) Malaria in childhood. *Advances in Paediatrics,* **19,** 319–340

SHANN, F., STACE, J. and EDSTEIN, M. (1985) Pharmacokinetics of quinine in children. *Journal of Pediatrics,* **106,** 506–510

SPENCER, H. C. (1985) Drug resistant malaria – changing patterns means difficult decisions. *Transactions of The Royal Society of Tropical Medicine and Hygiene,* **79,** 748–758

SWAI, A. B. M., PALLANGYO, K., KIHAM, C. M. and McLARTY, D. G. (1983) Clinical management of acute falciparum malaria in Tanzania. *Tropical Doctor,* **13,** 159–163

Tropical Disease Bulletin (1986) Controversy – quinine treatment for malaria. *Tropical Disease Bulleting,* **83,** 121–110

WARRELL, D. A. *et al.* (1982) Dexamethasone proves deleterious in cerebral malaria. *New England Journal of Medicine,* **306,** 313–319

WHITE, N. J. and WARRELL, D. A. (1983) Clinical management of chloroquine resistant Plasmodium falciparum malaria in South East Asia. *Tropical Doctor,* **13,** 153–159

WHITE N. J. *et al.* (1985) Pathophysiology and prognostic significance of cerebrospinal fluid lactate in cerebral malaria. *Lancet,* **i,** 776–778

WORLD HEALTH ORGANIZATION (1980) The clinical management of acute malaria. *WHO S.E. Asia Regional Publications No. 9,* New Delhi

WORLD HEALTH ORGANIZATION AND ROYAL SOCIETY OF TROPICAL MEDICINE AND HYGIENE (1986) 'Severe and Complicated Malaria' *Transactions of the Royal Society of Tropical Medicine and Hygiene.* **80,** Supplement, 30–32

Chapter 63

Cholera

D. H. Smith

Cholera is an acute, self-limiting gastroenteritis with a wide clinical spectrum ranging from mild or asymptomatic infection to severe forms presenting with profuse watery diarrhoea, progressive dehydration and metabolic acidosis terminating in early death. Classical *Vibrio cholera*, endemic especially in the Ganges and Brahmaputra deltas and responsible for previous pandemics has been replaced by the *Vibrio cholera, el Tor* biotype which, since 1961 has been responsible for the present pandemic notably in Asia and Africa.

Transmission is by the faecal–oral route either from contaminated water or food or direct contact. In epidemics, all age groups are susceptible whilst in endemic areas repeated exposure leads to increasing immunity, and clinical disease is then more common in children. Outbreaks may be explosive especially from common source infections whilst persisting endemicity is due to poor environmental sanitation. The el Tor vibrio is hardier than the classical organism; it survives longer in water sources; gives rise to more frequent mild and asymptomatic infections and a more prolonged carrier state. It is endemic in Asia and Africa where classical vibrios have never previously become established.

Pathogenic vibrios are virtually non-invasive. Gastric acidity provides a partial barrier to infection. Organisms multiply in the small intestine and pathogenicity is due to the liberation of an enterotoxin which stimulates adenylate cyclase activity causing an outpouring of protein free, isotonic fluid from the intact small intestinal mucosa, rich in bicarbonate and potassium. Infection is self-limiting and short lived and the majority are mild or asymptomatic. Morbidity is due to the rapidly progressive dehydration, hypovolaemic shock, metabolic acidosis and hypokalaemia. With adequate treatment the mortality should be reduced in severe cases to less than 1 per cent.

Recognition

After a short incubation period (average 2 days), the onset is abrupt with profuse diarrhoea which soon becomes watery (*rice-water stools*). Intestinal colic is absent initially although cramps in limbs and abdominal muscles occur in severe disease. Fever is rare in adults but not uncommon in children. Vomiting, which may be projectile and unaccompanied by nausea is common and follows the diarrhoea. In severe cases the alkaline diarrhoea rapidly leads to dehydration and acidosis. Fluid losses in adults may exceed 5 ℓ daily and proportionate amounts are lost in childhood. In moderate to severe cholera 5–10 per cent of the body weight or more is lost and within hours leads to hypovolaemic shock.

Fluid and electrolyte losses in adults are usually isotonic for sodium with increased concentration of potassium (15 mmol/ℓ) and bicarbonate (44 mmol/ℓ). In children, sodium losses are often less (100 mmol/ℓ) and potassium losses greater (25–30 mmol/ℓ). Hypoglycaemia occurs in children especially with prolonged dehydration and may contribute to the mental confusion, stupor, or coma associated with the metabolic acidosis. Hypokalaemia leads to weakness, cardiac arrhythmias and paralytic ileus, which may mask the extent of intestinal fluid losses, and in combination with the hypovolaemic shock contribute to development of acute tubular necrosis and renal failure. Convulsions and tetany may occur related to calcium and magnesium losses.

The diagnosis presents few difficulties during epidemics. Specific diagnosis is of particular importance at the start of an outbreak, to alert and mobilize medical resources. Stool microscopy shows numerous vibrios which are immobilized with specific group 01 antisera, and fluorescent microscopy using a fluorescein-conjugated cholera antiserum provides a rapid presumptive diagnosis. Faecal samples or rectal swabs for bacteriological examination should be collected into alkaline peptone water and plated onto selective media such as TCBS (thiosulphate–citrate–bile-salt–sucrose). Serum electrolyte estimation is of limited value but a measure of blood pH is of value in assessing acidosis.

Management

Cholera is a medical emergency. Immediate treatment of severe cases is essential and must NOT await a specific diagnosis or the results of laboratory investigation.

Assessment of severity

The first priority is to assess the severity of dehydration and acidosis. Moderate cases will have lost 5 per cent of their body weight (deficit of 50 ml/kg) and severe cases will have lost 10 per cent or more (deficit of 100 ml/kg or more). Dehydration is estimated from the general appearance, sunken eyes, skin turgor, depressed fontanelle and tissue shrinkage. Hypotension, tachycardia, or absent peripheral pulses with cold extremities denote hypovolaemic shock whilst respiratory rate and conscious level indicate the degree of metabolic acidosis (*see also* Acidosis and Electrolyte Disorders, Chapter 11).

Correction of fluid and electrolyte losses

The route of rehydration

In moderate and severe cases with losses of more than 5% of body weight and substantial dehydration, acidosis, or hypovolaemic shock, replacement is required intravenously initially. Milder cases can be effectively managed with oral replacement from the outset.

Initial intravenous rehydration

The aim is to replace 30–50 per cent of the estimated losses within 30 minutes and total rehydration within 2–3 hours. The collapsed child may need a temporary infusion into the jugular or femoral vein to establish peripheral circulation. A single IV replacement fluid for all patients has obvious advantages especially during epidemics and a number of suitable fluids are available; Ringer lactate, WHO IV Diarrhoea Treatment Solution, or Dacca 5.4.1 solution* (Dacca 5.4.1 contains Na^+ 133/mmol/ℓ, Cl^- 99 mmol/ℓ, K^+ 14 mmol/ℓ, and $HCO^-{}_3$ 48 mmol/ℓ). Dehydration in children may be isotonic or hypertonic and infusion with isotonic saline (NaCl 0.9%) alone may precipitate hypernatraemia. If hypotonic solutions are not available, rehydration should be more cautious and should be supplemented by increased glucose–water (5%) drinks as soon as possible. Failure to correct the metabolic acidosis during rehydration may lead to acute pulmonary oedema. Hypokalaemia may become evident clinically following rapid rehydration. Vomiting usually ceases once the acidosis is corrected.

Maintenance rehydration

Once initial fluid losses have been corrected, patients require maintenance fluids and electrolytes according to the continuing losses. With effective initial rehydration faecal fluid losses may increase to 20 ℓ per day in adults. Faecal fluid losses, vomitus and urine output as well as intake must be accurately recorded and maintenance rehydration adjusted to equal the combined losses plus an assessment of insensible losses. Oral or IV glucose should be included to prevent hypoglycaemia.

A cholera cot allows faecal losses to be collected and accurately measured via a central hole in the bed and rubber sleeve into a measured container. Oral replacement therapy (*see* Appendix 9) with the WHO oral rehydration solution should be started as early as possible and may be facilitated by using a nasogastric tube. Losses in excess of 15–20 ml/kg/hour require continuing IV therapy. Recovery is usually rapid and a light diet should be introduced early and helps to ensure a safe and adequate potassium intake.

Initial oral rehydration (see also Practical procedures, Chapter 93)

Oral replacement from the outset is successful in all but the more severe cases. Even children with moderate dehydration, diminished skin turgor, postural hypotension, and tachycardia respond to adequate oral replacement and vital IV fluids are thus conserved for more severe cases. Absorption of oral fluids and electrolytes is dependent upon maintaining glucose concentrations (glucose stimulated membrane transport). Suitable solutions include the WHO oral diarrhoea replacement solution (*see* Appendix 9). Oral therapy must be given frequently (every 1/4 to 1/2 hour) in amounts of 5–15 ml/kg/hour depending on clinical severity and continuing faecal losses.

* Refers to the number of grams per litre in the solution of NaCl (5), $NaHCO_3$ (4) and KCl (1) (Greenbough, Gordon and Benenson, 1964).

Antibiotics and other treatment

Several antibiotics, notably tetracyclines and chloramphenicol, reduce the volume and duration of diarrhoea and reduce the period of excretion of vibrios. Tetracycline resistance has been reported recently. Doxycycline does not have the renal toxicity associated with other tetracyclines. Antibiotics should be withheld until initial hydration is completed and continued for 48 hours or until diarrhoea has ceased. Chlorpromazine used to prevent vomiting also reduces the volume of diarrhoea.

Management of cholera outbreaks

Cholera occurs predominantly in rural populations remote from medical facilities, and epidemics are often explosive and widespread. The speedy provision of emergency treatment centres and mobile treatment teams dramatically reduces the mortality especially in epidemics. Vaccination plays no part in the management of cholera outbreaks; available vaccines provide only partial protection for 3–6 months and vaccination programmes divert resources from case detection and treatment, especially the provision of fluid replacement facilities. Nosocomial transmission is exceptional and simple hygiene including hand-washing is adequate protection for medical and nursing staff.

Reference

GREENBOUGH, W. B., GORDON, R. S. and BENENSON, A. S. (1964) Tetracycline in the treatment of cholera. *Lancet,* **i,** 355–357

Further reading

BURNA, D. and BURROWS, W. (eds) (1974) *Cholera* (includes discussion on Dacca solution). Philadelphia: W. B. Saunders

World Health Organisation (1976) *Treatment and Prevention of Dehydration in Diarrhoeal Disease. A Guide for Use at Primary Level.* Geneva: WHO

Chapter 64

Typhoid fever

Carol J. Rubidge

Deaths from typhoid fever in children may result from toxaemia or from one of its many complications. Not infrequently death occurs in the absence of diagnosis and appropriate therapy.

The diagnosis may be missed because of failure to recognize the following:

1. Typhoid has a world-wide distribution.
2. That no age is exempt.
3. Because typhoid causes a toxaemia and a septicaemia every organ in the body may be involved, leading to a wide variety of presenting symptoms, signs and complications.

Fever is the most constant of all clinical findings and typhoid should be excluded whenever fever remains unexplained in any patient, irrespective of age or geographical locality; but fever is not present in all cases on admission.

Emergencies in typhoid in children

Severe toxaemia – recognition

1. High fever.
2. Prostration.
3. Marked apathy.

Neurological manifestations – recognition

1. Delirium.
2. Meningism.
3. Stupor; all are indicative of severe illness.
4. In the very young, convulsions are frequent and may recur until appropriate antibiotic therapy is combined with anticonvulsants.
5. A wide range of neurological complications involving the central and peripheral nervous systems may be the presenting complaints.
6. The cerebrospinal fluid is usually normal, may show a mild pleocytosis and rarely may be frankly purulent, with typhoid bacilli present on culture.

Intestinal perforation

This very serious complication occurs in 3–5 per cent of children with typhoid and has a high mortality.

Recognition

1. Appropriate antibiotic therapy does not prevent its occurrence.
2. Early recognition and treatment are of the utmost importance but classical signs of acute peritonitis may not be obvious in the severely ill child.
3. Increasing pulse rate, restlessness, and vomiting are danger signals.
4. Paralytic ileus without perforation also occurs in typhoid and may be distinguished radiographically. Air in the peritoneal cavity indicates perforation. Air fluid levels without intraperitoneal air are seen in ileus. Patients with ileus require constant monitoring because ileus may progress to perforation.

Intestinal haemorrhage

Bleeding in typhoid is usually microscopic. In 2 per cent of children a large-bowel haemorrhage occurs.

Recognition

1. Blood may accumulate in the bowel lumen and symptoms and signs of shock with pallor, a rapid pulse, hypotension, and hypothermia may be the first indication of this catastrophe.
2. In endemic areas, the passage of moderate or large quantities of blood from the bowel is suggestive of typhoid.

Congestive cardiac failure in typhoid

This may be due to:

1. Anaemia.
2. Toxic myocarditis.
3. Fluid overload complicating acute glomerulonephritis.

Recognition

The diagnosis of typhoid is often missed because fever may be absent in the presence of severe anaemia (Mulligan, 1971).

Renal failure

This is a rare complication, and may necessitate dialysis. Causes include acute glomerulonephritis, acute tubular necrosis secondary to dehydration, and pyelonephritis (Buka and Coovadia, 1980).

Jaundice

Hepatitis was the probable cause of jaundice in 5 per cent of 1400 children with typhoid fever in Durban (Scragg, 1976). Haemolysis may account for some cases of jaundice.

Recognition

1. Typhoid hepatitis usually presents in seriously ill patients.
2. A high swinging fever should suggest the diagnosis of typhoid since this is an unusual feature of viral or toxic hepatitis.

Management

Antibiotic therapy

1. Chloramphenicol; 50 mg/kg daily in divided doses for 21 days. In the severely ill toxic patients, the dose should be doubled until improvement is obvious, when it may be reduced. When oral medication is impossible or contraindicated, chloramphenicol may be given intravenously. It remains the treatment of choice in many parts of the world. Resistant *Salmonella typhi* strains and potential toxic effects have led to use of other antibiotics.
2. Amoxycillin; 100 mg/kg daily in divided doses has proved an excellent alternative for the treatment of typhoid in children (Scragg, 1976). Intravenous therapy may be given if oral therapy is impractical for any reason.
3. Supportive therapy:
   (a) Fluid and electrolyte imbalance should be corrected without delay.
   (b) Blood transfusion may be life saving in the presence of severe bowel haemorrhage and is also indicated when severe anaemia of infection is present.
   (c) Corticosteroids (prednisolone 2 mg/kg daily for 3 days) have been recommended for severe toxaemia. They should be given in combination with antibiotic therapy.
   (d) Surgery is indicated where there is clear-cut evidence of recent acute perforation provided the general condition of the patient is satisfactory. Ileus without perforation or long-standing peritonitis complicating perforation are best managed conservatively with gastric suction, intravenous fluids, and parenteral antibiotics.

References

BUKA, I. and COOVADIA, H. M. (1980) Typhoid glomerulonephritis. *Archives of Disease in Childhood*, **55**, 305–307

MULLIGAN, T. O. (1971) Typhoid fever in young children. *British Medical Journal*, **iv**, 665–667

SCRAGG, J. N. (1976) Further experience with amoxycillin in typhoid fever in children. *British Medical Journal*, **ii**, 1031–1033

Further reading

SCRAGG, J. N. (1976) Typhoid fever and its management. *South African Journal of Hospital Medicine*, **ii**, 556–560

Chapter 65

Amoebiasis

Carol J. Rubidge

Emergencies in children include:

1. Fulminant amoebic colitis.
2. Perforation and peritonitis.
3. Intussusception.
4. Bowel haemorrhage.
5. Hepatic amoebiasis.

Fulminant amoebic colitis

This leads to destruction of the bowel wall from caecum to rectum and has a very high mortality. The onset may be insidious or abrupt.

Recognition

1. A history of bloody diarrhoea.
2. Generalized abdominal tenderness.
3. A severely ill, debilitated, and often dehydrated child.
4. The passage of many blood-stained mucoid stools which contain little or no faecal matter.
5. Extensive ulceration of bowel mucosa on proctoscopy or sigmoidoscopy.
6. The finding of haematophagous trophozoites microscopically, when fresh exudate from ulcers or mucoid faecal matter is mixed with a drop of saline and placed under a coverslip.

Management

1. Correction of dehydration and electrolyte imbalance.
2. IV plasma or blood transfusion if shock is present.
3. (a) Metronidazole 50 mg/kg daily in divided doses for 5 days by mouth.
   (b) Tinidazole 60 mg/kg in a single dose daily for 3 days, given by mouth (Scragg, Rubidge and Proctor, 1976).
4. Continuous monitoring of the child is essential: danger signals suggestive of impending peritonitis include:
   (a) Increasing abdominal distension.
   (b) Vomiting.
   (c) Worsening of the general condition.

Perforation and peritonitis

This most commonly complicates fulminant amoebic colitis when it is the result of slow leakage from many perforations. The onset is often insidious.

Recognition

1. Relatively painless increasing abdominal distension.
2. Vomiting.
3. Bowel sounds becoming infrequent and eventually absent.
4. More rarely a single amoebic ulcer may perforate and cause the dramatic picture of an acute abdomen followed by generalized peritonitis or occasionally a localized intraperitoneal abscess.

Management

1. IV metronidazole.
2. IV broad spectrum antibiotics.
3. IV fluid and electrolytes.
4. Continuous gastric suction.
5. (a) Surgery may be indicated for the repair of a single perforation provided the child's general condition is satisfactory.
   (b) The role of surgery in the presence of many perforations complicating fulminant amoebic colitis is controversial. Colonic resection in these severely ill children has a very high mortality.

Intussusception (see also Chapter 40, pages 368–369)

Although rare, intussusception complicating amoebic dysentery occurs more commonly in children than in adults. It is usually caecocolic.

Recognition

1. Attacks of abdominal colic.
2. Screaming attacks in infants.
3. Vomiting.
4. The finding of a sausage-shaped mass in line with the colon.
5. Barium enema may be hazardous in the presence of severe colitis.

Management

1. A spontaneous reduction may occur.
2. Surgical reduction should not be delayed if bowel resection is to be avoided.
3. Drug treatment and supportive therapy as for fulminant amoebic colitis.

Bowel haemorrhage

This uncommon complication is the result of the erosion of a vessel by amoebic ulceration.

Recognition

1. This may cause collapse due to shock.
2. The diagnosis is suggested by the passage of large quantities of blood per rectum.

Management

1. Replacement blood transfusion.
2. Drug therapy and supportive therapy as for amoebic colitis.

Hepatic amoebiasis

This complication may occur from 4 weeks of age and the peak incidence is in the first 3 years of life. Multiple abscesses are more common in children than in adults.

Recognition

A tender hepatomegaly is almost invariable and is frequently associated with:

1. Fever.
2. Anaemia.
3. Neutrophilia.
4. A visible and/or palpable mass in the liver area.
5. Elevation of the right diaphragm on chest radiograph.

Serological gel diffusion precipitin tests provide useful supportive evidence.

Ultrasound and radioactive liver scanning are of help in diagnosing the presence and number of abscesses and in their localization.

Management

1. Metronidazole or tinidazole as for amoebic colitis.
2. Aspiration at the point of maximum tenderness, prominence or fluctuation prevents rupture into adjoining spaces or organs, hastens recovery, and relieves pain. Repeat aspirations may be necessary.

Complications of amoebic liver abscess

Involvement of adjacent organs or spaces may be by extension or rupture of the liver abscess.

Recognition

Intra-abdominal rupture may be:

1. Intraperitoneal:
   (a) Often a gradual leak leading to chronic generalized or localized peritonitis.
   (b) Sudden massive rupture leading to shock and death is less common.
   (c) Into hollow organs, stomach or bowel; the abscess drains and may heal spontaneously or cause a fistula.

2. Intrathoracic. Right lobe abscesses on the superior surface of the liver may cause:
   (a) Right pleural effusion by extension.
   (b) If there is rupture through the diaphragm:
      (i) Right empyema.
      (ii) Hepatopleural fistula.
      (iii) Hepatobronchial fistula.
   (c) Blood spread to the lung may lead to amoebic lung abscess.
   Left lobe abscess may cause:
   (a) Pericardial effusion by extension with gradually increasing tamponade.
   (b) Sudden rupture into the pericardium leading to severe shock, distress and signs of acute tamponade.

Management

1. Metronidazole or tinidazole as for amoebic colitis.
2. Thorough drainage of pus from the pleural or pericardial spaces.
3. Surgical drainage of intraperitoneal pus and closure of fistulae where necessary.
4. Supportive therapy including correction of fluid and electrolyte disturbances and anaemia of infection by blood transfusion.

Reference

SCRAGG, J. N., RUBIDGE, C. J. and PROCTOR, E. M. (1976) Tinidazole in the treatment of acute amoebic dysentery in children. *Archives of Disease in Childhood,* **51,** 385–387

Further reading

RUBIDGE, C. J. (1984) In J. Forfar and G. C. Arneil (eds) *Textbook of Paediatrics* (3rd edn.), pp. 1484–1487. Edinburgh: Churchill Livingstone

Chapter 66

Haemorrhagic fever (dengue)

Wong Hock Boon

About 5 per cent of patients with dengue haemorrhagic fever (DHF) develop the shock syndrome, which constitutes one of the most important paediatric emergencies in South East Asia.

Recognition

Because DHF occurs in outbreaks, it can easily be diagnosed clinically, by the following features:

1. Fever lasting 3–10 days, usually low or medium grade.
2. Presence of the DHF rash on the third or fourth day. The rash starts on the trunk and spreads centrifugally; it may be macular or diffuse, and/or petechial.
3. Spleen usually palpable in affected children.
4. Leucopenia with mild thrombocytopenia.
5. Confirmation of diagnosis is serological, and rapid methods are now available.

However, the main problem is shock; but since 95 per cent are not in shock, it is important to recognize the pre-shock state in a predisposed patient and to start anti-shock measures early.

Pre-shock or shock

Common manifestations:

1. Shock, if it occurs, develops from the 3rd to 7th day of the illness.
2. The patient complains of abdominal pain and vomiting.
3. There is restlessness with clouding of consciousness.
4. There may be associated massive gastrointestinal bleeding.
5. The development of hypotension, ascites, pleural effusion (usually on the right).
6. Investigations may show:
   (a) A leucocytosis instead of leucopenia.
   (b) The platelets reduced to 50 000/mm^3 or less.
   (c) Signs of myocarditis in the ECG.
   (d) Hyponatraemia.

Pathophysiology of DHF shock

This may occur in the first or primary infection when the virus causes a direct vasculitis with exudation of fluid out of the intravascular space, and consequent shock. However, the majority of cases are secondary (i.e. have had a previous infection by other strains of dengue virus) as shown by the high serological titres found in DHF shock. Complement studies have shown that serum levels are inversely proportional to the severity of the illness, demonstrating that immunological mechanisms play a large part in DHF shock.

The shock state may be made worse by the development of disseminated intravascular coagulation (DIC; page 498). However, DIC plays a secondary rather than a primary role.

Whatever is the real cause of DHF shock, the important thing is that it evolves rapidly, and the patient can reach an irreversible stage in a short time.

Management

It is even more important to identify those patients who are going into shock rather than those who are already in shock. The chances of saving the former are much better than those of saving the latter.

Initial treatment

Intravenous fluids – NaCl 0.45% in glucose 2.5 or 5% should be given immediately at the rate of 40 ml/kg in the first 1–2 hours then at 10 ml/kg/hour depending on the state of the patient. Care must be taken not to overload the circulation (NaCl 0.45% in glucose 2.5% has been shown to be more effective in DHF than the 'standard' NaCl 0.9% in glucose 5%).

Observations to be made and recorded during treatment

1. Pulse rate.
2. Blood pressure.
3. Central venous pressure (CVP); IV fluids can be given if the CVP is less than 10 cm H_2O (7.6 mm Hg).
4. Respiration rate.
5. Chest X-ray (for pleural effusion).
6. Intake–output chart.
7. Haematocrit, WBC count, platelets.
8. Plasma sodium, potassium, bicarbonate, chloride, urea.

If facilities are available:

1. Blood gases and acid–base state.
2. Blood clotting studies and fibrin breakdown products (*see* page 498).

Further intravenous treatment

1. Blood transfusion need only be given if there is considerable loss of blood.
2. Plasma* can be given early in shock syndrome but care must be exercised in avoiding excessive dosage in the late stage as it may then initiate the shock lung syndrome.

* Or Plasma Protein Fraction (PPF), Dextran, etc.

3. Platelet transfusions may be useful if bleeding cannot be controlled, because of severe persistent thrombocytopenia.
4. Intravenous fluids and electrolytes should be given according to the results of serial electrolyte estimations.

Later progress

If the patient is going to respond, improvement usually occurs within 24–48 hours, when emergency measures may be relaxed. Over-treatment may be hazardous. Corticosteroids, antibiotics and heparin are of no proved value.

Reference

WONG, H. B. (1981) Dengue haemorrhagic fever in Singapore. *Annals of Academy of Medicine, Singapore,* **10,** 91–98

Further reading

WELLMER, H. (1983) Some reflections on the ecology of dengue haemorrhagic fever in Thailand. In N. D. McGlasman and J. R. Blunden (eds) *Geographical Aspects of Health.* London: Academic Press

Chapter 67

Viral haemorrhagic fevers

Susan Fisher-Hoch

Throughout the world there are a number of viruses which are natural animal parasites, often of rodents, but which can in certain circumstances infect man, in whom a non-specific febrile illness may progress to shock and haemorrhage, accompanied by acute renal failure. With the exception of dengue, exclusively a human virus (*see* Chapter 66), most of the recognized infections in endemic areas are in adults, but infections in children occur, particularly if they live in close contact with rodent reservoirs. Clinical infections will usually be encountered in the endemic areas, but with widespread travel imported cases are always possible.

The most important factor in recognition of these diseases is awareness of their existence and geographical distribution. Therefore, a brief summary of the more important viruses is given, but for a fuller account, the reader is referred to the review articles listed at the end of the chapter. In endemic areas local knowledge and specialist advice should also be sought.

The arenaviruses

The arenaviruses are common rodent viruses of which three are associated with severe haemorrhage in man: Lassa fever in Africa, and the Argentinian and Bolivian haemorrhagic fevers, Junin and Machupo. Lassa or related viruses probably occur throughout Africa, but the South American viruses seem to be more localized. All are common viruses of wild rodents with persistent infections with no immune response and little or no overt disease, and man as an accidental host. Only in Lassa fever has case-to-case transmission occurred, but tertiary cases are rare. Onset is insidious with malaise often accompanied by marked facial oedema and lymphadenopathy. Especially in Lassa, many mild or asymptomatic cases probably go unnoticed, but severe cases progress to shock and oliguria with haemorrhage, and death from hypoxia.

Marburg and Ebola

Marburg and Ebola are related viruses of a new group. The original outbreak of Marburg developed from imported laboratory monkeys, and Ebola was first seen in an outbreak in 1976 in the Sudan and Zaire. The viruses are apparently endemic in Sudan and Zaire and probably other parts of Africa, but the animal reservoir and mode of transmission are unknown. Onset is abrupt, with severe headache, prostration and high fever, maculopapular rash, painful conjunctivitis, watery diarrhoea, and generalized lymphadenopathy. Haemorrhages, proteinuria, and shock are common, with a high mortality rate. Case-to-case spread has been recorded, and is associated with close contact with blood from infected cases, as well as possible sexual transmission via semen.

Korean haemorrhagic fever with renal syndrome and nephropathia epidemica

Korean haemorrhagic fever with renal syndrome has been shown to be caused by a rodent bunyavirus (Hantaan virus), and a related agent is responsible for nephropathia epidemica in Scandinavia, and possibly also Balkan nephropathy. More than 3000 cases occurred in United Nations servicemen during the Korean War. Infections in man are a major problem in China and the USSR, and related viruses occur throughout temperate regions of the northern hemisphere in small wild rodents, possibly including the United Kingdom, but the extent of human disease is not yet known. The illness is biphasic with a prodrome of fever, headache, diarrhoea and vomiting, followed by acute renal failure with proteinuria and severe plasma loss into extravascular compartments. Bleeding is confined to infections with the Korean virus, and is usually minor.

Tick-borne haemorrhagic fevers

Several tick-borne viruses of wild animals produce fevers with severe haemorrhage in man and domestic animals such as Kyasanur Forest Disease in India, and Congo/Crimean haemorrhagic fever which occurs from South Africa, through the Middle East to the Balkans and South Russia, and as far as Pakistan. Congo/Crimean infections present with malaise, sore throat with oral ulceration, diarrhoea, vomiting, chest pains, petechial rash, and oedema of the face, neck and soft palate, and progress rapidly to severe haemorrhage in most cases. Inapparent human infections probably pass unnoticed in rural communities and little is known of its true extent.

Mosquito-borne haemorrhagic fevers

Yellow fever is the most important mosquito-borne haemorrhagic fever, now largely controlled by mosquito eradication and vaccination, though epidemics continue to occur in Africa. An incubation period of 3–6 days is followed by fever, rigors, headache, and backache. Nausea, vomiting, swollen lips and tongue and congested conjunctiva may be accompanied by haemorrhage and shock. Jaundice generally occurs only during the convalescent phase. Rift Valley fever virus is widespread throughout Africa, where it is mainly a veterinary problem, but an outbreak occurred in man in the Nile Delta of Egypt in 1977. Initial symptoms include headache, fever, conjunctival injection, diffuse myalgia and arthritis, and may progress to haemorrhage and death. Retinal damage may be a late sequel.

Recognition

The common treatable infections such as malaria and typhoid should be excluded. This can be difficult since the onset is non-specific and often insidious. The incubation period is short, so a good history, with clear evidence of recent rodent or case contact is the most valuable diagnostic pointer. Facial oedema, pharyngitis, oral ulceration, diarrhoea, rash or haemorrhage may help but variability of symptoms and signs make clinical diagnosis unreliable. Laboratory tests such as white cell counts are unhelpful, since both leucocytosis and leucopenia may occur sequentially in the same patient, with an early predominantly neutrophilic response. A high index of suspicion, and local knowledge are the most essential factors.

Specific diagnostic tests are available only in specialized laboratories. Diagnosis of Lassa can be made quickly (less than 24 hours) by virus isolation, but other rapid methods are not yet available. Diagnosis by serology is retrospective, using immunofluorescence. Information on diagnostic methods, suitable specimens and their correct and safe handling should be obtained from the nearest specialized laboratory (*see* list at end of chapter).

Prognosis

Mortality in Marburg and Ebola is high, but now that asymptomatic seroconversion and mild cases are recognized, some of the other fevers, such as Lassa, are losing some of their notoriety, the mortality rate in Lassa being probably only 2–10%. There is no evidence that the disease differs in subjects of different ethnic origin. Deterioration in severe cases is often rapid and death is usually due to hypovolaemic shock. Gross haemorrhage is unusual, particularly in Lassa, though ecchymoses are a feature of Congo/Crimean haemorrhagic fever. Central nervous system involvement including retinal damage should be excluded in South American haemorrhagic fever and Rift. Persistence of virus for several months occurs in Lassa and Marburg/Ebola.

Korean haemorrhagic fever with renal syndrome differs in that the illness is biphasic with anuria after subsidence of the original non-specific illness. The renal damage may be immunologically mediated. Frank haemorrhage is uncommon and with good supportive therapy chronic renal impairment is rare.

Management

Treatment with interferon and hyperimmune plasma has been advocated; there is no evidence that they are of major benefit and they may be actually detrimental. Ribavirin in the treatment of Lassa is effective.

Good supportive care is the most important factor of benefit to the patient and the reader is referred to the appropriate chapters in this volume. Dehydration from reduced fluid intake and the sometimes massive leakage of fluid and plasma proteins into extravascular compartments should be assessed and corrected. Impairment of renal function should be anticipated and managed appropriately. Hepatic function is usually disturbed, but not to the same degree as in fulminating viral hepatitis: jaundice is uncommon. Pulmonary oedema and occasionally interstitial pneumonitis may occur. Abnormal coagulation tests are usual, especially hypofibrinogenaemia and reduced platelet counts, even in the absence of frank bleeding. Disseminated intravascular coagulation appears to be a complicating, and often terminal event, rather than the central pathology of the bleeding disorder; prophylactic heparin has been advocated, but there is no evidence of any benefit. Efforts should be directed towards use of fresh blood products, especially platelets, prevention of hypovolaemic shock, and dialysis if required.

Case-to-case spread

Much of the notoriety of these fevers resulted from the publicity surrounding hospital outbreaks which involved relatives, nurses, doctors, and laboratory personnel. Mortality rates have been high in such outbreaks, and there is no doubt that Lassa, Marburg/Ebola and Congo/Crimean haemorrhagic fever in particular are a serious hazard to hospital staff. In developed countries strict regulations exist for containment procedures and care of cases, and reference should be made at once to these if a case is suspected. It is obvious that the degree of patient monitoring and management procedures advocated in this text present a hazard to personnel. Where they are available, portable isolators and specialized laboratories provide safe working conditions, but it is possible to monitor the more basic parameters for patient management with simple equipment, even in primitive surroundings as long as staff are suitably trained and equipped and fully aware of the nature of the hazards presented by specimens. In the major outbreaks of hospital or laboratory acquired disease reported, there was gross contamination of personnel with blood and secretions (for example, mouth-to-mouth resuscitation or needle sticks). On institution of simple, but properly conducted barrier nursing the outbreaks ceased abruptly.

Reference laboratories

Porton
The Director, Special Pathogens Reference Laboratory, PHLS Centre for Applied Microbiology and Research, Porton Down, Salisbury, Wiltshire SP4 0JG, England (Tel: 0980 610391).

Antwerp
Dr Guido van der Groen, Institut de Médecine Tropicale Prince Leopold, Nationalestraat 155, Antwerp B-2000, Belgium (Tel: Antwerp (03) 238 58 80).

Atlanta
Dr J. McCormick, Special Pathogens Branch, Virology Division, Centers for Disease Control, Atlanta, Georgia, 30333, USA (Tel: Atlanta (404) 329 3308).

Moscow
The Director, Institute of Poliomyelitis and Virus Encephalitides, P.O. Institute of Poliomyelitis, Moscow Oblast 142 782, USSR.

Johannesburg
Dr R. Swanepoel, Special Pathogens Unit, National Institute for Virology, Sandringham, Johannesburg, South Africa (Tel: Johannesburg 640 5031).

World Health Organization
Dr Fakhry Assaad, World Health Organization, 1211 Geneva 27, Switzerland (Tel: Geneva 91 26 60).

Further reading

CASALS, J., HENDERSON, B. E., HOOGSTRAAL, H., JOHNSON, K. M. and SHELOKOV, A. (1970) A review of the Soviet viral haemorrhagic fevers, 1969. *Journal of Infectious Diseases,* **122,** 437–453

GAJDUSEK, D. C. (1962) Viral haemorrhagic fevers. *Journal of Pediatrics,* **60,** 841–857

HALSTEAD, S. B. (1981) Viral haemorrhagic fevers. *Journal of Infectious Diseases,* **143,** 127–129

MONATH, T. P. (1974) Lassa fever and Marburg virus disease. *WHO Chronicle,* **28,** 212–219

SIMPSON, D. I. H. (1978) Viral haemorrhagic fevers of man. *Bulletin of the World Health Organization,* **56,** 819–832

World Health Organization (1978) Ebola haemorrhagic fevers in Sudan, 1976. Report of a WHO/International Study Team. *Bulletin of the World Health Organization,* **56,** 271–293

World Health Organization (1983) Haemorrhagic fever with renal syndrome: Memorandum from a WHO Meeting. *Bulletin of the World Health Organization,* **61,** 269–275

Chapter 68

Rabies

Dion R. Bell

Rabies is an enzootic infection, usually transmitted by the saliva of an infected animal during biting or the licking of an abrasion. Inhalation of virus can infect people exploring caves which harbour infected bats. Most human infections come from the bite of the domestic dog, and many occur in children. Ideally all cases of rabies in man and animals should be notified in accordance with the recommendations of the World Health Organization. Rabies is now a notifiable disease in Britain and many other countries but there is no uniformity of procedure.

Distribution and epidemiology

Wild animal or domestic dog reservoirs of rabies are found in most parts of the tropics, subtropics, the Americas and large parts of Europe. Man is not often affected directly from a rabid wild animal, although bat-transmitted outbreaks have occurred. Rabies in the European fox has spread into France and is at present moving south, and it is the fox-transmitted infection of a dog or cat smuggled into Britain that presents the greatest danger to the British Isles.

Recognition

Clinical

The diagnosis of human rabies during life is usually clinical. After an incubation period of from 2 weeks to more than a year, the onset is rapid. Early symptoms are fever, malaise, anxiety, and sometimes pain at the site of the original bite. Then follows reflex hyperexcitability of the nervous system, most typically manifest as painful cramps of the throat muscles when attempting to swallow, giving the disease the name 'hydrophobia'.

The reflex spasms, often accompanied by apnoea, become more and more frequent over the course of a day or two. Between spasms, the patient is conscious, and can often talk rationally. Restlessness, pruritus, and excessive salivation are common, and the patient typically spits abundant ropy saliva.

Hyperexcitability is often followed by progressive paralysis and the appearance of bizarre focal neurological signs. Death usually occurs within 7 days of onset, preceded by respiratory irregularities and cardiac arrhythmias.

Specific diagnosis

More specific diagnosis can be confirmed by specific immunofluorescent staining of corneal impression smears, but a negative result is indecisive, as the test is negative in more than 50 per cent of confirmed cases. Advice on the technique should be obtained from the Virus Reference Laboratory, Central Public Health Laboratory, Colindale Avenue, London NW9 5HT or from similar centres in other countries.

Management

Treatment of established rabies

Once rabies is diagnosed, treatment should be symptomatic. The single well-documented case of claimed survival from rabies (Hattick *et al.*, 1972) lacks the vital evidence of virus isolation, and could have been an atypical 'post-vaccinial encephalitis', as vaccine had been given. Rabies is an agonizing disease, and treatment with full doses of diamorphine, chlorpromazine and amylobarbitone together is effective. Conventional dosage must be exceeded if symptoms are not controlled. Whether heroic supportive measures are justified is a matter for the individual physician, but even in the most optimistic view, the prospects for recovery are infinitesimal.

Protection of staff in contact with rabid patient

Staff in contact with rabies must be protected by gowns, gloves, goggles, and masks, and cautioned about the special danger of saliva. Pre-exposure immunization is feasible now that human diploid cell vaccine is available.

Post-exposure prevention of rabies after the bite

Indications for post-exposure protection

When a child is seen who might have been exposed to rabies, the decision on what to do is often difficult, but detailed advice is given in the World Health Organization Report (1973). In general, if an animal is *well* 5 days after inflicting a bite, or *alive* 10 days later, it is extremely unlikely that it was infective at the time of biting. This information should always be sought. Where a bite was received in an area where rabies is endemic and there is no information about the animal (as in the case of one that attacks and then runs off) one must assume that exposure occurred. Factors that increase the likelihood of infection are: severe bites, proximal bites, and bites from wild animals. The incubation period is also shortened by all these factors, and with increasing youth.

Local treatment

If the child is seen within 12 hours of exposure, local treatment might be effective, although proof of this is confined to delays of up to 3 hours. Irrigation of superficial wounds or swabbing of deep puncture wounds with benzalkonium chloride 1% or soft soap solution 20% is recommended. Débridement and delayed primary suture are used when surgery is needed.

Antirabies serum

Passive immunity can be provided by injecting antirabies serum prepared from various animals, most commonly the horse. The dose is 40 iu/kg for heterologous, or 20 iu/kg for the scarce and costly human serum. One-half of the dose can be infiltrated into the wound site, the remainder given intramuscularly. The usual precautions with serum must be observed. In practice, serum is given where the risk of exposure is high and the incubation period likely to be short. Vaccine alone protects against mild exposure, and a difficult balance must be struck between risk and possible benefit. Up to 50 per cent of patients receiving horse serum will develop serum sickness. Serum is given at the same time as the first dose of vaccine, but at a different site.

Vaccination and its complications

Vaccination is started as soon as it is decided that exposure to rabies might have occurred. Duck embryo vaccine and the Semple type vaccines which are derived from the nervous tissue of infected animals, have both been superseded by the new human diploid cell vaccine manufactured by the Merieux Institute of Lyon. The only disadvantage of the new vaccine is its expense; its great advantages are its lack of side-effects and its extreme effectiveness in raising antibody levels in the vaccinees.

The normal regime for post-exposure vaccination is by 1 ml doses of reconstituted vaccine given by the deep subcutaneous route. Because of the small dose of the vaccine, it is no longer necessary to use the subcutaneous tissues of the abdomen. The normal regimen is to give injections on days 0, 3, 7 and 14, followed by booster doses on days 30 and 90. It is usual for antibodies to be detectable after the first two doses of vaccine have been given.

If a patient has been vaccinated previously within the last 12 months, and is re-exposed to rabies, it is normally only necessary to give one booster dose. If previous vaccination was more than 1 year previously, then two or three booster doses should be given at intervals such as days 0, 3 and 7.

Pre-exposure vaccination can be offered to those at special risk of rabies infection, such as veterinary surgeons and others at special risk in endemic areas. Effective levels of antibody are produced after two injections one month apart and the levels are increased by giving a booster dose one year later. Subsequent booster doses can be given every three to five years according to the risk of exposure.

So far, there have been no reports of neuroanaphylactic accidents with the human diploid cell vaccine. The only complication of diploid cell vaccine normally encountered is that the site of injection may become somewhat red and indurated. This is by no means as severe as the reaction that used to be produced by Semple vaccines or by the duck embryo vaccine.

To conclude: there is no stringent evidence that treatment of established rabies is effective. Aggressive therapy should be concentrated on efforts to produce immunity as soon as possible after exposure, and these efforts should not be relaxed just because there has been a long delay. The quickest way of doing this is by a combination of active and passive immunization.

With the advent of human diploid cell vaccine, pre-exposure vaccination of children is now feasible.

Centres where rabies vaccine and antiserum is available

England

Virus Reference Laboratory,
Central Public Health Laboratory,
Colindale Avenue,
LONDON NW9 5HT
Tel: 01 205 7041

Public Health Laboratory,
East Birmingham Hospital,
Bordesley Green East,
BIRMINGHAM B9 5ST
Tel: 021 772 4311 ext 680

Public Health Laboratory,
Church Lane,
Heavitree,
EXETER EX2 5AD
Tel: 0392 77833

Public Health Laboratory,
Bridle Path, York Road,
LEEDS LS15 7TR
Tel: 0523 645011

Public Health Laboratory,
Fazakerley Hospital,
Lower Lane,
LIVERPOOL L9 7AL
Tel: 051 525 2323

Public Health Laboratory,
Institute of Pathology,
General Hospital,
Westgate Road,
NEWCASTLE UPON TYNE NE4 6BE
Tel: 0632 38811 ext 297

Wales

Public Health Laboratory,
University Hospital of Wales,
Heath Park,
CARDIFF CF4 4XW
Tel: 0222 755944

Scotland

King's Cross Hospital,
Clepington Road,
DUNDEE DN3 8EA
Tel: 0382 85241

Central Microbiological Laboratories,
Western General Hospital,
Crewe Road South,
EDINBURGH EH4 2XU
Tel: 031 332 1311

Glasgow Royal Infirmary,
GLASGOW G4 0SF
Tel: 041 552 3535
Ruchill Hospital,
Bilsland Drive,
GLASGOW
Tel: 041 946 6491
Raigmore Hospital,
INVERNESS
Tel: 0463 34151

Northern Ireland
Belfast City Hospital,
Lisburn Road,
BELFAST
Tel: 0232 29241

For further advice in Britain ring Liverpool School of Tropical Medicine (Tel: 051 708 9393) or, out of hours, Liverpool Radio Page (Tel: 051 933 7977 and ask to contact unit 0939); or The London School of Hygiene and Tropical Medicine (Tel: 01 636 8636).

References

HATTICK, M. A., WEIS, T. T., STECHSCHULTE, J., BAER, G. M. and GREGG, M. B. (1972) Recovery from rabies: a case report. *Annals of Internal Medicine,* **76,** 931–942

World Health Organization Expert Committee on Rabies (1973) *WHO Technical Reports Series,* 523. Geneva: WHO

Chapter 69

Acute metabolic disorders in protein–energy malnutrition (Kwashiorkor; protein–calorie malnutrition, PCM)

B. Heyworth

Severe protein–energy malnutrition (PEM) should be regarded as a medical emergency. The mortality in PEM is very high in the first week after admission to hospital, particularly in the first 48 hours.

Septicaemia, especially with Gram-negative bacteria, severe anaemia, shock secondary to dehydration, and disseminated intravascular coagulopathy may all occur, requiring urgent detection and appropriate treatment in every new patient seen (*see* Shock and dehydration; Disseminated intravascular coagulation).

At the same time the following metabolic derangements, singly or in combination, are frequently encountered and must be treated promptly:

1. Hypothermia
2. Hypoglycaemia

} Often in combination.

3. Hyponatraemia
4. Hypokalaemia
5. Hypomagnesaemia
6. Acute cardiac failure

} In varying degrees, often in combination.

Hypothermia

In some countries where the ambient temperature is low, 20 per cent of children with severe PEM have a rectal temperature on admission at or below 35°C (95°F). The child who has to travel far, who may be in a fasting state, or who is exposed to the cool night air, will have a lower rectal temperature. Hypothermia may coexist with an infection.

Management

Unnecessary washing or exposure should be avoided. The child is wrapped in a blanket, but rapid heating with hot water bottles should be avoided. Bodily contact with the mother will be very helpful. Aluminium foil wrapped around the blanket will further conserve body heat.

Hypoglycaemia

This is often associated with hypothermia and may be the presenting feature on admission following a long journey, and is also associated with overnight fasting or infection. Symptoms include drowsiness or coma, but sweating, tremors, or convulsions caused by hypoglycaemia are unusual in PEM.

Management

If a Dextrostix shows a blood glucose value of under 2.5 mmol/ℓ (<45 mg/100 ml), confirmed if possible by the laboratory, even in the absence of symptoms, oral glucose feeds are necessary. If symptoms occur an immediate intravenous injection of glucose 25–50% at a dose of 1 g/kg should be given, followed by 10% glucose by a continuous drip to prevent rebound hypoglycaemia. These solutions are hyperosmolar and should be given slowly.

Only in the very severe case, with a tendency to persistence of the hypoglycaemia or comatose state, should hydrocortisone be given. In these cases, blood for culture should be taken and antibiotics started, and the child can then be given hydrocortisone 50 mg IV followed by predisone or prednisolone 0.5 mg/kg 6 hourly, orally.

Electrolyte disturbances are largely the result of chronic diarrhoea, but secondary hyperaldosteronism may also contribute (*see* Acute cardiac failure below).

Hyponatraemia (see also page 123)

The total body sodium is usually increased but hyponatraemia is common. Unless the serum sodium is ≤115 mmol/ℓ, sodium supplements should be avoided because of the risk of heart failure. The serum sodium will often rise when hypokalaemia is corrected, because of shift of sodium from the intracellular to the extracellular compartments.

Management

If the illness is associated with *peripheral circulatory failure*, IV therapy is given carefully with half-strength plasma (or PPF), 20 ml/kg to be given over 1–2 hours, then sodium chloride 0.45% in glucose 2.5% at 6 ml/kg/hour for 4–8 hours. The child should be examined frequently for signs of cardiac failure.

Hypokalaemia (see also page 127)

Total body potassium is usually grossly depleted in PEM, particularly in the presence of diarrhoea, but the serum potassium may be normal or only slightly reduced.

Management

Potassium should be given by mouth, if possible, when up to 10 mmol/kg daily can be given in divided doses. A solution of potassium *for oral use* containing 1 mmol/ml can be made up by dissolving 7.5 g KCl in 100 ml water.

Potassium can be given by *slow* IV infusion once the child is passing urine; the rate should be not more than 0.5 mmol/kg/hour. *Concentrations greater than 40 mmol/ℓ should be given with extreme caution.*

Hypomagnesaemia (see also page 138)

Because magnesium is mainly an intracellular ion, serum levels on admission may be relatively normal, but hypomagnesaemia is made worse when the high protein, phosphate, calcium, and potassium diet is started.

Recognition

Clinical evidence may not appear for a few days after admission. The signs and symptoms are irritability, carpopedal spasm, increased muscle tone, hyperreflexia and later, coarse tremors, or squirming movements (Waterlow, J. C., personal communication), and convulsions. Opposition of the thumb within a clenched fist is often an early sign of hypomagnesaemia in PEM. Chvostek's sign is often negative. If an ECG is available, shortening of the P-R interval and TV_5 depression are said to be specific. The serum magnesium is often low (≤0.7 mmol/ℓ).

Management

Treatment consists of intramuscular 50% magnesium sulphate 7 mg/kg (0.15 ml/kg) immediately and half this amount daily for 3–4 days. This is equivalent to 50 mg (1 ml) 50% $MgSO_4 \cdot 7H_2O$ (2 mmol magnesium) immediately and 25 mg (0.5 ml) magnesium sulphate daily, for a 7 kg infant.

Even in the presence of diarrhoea, magnesium hydroxide mixture (Milk of Magnesia) 10 ml three or four times daily (41–54 mmol daily) can be given orally after the first 3 or 4 days of intramuscular treatment. The usual preparation of magnesium hydroxide is an 8% solution containing 6.8 mmol magnesium in 5 ml.

Zinc depletion

It is now recognized that in malnutrition, particularly if associated with chronic diarrhoea, there may be considerable zinc depletion, which is of importance clinically. When zinc depletion is known to be present, or is suspected, the deficit should be replaced, using the oral route if possible. Of the available preparations, zinc gluconate and zinc acetate are better tolerated than is zinc sulphate. For children 0.5–1.0 mg/kg *zinc* should be given; 80 mg zinc gluconate contain 10 mg zinc, and 220 mg zinc sulphate contain 50 mg zinc (Arlette, 1983).

Acute cardiac failure (see Cardiac failure, page 263)

There is an excess of water in the body and in some cases an increased plasma volume, particularly in the presence of anaemia. Anaemia (Hb <7 g/100 ml) and a sodium intake of >1 mmol/kg daily increase the risk of heart failure. As oedema is lost there is a rapid shift of fluid from the tissues to the plasma. There may also be difficulty in excreting sodium at this stage. In some cases of PEM the serum aldosterone level is raised (author's unpublished observation). All of these factors contribute to heart failure.

Impending cardiac failure must be anticipated in a child losing peripheral oedema without losing weight. Increasing tachypnoea and increasing liver size are important signs.

Management

1. Oxygen should be given, at a rate of 5–8 ℓ/min.
2. Frusemide 5–10 mg IV may be given, (i.e. 1–1.5 mg/kg).
3. Spironolactone 3.0 mg/kg daily, in three divided doses, may help to remove oedema fluid without precipitating heart failure. It may also help to prevent urinary loss of potassium.
4. Digoxin 0.02 mg/kg (20 µg/kg) i.m. followed by 0.01 mg/kg (10 µg/kg) i.m. 6 and 12 hours later can be given, with a maintenance dose of 0.01 mg/kg (10 µg/kg) daily in two divided doses, i.m. or orally, providing that the child is receiving potassium. There is danger of digoxin toxicity because of the low serum potassium which is especially likely to occur when oedema fluid is lost and potassium moves back into the cells. The pulse rate and rhythm must be recorded carefully.

Evidence of hepatic damage

Elevation of serum alanine aminotransferase value and other liver enzymes and bilirubin are probably related more to enzyme leakage from liver cells than to true hepatic necrosis. Drowsiness, not related to hypoglycaemia, electrolyte disturbances, septicaemia or meningitis, will probably respond to rest and the normal diet for PEM.

References

ARLETTE, J. P. (1983) Zinc and the skin. *Pediatric Clinics of North America,* **30,** 583–586

Further reading

STAFF, T. H. E. (1968) Treatment of severe kwashiorkor and marasmus in hospital. *East African Medical Journal,* **45,** 399–406

WHITEHEAD, R. G. and ALLEYNE, G. A. O. (1972) Pathophysiological factors of importance in protein-calorie malnutrition. *British Medical Bulletin,* **27,** 72–78

Chapter 70

Acute toxic hypoglycaemia (ackee poisoning; vomiting sickness of Jamaica)

Colin G. Miller

The ackee (*Blighia sapida*) was introduced into Jamaica from West Africa in the eighteenth century. The fruit has always been enjoyed as a vegetable in Jamaica although in other parts of the West Indies and in Africa it has, until recently, been considered poisonous and not eaten. Tinned ackees have been exported from Jamaica in recent years and are available in Britain and other countries. The unripe fruit is three angled and about the size of an apple. On ripening it bursts open at the bottom revealing three shiny black seeds each embedded in a fleshy arillus. The arillus is usually eaten boiled or fried. If unripe fruit are opened and eaten or should seeds be accidentally cooked in the pot severe hypoglycaemia results (Stuart, Jelliffe and Hill, 1955).

The responsible toxin, hypoglycin, has been isolated in high concentration from the seed and unripe fruit (Hassall, Reyle and Feng, 1954) and shown to be an amino acid similar to leucine which appears to interfere with fatty acid oxidation (Senior and Sherratt, 1968; Senior, Robson and Sherratt, 1968). Milner and Wirdnam (1977) have also shown that hypoglycin stimulates insulin secretion but the clinical significance of this is uncertain.

Recognition

The sudden onset of vomiting and/or signs of cerebral depression occurring within a few hours of ingestion of a meal containing ackees is characteristic. Family involvement is common, the youngest members, particularly when undernourished, being most severely affected. A history of ingesting ackees is not always obtained as the young child may unknowingly open and eat unripe fruit. Vomiting does not always occur but clouding of consciousness leading to coma (often fluctuating in severity), fits, and death in severe untreated cases is typical. Fever, diarrhoea and obvious signs of infection are usually absent.

Reye's syndrome, ketotic hypoglycaemia and other acute poisonings are the main differential diagnoses, although viral encephalitis, pyogenic meningitis, and head injury must be considered.

The clinical picture is due to profound hypoglycaemia, blood and cerebrospinal fluid glucose levels frequently being unrecordable. Brain damage in survivors may result from prolonged coma.

Management

Prompt treatment is life saving. Blood glucose estimation using Dextrostix should be immediately performed and venous or capillary blood sent for confirmation and hypoglycaemia, and for urea and electrolyte estimation.

Immediately after the blood is taken and before obtaining laboratory confirmation of hypoglycaemia 50% glucose is injected intravenously in unconscious patients using a dose of 2 ml/kg body weight (1 g/kg body weight) to a maximum of 50 ml (25 g). This may result in the immediate return of consciousness in which case the blood glucose may be maintained by frequent glucose drinks, monitoring the level by hourly Dextrostix estimations for at least 24 hours. If the child vomits oral glucose or remains unconscious normal blood glucose levels must be maintained by an IV infusion of 10% glucose.

Where the diagnosis is in doubt lumbar puncture to exclude meningitis and estimation of blood ammonia and serum transaminase levels should be performed to exclude Reye's syndrome (*see* page 415). In severe cases with persistent coma intensive care with monitoring of intracranial pressure and the use of hyperventilation and intravenous mannitol when indicated may be necessary to prevent permanent brain damage or death (see page 295).

References

HASSALL, C. H., REYLE, K. and FENG, P. (1954) Hypoglycin A,B: biologically active peptides from *Blighia sapida. Nature,* **173,** 356–367

MILNER, R. D. G. and WIRDNAM, P. K. (1977) Hypoglycin stimulates insulin secretion. *Diabetologia,* **13,** 637–638

SENIOR, A. E. and SHERRATT, H. S. A. (1968) Biochemical effects of the hypoglycaemic compound pent-4-enoic acid and related non-hypoglycaemic fatty acids. *Biochemical Journal,* **110,** 499–509; 521–527

SENIOR, A. E., ROBSON, B. and SHERRATT, H. S. A. (1968) Biochemical effects of the hypoglycaemia compound pent-4-enoic acid and related non-hypoglycaemic fatty acids. *Biochemical Journal,* **110,** 511–519

STUART, K. L., JELLIFFE, D. B. and HILL, K. R. (1955) Acute toxic hypoglycaemia occurring in the vomiting sickness of Jamaica (clinical aspects). *Journal of Tropical Paediatrics,* **1,** 69–87

Part XVI

Neonatal emergencies

Chapter 71

Resuscitation of the newborn

M. F. Whitfield and J. A. Black

(For older children, *see under* Chapters 22 (Acute respiratory failure), 24 (Cardiac emergencies), 10 (Shock) and 6 (Drowning and near-drowning).)

Adequate resuscitation of the apnoeic or hypoxic infant is the most important and most urgent of all neonatal emergencies, comparable with a cardiac arrest in an older child or adult. Appropriate immediate action may save the infant from death or neurological damage, while delayed, inadequate, or inappropriate action may lead to death or permanent damage. The effectiveness of modern methods of infant resuscitation underline the necessity for adequate resuscitation facilities and available trained personnel wherever babies are delivered. Asphyxia presenting in the newborn originates *in utero*, and primary management should be prevention, by recognition of this fact, and active management of patients with fetal distress during labour.

The essentials for successful resuscitation are:

1. Good co-operation and communication between obstetrician and paediatrician at all levels.
2. Anticipation that an infant requiring resuscitation may be delivered.
3. Adequate resuscitation facilites in working order.
4. The presence of someone capable of intubation and other resuscitative procedures at all deliveries considered to be 'at risk'.

Apparatus (*see* Appendix 21 for list of recommended equipment). Basic requirements are:

1. A satisfactory working surface with a good light source.
2. A safe source of oxygen, suction and radiant heat.
3. Equipment for delivery of oxygen by mask or endotracheal tube.
4. Appropriate drugs immediately accessible.

Conditions requiring intubation

Severe hypoxia or apnoea at delivery ('white asphyxia')

Recognition

With complete apnoea, the oxygen content of the blood falls to zero within 3–4 minutes; the PCO_2 rises at 2.6 kPa (20 mm Hg) per minute and the pH falls by 0.1 units/minute (Swyer, 1975).

In most cases, fetal hypoxia ('fetal distress') will have been recognized before delivery, by cardiotochography and/or fetal scalp sampling.

Fig. 71.1

Apgar	*Appearance*	*0 Min immediate*	*2 Min*	*5 Min*	*10 Min*	*30 Min +*
0–2	Pale/Grey Limp Apnoea Heart <100	(1) Suck out (too vigorous sucking may cause bradycardia) (2) IPPV (intubation) (3) Na HCO_3 8.4% (5 ml IV over 1–5 min; 2–2.5 ml for baby <1.5 kg) (4) Score 0: ECM (*See* Note 3)	(1) Continue IPPV (2) Naloxone if previous opiate (Note 2) 0.04 mg IV (½ dose if baby <2.5 kg) (3) *Regular respiration for 2 min* Remove tube	(1) Continue IPPV (2) Repeat $NaHCO_3$ over 5–10 min (Dose as for 0 min) (3) Glucose 10% (3 ml IV over 1 min) (4) *Regular respiration for 2 min* Remove tube	(1) Continue IPPV (2) Adrenaline 1 in 10 000:1–2 ml into heart umbilical vein or down tube (3) Atropine (0.1 mg IV) (4) *Regular respiration for 2 min* Remove tube	*Apnoea* No circulation cease IPPV *Apnoea* Good circulation correct acidosis ventilator *Regular respiration* after 2 min Remove tube
			Apnoea ↑	Apnoea ↑	Apnoea ↑	Apnoea ↑
3–6	Blue/Grey Respiration; Gasping Weak Irregular Tone ± Response ±	(1) Suck out and wipe down (2) Insert airway (3) Oxygen: bag and mask	(1) IPPV (intubation) (2) $NaHCO_3$ (2 ml IV) (3) Naloxone if previous opiate 0.04 mg (½ dose if baby <2.5 kg) IV or i.m.	(1) Continue IPPV (2) Repeat $NaHCO_3$ over 5–10 min (2 ml IV) (3) Glucose 10% (3 ml IV over 1 min)	(1) Ventilator (2) Astrup $NaHCO_3$ as indicated	
			No change ↑ or apnoea ↘	No change ↑ or apnoea ↘	No change ↑ or apnoea ↘	

7–10	Pink Active Crying Regular Resp. at <1 min	Suck out and wipe down →		*Regular respiration for 2 min* warm towel mother or cot	*Regular respiration for 2 min* (1) Remove tube (2) Warm towel mother or cot	*Regular respiration for 2 min* (1) Remove tube (2) Incubator
Good condition at birth but apnoea at 1 min or stops breathing		*0 Min* Suck out and wipe down	*1 Min* (1) Insert airway (2) Oxygen bag & mask (3) Naloxone if previous opiate (0.04 mg) (½ dose if baby <2.5 kg) IV or i.m.	(1) IPPV (2) $NaHCO_3$ 8.4% (5 ml IV 2–2.5 ml if <1.5 kg over 1–5 min)	As for Apgar 3–6 (above)	As for Apgar 3–6 (above)
				Apnoea ⇡	Apnoea (Apgar 3–6) ⇡	Apnoea (Apgar 3–6) ⇡

⇡ (dotted) Deterioration or no change
→ Improvement

(1) Failure to go pink after IPPV for 1 min. Consider:
(a) Tube: oesophagus
(b) Tube: right main bronchus
(c) Tube: blocked
(d) Bronchi blocked
(e) ? Lung condition
? Heart condition
(2) Previous opiates: mother has received at <4 hours before delivery: pethidine, codein, heroin (diamorphine)
(3) External cardiac massage: use with IPPV if fetal heart was heard during second stage

Figure 71.1 Resuscitation scheme for paediatricians. Start clock for all deliveries

APPEARANCE

Such infants are:

1. Pale.
2. Limp.
3. Unresponsive.
4. Apnoeic.

The infant appears white because of severe acidaemia and circulatory collapse, and the heart rate is likely to be less than 60 per minute or inaudible.

OTHER CAUSES OF PALLOR AT DELIVERY (SEE TABLE 82.2, PAGE 672)

1. Shock from acute fetal blood loss immediately before or during delivery; these infants may not be apnoeic (*see* Chapter 82).
2. Severe chronic anaemia with heart failure (hydrops; *see* Chapter 84, page 679) which may be due to Rhesus isoimmunization, chronic blood loss *in utero*, or other causes.

Management (Figure 71.1) (see below for methods)

The important factors to have in mind at all times during a resuscitation are:

1. How long the resuscitation has been going on.
2. The baby's response to resuscitation, usually monitored by heart rate.
3. The adequacy of the airway.
4. Adequacy of the steps taken to maintain the baby's temperature.

PROCEDURE

1. At the time of delivery of the infant, start the clock on the resuscitation trolley.
2. Collect the infant from the obstetrician, in a warm towel, and transfer to the resuscitation surface under radiant heat.
3. Apply a stethoscope to the baby's chest to monitor heart rate.
4. Examine the larynx under direct vision and quickly suck out any obstructing material above and below the larynx.
5. Pass an oral endotracheal tube.
6. Inflate the lungs with intermittent positive pressure (IPPV) at a rate of 40 per minute with a prolonged inspiration time of 1 second and a peak pressure of 25 cm of water.
7. If the heart rate is under 40 per minute, start external cardiac massage.
8. If the heart beat remains absent for more than 2 minutes, inject 1 ml 1 in 10 000 adrenaline down the endotracheal tube or into the heart.
9. If there is a strong probability of depression by the morphine group of drugs, give naloxone (Narcan) into the umbilical vein (*see* page 617).
10. At 5 minutes if there is still apnoea, inject over 1–5 minutes 5 mmol $NaHCO_3$ and 5 ml 10% glucose.
    Dose: 5 mmol $NaHCO_3$ is a safe partial correction for a baby of 3–3.5 kg: for other weights use 1.5 mmol/kg. Several concentrations of $NaHCO_3$ are available:
    8.4% $NaHCO_3$ 1 mmol/ml.
    5% $NaHCO_3$ 0.6 mmol/ml.
    4.2% $NaHCO_3$ 0.5 mmol/ml.

11. At 5 minutes if the infant is showing a slow response to resuscitation, check that the endotracheal tube is correctly sited and that there is air entry on both sides of the chest (the tube may be down the right main bronchus or may be into the oesophagus).
12. At 10 minutes, if the infant will still not sustain spontaneous respiration but has a good heart beat, repeat bicarbonate and glucose.
13. At 15 minutes if the infant still shows a poor response to resuscitation with a slow heart beat and apnoea, carry out a quick physical examination of the infant to exclude major malformations.
14. At 30 minutes:
    (a) If there is no respiration or apex beat despite effective resuscitation for 30 minutes and the pupils are fixed and dilated, IPPV and formal resuscitation should cease, as the prognosis for such infants, if they survive, is extremely poor.
    (b) If there is no respiration but the heart beat is over 60 per minute with good colour and peripheral circulation and the pupils are of normal size, IPPV should continue while the blood gas is checked (the baby may have a severe metabolic acidosis and correction of this will initiate spontaneous respiration). At this stage consider also the possibility of acute haemorrhage before delivery; if so, the infant may improve following 20 ml O-Rhesus negative blood up to the umbilical vein.
    (c) If there is no respiration with IV $NaHCO_3$ but the infant's condition is otherwise satisfactory (*see* (b) above) the baby should be placed on a mechanical ventilator until an adequate assessment of the situation can be made.

Severe shock due to hypoxia

Recognition

The severely hypoxic infant, in a state of shock, may not respond to the conventional methods of resuscitation. In such cases, pallor and feeble or irregular respiration may persist; if practicable the blood pressure should be continuously recorded by an aortic arterial catheter with transducer system. A systolic blood pressure of less than 40 mm Hg (*see* Appendix 17) for normal range of blood pressures in the newborn) is an indication for measures to raise the blood pressure and improve tissue perfusion.

Management

In addition to external cardiac massage, if required, and IPPV, the following should be tried:

1. IV colloids. Plasma or other colloid solution should be given in a dose of 20 ml/kg over ½–1 hour, using the umbilical vein. If a colloid solution is not immediately available, one of the commonly used electrolyte solutions (not low sodium solutions such as 0.45% or 0.18% NaCl) such as 0.9% NaCl, Hartmann's Solution or Ringer Lactate can be used, but their effect on expansion of the blood volume is short compared with that of colloids.
2. If there is no improvement after IV colloid or electrolyte solution, dopamine should be given in a slow IV drip: for details of dosage, *see* Chapter 10, page 107.

Hypoxic cerebral birth injury (Hypoxic–ischaemic encephalopathy, HIE)

Recognition

There may be a history of intrapartum asphyxia or other risk factors (*see* Chapter 72). The Apgar score is not always low, and there may be evidence of trauma to the head or elsewhere. The infant may be hyperreflexic and hypertonic, with exaggerated primitive reflexes, and apathetic and hypotonic, with depressed and irregular respiration and apnoeic attacks. Seizures are likely from about 12 hours after birth and may be manifested by colour changes, irregular heart or respiratory rate, mouthing movements, smacking of the lips, fluctuating muscle tone, and extensor spasms. Extensor spasms may also be evidence of incipient 'coning'. Clonic jerking of the limbs and clonic blinking may indicate uncal seizures.

Management

In addition to the brain, the function of other organs may be affected by hypoxia:

1. *Neurological* – Cranial ultrasound should be performed in the first 24 hours if there is a possibility of a subdural haematoma. A CT scan at the age of 3–4 days gives the most prognostic information (Fitzhardinge *et al.*, 1981). Seizures should be controlled by phenobarbitone, with phenytoin if necessary (*see* page 704). Lumbar puncture in the presence of known or suspected raised ICP should NOT be done as it may precipitate 'coning'. Oral feeds should not be given.
2. *Respiratory* – Apnoeic attacks and meconium aspiration may necessitate IPPV. During ventilation the $PaCO_2$ should be kept low (3.5–4.0 kPa, 26–30 mm Hg) to prevent raised ICP. With meconium aspiration in persistent fetal circulation the $PaCO_2$ may have to be kept below 3.5 kPa (26 mm Hg) to maintain adequate oxygenation.
3. *Metabolic* – Hypocalcaemia should be corrected (*see* page 135) and the blood glucose maintained between 5 and 8 mmol/ℓ (90–150 mg/100 ml).
4. *Renal* – Acute tubular necrosis is common, with oliguric and red cells in the urine. Fluid intake should be reduced to 50 ml/kg/24 hours until urinary output improves (over 2 ml/kg/min). During the oliguria the serum potassium should be estimated daily.
5. *Circulation* – Plasma or blood should be given to correct hypovolaemia or hypotension; dopamine may be required to maintain blood pressure (*see* page 107) if there has been ischaemic myocardial damage.
6. *Disseminated intravascular coagulopathy* – Appropriate screening tests (*see* pages 498 and 677) should be done at early stages.
7. *Cerebral oedema (see also Chapter 26)* – Treatment is controversial, and a controlled study is needed. The normal ICP in the newborn is under 10 mm Hg. If active reduction of raised ICP is undertaken the pressure must be measured continuously using a non-invasive fontanelle transducer or a fine catheter inserted into the subarachnoid space via the anterior fontanelle (Levene and Evans, 1983). At the same time the arterial blood pressure should be continuously recorded. The aim is to keep the cerebral perfusion pressure (mean arterial pressure minus the ICP) within normal limits by maintaining the blood pressure and preventing an excessive rise in ICP. Levene and Evans (1985) suggest the following scheme:

(a) If the ICP is over 10 mm Hg for 2 hours dexamethasone 4 mg IV should be given and the ICP recorded over the next 6 hours.
(b) If, 6 hours after the dexamethasone, the ICP is still over 10 mm Hg, 20% mannitol 1 g/kg should be given over 20 minutes.

As yet, there has been no controlled study of the regimen, and it must be recognized that 'cerebral oedema' may, on occasion, represent swelling from necrosis and death of the neurones, and that cerebral perfusion may be governed by factors other than $PaCO_2$ and the cerebral perfusion pressure.

Delayed onset of respiration

Delayed respiration may be caused by:

1. Severe hypoxia (*see* above).
2. Drug depression, usually from morphine, pethidine (Meperidine, Demerol), codeine (diamorphine), or occasionally due to prolonged general anaesthesia or by heavy maternal sedation with barbiturates or benzodiazepines (diazepam) or magnesium sulphate if this is used for the treatment of severe pre-eclampsia. There is no specific treatment for the infant depressed after maternal general anaesthesia and it is rare for this to be a cause of apnoea.
3. No apparent reason.

Drug depression (morphine group)

Recognition

Some depression of the infant's respiration is likely if the mother has received one of this group of drugs within 4 hours of delivery. Such an infant is normally in good condition at birth but does not breathe immediately, or takes an initial gasp and then becomes apnoeic.

Management

1. If the probability of opiate drug depression is high, naloxone (Narcan) may be given either prophylactically (i.e. immediately after delivery) or after a predetermined period of apnoea under close observation. Naloxone (Narcan) is a specific opiate antagonist without depressant side-effects and is preferable to nalorphine (Lethidrone).
   Dose: the standard dose for naloxone is 0.01 mg/kg, but since the weight of the infant is not known at delivery, a standard dose of 0.04 mg (2 ml) for term infants and half this dose for infants under 2.5 kg is appropriate. The dose may be repeated, if necessary, after 10 minutes.
   Route: preferably intravenously.
   NOTE: the paediatric ampoules should be used; these contain 0.04 mg in 2 ml (0.02 mg/ml).
   Because the action of naloxone is short lived (sometimes as little as 30 minutes), the dose may have to be repeated after 30 minutes to 1 hour and, occasionally, several times during the first hours of life.
2. Failure to breathe at 1 minute, apparently due to opiate sedation uncorrected by early naloxone administration; proceed as for the severely asphyxiated group and intubate.

Delayed onset of respiration for no obvious reason

Whatever the Apgar score, if respiration does not start immediately after routine aspiration of the nose and mouth:

1. Oxygen should be given by mask and the heart rate monitored during the first 2 minutes after delivery.
2. If there is no respiratory effort by 2 minutes or if the infant's heart rate drops below 100, the infant should be intubated and treated as for the severely asphyxiated group.
3. The infant may require investigation of the cause of hypertonia (e.g. myopathy, dystrophia, myotonia, etc.).

Meconium aspiration

Recognition

It is not always possible to predict whether aspiration of meconium has occurred, even if the infant is covered with meconium at delivery or there is meconium-stained liquor. Infants with evidence of fetal distress before delivery and who are post-mature or small for gestational age are particularly at risk. Meconium aspiration syndrome is a common cause of respiratory difficulties with tachypnoea, cyanosis, indrawing and recession in the term infant.

Fetal hypoxia (fetal distress) in the preterm infant rarely causes the passage of meconium; the meconium-stained infant of less than 32 weeks is more likely to have suffered from intrauterine sepsis than asphyxia.

Management

1. If meconium-stained fluid has been draining before delivery, it is important that following delivery of the head, and before the infant has had an opportunity to take the first breath, the airway should be sucked out by the obstetrician supervising the delivery.
2. Following delivery, immediate direct laryngoscopy and suctioning of the airway should be done before IPPV is started. External cardiac massage may be required if the heart rate is less than 40 per minute.
3. If the membranes have been ruptured for longer than 48 hours, or the amniotic fluid is smelly, or the mother febrile, the infant should be given a 5 day course of antibiotics, normally gentamicin and penicillin, following a full infection screen.
4. If, despite adequate suctioning of the airway before resuscitation, the baby develops severe respiratory distress with tachypnoea, pallor and cyanosis, the umbilical artery should be catheterized, oxygen given initially in a concentration of 60 per cent or more and preparations made to transfer the infant to a regional neonatal intensive care unit.
5. For later management and complications *see* page 248.

Diaphragmatic hernia

Recognition

A term infant presenting with severe breathing difficulties at birth should be suspected of having a diaphragmatic hernia. The signs suggestive of this are a deviation of the apex beat to the right, sometimes into the right axilla, and a scaphoid abdomen. Bowel sounds will not be audible in the left side of the chest until the infant has swallowed air at delivery.

Management

1. If this problem is suspected, *under no circumstances* should mask IPPV be carried out as this will inflate the bowel in the left side of the chest.
2. Early intubation should be carried out and the baby given IPPV manually.
3. A large bore (8FG) nasogastric tube, preferably a Replogle tube, should be passed and connected to continuous suction to prevent inflation of the intestine in the left side of the chest.
4. The baby should be transferred for intensive care management in the regional neonatal surgical unit. Consider giving muscle relaxants (pancuronium 0.05 mg/kg) once the baby is effectively mechanically ventilated to prevent gasping and further entry of intestinal contents into the thorax through the hernia.

Methods of resuscitation (for apparatus *see* Appendix 21)

1. Oral endotracheal intubation (*see also* Chapter 22):
   (a) Flex the infant's neck and extend the head ('sniffing a flower'). Placing a rolled-up napkin under the neck may assist in adopting this position in the term infant, but may make intubation more difficult in very small preterm infants.
   (b) A straight-bladed infant laryngoscope should be used, with suction immediately available and an oral endotracheal tube of appropriate size (2.5, 3, or 3.5 mm) is passed. The tube is secured and connected to a source of humidifed oxygen with a means of providing IPPV and a safety blow-off at 25–30 cm H_2O. Occasionally, expansion of the lungs can only be obtained by using an initial pressure of as high as 60 cm H_2O, particularly in infants with severe hyaline membrane disease, but this pressure should not be sustained.
2. Bag and mask. This method can be used initially if intubation is not immediately required or in the infant with weak and gasping respirations. There are two types of bagging circuits:
   (a) A paediatric anaesthetic re-breathing bag and stop-cock; the valve should be open but the stop-cock shut.
   (b) A self-inflating bag with a pressure blow-off valve such as the Laerdal infant resuscitation bag. It is important that the mask fits adequately and that the chest moves with pressure on the bag. The position, which keeps the airway clear, is with the head extended. The procedure may be more effective if an infant oropharyngeal airway is used. Effective bag and mask IPPV requires considerable practice and experience.
3. Mouth-to-mouth inflation. This is indicated when no other method is available. The head is kept extended, and the nose and mouth of the infant covered by the operator's mouth. Inflationary pressure is applied only with the cheeks, NOT the chest, at 30–40 times per minute.
4. External cardiac massage (*see also* Chapter 24, page 276). The infant is placed on a firm, flat surface; the middle of the sternum is depressed 1–1.5 cm by the

index and middle fingers at 100–120 times per minute. Alternatively, the infant's chest is grasped by the operator's hands with the fingers at the back of the chest and the thumbs in the middle of the sternum; the sternum is then depressed sharply by squeezing between the thumbs and fingers. Good perfusion and blood pressure readings may be obtained in the newborn infant with effective external cardiac massage.

5. Injection of drugs into the umbilical vein. There are a number of dangers if an incorrect technique is used:
   (a) Haematoma and possibly injection into the artery; if a hypertonic substance is injected into the umbilical artery quickly, an area of sloughing may occur on the buttock.
   (b) The drug cannot be washed into the circulation and may therefore be ineffective.
   (c) The intima of the vein may be damaged by a hyperosmolar solution, causing thrombosis.

   The correct method is as follows:
   An umbilical catheter is attached to a 5 or 10 ml syringe; the catheter and half the syringe are filled with sterile 0.9% NaCl; the catheter is then inserted into the umbilical vein for about 5–7 cm until blood can be freely withdrawn. The catheter is then firmly pinched, and the syringe detached. The drug to be injected is aspirated into the syringe which now contains the drug diluted with 0.9% NaCl. The syringe is re-attached to the catheter excluding all air bubbles. Blood is now aspirated to fill the rest of the syringe and the whole contents are slowly injected. No drug should be injected more rapidly than over a period of 1 minute.

References

FITZHARDINGE, P. M., FLOODMARK, O., FITZ, C. R. and ASHBY, S. (1981) The prognostic value of computed tomography as an adjunct to an assessment of the full term infant with post-asphyxial encephalopathy. *Journal of Pediatrics*, **99**, 777–781

LEVENE, M. I. and EVANS, D. H. (1983) Continuous measurement of subarachnoid pressure in the severely asphyxiated newborn. *Archives of Disease in Childhood,* **58,** 1013–1015

LEVENE, M. I. and EVANS, D. H. (1985) Medical management of raised intercranial pressure after severe birth asphyxia. *Archives of Disease in Childhood,* **60,** 12–16

SWYER, P. R. (1975) *The Intensive Care of the Newly Born,* p. 75. Basle: S. Karger

Further reading

OSTHEIMER, G. W. (1982) Resuscitation of the newborn infant. *Clinics in Perinatology,* **9,** 177–189

SWYER, P. R. (1975) *The Intensive Care of the Newly Born.* Basle: S. Karger

TING, P. and BRADY, J. P. (1975) Tracheal suction and meconium aspiration. *American Journal of Obstetrics and Gynecology,* **122,** 767–771

THOMPSON, A. J., SEARLE, M. and RUSSELL, G. (1977) Quality of survival after severe birth asphyxia. *Archives of Disease in Childhood,* **52,** 620–626

Chapter 72

Birth trauma and accidents related to delivery (including intraventricular haemorrhage)

M. F. Whitfield and J. A. Black

The risks of delivery are minimized by a controlled vertex delivery, where possible. During this process, the infant is subjected to a degree of hypoxia, moulding of the head, and formation of caput and some bruising of the presenting part. There may also be trauma to the head due to fetal blood scalp sampling and at the site of attachment of an electrode used for electronic fetal monitoring. These are the normal effects of labour on the infant. Risks to the infant are increased by other routes of delivery and an accurate knowledge of the complications associated with the various types of delivery assists in early diagnosis and treatment. Only complications requiring urgent treatment are considered here.

Precipitate vertex delivery

Infants born by precipitate vertex delivery frequently have almost confluent petechiae on the face and head ('traumatic cyanosis') which may be mistaken for central cyanosis. Such infants usually also have subconjunctival haemorrhages and are irritable and 'screechy' for some time after delivery. Serious trauma from precipitate vertex delivery may include tearing of the venous sinuses in the tentorium cerebelli or falx cerebri, with resulting acute subdural haemorrhage.

Breech delivery

The risks related to breech delivery are greater if the baby's head is extended *in utero*. Rapid delivery of the unprotected head may cause a tear of the tentorium or falx as described above. Brachial plexus injury is common in difficult breech delivery but constitutes an emergency only when injury to the phrenic nerve causes diaphragmatic paralysis. Cervical fracture–dislocation may occur from over-extension of the neck during delivery of the head, and fractures of the clavicle, humerus, or femur are not uncommon. Shock may occasionally develop from massive bleeding into the soft tissues of the buttocks or from intra-abdominal blood loss due to internal abdominal injuries.

Infants born by breech delivery, owing to the increased degree of bruising to which they are subjected, frequently become significantly jaundiced within the first week of life and may require treatment.

Face delivery

An infant presenting by the face can be delivered vaginally. A goitre may be the cause of the malpresentation and the neck should be examined carefully after delivery. Spinal anomalies (e.g. iniencephaly) may also cause face presentation. Direct pressure of the larynx against the symphysis pubis may occasionally cause glottic oedema or dislocation of the cricothyroid or cricoarytenoid articulations.

Brow delivery

In infants presenting in the brow position, the head usually cannot pass through the pelvis and if a vaginal delivery is persisted with, severe asphyxia and considerable cranial trauma usually ensue. Bilateral temporomandibular joint dislocation with consequent difficulty of intubation for resuscitation may occur in infants who have been permitted to continue in the brow position for some time.

Forceps delivery

Although the use of forceps *per se* is not intrinsically dangerous, the requirement to use forceps marks such a delivery as being at relatively high risk. Cephalhaematoma is common in forceps deliveries and subaponeurotic haemorrhage may develop, particularly in infants of African race. In traumatic forceps deliveries, acute subdural haemorrhage may result from rupture of the communicating veins or from a torn venous sinus. Direct trauma to facial structures may occur from misapplication of the blade. 'Lift out' forceps delivery associated with epidural anaesthesia is rarely a traumatic procedure.

Vacuum (ventouse) extraction

Although ventouse extraction can be an effective atraumatic method of assisting delivery of an uncompromised infant during maternal exhaustion in labour, it creates a large caput, sometimes complicated by scalp necrosis and permanent hair loss, if the suction cup is inexpertly applied. The ventouse is not a rapid means of delivering an asphyxiated infant and its use in this situation will result in a severely depressed infant at delivery. A subaponeurotic haemorrhage is an occasional complication.

Caesarean section

The risks of caesarean section are related mainly to the indication for which the operation was carried out. Acute fetal haemorrhage, which is easily overlooked at operation, may be due to fetal bleeding in addition to maternal bleeding in antepartum haemorrhage, incision of a fetal vessel at operation, accidental incision into the scalp or elsewhere, or draining of blood out of the infant into the placenta by holding the infant above the placenta without first clamping the cord. Caesarean section for delivery of the premature infant following prolonged ruptured membranes and drainage of the liquor may present severe problems in the delivery of the fetal head and result in an asphyxiated infant requiring urgent resuscitation.

Multiple pregnancy

Nearly all multiple pregnancies are now diagnosed in the antenatal period, by ultrasound examination. Any multiple delivery is a high-risk delivery and requires full neonatal resuscitation facilities with sufficient experienced resuscitators to cope with the number of fetuses anticipated. Prematurity is more common in multiple pregnancies and respiratory difficulties must be anticipated. Fetofetal (twin-to-twin) transfusion may occur in monozygotic twins (*see* pages 671 and 679), and malpresentation and cord accidents are relatively frequent with vaginal delivery. Most authorities consider that multiple pregnancies delivering at 32 weeks gestation or less should be delivered by caesarean section because of the risks to the second premature twin of a vaginal delivery.

Antepartum haemorrhage

Antepartum bleeding may include blood from the fetal circulation as well as the maternal circulation and may be due to placenta praevia or placental abruption. The infant born following a major placental abruption may suffer from severe intrapartum hypoxia in addition to haemorrhagic shock. Maternal blood swallowed by the fetus may be vomited after delivery or passed in the stools (*see also* page 676).

Prolapsed cord

Cord prolapse is associated with rapid reduction in fetoplacental circulation and frequently the birth of a severely hypoxic infant who may have meconium aspiration.

Local (regional) anaesthesia

In general, the fetus is benefited by the use of regional anaesthesia because of the avoidance of the depressant effects of opiates. The fetus may be affected, however, by local anaesthetic agents indirectly due to maternal hypotension, or directly by high blood levels of local anaesthetic.

Shoulder dystocia

Shoulder dystocia usually occurs in large infants and may result in an infant subjected to sudden acute asphyxia, with brachial plexus injury and clavicular fracture.

Recognition and management of the emergencies

Cerebral birth injury

Recognition

This general term covers the effects of cerebral hypoxia before, during and immediately after delivery, and of intracranial bleeding resulting from direct trauma or deformation of the skull due to a precipitate, prolonged or difficult delivery. The clinical picture may be confused by the coexistence of hypoxic–ischaemic encephalopathy (HIE) with intracranial haemorrhage. In addition, the effects of drugs given during labour may have to be considered.

The recognition and management of HIE are considered in detail in Chapter 71 (page 616). Intracranial haemorrhage may be subdural (*see* below), intraventricular (*see* pages 626–629) or more rarely, solely subarachnoid.

Symptoms of cerebral birth injury are often non-specific, and an accurate diagnosis depends initially upon non-invasive methods, such as ultrasound and CT scans. A purely clinical diagnosis of raised intracranial pressure is difficult, since initially the fontanelle may be both tense and bulging. On a scan, in raised intracranial pressure the lateral ventricles are seen to be narrowed or slit like; localized collections of blood can also be detected by scanning techniques.

Management

Apart from the treatment of shock and the effects of cerebral hypoxia (*see* page 616) management depends upon an accurate diagnosis, as described above. Lumbar puncture should not be done in the presence of suspected or known raised intracranial pressure. The only exceptions to this rule are the possibility of meningitis already present before delivery (*see* page 651) and the necessity for distinguishing between subarachnoid haemorrhage and meningitis.

Acute fetal haemorrhage from any cause

See page 671.

Acute subdural haemorrhage

Recognition

The infant becomes shocked within a few hours of delivery, with apnoeic attacks or fits and a tense or bulging fontanelle. Ultrasound or CT scan examinations will confirm the presence of a subdural haemorrhage.

Management

Blood may be aspirated by subdural taps at the lateral angles of the anterior fontanelle and the opinion of a neurosurgeon should be sought. A posterior fossa haematoma cannot be removed by subdural taps and may require surgical intervention.

Subaponeurotic haemorrhage

Recognition

An obvious swelling of the head develops at 24–36 hours after delivery. There is pitting oedema of the scalp which may extend as far as the attachment of the aponeurosis to the superior nuchal line or forwards into the frontal region and bruising may be visible in the upper eyelids.

Management

A large supaponeurotic haemorrhage may contain almost half the infant's circulating blood volume and an urgent transfusion may therefore be required. Vitamin K_1 (1 mg) should be given i.m. or IV if a coagulation disorder is suspected. In every case, the infant should be investigated for thrombocytopenia and coagulation defect.

Fetal scalp haemorrhage

Recognition

It is frequently difficult to recognize this condition unless blood has collected in the oedematous tissues of the caput.

Management

Blood transfusion may be required and investigation should be initiated to rule out coagulation defects.

Direct injury to the larynx

See page 622.

Diaphragmatic paralysis with brachial plexus injury

See pages 250 and 621.

Effects of local anaesthesia

Recognition

Fetal bradycardia followed by the delivery of a depressed and possibly apnoeic infant following local anaesthesia (particularly paracervical, caudal, perineal or pudendal block) should suggest the possibility of the effect of high fetal blood levels of the local anaesthetic. Convulsions occur in severely affected infants.

Management

The apnoeic or hypoxic infant should be resuscitated in the usual way. Metabolic acidosis is common and should be treated with intravenous bicarbonate (*see* page

119). Convulsions should be treated with phenobarbitone (*see* page 703). Severely affected infants who show no improvement on the above treatment may require an exchange transfusion or ventilation.

Rupture of liver or spleen

See page 674.

Adrenal haemorrhage

See pages 674–675.

Renal vein thrombosis

See pages 674–675.

Cerebral intraventricular haemorrhage

Cerebral intraventricular haemorrhage (IVH) occurs in 30–40 per cent of premature infants of 1.5 kg birth weight (32 weeks gestation) or less. Unlike other forms of intracranial haemorrhage in the newborn, IVH does not appear to be due to birth trauma *per se* and is almost entirely confined to small premature infants, particularly those who have been subjected to perinatal asphyxia, or who have severe hyaline membrane disease complicated by pulmonary interstitital emphysema and pneumothorax. The susceptibility of small premature infants to IVH appears to be due to:

1. A tendency at this stage of development of the cerebral circulation to bleeding from the germinal eminence adjacent to each lateral ventricle.
2. A lack of 'autoregulation' of the cerebral circulation in response to changes in blood pressure, which permits exposure of the brain to sudden fluctuations in blood pressure.

Table 72.1 Classification of intraventricular haemorrhage

Grade 1	Isolated germinal matrix haemorrhage
Grade 2	Intraventricular haemorrhage with normal ventricular size
Grade 3	Intraventricular haemorrhage with ventricular dilatation
Grade 4	Intraventricular haemorrhage with parenchymal haemorrhage

From Papile *et al.*, 1978.

3. A high risk of severe respiratory disease, requiring high ventilation pressures, and periodic unpredictable catastrophies such as pneumothorax which have been correlated with major blood pressure fluctuations and intraventricular haemorrhage. The tendency to intraventricular haemorrhage appears to be confined to the first 2–3 weeks of life, with 80 per cent of IVHs occurring in the first 7 days of life.

Table 72.2 Early childhood neurological handicap after intraventricular haemorrhage in infants of 1500 g birth weight or less

	No. in grade	*Normal (%)*	*Handicap n (%)*		
			Minor	*Major*	*Multiple**
No IVH	116	57 (49)	46 (41)	12 (11)	7
Grade 1	33	16 (48)	14 (42)	3 (9)	2
Grade 2	18	9 (50)	7 (39)	2 (11)	0
Grade 3	14	2 (14)	7 (50)	5 (36)	4
Grade 4	17	2 (12)	2 (12)	13 (76)	10

* No. of infants in major handicap column whose handicaps were multiple.
From Papile *et al.*, 1983.

Bleeding starts in the germinal eminence and may initially be confined to the germinal layer by the ependyma (subependymal or germinal layer haemorrhage). Extension through the ependyma into the lateral ventricle constitutes true intraventricular haemorrhage which may be associated with ventricular dilatation. In addition, there may be extension directly into the cerebral substance; or areas of haemorrhagic cerebral infarction may develop adjacent to or remote from the initial IVH. Papile's grading system of IVH (*Table 72.1*), despite some shortcomings, is the most commonly used and is of some predictive value in

Table 72.3 Outcome in infants with Grade 3 or 4 IVH with or without post-haemorrhagic hydrocephalus (PHH)

	No. of subjects	*Normal (%)*	*Handicap (%)*		
			Minor	*Major*	*Multiple**
No PHH	14	3 (21)	3 (21)	8 (57)	4
PHH	17	1 (5)	6 (35)	10 (58)	10

* No. of infants in major handicap column whose handicaps were multiple.
From Papile *et al.*, 1983.

anticipating complications and outcome (*see Tables 72.2* and *72.3*). However, factors other than size or location of IVH are also important determinants of neurodevelopmental outcome (asphyxia, severe acidaemia, hypoglycaemia, birth weight, sex, social class).

Recognition

Clinical signs of IVH are usually subtle or absent except in a large IVH where the size of the haemorrhage leads to a significant drop in circulating blood volume. Clinical signs may include:

1. Sudden unexplained deterioration in circulation with cold pallor, blotchiness, sometimes hypotension, and a drop in haematocrit.

2. Neurological deterioration including reduction in spontaneous movements, apathy, seizures, and apnoea.
3. Tense fontanelle.
4. Biochemical changes; reduced glucose tolerance if receiving parenteral nutrition, severe recurrent unexplained metabolic acidosis, coagulopathy.

A presumptive diagnosis may be made on the basis of the above findings. Cranial ultrasound using a sector scanner with views through the fontanelle, provides a quick, easy non-invasive method of diagnosis using portable equipment which causes little disturbance to the infant or to his treatment. Because of the lack of signs in many cases, most neonatal intensive care units have a standard protocol for ultrasound examinations in small infants. For example, infants of 1.5 kg birth weight or less are routinely scanned at 3–4 days, 14 days, and 2–4 weekly thereafter until ventricular size is stable and there is resolution of the intraventricular clot. Larger infants are scanned if there has been asphyxia, severe respiratory disease or pneumothorax.

Management

1. There is no specific treatment for IVH once it has occurred.
2. Blood transfusion may be required to correct anaemia and support blood pressure and perfusion. Transfusions should be given slowly to avoid sudden surges in blood pressure (*see* below).
3. Ventilation may have to be altered to correct acidosis and hypoxia. Bicarbonate may be required if there is a persistent metabolic acidosis after readjustment of ventilation, and should be given slowly over several hours.
4. Glucose infusion rate may have to be reduced if the blood glucose value rises above 11 mmol/ℓ (200 mg/100 ml), and the glucose level should be monitored.
5. Platelet count and coagulation status should be reviewed and appropriate corrective treatment given. Ethamsylate may be useful in correcting abnormal platelet adhesion.
6. Cranial ultrasound should be repeated and compared with previous scan results.
7. Seizures should be treated with phenobarbitone (*see* page 703).
8. Occasionally, in the days following major IVH, the clinical status of the infant and the ultrasound findings may require to serious consideration about the desirability or otherwise of continued active medical management. Death due to IVH alone, however, is extremely rare.

Complications

1. 'Transient ventriculomegaly'. Transient mild ventricular dilatation is a frequent finding on serial cranial ultrasound examinations during the first 2–3 weeks after IVH. This appears to be relatively benign but probably represents the mildest self-limiting form of post-haemorrhagic hydrocephalus.
2. Post-haemorrhagic hydrocephalus (PHH). The development of progressive hydrocephalus following IVH is most common in Grade 3 or 4 IVH. In Papile's study, no infants who had Grade 2 or less IVH developed PHH while in the 42 infants with Grade 3 or 4 IVH, 22 (52 per cent) developed this complication.

Recognition:
(a) Progressive ventricular dilatation on serial cranial ultrasound.
(b) Fullness of the fontanelle with widening of the sutures.
(c) Excessive growth in occipitofrontal circumference.
Management:
(a) In a few cases, the hydrocephalus arrests spontaneously.
(b) In some cases, attempts to reduce CSF production may be successful in slowing or halting progressive ventricular enlargement, using glycerol, isosorbide, or carbonic anhydrase inhibition with acetazolamide.
(c) In most cases, repeated removal of 15–20 ml CSF 2–14 times per week may be required, by lumbar puncture in communicating, or ventricular drainage reservoir in non-communicating hydrocephalus.

Repeated CSF removal and glycerol or other osmotherapy may cause major problems in sodium and water balance, and acetazolamide may cause a severe metabolic acidosis. Although in individual cases, (b) and (c) (above) appear to have avoided the necessity for ventriculo-peritoneal shunting, this does not appear to be the case in the majority of infants, and repeated LP or reservoir drainage constitutes a significant infection risk.
(d) Ventriculo-peritoneal shunting should be carried out in infants with progressive hydrocephalus once the CSF is clear of blood and has a low protein content (to avoid shunt blockage) and the infant is considered large enough and stable enough for the operation.

3. *Microcephaly and cerebral atrophy* – Extensive IVH and cerebral infarction may lead to enlarged ventricles with cystic degeneration in the white matter (periventricular leucomalacia (PVL)), and porencephalic cysts visible on cranial ultrasound. The poorly growing head helps to differentiate this situation from progressive hydrocephalus, and drainage procedures are not indicated. The neurodevelopmental outlook for such infants is very poor with multiple major handicaps.
4. *Neurodevelopmental handicap* – Intraventricular haemorrhage is a major indication of future neurodevelopmental handicap in small premature infants (*Table 72.2*) and the risks are further increased in infants with PHH (*Table 72.3*). Major handicaps include mental retardation, cerebral palsy, microcephaly, sensory deficits and seizure disorder. On present evidence the risk of handicap does not appear to be significantly increased in infants with Grade 1 or 2 IVH compared with infants with no IVH. Grades 3 and 4 IVH are associated with a high incidence of handicap (*Table 72.2*). In most instances, however, the neurological damage is not due to the IVH *per se*, but to the reduction in cerebral perfusion at the time of IVH, leading to ischaemic damage to the white matter (PVL). Thus PVL may be observed on cranial ultrasound as hyperechogenic areas which over a number of weeks become cystic. Similar observations have also been made in the absence of IVH.

Prevention

Current theories of the genesis of IVH and the susceptibility of the immature brain to fluctuations in blood pressure suggest that avoidance of blood pressure fluctuations and pneumothorax in particular are important in managing small infants at risk of intraventricular haemorrhage.

References

PAPILE, L.-A., BURSTEIN, J., BURSTEIN, R. and KOFFLER, H. (1978) Incidence and evolution of subependymal and intraventricular haemorrhage. A study of infants of birth weight less than 1500 grams. *Journal of Pediatrics,* **92,** 529–534

PAPILE, L.-A., MUNSICK-BRUNO, G. and SCHAEFER, A. N. (1983) Relationship of cerebral intraventricular haemorrhage and early childhood neurological handicaps. *Journal of Pediatrics,* **103,** 273–277

Further reading

VOLPE, J. J. (1983) *Neurology of the Newborn.* Philadelphia: W. B. Saunders

PAPE, K. E. and WIGGLESWORTH, J. S. (1979) *Haemorrhage, Ischaemia and the Perinatal Brain.* Philadelphia: Lippincott

Chapter 73

Transport of the sick neonate

M. F. Whitfield

Management

The survival and morbidity statistics for sick and for low birth weight infants are better if the infant is cared for in a Neonatal Intensive Care Unit (NICU) than in the referring hospital Special Care Baby Unit (SCBU) where it may not be possible to provide appropriate equipment and experienced round-the-clock staffing. The transport of high-risk or potentially high-risk patients is a major concern in modern paediatric practice. Neonatal intensive care of the high-risk neonate is only one arm of the high-risk obstetric/neonatal combined approach and the best results are obtained by co-operation at all levels between obstetric and neonatal staff, both in the referring hospital and in the neonatal intensive care unit hospital.

Maternal transport

Whenever possible, a mother whose infant may require full intensive care facilities in the newborn period should be transferred with the infant *in utero* to the High-Risk Obstetric Unit in the neonatal intensive care unit hospital. The decision to transfer the mother should be a joint one involving the paediatric and obstetric staff in the referring hospital and the staff of the regional perinatal unit. Although each patient presents a different problem, variables such as bed space and bad weather may affect timing of the transfer, the following are indications for possible transfer to the regional perinatal centre:

1. The onset of premature labour in a pregnancy of 33 weeks gestation or less.
2. Multiple pregnancy.
3. Serious complications of pregnancy, such as significant antepartum haemorrhage or pregnancy induced hypertension.
4. Serious coincidental maternal disease, e.g. heart disease, renal disease, and diseases that may affect the fetus such as myasthenia, idiopathic thrombocytopenic purpura or disseminated lupus erythematosus.
5. Previously recognized fetomaternal problem such as severe Rhesus isoimmunization.
6. Poor intrauterine growth as shown by clinical assessment or sequential ultrasound measurements.
7. Identified fetal anomaly on ultrasound, possibly amenable to intrauterine treatment (e.g. obstructive uropathy) or requiring urgent management following delivery (e.g. diaphragmatic hernia).

Contraindications to maternal transfer

The pregnancy must be in a reasonably stable state before transfer. The mother should not be transferred if the blood pressure is out of control or if there is active bleeding. Rapidly advancing labour constitutes a major contraindication to transfer as it may lead to delivery *en route*, to be avoided at all costs. The situation should be assessed and the mother stabilized before transfer, in discussion with the obstetrician in the regional High Risk Obstetric Centre. Immediately before transfer, the degree of cervical dilatation should be assessed to reduce the risk of delivery before arrival at the regional centre.

Neonatal transport

Sometimes delivery in the referring hospital is inevitable because of the advanced stage of labour of the mother on arrival, continuing antepartum haemorrhage or fulminating pregnancy-induced hypertension. In this situation, the route of delivery should be decided upon by the obstetric staff in the referring hospital and the Regional Centre, and the best facilities provided for delivery of the infant, resuscitation after delivery, and subsequent stabilization before transfer.

The Regional Neonatal Intensive Care Unit provides transport for infants needing to be transported to the Regional NICU. The regional transport team acts as an extension of the Neonatal Intensive Care unit, providing similar facilities. The facility used by the Neonatal Transport Team may be in the form of a specially modified intensive care transport incubator or may be a specially modified ambulance or aircraft. The transport must provide:

1. Adequate temperature homeostasis, with a transport incubator with heater output and ability to maintain the body temperature of an infant of less than 1 kg in whatever environmental temperature is likely to be met. This may be a traditional convected air incubator, preferably with a double wall, or it may be a unit using radiant heat. In a convection incubator, it may be desirable to wrap the infant in warmed Gamgee or kitchen aluminium foil to prevent radiant heat loss.
2. Self-contained infant ventilator with adequate supply of oxygen and air and a suitable gas mixture.
3. Continuous monitoring facilities for heart rate, core temperature, and inspired oxygen concentration. A recent useful addition to neonatal transport equipment is a portable battery powered transcutaneous oxygen monitor.
4. Equipment for resuscitation, ventilator connection, intravascular infusion, chest drains, and chest drain valves, and Dextrostix. Intravascular infusions must be controlled by a battery powered infusion pump, either a syringe pump or peristaltic pump.
5. Drugs; sodium bicarbonate, digoxin, antibiotics, anticonvulsants, glucose 10% and other IV infusion fluids.

The neonatal transport equipment must be fully battery powered but able to run off the mains electricity supply (240 or 110 volts a.c.) or 12 volts d.c., as is available in most ambulances. The equipment should also be adapted to run off 24 volts d.c., as this is the voltage frequently provided in aircraft. The equipment must be checked and be in a state of readiness at all times.

Staff should be able to 'trouble-shoot' the equipment (provided by a respiratory technician, an ambulance attendant, a doctor or a nurse) and assess and treat the infant (a doctor, a specially trained nurse, or a specially trained ambulance attendant). The person responsible for the management of the infant must be highly skilled and fully conversant with clinical assessment of the infant, and X-ray and blood gas interpretation.

Indications for transfer

Discussion about transfer to a NICU is indicated in the following situations:

1. Low birth weight: less than 1.5 kg. Although not all infants of 1.5 kg birth weight become seriously ill, many develop nutritional and respiratory problems requiring intensive management, which may be only possible in the Regional Neonatal Intensive Care Unit. The smaller the infant, the greater the chance of significant problems. The improvement in survival and morbidity in infants of 1 kg or less at birth depends on regionalized management.
2. Hyaline membrane disease, meconium aspiration syndrome, pneumothorax and other forms of displaced air. If blood gas analysis is not available, infants with relatively mild respiratory problems requiring FiO_2 greater than 0.30 (30% oxygen) to abolish cyanosis should be transferred in order to provide adequate blood gas monitoring. Infants with hyaline membrane disease requiring FiO_2 in excess of 0.6 in order to maintain a PaO_2 of 8.0 kPa (60 mm Hg) should be transferred to the Regional NICU because of the high incidence of ventilatory failure and requirement for ventilatory assistance and posssible pneumothorax. Infants with significant meconium aspiration requiring increasing FiO_2 greater than 0.30 should be transferred, as they are likely to develop severe ventilatory problems in the first 48 hours due to persistent fetal circulation (*see* pages 250 and 259).
3. Life-threatening congenital abnormalities which may require urgent surgical management, e.g. diaphragmatic hernia, congenital heart disease, gastroschisis, oesophageal atresia with tracheo-oesophageal fistula, neonatal intestinal obstruction.
4. Diagnostic problems.
5. Other management problems in the sick neonate, e.g. neonatal seizures, intolerance of feeds, severe jaundice requiring diagnosis and/or exchange transfusion, metabolic abnormalities.

The best management of the infant should be discussed by the referring hospital staff and the NICU staff; the infant's condition should be stabilized after delivery and before the arrival of the neonatal transport team. The aim of stabilization before transfer is to improve the baby's condition and to avoid problems *en route*. This involves prevention or correction of hypoxia, hypercapnia, acidaemia, hypoglycaemia and shock. The infant usually requires an intravenous line and intravenous glucose at 60 ml/kg/24 hours and will benefit from blood gas monitoring and appropriate manipulation of FiO_2 and ventilatory assistance if indicated.

The neonatal transport team should reach the referring hospital as quickly as possible, as the infant may continue to deteriorate after the original telephone call. On arrival, the neonatal transport team assesses and consolidates stabilization of the infant. The need for appropriate ventilation should be confirmed by blood gas analysis before transfer. Endotracheal tubes must be securely fixed for transport, and if possible a chest X-ray should be carried out before transfer to confirm the position of the endotracheal tube and to exclude a pneumothorax, particularly if air transfer in unpressurized aircraft is contemplated, as a pneumothorax increases in size with decreasing external barometric pressure.

Before departure from the referring hospital, the neonatal transport team collect all relevant documentation about the mother, the pregnancy, the delivery, and the hospital course before their arrival. They should also collect the placenta, if available, and a sample of maternal blood and any available X-rays. The situation must be discussed with the parents and they should have an opportunity to see the baby before departure.

In transit, the neonatal transport team must monitor the heart rate, respiratory rate, colour, temperature, and activity of the infant and the functioning of the equipment, the adequacy of the battery pack and of the inspired gases. If the transport involves a flight in unpressurized aircraft, the FiO_2 will have to be increased considerably in order to maintain the same PaO_2 (*Table 73.1*). In pressurized aircraft, it may be necessary to request for lower equivalent altitude pressurization than usual in order to improve oxygenation.

Table 73.1 Table of equivalent oxygen concentrations at different altitudes

Altitude (feet)								
Sea level	21	30	40	50	60	70	80	90
				Equivalent O_2 concentration (%)				
2000	23	32.5	43	55	65	75	86	98
4000	25	35	47	59	70	81	94	
6000	27	38	51	63	76	88	>100	
8000*	29	42	55	68	82	96		
10 000	31	45	60	75	90	>100		
12 000	34	49	65	82	100			

* Assume this altitude in pressurized commercial jets unless pilot states otherwise.

Data calculated from Liebman *et al.* (1976).

On arrival in the regional NICU, the neonatal transport team hand the infant over to the intensive care staff, ensuring transfer of all relevant data, and inform the parents of the infant's safe arrival.

The involvement of the paediatrician in the referring hospital during the baby's stay in the Regional Neonatal Intensive Care Unit is of considerable importance and early transfer back to the referring hospital should be arranged as soon as the infant is no longer in need of intensive care management.

Special situations

Diaphragmatic hernia

Infants with diaphragmatic hernia frequently present with severe respiratory insufficiency in the first hours after delivery; it is aggravated by gaseous distension of the bowel in the left hemithorax and the infant's vigorous respiratory efforts which frustrate effective ventilation, and due to high negative intrapleural pressure excursions encourage further passage of bowel into the left hemithorax. It is important NOT to give IPPV by mask as this inflates the intestine; as soon as the condition is recognized, a large-bore Replogle tube size 8FG should be passed into the stomach and attached to continuous suction. Before transfer, the baby should be intubated and IPPV started, and it may be desirable to secure muscle relaxation by paralysis with pancuronium (0.1 mg/kg per dose).

Gastroschisis (or exomphalos)

A major gastroschisis is obvious at delivery. The exposed bowel provides surface area for heat and fluid loss. This can be prevented by covering the bowel with sterile Gamgee or swabs soaked in warmed saline, and covering the swabs with polythene cooking foil such as Saran wrap. In addition, a nasogastric tube should be passed and attached to continuous suction, as inflation of the exteriorized bowel by swallowed air makes replacement at operation much more difficult.

Tracheo-oesophageal fistula with oesophageal atresia

In the most common form of tracheo-oesophageal fistula, the diagnosis may be suspected antenatally by polyhydramnios, and confirmed at delivery by inability to pass a nasogastric tube beyond 10 cm in a term infant. In general, this lesion is readily operable but there is a risk of inhalation of saliva from the upper gastrointestinal tract and of reflux of gastric contents via the lower end of the oesophagus through the fistula and into the respiratory tract. Adequate suctioning of the pharynx is important to prevent aspiration of saliva and the baby should be kept in a head-up position lying semiprone on the right side to encourage the downward passage of gastric contents.

References

LIEBMAN, J., LUCAS, R., MOSS, A., COTTON, E., ROSENTHAL, A. and RUTTENBERGER, H. (1976) Airline travel for children with chronic pulmonary disease. *Pediatrics,* **57,** 408–410

Further reading

BLAKE, A. M., McINTOSH, N., REYNOLDS, E. O. and ST. ANDREW, D. (1975) Transport of newborn infants for intensive care. *British Medical Journal,* **iv,** 13–17

CHANCE, G. W., O'BRIEN, M. J. and SWYER, P. R. (1973) Transportation of sick neonates, 1972; an unsatisfactory aspect of medical care. *Canadian Medical Association Journal,* **109,** 847–851

CHANCE, G. W., MATTHEW, J. D., GASH, J., WILLIAMS, G. and CUNNINGHAM, K. (1978) Neonatal transport: a controlled study of skilled assistance. *Journal of Pediatrics,* **93,** 662–666

GREENE, W. T. (1980) Organization of neonatal transport services in support of a regional referral centre. *Clinics in Perinatology,* **7,** 187–195

Chapter 74

Care of the infant of very low birth weight (under 1.5 kg)

M. F. Whitfield

Low birth weight is a major cause of neonatal death. With increasing understanding of neonatal physiology and the development of techniques to support such infants, the mortality and morbidity rates for small infants have greatly improved. With a high standard of care, the majority grow into normal children and adults.

An infant may be of low birth weight because he is:

1. Born early ('preterm'): probably less than 32 weeks gestation.
2. Poorly grown for the number of weeks spent *in utero* due to:
   (a) Placental insufficiency.
   (b) Lack of growth potential due to some intrinsic growth defect in the infant such as major multiple congenital anomalies or intrauterine infection.
3. Both born early *and* undernourished *in utero*.

An infant anticipated antenatally to be of very low birth weight should be born in the maternity unit serving the Regional Neonatal Intensive Care Unit. However, it is not always possible to transfer the mother to the Regional Neonatal Intensive Care Unit Hospital (*see* page 631) and preparations have to be made for delivery, resuscitation, and stabilization in the local maternity unit. A very small infant born in a maternity unit with less than appropriate neonatal intensive care facility should be transferred to a larger, better equipped and better staffed unit.

Recognition

Size

The infant's small size is obvious but this must be accurately documented by measurements of weight, length, and head circumference soon after birth, preferably before the infant becomes attached to monitoring equipment and intravenous lines and so becomes difficult to weigh accurately. Allowance should be made for the weight of the metal cord clamp in assessing the true weight as the birth weight is an important predictor of the infant's survival.

Gestational age

This may be assessed by a combination of:

1. Obstetric dates.
2. Corroboration of obstetric dates by clinical examination and ultrasound measurement of biparietal diameter early in pregnancy.

3. Clinical examination of the infant and the determination of gestational age by a systematic scoring system for assessing neurological and physical characteristics, such as the Dubowitz scheme.

Growth in relation to gestational age

By plotting the growth against the best estimate of gestational age on a suitable intrauterine growth chart (e.g. Gairdner and Pearson, 1971), the infant's appropriateness of growth may be assessed against his gestational age. A small for gestational age infant (SGA) has a weight below the 10th percentile for gestational age, and such an infant may be of term gestation (between 37 and 41 completed weeks), post-term (beyond 41 weeks' gestation) or preterm (of less than 37 completed weeks). Although the SGA infant is more mature for his weight than a normally grown infant of the same weight, the small infant is less liable to develop severe respiratory distress syndrome but is more likely to be severely asphyxiated at delivery, with meconium aspiration, to require resuscitation, and to develop hypoglycaemia. SGA infants show behavioural anomalies for several months after delivery and are at increased risk for residual neurological damage such as hyperkinesis, 'minimal brain damage syndrome' and educational problems. The avoidance of asphyxia and hypoglycaemia and prompt resuscitation at delivery are likely to reduce the incidence of neurological sequelae.

Management

Optimal life support of the low birth weight infant depends upon four separate factors.

1. Prevention of asphyxia and prompt resuscitation at delivery.
2. Respiratory support and blood gas management.
3. Temperature homeostasis.
4. Nutrition and fluid balance.

Avoidance of asphyxia and prompt resuscitation after delivery (*see* page 611)

The delivery of a preterm or SGA infant requires special attention to the avoidance of asphyxia by selecting the optimal time and route of delivery and by fetal monitoring techniques such as cardiotochography and fetal scalp sampling when indicated. At delivery, a small infant requires appropriate resuscitation equipment, and a low threshold for intervention.

Respiratory support

An infant of 1.5 kg or less may develop some degree of ventilatory failure in the first 24 hours of life. The most likely causes are:

1. Neonatal pulmonary oedema ('wet lung'), transient tachypnoea of the newborn.
2. Surfactant-deficient hyaline membrane disease (Idiopathic Respiratory Distress Syndrome, RDS).
3. Pulmonary and systemic infection (most likely due to group B streptococcal infection).

To assess the adequacy of the infant's respiratory status, it is necessary to carry out repeated blood gas estimations on arterial or free-flowing capillary blood if harmful degrees of hypoxia or hyperoxia, or hypercapnia are to be avoided. An umbilical arterial catheter or an indwelling radial arterial catheter provides ready access to arterial sampling with minimal disturbance of the infant.

The aim is to maintain the infant's arterial PO_2 between 6.7 and 11.0 kPa (50–85 mm Hg) and a blood pH over 7.20, by the administration of oxygen, ventilatory assistance as CPAP or IPPV and the giving of bicarbonate. Avoidance of hypoxia, hypoglycaemia, acidaemia and hypothermia favour optimal surfactant synthesis and avoidance of the downward hypoxia-acidaemia spiral.

Temperature homeostasis

The small immature infant loses heat very rapidly due to large surface area:mass ratio and inadequate thermogenesis.

A small infant in an incubator with a radiant heat shield requires an air temperature of 36°C (97°F) to maintain a core temperature between 36.5°C (98°F) and 37°C (98.6°F). Infants of less than 1 kg birth weight often require incubator temperatures of 37°C (98.6°F) or more because of very low endogenous heat production and large transcutaneous water losses. In such infants, maintenance of a high humidity level inside the incubator reduces further heat loss. A skin temperature more than 0.5°C (1°F) below core temperature suggests that an infant is at the lower end of the thermoneutral zone and is having to catabolize metabolic fuel to maintain his body temperature. A drop in core temperature below 36°C (97°F) for more than a few hours is associated with progressive acidaemia and hypoglycaemia and poorer survival. While infra-red overhead heater intensive care tables provide ready access to the infant for procedures and maintain the temperature well, they are unsuitable for the care of the very small infant for more than a few hours as they double insensible water loss (to over 100 ml/kg daily) particularly in the very small infant with gelatinous skin (usually less than 27 weeks' gestation). At the present time, a double-walled incubator with a proportional servo-control heater pack usable to servo-control air temperature or infant's temperature, providing at least 70 per cent humidity, is the most suitable equipment.

Nutrition and fluid balance

An adequate nutritional intake is most important. The absence of co-ordinated sucking and swallowing make the enteral feeding of small infants hazardous, since gastric emptying may be delayed and intestinal motility reduced. Gastrointestinal absorption of food, particularly as fat, is unreliable during the early weeks of life. Electrolyte and blood gas disturbances, serious respiratory problems, and possibly the presence of an umbilical arterial catheter delay the appearance of peristalsis. Events in the perinatal and neonatal course of the infant may predispose it to necrotizing enterocolitis. For these reasons, fluid and calorie requirements may have to be given totally by the parenteral route. A low birth weight infant needs around 65 ml/kg fluid in the first 24 hours but this requirement may be more than doubled by the effects of phototherapy, tachypnoea, pyrexia, inadequately humidified respiratory gases, and transcutaneous water loss. A urine osmolality of 200 mosmol/kg or less indicates adequate hydration. Glucose 10% via peripheral vein or umbilical catheter usually provides the bulk of the infant's food requirements over the first 48 hours, although small volumes (1–2 ml/hr increasing) of expressed human milk or formula may be tolerated by intermittent or continuous nasogastric infusion, with 3 hourly aspiration of the stomach to prevent accumulation of gastric contents and the risk of feed aspiration. Glucose 10% orally delays gastric emptying and is tolerated less well than human milk, if aspirated into the lungs.

Glucose (10%, 65 ml/kg daily) provides between one-third and one-half of the infant's calorie requirements and if the infant cannot tolerate adequate amounts of milk by the enteral route by 72 hours of age, consideration should be given to total or supplementary parenteral nutrition with carbohydrate, aminoacids, and fat emulsions. In the first weeks of life inadequate nutrition delays the resumption of growth, while overenthusiastic feeding may result in pulmonary milk aspiration, abdominal distension, and apnoeic attacks, and may increase the incidence of necrotizing enterocolitis. In infants recovering from respiratory problems in the newborn period, a bolus size of more than 5 ml/kg delivered into the stomach may affect pulmonary mechanics and the respiratory status of the baby. Some infants tolerate continuous infusion of milk into the stomach, duodenum or jejunum when they will not tolerate bolus feeding into the stomach.

The appearance of abdominal distension, blood in the stools, disappearance of bowel sounds, and bilious gastric aspirates suggest the onset of necrotizing enterocolitis (*see* page 367), and enteral feeds should be stopped for several days and the infant supported by parenteral nutrition (*see* Appendix 6).

Timetable for management of the low birth weight infant

Aim to maintain the infant in the best possible respiratory, blood gas, thermal, metabolic and nutritional status at all times.

Before birth

Preparation; liaison with obstetric staff; consideration of the possibility of fetal therapy and the timing and route of delivery.

Medical staff

Close liaison with the obstetric staff is necessary in order to be aware of antenatal problems, adequacy of intrauterine growth, the absence of fetal distress and the choice of route of delivery. Ultrasound information may be available about the infant's growth throughout pregnancy, and amniocentesis may have been carried out to determine the appearance of lung maturity (by lecithin:sphingomyelin ratio, or the presence of phosphatidyl glycerol).

A low lecithin:sphingomyelin ratio (< than 2:1) and a maturity of less than 34 weeks should suggest the giving of dexamethasone or betamethasone to the mother, and attempts should be made to delay delivery pharmacologically.

Signs of infection in the mother, particularly if the membranes have been ruptured for more than 48 hours, usually indicate prompt delivery. The factors involved in the delivery should be discussed with the parents, both by obstetric and paediatric staff.

Nursing staff

Assemble and check the equipment likely to be used in the stabilization of the infant after delivery:

1. Double walled servo-controlled incubator or single walled servo-controlled incubator with a Perspex semicylindrical radiant heat shield. The incubator must be prewarmed and set at maximum humidity.
2. Cardiorespiratory monitoring equipment.
3. Oxygen analyser to measure inspired oxygen concentration.
4. Check oxygen cylinders, if no piped oxygen.
5. Tray for umbilical catheterization.
6. Resuscitation equipment and laryngoscope (check light).
7. Neonatal ventilator checked and ready for use.
8. Head box oxygen hood.
9. Adequate lighting.
10. Baby scales.

Birth to 2 hours

Birth; resuscitation; transfer to SCBU/NICU.

Medical staff

Adequate prompt resuscitation with low threshold for intervention; baby may need glucose (3 ml 10%) and sodium bicarbonate (2 mmol/ℓ) via umbilical vein if there has been documented fetal acidosis.

Dry infant all over with a towel early in resuscitation to prevent heat loss. Resuscitation must be done under a radiant overhead heater.

When the infant is breathing spontaneously, he should be transferred as soon as possible to NICU/SCBU having first been shown to the mother. A mother may hold even a small infant at this stage, providing the infant is adequately wrapped and constantly observed by the resuscitation staff.

Nursing staff

The infant requires the full attention of an experienced neonatal nurse. The baby should be weighed at the time of transfer from the resuscitation equipment to the incubator and then connected to cardiorespiratory monitoring equipment:

1. Give 30% oxygen if cyanosed.
2. Monitor heart rate, respiratory rate, colour and temperature, and the development of signs of respiratory distress (nostril flaring, grunting, chest recession, tachypnoea and tachycardia).
3. An intravenous infusion of glucose (10% 65 ml/kg daily) should be started, to prevent hypoglycaemia.
4. The infant, when settled, must be handled as little as possible and be in a good light so that any change in colour can be readily appreciated.
5. Suck out the mouth if mucousy.
6. Call the doctor if the infant's condition is deteriorating or if cyanosed in FiO_2 of 0.30–0.35 (30–35%) before 1–1.5 hours of age.

Medical staff

Reassess after 1–1.5 hours. Is the baby getting better or worse on the basis of:

1. Colour.
2. Oxygen requirement.
3. Development of signs of respiratory distress.
4. Air entry on auscultation.
5. Stability of observations?

A transcutaneous oxygen monitor may be of use in establishing requirements. If there are signs of respiratory distress and a requirement of more than FiO_2 of 0.30 (30%), the baby needs:

1. An arterial line for blood gas sampling. This may be either an umbilical arterial catheter (open-ended PVC 3.5 FG with radio-opaque tracer) or a radial or posterior tibial arterial line inserted with the aid of transillumination to locate the artery.
2. Chest X-ray including most of the abdomen:
   (a) To define the cause of the respiratory difficulty and the radiological degree of hyaline membrane disease.
   (b) To define the position of the arterial catheter. The tip may be located just above the aortic bifurcation at around L3/4 or above the diaphragm in the thorax.
3. Blood gases from the arterial line.
4. Glucose 10% intravenously via the umbilical catheter (60 ml/kg daily).
5. A nasogastric tube may be passed into the stomach to aspirate stomach content; this may be left *in situ*, provided the nasal airway is not obstructed.

2–12 hours: developing respiratory failure, fluid and calorie provision

If the infant is developing respiratory difficulty, blood gases and blood glucose or Dextrostix should be monitored 4 hourly and action taken, if necessary, to maintain the blood gas status by ventilatory assistance (CPAP or IPPV) and half correction of metabolic acidosis with intravenous bicarbonate (1/6 × base deficit × body weight equals number of mmol required for half correction of the metabolic component of the acidosis). The blood glucose should be maintained above 1.7 mmol/ℓ (>30 mg/100 ml). An approximate account of urine output can be kept by the weight increase of preweighed disposable napkins, or urine may be collected directly in males. The urine output is usually low in the first 12 hours in newborn infants and particularly in infants with respiratory difficulties (less than 2 ml/kg/hour). It is best not to feed an infant with respiratory difficulties enterally in the first 12–24 hours of life as hyaline membrane disease tends to worsen during this time, and pulmonary aspiration of feed must be avoided.

Because of the difficulty in excluding the possibility of group B streptococcal pneumonia and septicaemia as a component of the infant's respiratory difficulty, some units give prophylactic ampicillin (100 mg/kg daily) in infants with respiratory distress after blood culture, gastric aspirate, and differential white count have been taken. Ampicillin may be stopped if the culture report is negative.

An infant who has respiratory problems in the first 2–3 hours of life and is requiring an increasing FiO_2 is likely to go on to require respiratory assistance, and if these facilities are not available in the hospital where the infant is being managed, contact with the Regional Intensive Care Unit should be made at once.

If the infant does not have respiratory difficulty and does not require umbilical catheterization, feeds may be started cautiously by the nasogastric route, either as a continuous nasogastric infusion of 1–2 ml/hour with 3-hourly nasogastric aspiration or as intermittent bolus feeds at 1 or 2-hourly intervals of a similar volume of milk. Infants of 34 weeks' gestation or more who are appropriately grown can usually tolerate enteral feeding and may manage without the insertion of an intravenous infusion. Infants below this gestational age are better managed with a glucose infusion to maintain the blood glucose and to reduce the chance of excessively rapid enteral feed administration.

12–48 hours – stabilization; fluid, calorie and electrolyte balance; possibility of apnoeic attacks

Medical staff

Check on and assess the following.

1. FLUID INTAKE AND URINE OUTPUT

The baby's fluid intake can be expected to be around 90 ml/kg/24 hours by 48 hours of life. If the infant did not require an umbilical arterial catheter, supplementary parenteral fluids must be provided by peripheral vein infusion unless the nasogastric intake is adequate. An infant who is totally maintained on intravenous fluids should receive sodium chloride 2.5 mmol/kg/24 hours, potassium chloride 2 mmol/kg/24 hours and calcium gluconate 2 mmol/kg/24 hours in addition to fluid and glucose.

2. TEMPERATURE HOMEOSTASIS

3. VENTILATORY STATUS

Oxygen requirement and adequacy of respiratory support must be assessed. Infants with mild hyaline membrane disease are usually recovering by this stage as shown by reducing oxygen requirement and a reduction in respiratory difficulty. In infants requiring IPPV, pneumothorax is more likely to occur at this stage when lung compliance is improving; sudden collapse of the infant may be due to this cause. Infants of less than 34 weeks are likely to develop apnoeic and bradycardic episodes at this stage, these episodes usually responding to stimulation; but some infants may eventually require ventilatory assistance with low pressure CPAP (3 cm H_2O) or IPPV. Ventilatory assistance may be avoided in some infants by the use of intravenous aminophylline (loading dose 7 mg/kg IV over 20 minutes followed by 1.4 mg/kg 8-hourly intravenous maintenance; blood level should be maintained at 8–11 μg/ml).

4. NEUROLOGICAL STATE OF THE INFANT

5. CAN THE ARTERIAL CATHETER BE REMOVED?

6. CHEST X-RAY TO ASSESS PROGRESS OF PULMONARY DISEASE AND METHOD OF NUTRITION

Feeding can usually be started cautiously by the nasogastric route by about 48 hours of life in infants who are recovering from respiratory distress. Small frequency feeds or continuous feeding are most likely to succeed. A bolus size in excess of 5 ml/kg per feed has been shown to affect adversely the respiratory status of infants recovering from respiratory distress.

Nursing staff

The infant with developing apnoeic attacks requires careful observation and vigilance and is a worrying prospect in an understaffed nursery. Although most apnoeic attacks respond to stimulation, facilities for IPPV by mask (e.g. using a Laerdal infant resuscitator) must be available in the incubator. Infants who have required respiratory assistance and intubation during the first 48 hours of life become progressively more of a problem if the endotracheal tube cannot be removed early, due to increasing volume and viscosity of secretions.

Survival rates in excess of 80 per cent should be expected in the Tertiary Intensive Care Nursery environment for infants of between 750 and 1000 g at birth. A significant number of infants may also be expected to survive below this birth weight in optimal circumstances. The management of these infants is a very specialized problem, and if avoidable mortality and morbidity are to be prevented they must be transferred, preferably *in utero*, for tertiary care. Such infants present challenging problems in fluid and electrolyte balance and nutrition, are likely to develop bronchopulmonary dysplasia and have a high risk of significant intraventricular haemorrhage.

Reference

GAIRDNER, D. and PEARSON, J. (1971) A growth chart for premature and other infants. *Archives of Disease in Childhood,* **46,** 783–787

Further reading

AULD, P. A. M. (1980) Symposium on neonatal intensive care. *Clinics in Perinatology,* **7,** 1–221

DWECK, H. S. (1977) Symposium on the tiny baby. *Clinics in Perinatology,* **4,** 213–429

VOHR, B. R. and HACK, M. (1982) Developmental follow up of low birth weight infants. *Pediatric Clinics of North America,* **29,** 1441–1454

Chapter 75

Hypothermia

M. F. Whitfield and J. A. Black

Transient hypothermia after delivery

Even term infants can become hypothermic at delivery owing to transient factors operating at that time. The following precautions should be taken to minimize the risk in the delivery room (*see also* page 614):

1. An infant requiring resuscitation should be resuscitated under a radiant overhead heater, and drafts minimized as much as possible. If no radiant overhead heater is available, the room temperature should be above 26°C (79°F).
2. The baby should be placed in a warm, dry towel.
3. During the immediate resuscitation period the infant should be dried as soon as possible.
4. Prompt resuscitation of asphyxiated infants will stabilize the body temperature.
5. In the hours after delivery the baby should be kept well wrapped up and should not be subjected to repeated examinations and should not be bathed within the first 6 hours.

Infants most at risk of significant perinatal hypothermia are:

1. Infants of low or very low birth weight, because of the unfavourable mass to surface area ratio.
2. Infants who are asphyxiated or shocked.
3. Infants affected by maternally administered opiates given for therapeutic reasons.

Recognition

In mild hypothermia, the extremities are cold and there is peripheral cyanosis but the face and trunk are warm and pink. The rectal temperature is below 36°C (97°F).

Management

The infant should be warmed in an incubator set up between 34°C (93°F) and 37°C (98.6°F) depending on the size of the infant, and the rectal temperature should be monitored as it returns to 37°C (98.6°F). Failure of the temperature to rise above 36.5°C (98°F) in 2 hours, suggests that other factors may be involved and the infant should be investigated and managed as for secondary hypothermia (*see* below).

Secondary hypothermia

An infant who has previously been able to maintain temperature adequately, and then becomes hypothermic may have an underlying cause such as:

1. Severe systemic illness usually with acidosis:
   (a) Septicaemia is the most likely.
   (b) Severe heart failure.
   (c) Respiratory problems complicated by hypoxia.
2. Growth and maturity:
   A large but preterm infant (34–37 weeks) if cot nursed in the first few days of life may be unable to maintain temperature; a term but small for gestational age (e.g. 40 weeks but only 2.3 kg at birth) similarly may not be able to maintain temperature and also is likely to be hypoglycaemia (*see* below).
3. Post-exchange transfusion:
   In all cases of hypothermia, hypoglycaemia should be suspected. Hypoglycaemia may be the cause of hypothermia and hypothermic infants frequently become hypoglycaemic. Infants with severe systemic illness, however, may also become hyperglycaemic.

Severe acute hypothermia

Sustained exposure to low temperature for several hours, as may happen in a home delivery, delivery in transit, delivery into the lavatory, or with unrecognized malfunction of an incubator may cause severe acute hypothermia.

Recognition

The infant is lethargic with reduced heart rate and respiratory rate. The trunk and extremities are cold and have a blotchy marbled white and blue appearance. The core temperature is usually less than 29°C (84°F).

Management

Exposure to cold for not more than 6 hours is unlikely to cause cold injury and therefore rapid rewarming should be safe. The infant should be placed in an incubator between 34°C and 36°C (93–97°F) depending on the infant's weight. Blood glucose and blood gases should be monitored during the recovery phase.

Cold injury

This is the most serious form of hypothermia. It is usually confined to the first month of life, although older children, especially those in poor social circumstances, may also be affected. Cold injury results from slow cooling over a long period.

Recognition

A history of adverse socioeconomic conditions should be sought; inadequate heating at night is frequently a contributory factor during cold spells. Infection and undernutrition are important predisposing causes. The infant has a misleadingly healthy appearance with pink extremities and nose but there is little spontaneous movement and the face is expressionless. The diagnosis is obvious as soon as the frog-like coldness of the trunk and limbs is felt. Both heart and respiration rate are slow and the metabolic rate is low.

Management

1. Slow warming is probably safer than rapid warming. The environmental temperature should be maintained at 1°C (2°F) above the rectal temperature and this should be raised by 1°C (2°F) every 4 hours.
2. During re-warming, the blood gases and plasma glucose should be monitored and an infusion of 10% glucose given at a rate which does not cause hyperglycaemia.
3. It should be assumed that the infant is infected and a septic work-up carried out and antibiotics started. Caution should be exercised in using aminoglycosides because of depressed renal function.

Chapter 76

Sudden collapse in the newborn

M. F. Whitfield and J. A. Black

General considerations

1. If there is no evidence of a respiratory or abdominal emergency an acute infection should be considered, and a complete infection screen should be done (blood culture, lumbar puncture, surface swabs from throat, umbilicus and rectum and any superficial septic lesions, suprapubic urine aspiration, chest X-ray, and white cell count and differential).
2. In infants with either respiratory or abdominal emergencies (or both) an X-ray of both chest and abdomen should be done since it is not always possible to distinguish whether the problem is above or below the diaphragm.
3. The most common biochemical cause of acute collapse is hypoglycaemia.
4. In small ventilated infants, sudden deterioration shown by bradycardia, cyanosis and circulatory deterioration is most likely to be due to:
   (a) Inadequate ventilation due to disconnection or kinking of ventilation tubing, blockage of the endotracheal tube by secretions, or ventilator malfunction.
   (b) Increased ventilation requirements, pulmonary interstitial emphysema, atelectasis, pneumonia, major ductal shunting due to patent ductus arteriosus.
   (c) Air leak, pneumothorax, pneumomediastinum, pneumopericardium, pneumoperitoneum; in infants under 2 kg transillumination with a fibreoptic light provides accurate, rapid diagnosis and treatment without waiting for an X-ray.
   (d) Other acute complications of prematurity; necrotizing enterocolitis, massive intracranial haemorrhage, septicaemia.

Table 76.1 Causes of sudden collapse in the newborn

	Possible clues	*Diagnostic investigation*
Abdominal conditions		
Rupture of the liver (*see* page 674)	Large infant, 36–72 hours after difficult delivery; shock. Rhesus isoimmunization	Ultrasound and X-ray of abdomen. Aspiration of peritoneal cavity
Rupture of spleen (*see* page 674)	Rhesus isoimmunization and shock	As above
Rupture of umbilical vein	Clue: exchange transfusion	As above
Adrenal haemorrhage (*see* page 674)	Lumbar masses	Abdominal ultrasound
Necrotizing enterocolitis (*see* page 367)	Pre-term, small for gestational age, or term and asphyxiated; abdominal distension, blood in the stools, bilious vomiting	Erect and supine abdomen X-ray
Gastric perforation	Sudden collapse and distension, usually with nasogastric tube in place 1st–5th day of life	Erect X-ray of abdomen
Acute intestinal bleeding (*see* page 371)	End of the 1st week; shock	Blood in stool
Intrathoracic conditions		
Tension pneumothorax (*see* page 245)	Meconium aspiration, respiratory distress syndrome, pulmonary hypoplasia, IPPV	Transillumination with fibreoptic intense light source, chest X-ray, needle aspiration of the chest
Pneumomediastinum Pneumopericardium (*see* page 245)	Usually preceding pulmonary interstitial emphysema and associated with pneumothorax	Transillumination, X-ray of chest
Oesophageal perforation	Pre-term infants; spontaneous or related to tube feeding	Chest X-ray may show pneumothorax or displaced nasogastric tube
Massive pulmonary haemorrhage (*see* pages 215 and 251) Haemorrhagic pulmonary oedema	Pre-term or asphyxiated; dyspnoea with copious frothy blood-stained secretions in the pharynx and larynx	X-ray of chest
Acute pneumonia (*see* page 247)	Deterioration on IPPV	X-ray of chest
Acut atelactasis	Sudden deterioration on IPPV	X-ray of chest
Cardiovascular conditions		
Arrhythmia (*see* page 269)	Exchange transfusion; Electrolyte disturbances; Fetal Hydrops	ECG
Air embolus (*see* page 694)	Exchange transfusion; pulmonary interstitial emphysema, necrotizing enterocolitis	Chest and abdominal X-ray
Cardiac failure (*see* page 259)	Murmur, cyanosis, hepatomegaly, especially hypoplastic left heart syndrome with shock in first week	X-ray chest, ECG
Neurological conditions		
Intraventricular haemorrhage (*see* page 626)	Prematurity, respiratory distress syndrome, pneumothorax	Sudden drop in hematocrit, cranial ultrasound
Biochemical conditions		
Hypoglycaemia (*see* page 459)	Infant or diabetic mother; Small for gestational age infant Pale, lethargic, with or without fits	Dextrostix or blood glucose

Chapter 77

Acute infections

M. F. Whitfield and J. A. Black

The infant may become infected *in utero*, during birth, or after delivery. Only the emergency aspects of fetal and neonatal infection are considered here.

Infections during pregnancy ('congenital infections', transplacental infections)

These infections are acquired across the placenta, secondary to maternal infection and include cytomegalovirus (CMV), rubella, toxoplasmosis, syphilis, enterovirus infections, South American trypanosomiasis (Chagas' disease), malaria, tuberculosis, varicella (chickenpox) and acquired immune deficiency syndrome (AIDS).

Recognition

1. There may be a history of an infectious illness during the pregnancy.
2. Clinical signs are not clearly specific for the infecting organism; hepatosplenomegaly, thrombocytopenia and neurological symptoms are the most frequent findings. Relatively specific signs are given in *Table 77.1.* CMV, rubella, toxoplasmosis and South American trypanosomiasis may present a clinical appearance similar to Rhesus isoimmunization, with hepatosplenomegaly, purpura, thrombocytopenia, jaundice, and anaemia with or without hydrops.
3. Some infants are markedly growth retarded for gestational age having symmetrical stunting affecting weight, length and head circumference equally. Such infants usually have other signs of congenital infection however.

Diagnostic investigations

1. Placental histology.
2. Cord blood IgM and agent-specific IgM.
3. Urine and pharyngeal secretions for virus culture, samples being sent three times (CMV and rubella).
4. Sequential maternal and neonatal serology from birth to 3 months (falling maternal titre and rising infant titre suggest infection).
5. Neonatal retinal examination by an ophthalmologist.
6. Skull and long bone X-rays for intracranial calcification and abnormalities of ossification of the long bones.

7. Specific disease investigation:
   (a) Toxoplasmosis: serial determination of IgG, isolation of *T. gondii* from placenta, CSF, and blood.
   (b) Syphilis: reagin (VDRL) and fluorescent antibody tests, dark field microscopy of smears from mucocutaneous lesions.
   (c) Malaria (usually falciparum): placental histology, thick blood smears from mother and infant.
   (d) South American trypanosomiasis: blood film or thick drop preparation and other special tests (Bittencourt, 1976).
   (e) Tuberculosis: placental histology, maternal investigations; look for miliary and tuberculous meningitis in infant.
   (f) Perinatal chickenpox: history and vesicular rash, electron microscopy of vesicle fluid, serology.

Table 77.1 Some relatively agent-specific features of the commoner types of congenital and intrapartum acquired infections

Cytomegalovirus	Microcephaly with periventricular calcification. Thrombocytopenia, petechiae and hepatosplenomegaly
Toxoplasmosis	Hydrocephalus with generalized intracranial calcification. Choroidoretinitis
Rubella	'Blueberry muffin' syndrome. Vertical striations of long bones ('celery stalking'). Cataracts, retinal pigmentation. Peripheral pulmonary arterial coarctation or stenosis
Syphilis	Mucocutaneous lesions ('syphilitic snuffles'). Periostitis, osteochondritis, and bone pain
Herpes	Skin vesicles. CNS and liver symptoms
Enterovirus	CNS and liver symptoms. Myocarditis

Adapted from Stagno (1981).

Management

Specific management of these conditions is unsatisfactory as considerable damage may have been sustained by several organs, and specific cures are for the the most part not available. The following considerations are of importance, however:

1. Infectivity:
   (a) Infants with CMV and rubella excrete virus in large quantities in urine and other secretions and are an infective risk to pregnant staff.
   (b) Congenital syphilis: the infant should be isolated and handled with rubber gloves.
2. Anaemia and jaundice: this may be a major problem and should be managed as described elsewhere (*see* page 658). If exchange transfusion is required care must be taken to obtain all diagnostic samples before the exchange transfusion.
3. Thrombocytopenic DIC: may require platelet transfusions and treatment for DIC including exchange transfusion (*see* page 697).

4. Specific treatment:
   (a) Syphilis; benzylpenicillin 150 000 u/kg/24 hours (90 mg/kg/24 hours) in three divided doses i.m. or IV for 15 days.
   (b) Toxoplasmosis: treatment is unsatisfactory; pyrimethamine 2 mg/kg/24 hours for the first day then 1 mg/kg/24 hours orally in two divided doses for 30 days plus sulphadiazine 150 mg/kg/24 hours in four divided doses for 30 days plus folinic acid 1 mg/kg/24 hours orally to reduce marrow toxicity of pyrimethamine. Prednisolone should probably be added if there is chorioretinitis.
   (c) Trypanosomiasis: treatment is unsatisfactory. Nifurtimox (Lampit, Bayer; Alvarez and Cob Sosa, 1976) 25 mg/kg/24 hours for 15 days then 15 mg/kg/24 hours for a total of 3 months plus metronidazole 20 mg/kg/24 hours for 1 month.
   (d) Tuberculosis: isoniazid, with rifampicin if resistant organism.
   (e) Malaria: chloroquine i.m. for 5 days (*see* page 572 for dosage).
   (f) Chickenpox: zoster immune globulin i.m. particularly in infants who have not developed the rash at delivery because of the lack of protective maternal antibodies.
   (g) There is no proved treatment for rubella or CMV.

Infection acquired during labour

Infection may be acquired during labour as:

1. A transplacental infection resulting from maternal bacteraemia (e.g. pyelonephritis, appendicitis). Infection is usually with a Gram-negative bacillus and the fetus may develop septicaemia with or without meningitis.
2. Ascending infection following prolonged rupture of the membranes usually greater than 48 hours and usually heralded by maternal pyrexia and leucocytosis. Organisms implicated are most likely to be:
   (a) Streptococci: group B streptococcus, *Streptococcus pneumoniae.*
   (b) *Listeria monocytogenes.*
   (c) Gram-negative bacilli.
   (d) *Haemophilus influenzae.*
   (e) Anaerobes (e.g. bacteroides).
   (f) Herpes simplex if there is an active lesion in the genital tract.

Recognition

The infant may appear lethargic and respond poorly at delivery, with poor perfusion, and developing respiratory problems, or may appear normal for 3–4 hours before developing signs of respiratory distress and rapid downhill course with acidaemia, hypoxaemia and persistent fetal circulation requiring heroic ventilator management. In herpes simplex infection, the course is the same as with the infection acquired during delivery (*see* page 652).

Management

1. A full infection screen should be carried out (*see* page 655) and the infant started on an antibiotic regimen to cover the above organisms (e.g. ampicillin and gentamicin IV). A vaginal swab should be taken from the mother in addition.
2. Full supportive management may be required to counter major metabolic and acid base disturbance.

Infections acquired during delivery

Not all such infections cause acute illness but the following require special attention.

Gonococcal conjunctivitis (gonococcal ophthalmia) (see also Chapter 12, page 150)

Recognition

This should be suspected with any severe purulent conjunctivitis developing within the first week (usually within 48 hours of delivery). A Gram film of the pus should be examined for Gram-negative intracellular diplococci and the pus cultured on appropriate media, *usually plated out at the bedside.* Gonococci will not tolerate a prolonged journey on a dry swab to the bacteriology laboratory using the hospital messenger systems.

Management

1. Systemic benzylpenicillin 200 000 units (120 mg), 4 hourly i.m. or IV accompanied by local hygiene to the eyes and irrigation with penicillin eye drops 20 000 units/ml (12 mg/ml).
2. Failure to improve within 24–48 hours suggests the possibility of a resistant organism, in which case use of erythromycin or spectinomycin should be considered.
3. The mother, her consorts, and any other sexual contact should be traced, investigated, and treated and blood sent from mother and infant for VDRL.

Chlamydial conjunctivitis ('Inclusion Body Conjunctivitis')

Infection is by the same route as for gonococcal ophthalmia but chlamydia produces a persistent low-grade conjunctivitis which may cause conjunctival scarring but is of particular importance as there is a significant incidence of chlamydial pneumonitis during the first 6 months of life in infants infected with chlamydia at birth.

Recognition

Low-grade conjunctivitis developing between 5 and 10 days of age. Special culture techniques are required to isolate and identify the organism.

Management

Erythromycin eyedrops and systemic erythromycin for 2 weeks.

Herpesvirus hominis

This is a potentially fatal infection acquired from active maternal genital herpes lesions. If an active lesion is recognized before delivery, the infant should be delivered by caesarean section if the membranes have not been ruptured.

Recognition

A disseminated form develops about 5–10 days after delivery. There may or may not have been an obvious active lesion in the maternal birth canal, and the baby may or may not have one or more vesicular lesions. Occasionally the disease remains localized as a skin eruption but usually the illness takes the form of a fulminating infection with respiratory, cerebral and hepatic manifestations. The virus can be identified on electron microscopy of vesicle fluid and can be cultured. There is usually CSF pleocytosis (up to 200 cells/mm^3) and high CSF protein level (5–10 g/ℓ).

Management

1. Isolation to protect other infants.
2. General supportive measures including respiratory support, control of seizures, and management of liver failure if this develops (*see* Chapter 47).
3. At the present time there is no proved specific treatment. Vidarabine (30 mg/kg/24 hours IV) has been used with variable results; acyclovir (10 mg/kg daily IV) appears promising but has not yet been adequately evaluated. The prognosis in severe systemic infection with herpesvirus hominis is very poor.

Enterovirus infection

Enterovirus infection may be acquired transplacentally following acute infection in the mother just before delivery but presents a somewhat similar clinical pattern to herpesvirus hominis infection and therefore is considered here. The organisms most likely to be implicated are Coxsackie B, or Echovirus of different types (Speer and Yawn, 1984).

Recognition

The mother may develop a rash around the time of delivery accompanied by influenza-like symptoms. At 5–7 days the infant develops:

1. Signs of severe systemic infection with fever, poor feeding, diarrhoea, jaundice and rash. This illness is usually self-limiting but sometimes liver failure develops due to massive hepatic necrosis sometimes with adrenal necrosis, also associated with a poor prognosis; DIC may complicate the picture. The initial symptoms may suggest an abdominal emergency (Speer and Yawn, 1984).
2. Heart failure due to myocarditis and seizures are accompanied by signs of severe systemic infection; also associated with a high mortality rate.

Management

1. There is no specific treatment.
2. Isolation of the infant to protect other infants, and the careful observation for signs of infection.
3. General supportive measures.

Listeria monocytogenes

This infection may present as:

1. A transplacentally acquired septicaemic illness with hepatosplenomegaly, respiratory features and in a few cases, small reddish-grey skin papules.
2. An infection acquired during delivery with respiratory features and septicaemia within the first week. Meningitis is common.

Management

See listeria meningitis (*see* page 338).

Hepatitis B

Acute hepatitis due to hepatitis B virus (HBV) may occur during pregnancy with a high transmission rate to the infant, particularly if the disease occurs during the third trimester; or the mother may be a carrier of the virus and the infant may come into contact with infected secretions or maternal blood during delivery. Acquisition of the virus by the infant is detected as Hepatitis B surface antigen (HBsAg) in the infant.

The transmission rate from asymptomatic carriers to their infants is particularly high in mothers of Oriental origin and in individuals with the e antigen and no anti e antibodies. Infected infants become HBsAg positive between 2 and 5 months of age, this period presumably reflecting infection at delivery followed by the incubation period, and may develop jaundice and hepatosplenomegaly and chronic hepatitis.

Recognition (in neonatal period)

Mother has HBsAg; usually detected on screening of high-risk groups (*see* above).

Management

1. The infant should receive hepatitis B hyperimmune globulin 0.5 ml (200 i.u., 200 mg) i.m. at birth or in any case within 48 hours of delivery, in an attempt to reduce the risk of infection from contact with the virus at delivery. If available, HBV vaccine (0.5 ml, 10 μg) should be given i.m. at the same time as the immunoglobulin, and second and third doses should be given 1 and 6 months after the first one.
2. There is doubt about the advisability of breast feeding but insufficient evidence is available to contraindicate it.
3. Hepatitis serology should be repeated at 6 months to establish whether or not the infant has been infected or is a carrier.
4. The infant is probably not infectious in the neonatal period but it is advisable to take hepatitis precautions with blood samples.

Acute postnatal infections

Newborn infants, particularly prematures, are more susceptible to generalized infections than older children and may be considered relatively immunocompromised. Local infections become disseminated very quickly, although metastatic lesions may develop during a period of bacteraemia (e.g. osteomyelitis). Occasionally also, term infants appear to develop a localized pyelonephritis.

Acute septicaemia

Recognition

Symptoms requiring immediate investigation include:

1. A sudden change in behaviour or appearance, such as grey pallor, lethargy, deterioration in feeding. These are more likely to be noticed by the mother or nurse.
2. A rise or fall in temperature.
3. Apnoeic attacks, tachypnoea, dyspnoea or cyanosis.
4. Abdominal distension.
5. Exacerbation of jaundice with or without hepatosplenomegaly.
6. Sudden diarrhoea or vomiting.
7. Sudden shock.
8. Bleeding or oozing from puncture sites (possibility of DIC).

It should be remembered, however, that similar symptoms including jaundice may also be due to various inborn errors of metabolism (*see* Chapter 91).

Investigation

Full infection screen. A standard plan of investigation should be used in all cases and should be completed even after one of the investigations is found to be abnormal:

1. Blood culture: taken with full aseptic precautions from a vein or artery, not from a catheter.
2. Lumbar puncture with examination of the fluid for glucose, protein, cell count and Gram film. Counter-immunoelectrophoresis or coagglutination tests may be available for specific organisms.
3. Urine: because of the difficulty in obtaining a clean specimen, suprapubic bladder tap should be carried out, any growth indicating infection.
4. Chest X-ray.
5. Surface swabs: throat, umbilicus, and rectum are most fruitful sites to swab in addition to any clearly infected lesions.

Management of infections in general

1. Shock: this usually occurs in any septicaemic illness and is best treated with colloids such as fresh frozen plasma, albumin, or whole blood (20 ml/kg; the first 10 ml/kg given over 30 min), with monitoring of blood pressure.

2. Antibiotics: the initial antibiotic choice depends on the policy in the nursery. The combination should cover Gram-positive organisms including streptococci and staphylococci, haemophilus influenzae, and Gram-negative bacilli. The choice depends on the local bacterial flora, but penicillin or ampicillin combined with gentamicin usually provide adequate cover. Cloxacillin should be added if there is a chance of deep-seated staphylococcal infection with a penicillinase producer. In meningitis, the initial choice could bc chloramphenicol and gentamicin, or ampicillin, gentamicin and cefotaxime, one of the third-generation cephalosporins which penetrates CSF well. Antibiotic choice will be modified following culture results and sensitivity.
3. Ventilatory support where blood gases are abnormal.
4. Careful fluid and electrolyte balance and maintenance of the haemoglobin.
5. Where these measures appear to be unsuccessful, exchange transfusion, transfusion with fresh frozen plasma, or granulocyte transfusions should be considered.

Any baby with a positive blood culture must have a lumbar puncture to exclude meningitis.

Infections requiring special attention

1. Meningitis (*see* page 334).
2. Pneumonia (*see* page 247).
3. Skin infections (*see* page 506).

Group B β-haemolytic streptococcal infections

This may present as:

1. A fulminating septicaemic illness with pneumonia and respiratory symptoms in the first 12 hours of life (*see* page 651), the organism having been acquired from the birth canal.
2. Isolated meningitis between 1 and 12 weeks of age. Infants with Group B streptococcal infection may also develop arthritis, osteitis and empyema. Many infants, however, are merely colonized with Group B streptococci at delivery and suffer no ill effects. It appears that these infants are protected by transferred maternal antibodies.

Management

1. Prophylaxis: Group B streptococcal disease occurs so soon after delivery, can be so devastating, and is so difficult to differentiate from other more benign forms of respiratory distress that some have advocated the use of prophylactic ampicillin 100 mg/kg/24 hours IV in any infant with respiratory symptoms, after an initial blood culture, gastric aspirate, and white count have been sent. This appears to prevent the development of fulminating streptococcal disease in most infants at risk. The ampicillin can then be stopped if the cultures are negative after 48 hours.

2. Infants strongly suspected or who have been proved to have streptococcal septicaemia should be treated with ampicillin 200 mg/kg daily and an aminoglycoside intravenously for 10 days to 3 weeks.
3. Supportive treatment is important in preventing or treating shock.
4. The infant is likely to develop persistent fetal circulation and to require energetic ventilator treatment.

Osteitis (osteomyelitis)

Osteitis in the newborn differs from osteitis in other age groups in four ways:

1. Infection of the upper metaphysis of the humerus or femur may involve the shoulder and hip joints, respectively, causing a septic arthritis.
2. More than one bone may be involved.
3. Unusual sites may be infected (e.g. the maxilla or premaxilla).
4. Numerous organisms may cause osteitis, the commonest being the staphylococcus; less common are Gram-negative bacilli, streptococci, pneumococci, gonococci, and meningococci.

Recognition

1. The initial symptoms may be those of a septicaemia and evidence of bone involvement may only become apparent later. When osteitis is suspected a complete X-ray skeletal survey should be done.
2. Localizing symptoms are those of swelling and loss of movement, or crying when the affected area is touched or moved.
3. Infection of the shaft of the long bones is usually obvious because of the swelling, but infection of the upper end of the humerus or femur is less obvious since swelling occurs later. It should be remembered that infection of the femoral head or hip joint may be a complication of femoral vein puncture.
4. Confirmation of the diagnosis may be provided by aspiration and culture of pus from an obvious swelling, or from blood culture. Aspiration of the shoulder or hip joint should be done by an orthopaedic surgeon.

Osteitis at special sites

Sites which are difficult to detect

1. The vertebrae: osteitis of the vertebrae is particularly difficult to detect clinically. Infection of a cervical vertebra may cause torticollis in an infant, with or without swelling due to an abscess.
2. Sacrum or sacroiliac joint: infection may only become obvious at a very late stage unless it is detected in a skeletal survey.

Osteitis of the maxilla

This infection is rarely seen outside the neonatal period. It may present with swelling of the cheek, with periorbital oedema, proptosis, or chemosis of the conjunctiva. Pus may be discharged at the inner or outer canthus of the eye, the mid-point of the lower lid, the outer surface of the alveolar margin near the site of the first milar, through the hard palate, or through the nose on the affected side. The condition may be mistaken for orbital cellulitis. Radiography is rarely helpful, but culture of the blood or pus usually yields a growth of staphylococcus. Early diagnosis and treatment will avoid damage to the first dentition and facial asymmetry.

Osteitis of the premaxilla

This causes similar symptoms but the first sign is swelling of the upper alveolar margin near the midline. Infection is usually confined to the premaxilla but may spread to the maxillary sinus.

Investigation is as for maxillary osteitis.

Management

1. In the absence of contrary evidence it should be assumed that the infection is staphylococcal. An orthopaedic surgeon should be asked to see infections involving the long bones or joints, and a dental surgeon to see infections of the maxilla and premaxilla.
2. Antibiotics: treatment should be started with cloxacillin with gentamicin in addition if the organism is not known. There is no justification in using benzylpenicillin initially since the likelihood of a penicillinase-producing staphylococcal infection is high. In staphylococcal infections which do not respond to cloxacillin, erythromycin, sodium fusidate (Fucidin), lincomycin or clindamycin may have to be considered.
3. Duration of treatment: antibiotic treatment should be continued for a minimum of 2 weeks after all signs of activity (return of WBC count and ESR to normal) have disappeared and in any case for not less than 4 weeks. There is no need to continue treatment until the X-ray appearance is normal.

Pyelonephritis

Acute pyelonephritis in the newborn may develop in two ways:

1. As part of a septicaemic illness in which infection of the renal tissue occurs as part of the septicaemia. The renal tract is usually normal, but an IVP should nevertheless be done.
2. As a primary infection in an abnormal tract, often with a secondary septicaemia. In either case jaundice may be the presenting feature.

Recognition

Unless there is a palpable renal mass, hypertrophied and palpable bladder, or an obviously defective urinary stream, it is often impossible to distinguish clinically between (1) and (2) above. The urine should be examined by microscopy and both blood and urine should be cultured. Since the infection is usually a generalized septicaemia a full 'infection screen', including lumbar puncture, should be done.

Management

1. When it has been established that the urine is infected, the plasma urea and electrolytes should be estimated. Even with a normal renal tract the plasma urea level is usually slightly raised during the acute phase of the illness. An initially high plasma urea (>16 mmol/ℓ, >100 mg/100 ml) which remains high after adequate treatment suggests an abnormal tract.
2. Antibiotics: gentamicin (reduced dose with a raised blood urea value) and benzylpenicillin should be used in the treatment of an initial septicaemic illness without meningitis, and ampicillin should be used in an infection confined to the renal tract. Treatment should be continued for 2 weeks.
3. All infants should have an IVP or ultrasound after recovery: a micturating cystogram may also be required.
4. Infants with an anatomical abnormality of the renal tract should be treated with a maintenance dose of an appropriate antibiotic while surgical correction is being considered.

AIDS in infants

Present evidence suggests that AIDS can be acquired from an infected mother, transplacentally, during the delivery, or post-natally, possibly through breast milk (Scott *et al.*, 1984; Ziegler *et al.*, 1985). Infection from blood transfusions during the neonatal period has also occurred.

There appears to be a latent period of from 1 to 6 months after birth before symptoms develop. The commonest presenting symptom is severe failure to thrive, with recurrent attacks of pneumonitis, or chronic diarrhoea. Mild atopic eczema is common, and generalized lymphadenopathy with hepatosplenomegaly are found in about one third of the cases. The symptoms are due to infection with opportunistic organisms, commonly *Pneumocystis carinii* in the lungs, but infection with herpes virus, Epstein–Barr virus, and less commonly herpes zoster may also occur. Additional infection with bacteria such as *Strep. pneumoniae, Staphylococcus epidermidis, E. coli* or *Pseudomonas aeruginosa* may also develop. Mortality during the months after the onset of symptoms is around 30 per cent, but no long-term follow-up of recognized cases has yet been possible. Kaposi's sarcoma has not been observed in infants with AIDS, but at autopsy cells resembling those of the Kaposi sarcoma have been found in the lymph nodes and spleen. Treatment of the opportunistic infection and secondary bacterial invaders is essential.

Pre-symptomatic diagnosis is unlikely to be successful and screening of newborn infants born to women with AIDS, or belonging to the at-risk groups is not likely to be useful, since antibodies to the HLV3 (Human T-Cell Lymphotropic Virus type 3) virus may not be present during the neonatal period even in children who subsequently become clinically ill and serologically positive. Nevertheless, infants born to mothers with AIDS and to those in high-risk groups should be carefully followed up, possibly for as long as a year. Obviously screening of the at-risk mothers before delivery should identify those likely to infect their children, though the presence of the antibody to HTLV3 does not indicate infectivity and the currently used antibody test may give either false negative or false positive results. The distribution of at-risk groups in the United Kingdom is not identical with that in the United States. In general, however, the women at risk are:

1. Sexual partners of men known to have AIDS or to have antibodies.
2. Known IV drug users (at present a relatively small group in Britain).
3. Recipients of multiple blood transfusions.
4. Women known to have a bisexual male partner.
5. In the United States there is an increasing number of cases in women who have had sexual contact with men with previous heterosexual relations in Central Africa or the Caribbean.
6. Women of African origin who have had intercourse in Africa.

Clearly such details of the sexual history of women and their male partners are unlikely to result from a routine history, but when symptoms in the mother or child suggest the possibility of AIDS, it is particularly important to obtain a full history and in particular to enquire about the mother's contact with a bisexually active male partner, as this appears to be the group with the greatest risk of being infective.

Acute gastrointestinal infections

This may be due to distinguishable types of enteropathogenic *E. coli*, campylobacter, rotavirus, shigella, or salmonella and occasionally an intestinal staphylococcal infection.

Recognition

The sudden onset of frequent, loose stools with vomiting or deterioration in feeding raises the possibility of acute gastroenteritis. Blood and mucus in the stool may occur with campylobacter, shigella, or salmonella but are rare in *E. coli* infections. Other conditions which must be considered are:

1. Mismanagement of feeds with underfeeding.
2. Profuse diarrhoea within a few hours of starting milk due to lactose intolerance.
3. Necrotizing enterocolitis or intussusception.
4. Diarrhoea with abdominal distension preceded by delayed passage of meconium due to Hirschsprung's disease.
5. Cows' milk allergy.
6. Acute adrenal failure due to adrenogenital syndrome (adrenal hyperplasia).
7. Orally administered drugs which might cause frequent stools (e.g. ampicillin, ferrous sulphate, calcium gluconate).
8. Incarceration of an inguinal hernia.
9. A septicaemic illness may present with abdominal distension and diarrhoea.

Management

1. Isolation and collection of stool for bacteriological analysis. A full 'infection screen' should be carried out if the infant appears unwell.
2. If there is moderate to severe dehydration or the infant is not tolerating feeds, intravenous fluids should be started.
3. In term infants with mild dehydration who can tolerate feeds, oral replacement can be attempted.

4. Choice of oral fluids: In early cases, such as are frequently encountered in the newborn, one of the standard oral glucose electrolyte solutions can be used (*see* Chapter 46 and Appendix 9). Alternatively, 0.45% NaCl in 2.5% glucose may be used.
5. Antibiotic: In salmonella infections amoxycillin should be given; shigella infections are often resistant to amoxycillin and ampicillin; the most appropriate antibiotic depends upon the sensitivities. In most salmonella and shigella infections antibiotics are not indicated unless there is evidence of septicaemia or meningitis. Antibiotics are not indicated in viral gastroenteritis and are not of proved value in gastroenteritis due to enteropathogenic *E. coli.*

Administrative aspects of infective gastroenteritis in a maternity unit

Single cases

1. An infant developing sudden diarrhoea should be regarded as potentially infective, transferred to an isolation cubicle, and investigated. Once the infection is confirmed, the baby should be transferred to the isolation ward of the nearest paediatric unit. The baby's survival depends on neonatal intensive care unit technology; the baby must be barrier nursed.
2. A search to find the source of the infection must be initiated including all contacts of the infant during the previous 10 days. All staff with a positive culture should be put off duty until they have produced 3 consecutive negative cultures. An infective mother should be isolated and sent home as soon as possible.
3. Stool specimens should be sent from infants nursed in the same room as the index case and no further infants admitted to that room until the stool samples have come back negative. Any infant developing diarrhoea must have a stool sample sent immediately and be isolated.
4. In presumed viral infection a period of 10 days without symptoms in a contact should be regarded as evidence of non-infectivity.

More than one case occurring simultaneously

This is likely to be caused by infected feeds originating from a common source or to widespread infection from an undetected case. In these circumstances there is little choice but to close the unit to further admissions until the outbreak can be brought under control.

Antibiotics policy in the newborn

1. Local applications should not contain any antibiotic which could be used systemically, because of the risk of inducing resistant organisms.
2. In general, the following antibiotics are *contraindicated* in the newborn: bacitracin, co-trimoxazole, neomycin, novobiocin, polymyxin, tetracyclines; and sulphonamides in the presence of jaundice. Chloramphenicol should normally be used only for the treatment of meningitis due to Gram-negative bacilli. Tobramycin may be useful in infections, particularly with Pseudomonas.
3. In neonatal units there should be continuous monitoring of the bacterial flora to detect the emergence of resistant strains and in the knowledge of the local flora, there should be a definite policy as to the first choice antibiotic combination.

Antimicrobial drug dosage

See Table 77.2

Table 77.2 Neonatal antibiotic dosage/kg/24 hours

Antibiotic	*Age <7 days*	*Age 7–28 days*
Benzylpenicillin (penicillin G)	50 000–100 000 units (30–60 mg) in two doses	100 000–250 000 units (60–150 mg) in three doses
Cloxacillin	50–100 mg in two doses	100–200 mg in three doses
Ampicillin	100 mg in two doses	200–300 mg in three doses
Gentamicin	5 mg in two doses	7.5 mg in three doses
Kanamycin	15 mg in two doses	15 mg in two doses
Tobramycin	4 mg in two doses	6 mg in three doses
Chloramphenicol	25 mg premature 25 mg term in two doses	25 mg premature 50 mg term in two doses
Vancomycin	30 mg in two doses	45 mg in two doses
Cefotaxime	150 mg in three doses	150 mg in three doses
Levels	Gentamicin and tobramycin	Peak 5–10; trough <2 μg/ml
	Kanamycin	Peak 15–25; trough <2 μg/ml
	Chloramphenicol	Peak 15–25; trough <2 μg/ml

References

ALVAREZ, R. and COB SOSA, C. (1976) Enfermedades parasitarias. In Jaimes E. Calderón and M. Salas Alvarado (eds) *Conceptos Clinicos de Infectiologia* (3rd edn.), p. 454. Mexico: Mendez Cervantes

BITTENCOURT, A. L. (1976) Congenital Chagas' disease. *American Journal of Diseases of Children,* **130,** 97–103

SCOTT, G. B., BUCK, B. E., LETERMAN, J. G., BLOOM, F. L. and PARKS, W. P. (1984) AIDS in infants. *New England Journal of Medicine,* **310,** 76–81

SPEER, M. E. and YAWN, D. H. (1954) Fatal hepatoadrenal necrosis associated with Echovirus Types 11 and 12 presenting as a surgical emergency. *Journal of Pediatric Surgery,* **19,** 591–593

STAGNO, S. (1981) Diagnosis of viral infections in the newborn infant. *Clinics in Perinatology,* **8,** 582–589

ZIEGLER, J. B., COOPER, D. A., JOHNSON, R. D. and GOLD, J. (1985) Post-natal transmission of AIDS associated retrovirus from mother to infant. *Lancet,* **i,** 896–898

Further reading

CAMPBELL, A. N., O'DRISCOLL, M. C., ROBINSON, D. L. and READ, S. E. (1983) A case of neonatal herpes simplex with pneumonia. *Canadian Medical Association Journal,* **129,** 725–726

PLOTKIN, S. A. and STAR, S. E. (1981) Symposium on perinatal infections. *Clinics in Perinatology,* **8,** 395–637

Chapter 78

Apnoeic attacks in the newborn

M. F. Whitfield

Recognition

The premature newborn and to a lesser degree the term newborn have periodic respiration. Prolonged apnoea greater than 20 seconds, however, is likely to be associated with bradycardia of less than 100 beats per minute and transient pallor and cyanosis. Although the infant may respond to gentle stimulation, the apnoeic attacks may become sufficiently bad to require full-scale resuscitation including intubation. Sometimes bradycardia precedes apnoea or the infant may breathe against a closed glottis ('obstructive apnoea'). In the preterm infant (particularly less than 34 weeks' gestation) apnoeic attacks may be an almost physiological phenomenon (apnoeic attacks of prematurity) or may be the first indication that incipient pathology is developing, requiring urgent attention. In the term infant, apnoeic attacks are usually an indication of underlying illness. The most likely causes to be considered include:

1. Preterm:
   (a) Anaemia.
   (b) Hypoxia.
   (c) Acidaemia.
   (d) Septicaemia and/or meningitis.
   (e) Hypo- or hyperthermia or wide fluctuations in incubator temperature.
   (f) Hypoglycaemia.
   (g) Nasal obstruction by secretions or feeding tube.
   (h) Heart failure (e.g. due to patent ductus arteriosus).
   (i) Pulmonary milk aspiration.
   (j) Developing necrotizing enterocolitis.
   (k) Progressive atelectasis, pulmonary secretion retention, or pneumonia.
   (l) Fluid or electrolyte imbalance.
   (m) Seizures which have not yet been recognized as such.
2. Term:
   (a) Septicaemia.
   (b) Seizures due to hypoxic ischaemic encephalopathy, meningitis, or intracranial malformation (*see* page 702).
   (c) Hypoglycaemia.
   (d) Major pulmonary abnormality.
   (e) Major cardiac abnormality with heart failure.

Management

1. Investigations should be done to discover the cause of the apnoeic attacks; these may include an infection screen, a chest X-ray, blood glucose, electrolytes, and blood gases, a haemoglobin level, and the exclusion of airway obstruction. Feeds may have to be stopped until the situation has been fully evaluated.
2. The infant requires intensive nursing and monitoring; a transcutaneous PO_2 monitor is extremely useful in this situation. Many infants have fewer apnoeic attacks in the prone position with the head of the incubator tray raised. Attacks should be treated by:
   (a) Stimulation.
   (b) IPPV by bag and mask, with intubation if the baby does not respond. Apnoeic attacks requiring more than stimulation should be an indication for initiating either CPAP at 3–5 cm H_2O, by nasal catheter, a nasopharyngeal tube, or endotracheal tube, or the administration of aminophylline (loading dose 7 mg/kg IV followed by 1.25 mg/kg 8 hourly IV to reach a serum level of 6–11 μg/ml). Infants with obstructive apnoea respond to intubation and CPAP.
3. Intubation and IPPV may be required. Evidence linking significant apoeic attacks with cerebral hypoperfusion and subsequent periventricular leukomalacia have led to a more active approach to the treatment of apnoeic attacks.

Chapter 79

Cyanosis in the newborn

M. F. Whitfield and J. A. Black

Recognition

Persistent cyanosis in the newborn requires urgent investigation.

Peripheral cyanosis

1. 'Traumatic cyanosis of the head'; an appearance caused by confluent petechiae on the head may be due to the cord tightly around the neck, delay in delivery due to shoulder dystocia, or uncontrolled rapid delivery of the head. Such infants may also have subconjunctival haemorrhages. No treatment is required apart from reassurance of the mother.
2. Peripheral cyanosis in a vigorous infant with warm extremities is of no consequence and usually disappears after 2–3 days. It may also occur transiently due to moderate chilling after delivery.
3. Peripheral cyanosis may be a sign of circulatory failure and shock from any cause (*see* page 672) or in hypothermia (*see* page 644).

Central cyanosis

The most common causes of persistent central cyanosis are:

1. Cardiac (*see* page 259).
2. Respiratory (*see* page 240).
3. Polycythaemia; infants of diabetic mothers, SGA infants, cases of twin-to-twin transfusion, and infants in whom cord clamping has been delayed with the infant held lower than the placenta frequently have haematocrits greater than 65 per cent. The high blood viscosity may lead to venous sinus thrombosis, circulatory problems, an increased risk of necrotizing enterocolitis, and persisting neurological and behavioural abnormalities. Current evidence suggests that infants with a venous haematocrit greater than 65 per cent should be subjected to dilutional exchange transfusion with dextran or plasma (*see* page 697).
4. Severe acidaemia.
5. Hypoglycaemia.

6. Congenital or acquired methaemoglobinaemia; in this condition, blood fails to turn red when exposed to oxygen and remains a chocolate brown colour. Diagnosis is by haemoglobin spectroscopy and chromatography.

Management of cyanosis

The management of the commoner causes of cyanosis is considered under the causes. Methaemoglobinaemia may be abolished (temporarily in the congenital forms) by the IV injection of methylene blue (1%; 10 mg/ml) in a dose of 1–2 mg/kg. Ascorbic acid 100 mg three to four times daily can be given orally. This acts more slowly but can be used as maintenance treatment.

Chapter 80

Stridor in the newborn

J. A. Black

Recognition

The noise made by an infant with stridor may be loud and rasping or it may be a loud wheeze or a soft purr like a vibration. In making a preliminary assessment it is necessary to determine: (1) the probable site of obstruction; (2) the severity.

The site

1. Inspiratory stridor alone is invariably due to an obstruction in or near the larynx.
2. A hoarse or absent cry indicates involvement of the vocal cords. An exception is severe subglottic stenosis in which the expiratory flow is insufficient to produce a cry.
3. Inspiratory and expiratory ('to-and-fro') stridor indicates tracheal obstruction.
4. Stridor which varies with position, particularly if reduced or absent in the prone position, indicates either an 'infantile' larynx (as in congenital laryngeal stridor) or obstruction due to the tongue falling back in the supine position, or upper respiratory infection.
5. Stridor accompanied by extension of the head may be due to a goitre, tracheal compression by a vascular ring, or (rarely) injury to the larynx in the course of a face delivery: the extension of the head after face delivery is merely a persistence of the intrauterine position.
6. Expiratory stridor alone is likely to be due to bronchial obstruction, as in lobar emphysema, lung cyst, or mediastinal displacement.

Severity

1. Stridor which is intermittently present or is absent during quiet breathing usually indicates a mild degree of obstruction.
2. Continued stridor with marked in-drawing and recession indicates a moderate-to-severe obstruction.
3. Stridor with cyanosis or pallor and restlessness requires immediate relief.

The development of stridor in a low birth weight infant recovering from a period of intensive care management

This is most likely due to one of the following:

1. Damage to the larynx due to prolonged endotracheal intubation producing subglottic stenosis of granulomata.
2. Damage to the recurrent laryngeal nerve on the left, if the baby required ligation of a patent ductus arteriosus.

Management of severe obstruction with stridor

Urgent direct laryngoscopy in the theatre by an experienced ENT surgeon is necessary; facilities for intubation or tracheostomy must be available.

Inspiratory stridor with normal cry

This may be due to:

1. 'Congenital laryngeal stridor', or the Pierre–Robin syndrome: nursing in the prone position is usually all that is required.
2. Where change in posture makes no difference, the cause may be a goitre (*see* page 477), subglottic stenosis, or haemangioma.

Inspiratory stridor with weak, hoarse or absent cry

This may be due to:

1. Traumatic injury to the cords during resuscitation, or post-intubation oedema.
2. Cyst, haemangioma of the cords, or laryngeal web.
3. Unilateral or bilateral recurrent laryngeal palsy; rare except on the left side after ligation of a patent ductus arteriosus.
4. Direct injury to the larynx at delivery (rare).

In (1), relief of the obstruction is usually unnecessary; a short course of corticosteroids may reduce the oedema, or in some cases reintubation with a loosely fitting endotracheal tube may be necessary.

In (2), tracheostomy is usually required, followed by appropriate treatment of the obstruction at the time of tracheostomy or later.

In (3), a bilateral cord paralysis may require tracheostomy, but a unilateral paralysis seldom needs it.

Inspiratory and expiratory stridor

This is rarely an emergency in the immediate neonatal period, though obstruction may suddenly increase later, possibly due to oedema from an upper respiratory infection. All cases should be thoroughly investigated *before* the obstruction becomes severe.

Expiratory stridor

Chest X-ray may indicate the probable cause of the bronchial obstruction; bronchoscopy may be required. For management of lobar emphysema, and lung cyst *see* page 248.

Chapter 81

Nasal and nasopharyngeal obstruction

M. F. Whitfield and J. A. Black

Most newborns are obligatory nose-breathers during the first 3 months of life, and minor degrees of nasal airway obstruction are common, due to the small size of the airway and the significant increase in airway resistance caused by even small amounts of secretions or crusts. A coryzal illness in a normal infant with a small dose may produce considerable problems due to airway obstruction particularly during feeding, and the ingestion of a considerable amount of swallowed mucus. Unilateral nasal or nasopharyngeal obstruction does not cause severe symptoms and may go unrecognized until unilateral mucupurulent nasal discharge develops on the affected side. Bilateral nasal obstruction, however, causes early symptoms and can be fatal if not recognized and treated.

Recognition

1. Complete bilateral nasal obstruction causes severe inspiratory in-drawing and recession with cyanosis, but without stridor. The signs may be initially difficult to distinguish from other causes of respiratory distress in the newborn (*see* page 241); they are instantly relieved when crying causes the infant to breathe through the mouth, or by the insertion of an oropharyngeal airway. The commonest cause is choanal atresia.
2. Incomplete or intermittent nasal obstruction, particularly if it varies with the position of the patient, is likely to be due to a nasopharyngeal tumour or nasal encephalocele. If the obstruction is incomplete, inspiration is likely to be accompanied by a snoring or snorting noise. These tumours are often pedunculated and asymmetrically placed and usually produce variable symptoms.
3. Mild nasal obstruction developing after birth is usually due to an upper respiratory infection, or to oedema and infection from an indwelling nasal tube.
4. Nasal obstruction may occur with a nasal tube *in situ* if the 'free' nasal airway becomes obstructed by secretions or oedema.

Management

Bilateral choanal atresia is an emergency which requires experienced operative intervention. Temporary relief can be obtained by the insertion of an oropharyngeal airway provided this is adequately fixed with adhesive tape to prevent rejection by the infant. Suspected tumours may require similar management and should be referred to a specialist as an emergency.

The obstruction due to nasopharyngitis can usually be relieved by giving vasoconstrictor nose drops; crusts should be softened by cotton wool soaked in warm, sterile normal saline. Suitable nose drops are 0.5% ephedrine in 0.9% sodium chloride and should be instilled 10–20 minutes before each feed in order to relieve nasal obstruction during feeding. This treatment should not be continued for longer than 7–10 days.

Chapter 82

Acute blood loss at or after delivery

J. A. Black

Acute blood loss in the newborn may occur during pregnancy, during labour, during delivery, or after delivery. If blood loss has occurred before the infant was delivered, shock may be present at birth and this must be distinguished from hypoxia (asphyxia) (*Table 82.1*).

Acute blood loss up to delivery

Recognition

Fetal tachycardia or bradycardia already recognized during labour may be attributed to hypoxia (fetal distress). However, *shock from haemorrhage does not*

Table 82.1 Acute blood loss up to delivery

Time	*Cause*	*Diagnostic investigation*
During pregnancy	Fetomaternal bleed (acute) Fetofetal bleed (acute) in twins	Kleihauer on maternal blood Hb on both twins: appearance of twins and placenta
	Injury at amniocentesis, intrauterine transfusion or fetal blood sampling	Blood-stained amniotic fluid
	Fetal bleeding in placenta praevia or accidental haemorrhage	Clinical features
During labour or delivery	Injury to fetal vessels at caesarean section, rupture of fetal vessels in vasa praevia, velamentous insertions, or accessory lobe of placenta	Examination of placenta and fetal vessels
	Puncture or tear by monitor electrode or fetal-blood sampling	Examination of the infant
During delivery	Rupture of umbilical vessels from: short or entangled cord, cord round the neck, precipitate or unattended delivery	Appearance of cord
	Draining blood into placenta at caesarean section	

usually cause primary apnoea (*Table 82.2*). In shock from haemorrhage, attempts at conventional resuscitation are unlikely to produce any clinical improvement. The infant appears pale and hypotonic, with cool greyish-blue extremities, is unresponsive to stimuli and may be semiconscious, with rolling eyes. The cord is collapsed, with weak or absent pulsation. The brachial pulse is rapid and feeble or impalpable and the heart sounds are weak: the heart rate is rapid (>160) or slow (<60) in a preterminal (but recoverable) state. Respiration is shallow and irregular, or gasping (apnoea or apnoeic attacks may also occur (*see Table 82.2* for differential diagnosis of pallor at delivery).

Table 82.2 Pallor at delivery: differential diagnosis

	Severe hypoxia	*Acute blood loss*	*Severe chronic anaemia**
Fetal tachycardia	+	Depends on the cause	May occur
Apnoea	+	Not primary	Only in hydrops
Pallor	+	+	++
Cyanosis	++	++	No
Cord	Collapsed	Collapsed	Distended
Cord pulsation	Feeble or absent	Feeble or absent	Normal
Heart rate	Slow	Rapid to slow	Rapid
Brachial pulse	Feeble or impalpable	Feeble or impalpable	Normal or feeble
Hypotonia	++	+	No
Abdomen	Normal	Normal	Distended (hepatosplenomegaly)
Skin haemorrhage	No	No	In severe Rhesus isoimmunization

* Severe Rhesus isoimmunization, or chronic fetomaternal or fetofetal bleeding, homozygous α-thalassaemia.

Management

Restoration of the plasma volume is the most urgent consideration, and should precede attempts to discover the cause of the blood loss. In nearly every case, when bleeding has occurred before or during delivery, the blood loss will have ceased as soon as the cord has been clamped. An Hb level estimated during early shock may give a misleadingly normal or near normal level; nevertheless blood should of course be taken from the infant for Hb (base-line) and grouping, and from the mother for cross-matching. The severity of shock can be assessed and the amount required to the transfused can be estimated by blood pressure recording (*see* Appendix 17).

Acute blood loss at or after delivery

1. Extreme urgency, (i.e. the infant appears likely to be die within the next few minutes). An IV drip should be set up immediately, using the umbilical vein and taking a blood sample at the same time.
   (a) Any of the immediately available IV fluids or plasma expanders (including O Rh negative blood) can be used provided that the fluid is NOT cold from refrigeration, since this may produce arrhythmias. The IV fluid should be given at a rate of 20–30 ml/kg/hour until emergency cross-matched blood

becomes available; this should be possible within 20–30 minutes of its request; at the same time a formal cross-matching should be set up, taking between 1 and 2 hours.

(b) Blood when available should NOT be given cold (*see* above); a warming coil should be used, as for an exchange transfusion (*see* page 693). It should be assumed that an infant has lost 20–30 ml/kg blood (i.e. about 25–30 per cent of its blood volume). Undertransfusion is a more likely error than overtransfusion. The newborn infant in any case is very tolerant of large additions to its blood volume (as in the placental transfusion in delayed clamping of the cord) but is intolerant of blood loss.
Rate of transfusion:
0–30 minutes: (electrolyte solution or plasma expander): 10 ml/kg.
30–60 minutes: blood, 10 ml/kg.
60 minutes onwards: blood, 10–20 ml/kg/hour until shock is relieved.
Blood pressure monitoring is helpful as a guide to the severity of the shock and as an indication of progress. Systolic blood pressure of under 40 mm Hg is an indication for urgent transfusion, preferably with blood (*see* above). Dopamine may be useful (*see* page 107 for dosage) if IV colloids or blood fail to raise the blood pressure (*see* Appendix 17 for normal blood pressure in the neonatal period).

2. In less urgent cases, all preparation should be made for transfusion through the umbilical vein, but the actual transfusion can be delayed until grouped and cross-matched blood is available. If the infant begins to deteriorate during this period, an IV drip should be started as in (1) above. The respiration rate, heart rate and blood pressure should be monitored continuously while waiting for the blood.
3. If the infant appears shocked but the diagnosis of blood loss is uncertain it is safer to give blood empirically as in (1) or (2) according to the degree of urgency.

Acute blood loss after delivery

The commoner causes of acute postnatal bleeding are given in *Table 82.3*. The reabsorption of blood from an enclosed cavity or damaged tissues may contribute to the development of hyperbilirubinaemia, particularly in the pre-term infant.

Table 82.3 Acute blood loss after delivery: commoner causes

0–24 hours	*24–36 hours*	*36–72 hours*	*2–7 days*	*At any time*
Fetal scalp-sampling site Cord haemorrhage Cephalhaematoma	Rupture of liver Rupture of spleen (Rh cases only) Subaponeurotic haemorrhage Muscle and soft-tissue bleeding (breech) Pulmonary haemorrhage	Adrenal haemorrhage Intracranial haemorrhage Bleeding into the mesentery of the intestine	Haemorrhagic disease Intracranial haemorrhage in RDS (IVH)	Renal vein thrombosis Bleeding into giant haemangioma with thrombocytopenia

Recognition

Intracranial haemorrhage

1. Intraventricular haemorrhage (IVH) (*see* page 626): this occurs mainly in pre-term infants with respiratory distress syndrome and is indicated by fits, or apnoeic spells, with or without a bulging fontanelle. The CSF is heavily blood stained. This type of bleed is frequently fatal. It can usually be detected by ultrasound (*see* page 628).
2. Acute subdural haematoma (*see* page 624).
3. Subarachnoid haemorrhage: this occurs mainly in term infants or may accompany a bacterial meningitis (*see* page 336).

Cephalhaematoma

Shock or anaemia requiring transfusion are rare and reabsorption of blood is so slow that it very rarely contributes to the development of hyperbilirubinaemia.

Subaponeurotic haemorrhage

See page 625.

Massive pulmonary haemorrhage

See pages 215 and 251.

Intraperitoneal haemorrhage

1. Rupture of the liver: this occurs more commonly in large term infants after a latent period of 24–36 hours. A definite diagnosis is difficult to make but should be suspected in any infant developing sudden shock (symptoms as described on page 672); there may be slight abdominal distension and an erect X-ray of the abdomen may show a fluid level of blood in the pelvis, with the bowel above it. Confirmation of intraperitoneal bleeding is by aspiration of blood from the peritoneal cavity on the introduction of a wide-bore needle into the left flank.
2. Rupture of the spleen: this is only likely to occur in Rhesus isoimmunization. The symptoms and signs are the same as in rupture of the liver.

Retroperitoneal haemorrhage

1. Renal vein thrombosis produces a large accumulation of blood into one or both kidneys; there is a large mass in the flank, usually with obvious or microscopic haematuria (*see Table 82.4* for distinction from massive adrenal haemorrhage).
2. Adrenal haemorrhage: the physical signs are similar to those of renal vein thrombosis, but shock is severe if both adrenals are involved (*see Table 82.4* and page 470).

Gastrointestinal haemorrhage

1. For haematemesis and the effects of swallowed maternal blood *see* pages 371 and 386.
2. Haemorrhagic disease: *see* page 678.
3. Bleeding into the mesentery of the intestine produces a mobile mass in the abdomen. An X-ray may show the intestines to be displaced laterally.

Table 82.4 Adrenal haemorrhage and renal vein thrombosis: differential diagnosis

	Adrenal haemorrhage	*Renal vein thrombosis*
Predisposing maternal conditions	Anticoagulant treatment except heparin. Drugs causing thrombocytopenia	Usually none: maternal diabetes
Age of onset	36–72 hours	Any time in infancy
Septicaemia	Common	Rare
Shock	Usually	Sometimes
Anaemia	Always	Sometimes
Haematuria	None or a few RBCs	Usually obvious
Proteinuria	None or trace	Marked
IVP or ultrasound	Kidney on affected side displaced downwards, with flattening of the upper calyces	Affected kidney does not excrete

Bleeding into a haemangioma

See page 509.

Soft-tissue haemorrhage in a breech delivery

See page 621.

Management

1. Investigation: if there is any possibility of DIC, coagulation disorder or thrombocytopenia, the appropriate investigations should be done (*see* page 677).
2. If an exploratory laparotomy (e.g. for a ruptured liver) is required, Vitamin K_1 (phytomenadione) should be given i.m. (or IV if a coagulation defect is present) in a dose of 1–2 mg.
3. Shock: the treatment is as described on page 672.

Chapter 83

The bleeding neonate

Judith M. Chessells

Haemorrhage in the newborn infant may be due to local causes (e.g. slipped cord clamp) or to a generalized bleeding disorder; bleeding from one site may be due to either. In management of the bleeding newborn infant three problems must be faced:

1. Emergency treatment of acute blood loss (*see* page 672).
2. In the case of apparent gastrointestinal loss, could this be maternal blood? Do the Apt test (*see* Appendix 18).
3. Is the bleeding a manifestation of haemostatic failure? Blood is taken for Hb, PCV, film, platelet count and screening tests of coagulation (PT, PTTK, TT) before transfusion. If disseminated intravascular coagulation (DIC) is suspected be sure to take sample for fibrin degradation products (FDP) into EACA or other fibrinolytic inhibitor. If the baby has not received vitamin K give 1 mg IV phytomenadione.

Normal values in the neonatal period

In pre-term and mature infants the platelet count and factors V, VIII, and fibrinogen are in the normal adult range. Prothrombin and factors VII, IX and X are low at birth (so the PT and PTTK may be prolonged even in a normal newborn) and drop further at 3–4 days *unless* the baby is given vitamin K. The thrombin time is moderately prolonged but should not exceed twice that of the control.

Clinical clues to the type of bleeding disorder

The baby – Breast or bottle fed? Has vitamin K been given? Is there evidence of respiratory distress, hypothermia, infection, or hepatosplenomegaly? If so, this suggests DIC. Has the bleeding followed trauma, e.g. circumcision in a well baby? If so consider haemophilia or Christmas disease. Late cord bleeding is seen in the (very rare) deficiencies of fibrinogen or factor XIII. Extensive purpura in an otherwise well baby suggests immune thrombocytopenia. Presence of congenital anomalies may indicate a genetically determined thrombocytopenia.

The mother – History of bruising or drugs which may cause thrombocytopenia (rare, e.g. quinidine, thiazides) or affect platelet function (common, e.g. aspirin). The WR result should be checked. Blood is taken for platelet count and film.

By assessment of these points and results of screening tests (*Tables 83.1* and *83.2*) a diagnosis may be made.

Table 83.1 Screening tests of haemostasis in the newborn

Disorder	*Platelets*	*PT*	*PTTK*	*TT*
Immune thrombocytopenia*	ABN	N	N	N
Disseminated intravascular coagulation	ABN	ABN	ABN	ABN
Vitamin-K deficiency	N	ABN	ABN	N
Afibrinogenaemia	N	ABN	ABN	ABN
Factor XIII deficiency†	N	N	N	N
Haemophilia	N	N	ABN	N
Liver disease	N	ABN	ABN	ABN

N = normal result; ABN = result usually abnormal; PT = prothrombin time; PTTK = partial thromboplastin time with kaolin; TT = thrombin time.

* *See Table 83.2*

† Special screening test needed

Table 83.2 Thrombocytopenia in the newborn

Mechanism	*Examples*
Platelet production decreased or abnormal	Thrombocytopenia with absent radius. Wiskott–Aldrich syndrome. Infections
Immune thrombocytopenia	
Passive	Maternal ITP. Maternal systemic lupus erythematosus. Maternal drug ingestion.
Active	Isoimmune neonatal thrombocytopenia.
Intravascular coagulation	
Generalized	Asphyxiated, hypothermic, acidotic infants. Erythroblastosis fetalis (Rhesus isoimmunization). Respiratory distress syndrome. Congenital infections: syphilis, rubella, cytomegalovirus, herpes simplex. Acquired infections.
Localized	Cavernous haemangioma. Renal vein thrombosis. Catheter thrombus.

Management of individual disorders

Thrombocytopenia with no clotting defect

Immune thrombocytopenia is most likely; for other rare causes *see Table 83.2*. Problems in immune thrombocytopenia are most likely in the first few hours of life. If bruising is the only problem no treatment is needed. If bleeding is severe, platelet concentrate (from one unit of blood is sufficient) should be given but may not be effective. Exchange transfusion should be considered using fresh heparinized blood to remove antibody and (in isoimmunization) subsequent infusion of washed maternal platelets. Recently, isoimmune thrombocytopenia in the newborn has been successfully treated with IV immunoglobulin (Sandoglobulin) in a dose of 400 mg/kg/day for 5 days (Derycke *et al.*, 1985) (*see* also page 495).

Vitamin K deficiency

See Table 83.1. This is manifested by bleeding, usually on days 3 or 4 in breast-fed babies who have not received vitamin K, and it may also exacerbate subaponeurotic haemorrhage after vacuum extraction. It may also occur in infants of mothers on anticonvulsants. This is the *only* condition in which vitamin K stops bleeding and restores normal clotting factors. If vitamin K does not work the diagnosis should be reconsidered, e.g. DIC. Vitamin K responsive haemorrhage after the first few days of life may occur in diarrhoea or after antibiotic administration but may also be the first manifestation of serious underlying liver disease, e.g. biliary atresia or associated with α-1-antitrypsin deficiency, galactosaemia, or fructose intolerance.

Failure of synthesis of clotting factors

This can occur in neonatal hepatitis, or metabolic disorders. The cause should be found and treated where possible. Fresh frozen plasma 10–15 ml/kg will replace clotting factors.

Congenital clotting-factor deficiencies

Replacement therapy as detailed on page 496.

Disseminated intravascular coagulation (see page 498)

For common causes in the newborn *see Table 83.2*. The cause should be found and treated: DIC in the newborn is often self-limiting. If bleeding is a continuing problem, platelet concentrate must be given and FFP as detailed above; heparin is rarely indicated except when thrombosis is the main problem. The dose of heparin is as on page 498.

Identification of groups at risk and prevention of haemorrhage

Routine administration of vitamin K_1 (phytomenadione) to all babies at birth will prevent vitamin K responsive bleeding. Prompt correction of neonatal hypoxia, shock and hypothermia, and treatment of infection, will help in prevention of DIC.

Reference

DERYCKE, M., DREYFUS, M., ROPERT, J. C. and TCHERNIA, G. (1985). Intravenous immunoglobulin for neonatal isoimmune thrombocytopenia. *Archives of Diseases in Childhood,* **6**, 667–669

Further reading

OSKI, F. A. and NAIMAN, J. L. (1982) Blood coagulation and its disorders in the newborn. In *Hematologic Problems in the Newborn Infant* (3rd edn.), pp. 137–174. Philadelphia: W. B. Saunders

OSKI, F. A. and NAIMAN, J. L. (1982) Disorders of the platelets. In *Hematologic Problems in the Newborn Infant* (3rd edn.), pp. 175–222. Philadelphia: W. B. Saunders

Chapter 84

Anaemia in the newborn

J. A. Black

Acute anaemia is considered under Acute blood loss, page 671. Severe chronic anaemia in the newborn results from a continued blood loss or haemolysis. Either of these may occur before or after delivery but haemolysis may continue after delivery. A clinical picture similar to that of chronic anaemia is also produced by a number of intrauterine infections (*see* page 649).

At delivery

Continued blood loss

Fetomaternal haemorrhage

The acute form may cause shock (*see* page 671); more commonly the bleeding occurs slowly or recurrently.

RECOGNITION

The infant is pale, with hepatosplenomegaly (occasionally hydropic) and closely resembles an infant with severe Rhesus isoimmunization, except that jaundice does not develop within 1–4 hours of delivery. The Hb level is usually 7–10 g/100 ml, with numerous nucleated cells in the blood film. Confirmation of the diagnosis is made by a Kleihauer test on the mother's blood.

Fetofetal ('twin-to-twin') haemorrhage

This may also occur in an acute form (*see* page 671), but more commonly as a severe anaemia in one twin and plethora in the other.

RECOGNITION

The anaemic twin has the same appearance as in fetomaternal haemorrhage; the plethoric twin has a reddish-blue appearance, often with cyanosed extremities. The difference between their Hb levels is at least 3 g/100 ml, and often more.

Continued haemolysis

This is almost invariably due to Rhesus isoimmunization, but may be due to other blood group incompatibilities. ABO incompatibility very rarely causes anaemia during fetal life (*see* page 689 for Rhesus isoimmunization, etc.).

Severe haemoglobinopathy

Homozygous α-thalassaemia (Chinese and Far Eastern races) causes hydrops in the newborn which appears to be incompatible with survival. Very rarely, homozygous sickle cell disease presents in the neonatal period, with jaundice and anaemia (Hegyi *et al.,* 1977).

Intrauterine infection

A number of chronic intrauterine infections cause moderate anaemia with hepatosplenomegaly and rapidly developing jaundice, with or without thrombocytopenia, and may be mistaken for some form of blood group incompatibility. For further consideration of these conditions (syphilis, toxoplasmosis, cytomegalovirus infection, rubella, malaria, Chagas' disease) *see* pages 649–651.

Malignancy

Very rarely, congenital leukaemia or neuroblastoma may present with severe anaemia.

Management

RHESUS AND ABO HAEMOLYTIC DISEASE

See page 689.

FETOMATERNAL AND FETOFETAL BLEEDING

Infants in a state of hydrops (cardiac failure with ascites and pleural effusion) and an Hb under 7 g/100 ml require a partial exchange transfusion (*see* page 000) as described under Rhesus isoimmunization. Infants with an Hb of 7–10 g/100 ml without hydrops should be transfused by slow drip with packed or concentrated red cells.

1. Volume of packed of concentrated cells; *see* page 499 for calculation.
2. Duration of transfusion: normally this should be given *slowly*, over at least 4 hours. A careful watch should be kept on the respiration and heart rate and the size of the liver. Dyspnoea and tachypnoea with rapid enlargement of the liver indicate cardiac failure; the transfusion should be temporarily stopped and frusemide should be given IV or i.m. The transfusion can be restarted or completed when the infant has recovered.

THE PLETHORIC TWIN IN FETOFETAL BLEEDING (SEE ALSO PAGE 697)

Normally no treatment is required, though the development of cardiac failure with a raised venous pressure may require a venesection of 10 ml/kg. Frusemide should NOT be given because of the danger of thrombosis. The serum bilirubin should be estimated at least daily until it is clear that there is no risk from hyperbilirubinaemia. A dilutional exchange transfusion has been used to lower the haematocrit if there is considered to be a risk of cerebral or renal vein thrombosis or necrotizing enterocolitis from hyperviscosity. The critical level for thrombosis appears to be a haematocrit of over 65 per cent; an exchange transfusion of 15 ml/kg using plasma or dextran as the donor fluid should lower the haematocrit to 60 per cent.

Anaemia developing postnatally

This may be due to:

1. Missed Rhesus or ABO haemolysis (*see* page 689).
2. Missed fetomaternal haemorrhage (*see* page 679).
3. Congenital haemolytic anaemias (*see* page 685).
4. Intrauterine infections (*see* page 649).
5. Congenital hypoplastic anaemia (*see* page 689).
6. Early or late anaemia of prematurity.
7. β-thalassaemia at 3–4 months or homozygous sickle-cell disease (*see* page 680).

Anaemia of prematurity

Early anaemia

A slowly developing anaemia may occur in very low birth weight infants (<1.5 kg) in the first 6–8 weeks.

Iron deficiency anaemia

An iron deficiency anaemia may develop at 4–5 months which may be so severe (before recognition) that the Hb is 4–5 g/100 ml; this is particularly likely to occur in twins or multiple births.

Early anaemia

A transfusion should be given when the Hb value falls below 8 g/100 ml, using concentrated cells.

Late anaemia

Normally this does not constitute an emergency and can be treated with an oral iron preparation. A transfusion is indicated at Hb levels of 7 g/100 ml, if the infant is not thriving, or to expedite return home.

Reference

HEGYI, T., DELPHIN, E. S., BANK, A., POLIN, R. A. and BLANC, W. A. (1977) Sickle-cell anaemia in the newborn. *Pediatrics,* **60,** 213–216

Chapter 85

Jaundice

M. F. Whitfield and J. A. Black

Jaundice may present as an emergency in three ways:

1. In the management of a haemolytic anaemia of known cause (e.g. Rhesus or ABO isoimmunization, G-6PD deficiency, etc. *see* pages 688 and 689).
2. Early onset jaundice presenting within the first 24 hours after delivery.
3. Rapidly increasing jaundice of unknown cause.

Dangers of hyperbilirubinaemia

1. Kernicterus.
2. Unrecognized septicaemia (*see* page 649).
3. Unrecognized metabolic disorder (*see* page 684).

Factors that may contribute to hyperbilirubinaemia

Although in some infants one predominant factor can be identified as the cause of neonatal jaundice, frequently there are many other factors. The commonest of these are:

1. Prematurity.
2. Asphyxia (hypoxia).
3. Enclosed haemorrhage or soft-tissue bruising.
4. Infection (congenital or acquired).
5. Haemolysis from any cause.
6. Infant of the diabetic mother.
7. Dehydration.
8. Delayed enteral feeding.
9. Polycythaemia.
10. The conjugation inhibitor found in the breast milk of some mothers.
11. Hypothyroidism.

Difficulties in estimating severity

Although it is easy to identify most infants who are significantly jaundiced and it may be possible to make a reasonable clinical estimate of the bilirubin level, the clinician should be wary of the following factors:

1. Infants becoming jaundiced in the first 24 hours frequently appear to be less jaundiced than the bilirubin level actually indicates them to be.
2. Artificial light.
3. Infants who are plethoric.
4. Infants with dark skin.
5. After phototherapy.

Jaundice developing in the first 24 hours after delivery

The fact that an infant looks clinically jaundiced within the first 24 hours of delivery, implies a rapid rate of rise of the bilirubin level and requires urgent investigation to establish the bilirubin level and the cause of the jaundice. If the situation is neglected the infant may reach potentially toxic bilirubin levels before an exchange transfusion can be carried out. The probable causes are:

1. Missed Rhesus isoimmunization due to inadequate antenatal screening, inadequate application of the Rhesus prevention programme, or the development of Rhesus antibodies late in pregnancy due to third trimester fetomaternal haemorrhage (amniocentesis may be a cause).
2. Rhesus isoimmunization against Rhesus groups other than D (e.g. E, e, or c).
3. Severe ABO incompatibility.
4. Isoimmunization against rare blood groups (e.g. Duffy, Kell etc.).
5. Chronic intrauterine infections (*see* page 649).

Recognition

1. Early onset clinical jaundice may be difficult to recognize (*see* above), or easy to recognize if the infant is also anaemic.
2. Investigations:
   (a) Blood should be sent from the infant for haemoglobin and reticulocyte count, ABO and Rhesus grouping, direct and indirect Coombs' test, and where appropriate circulating immune anti-A or anti-B in the infant's serum and on the red cells.
   (b) From the mother for ABO and Rhesus testing, antibody screening, and where appropriate immune anti-A or anti-B in the serum. Sufficient blood should be retained for use in compatibility testing of the infant's red cells and for cross-matching purposes.

If there is no evidence of isoimmunization and the cause of the jaundice is obscure, 10–20 ml blood should be taken for subsequent investigation, should an exchange transfusion need to be carried out.

Management

The main aim of treatment is to prevent kernicterus (*see* page 691):

1. Serum bilirubin increasing at greater than 8.5 μmol/ℓ (over 0.5 mg/100 ml) per hour will probably necessitate an exchange transfusion (*see* page 691).
2. Phototherapy should also be used (*see* page 686).

Rapidly increasing jaundice of unknown cause (excluding the first 24 hours)

In addition to the causes of jaundice occurring in the first 24 hours the following should also be considered:

1. Septicaemia.
2. Metabolic disorders.
3. Chronic intrauterine infection.
4. Haemolytic anaemia due to a genetically determined intrinsic red cell defect (e.g. glucose 6-phosphate dehydrogenase deficiency).

Septicaemia

Recognition

1. The perinatal circumstances surrounding the birth of the infant may suggest infection; the infant appears ill with signs suggestive of infection (*see* page 655). Although the bilirubin will be unconjugated there is also likely to be a significant conjugated fraction.
2. A complete infection screen should be carried out on the infant (*see* page 655) and consideration given to starting intravenous antibiotics (*see* page 656).

Metabolic disorders

Recognition

Galactosaemia

The infant appears ill, vomits, and may already have lost a considerable amount of weight. The liver is usually greatly enlarged and there is elevation of both conjugated and unconjugated bilirubin fractions. The urine is Clinitest positive and Clinistix negative and laboratory investigation confirms the presence of galactose in blood and urine, and the blood glucose is usually at hypoglycaemic levels. If the infant is receiving intravenous fluids only, galactose may not be detected but the red cell screening test will be positive provided an exchange transfusion has not yet been carried out. As *both* glucose and galactose may be present in the urine, a positive Clinistix test does not exclude the diagnosis (*see* also page 712).

Fructose intolerance

Clinically, this condition is similar to galactosaemia but does not occur until the infant has received fructose (either in the form of sucrose or fructose, sometimes included in parenteral nutrition infusions). The urine should be tested with Clinitest and Clinistix and reducing sugars identified by the laboratory, and plasma fructose levels measured. There is no specific early test to confirm the diagnosis of fructose intolerance until the infant has improved with empirical treatment, by exclusion of sucrose and fructose from the diet (*see also* Chapter 91).

Chronic intrauterine infection

Recognition

Infants with jaundice due to chronic intrauterine infection (*see* page 649) usually have marked hepatosplenomegaly, with moderate anaemia, frequently have thrombocytopenia, and both fractions of bilirubin are increased. The infant may be poorly grown for the gestational age and the IgM will be increased.

Haemolytic anaemia due to a red cell defect

Recognition

1. There may be a family history of jaundice, anaemia and splenectomy or of drugs recently given to the mother or infant.
2. The infant is usually anaemic but splenomegaly is frequently absent.
3. The conditions to be considered are:
   (a) Hereditary spherocytosis (most common in Caucasians).
   (b) G-6PD deficiency, and other less common red cell abnormalities (e.g. pyruvate kinase deficiency).
   (c) Homozygous sickle cell disease (very rare) (*see* page 680).
4. Isoimmunization is first excluded by ABO and Rhesus grouping and a Coombs' test; the reticulocyte count is usually high. Spherocytosis is inherited as a dominant, but there is a significant spontaneous mutation rate or the affected parent may not have been detected. Even though the blood film may show numerous microspherocytes and there may be increased osmotic fragility, the results of these tests may be very difficult to interpret in the newborn period and the precise diagnosis may have to await further investigation after 3 months of age.
5. G-6PD deficiency (*see also* page 485) should be considered in infants of the following racial groups or origins:
   (a) African or West Indian origin.*
   (b) Mediterranean basin.**
   (c) Chinese,** especially from South China (Canton (Guanzhou) and Hong Kong) (Chan, Dodd and Tso, 1976).
   (d) Thailand.**
   (e) Hawaii.**
   (f) Israel.*
6. The infant with clinical haemolysis due to G-6PD deficiency may have a normal or low haemoglobin value. The reticulocyte count is usually raised but may be normal and the maximum bilirubin level occurs between the 2nd and 5th day of life but may be as late as the second week.

* Spontaneous haemolysis (i.e. haemolysis occurring without drugs) appears *not* to occur in these groups, though there is a high incidence of hyperbilirubinaemia in G-6PD-deficient preterm and occasionally term infants of African origin.
** These forms have spontaneous haemolysis in the neonatal period.

Management

1. An exchange transfusion may be necessary, whatever the diagnosis, for severe hyperbilirubinaemia, to prevent kernicterus.
2. Septicaemia: if proved or suspected, the infant should be treated with appropriate antibiotics by injection (*see* page 656).
3. If a metabolic disorder is suspected, all sugars metabolized to galactose or fructose should be excluded (i.e. lactose, sucrose and fructose). An infant maintained on oral or intravenous glucose with electrolytes, meets this criterion. Feeds should be resumed with an appropriate synthetic milk (*see* page 711).
4. Chronic intrauterine infections require supportive management (*see* page 650).
5. Haemolysis due to intrinsic red cell defect:
   (a) In G-6PD deficiency, all drugs likely to induce haemolysis should be avoided (*see Table 54.3*). Vitamin K_1 should not be given in a dose greater than 1.0 mg.
   (b) Exchange transfusion may be required particularly in preterm infants in whom there is an hereditary red cell defect. Phototherapy may be adequate in mature infants.

Phototherapy

Exposure of the infant to blue light photo-oxidizes bilirubin and increases the excretion rate of bilirubin, thereby slowing down the rate of rise of serum bilirubin and reducing the height of the peak level. Phototherapy prevents the need for exchange transfusion in term infants with exaggerated physiological jaundice but is no substitute for exchange transfusion in infants with active haemolysis. It may prevent the necessity for subsequent exchange transfusions in infants with severe haemolysis.

There is no indication to start phototherapy until the infant is clinically jaundiced. Phototherapy is usually started before the infant is expected to reach the level at which exchange transfusion would be indicated; phototherapy may be started at 50 per cent, or 85 μmol/ℓ (5 mg/100 ml) less than the exchange transfusion level, e.g.:

At term: start at 255 μmol/ℓ (15 mg/100 ml).
34 weeks: start at 188 μmol/ℓ (11 mg/100 ml).
30 weeks: start at 120 μmol/ℓ (7 mg/100 ml).

Management

1. The use of phototherapy does not preclude the necessity of reaching a diagnosis.
2. The babies should be protected by a safe and effective eye shield.
3. The procedure should be explained to the mother before phototherapy is started.
4. The infant's temperature should be carefully monitored every 4 hours.
5. An additional 10 per cent of extra fluid should be given to make up for increased insensible water losses and increased water loss in the stool.
6. Phototherapy should be stopped once the bilirubin level is demonstrably falling.

Conjugated hyperbilirubinaemia

Conjugated hyperbilirubinaemia with bile in the urine in the newborn period is always pathological and requires investigation.

Recognition

Conjugated hyperbilirubinaemia is usually an indication of significant liver disease, but the underlying cause may include:

1. Metabolic or endocrine disorders:
   (a) Galactosaemia.
   (b) Fructose intolerance.
   (c) Tyrosinaemia.
   (d) Hypopituitarism, often associated with septo-optic dysplasia (Kaufman *et al.*, 1984); micropenis in males.
2. (a) Chronic congenital infection.
   (b) Neonatal hepatitis.
3. Genetic:
   (a) α-1 antitrypsin deficiency.
   (b) Conjugated hyperbilirubinaemia of the North American Indian.
4. Biliary obstruction:
   (a) Biliary atresia.
   (b) Liver damage associated with total parenteral nutrition.
   (c) Choledochal cyst.

Management

Diagnosis and management of this situation is outside the scope of this book; because of the degree of liver disease usually involved parenteral vitamin K_1 is required to avoid the development of a haemorrhagic state.

References

CHAN, T. K., DODD, D. and TSO, S. C. (1976) Drug-induced haemolysis in glucose-6 phosphate dehydrogenase deficiency. *British Medical Journal,* **ii,** 1227–1229

KAUFMAN, F. R., COSTIN, G., THOMAS, D. W., SINATRA, F. R. and ROE, T. F. (1984) Cholestasis and hypopituitarism. *Archives of Disease in Children,* **59,** 787–789

Further reading

LEVINE, R. L., FREDERICKS, W. R. and RAPOPORT, S. I. (1982) Entry of bilirubin into the brain due to opening of the blood–brain barrier. *Pediatrics,* **69,** 255–259

LUCEY, J. F. (1982) Bilirubin and brain damage: a real mess. *Pediatrics,* **69,** 381–382

MAISELS, M. J. (1981) Neonatal jaundice. In G. P. Avery (ed.) *Neonatology,* pp. 474–544. New York: J. B. Lippincott

RITTER, D. A., KENNY, J. D., NORTON, H. J. and RUDOLPH, A. J. (1982) A prospective study of free bilirubin and other risk factors in the development of kernicterus in premature infants. *Pediatrics,* **69,** 260–266

SCHREINER, R. L. and GLICK, M. R. (1982) Interlaboratory bilirubin variability. *Pediatrics,* **69,** 277–281

TURKEL, S. B., MILLER, C. A., GUTTENBERG, M. E., MOYNES, D. R. and HODGMAN, J. E. (1982) A clinical pathological reappraisal of kernicterus. *Pediatrics,* **69,** 267–272

Chapter 86

Rhesus and other forms of isoimmunization

M. F. Whitfield and J. A. Black

Rhesus incompatibility

Recognition

Antenatally

All Rhesus negative women should be screened for antibodies early in pregnancy and from time to time throughout pregnancy; amniocentesis should be carried out in those with antibodies. If this policy is followed a reasonably accurate prediction of the occurrence and the severity of the haemolytic process will be made in all cases.

At delivery

The infant may have the following clinical appearance:

1. An apparently normal infant, usually with moderate hepatosplenomegaly.
2. An infant with jaundice in the first 24 hours (*see* page 683).
3. A severely affected infant with marked hepatosplenomegaly and pallor. Such infants may pose resuscitation problems because of anaemia.
4. Isoimmune hydrops with severe pallor, generalized oedema, with pleural effusion and ascites; such an infant may be difficult to resuscitate, requiring emergency abdominal paracentesis and thoracocentesis before responding (*see* page 700).

Confirmation of the diagnosis and prediction of severity

Confirmation of the diagnosis of Rhesus isoimmunization hinges on the result of the blood group, Coombs' test, haemoglobin and reticulocyte count and bilirubin tests, carried out preferably on cord blood, as this has specific predictive value. *Table 86.1* gives accepted criteria for management in term infants in whom there are no other contributory factors (*see* page 682).

Problems in the interpretation of cord blood results

1. A poor cord sample may give a falsely low haemoglobin reading due to haemolysis, clotting, or the inclusion of Wharton's jelly.

Table 86.1 Classification of infants by means of cord blood results

Rhesus group	*Coombs' test*	*Hb* (g/100 ml)	*Serum bilirubin* (μmol/ℓ (mg/100 ml))	*Category*	*Treatment*
Negative	Negative	Not required	Not required	Unaffected	None
Positive	Negative	Not required	Not required	Unaffected	None
Positive	Positive	>14, and →	50 (3) or less	Mild	Observe and repeat bilirubin at 4 hours and at intervals if jaundice develops
Positive	Positive	7–14 and →	>50 (>3)	Moderate to severe	Exchange transfusion within 4–6 hours
Positive	Positive	<7 or clinically hydropic	>50 (>3)	Very severe	Modified exchange

2. A false negative Rhesus result and a false negative direct Coombs' test may occur in some severely affected infants, or following intrauterine transfusions.
3. If maternal plasmaphoresis has been used to control maternal antibody level antenatally the predictive value of the cord results is not well established, particularly in infants where intrauterine transfusion has been used in addition. In this circumstance, some infants are still severely affected, while other infants, despite being Rhesus positive, appear to have very mild disease.

Assessment of an affected infant in the absence of a cord blood specimen

The tests indicated above should be carried out on a venous blood sample and sequential serum bilirubin estimations should be plotted against time to determine the rate of rise and timing of exchange transfusion if necessary (*see* pages 691–692).

MANAGEMENT

Supportive treatment – Steps should be made to reduce the effect of other factors likely to contribute to the severity of hyperbilirubinaemia (*see* page 682).

Phototherapy – This should never be relied upon to control the rise of serum bilirubin in severe Rhesus isoimmunization but may help mildly affected cases.

Exchange transfusion – *see* Chapter 87.

ABO incompatibility

ABO isoimmunization occurs in mother and baby pairs who are ABO incompatible, in whom the mother has IgG anti-A or anti-B haemolysins. ABO isoimmunization is not as severe as Rhesus isoimmunization, rarely causes jaundice in the first 24 hours, and the degree of jaundice is not usually severe enough to warrant exchange transfusion, although this may be required in preterm infants or infants with other aggravating factors.

Recognition

The mother is usually group O and the baby A,B, or AB. The infant has a normal haemoglobin or slight anaemia with a mild reticulocytosis; anti-A or anti-B hemolysins can be detected in maternal serum or coated onto the infant's red cells.

Management

Phototherapy

This is effective in the majority of cases.

Exchange transfusion

This may be required in severe cases and low birth weight infants. The blood to be used is often of a Rhesus group appropriate for the baby, but of group O; washed packed cells resuspended in fresh frozen plasma from AB blood eliminates the infusion of IgM anti-A and anti-B during the exchange.

Chapter 87

Exchange transfusion

M. F. Whitfield and J. A. Black

Although exchange transfusion is usually carried out for hyperbilirubinaemia, it may also be indicated in acute poisoning, inborn errors of metabolism, septicaemia and sclerema, polycythaemia with hyperviscosity syndrome, and in cases of severe anaemia with heart failure when the patient is felt to be incapable of tolerating any further circulatory volume load.

An exchange transfusion is a potentially dangerous procedure involving major fluid shifts and metabolic disturbances, and carries a significant morbidity rate and a 1–2 per cent incidence of sudden unexpected cardiac arrest even in experienced hands.

Indications for exchange transfusion in hyperbilirubinaemia

1. Rhesus isoimmunization based on cord blood predictions (*see* page 689).
2. On postnatal blood samples based on:
   (a) The serum bilirubin level exceeding an absolute critical value (*see* below).
   (b) The prediction that the serum bilirubin will exceed the critical value within 4 hours.
   (c) The rate of rise of serum bilirubin based on three estimations is greater than 8.5 μmol/ℓ (greater than 0.5 mg/100 ml/hour) or
   (d) Based on the predictive chart of Allen and Diamond (1958) (*Figure 87.1*).
3. Clinical evidence of kernicterus irrespective of the level of serum bilirubin.

One commonly accepted set of critical values for exchange transfusion (Swyer, 1975) is as follows:

At term: 340 μmol/ℓ (20 mg/100 ml).
At 36 weeks: 306 μmol/ℓ (18 mg/100 ml).
At 34 weeks: 272 μmol/ℓ (16 mg/100 ml).
At 32 weeks: 238 μmol/ℓ (14 mg/100 ml).
At 28–32 weeks: 205 μmol/ℓ (12 mg/100 ml).

The bilirubin levels given here refer to unconjugated bilirubin only, and it can be assumed that only in haemolytic conditions and in hepatic immaturity will the total bilirubin measured be wholly unconjugated. In infants severely affected by Rhesus isoimmunization there is occasionally a significant amount of conjugated bilirubin in the cord blood, or the amount of conjugated bilirubin may rise rapidly after delivery; in such cases unconjugated *and* conjugated bilirubin should be estimated

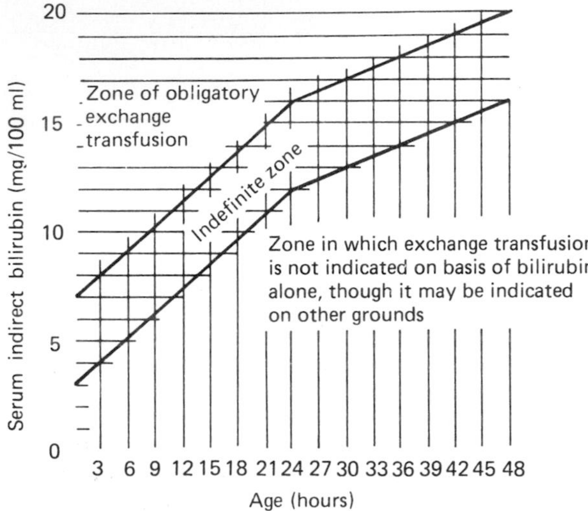

Figure 87.1 Guide to the use of serum indirect bilirubin as the sole criterion for exchange transfusion in mature infants. *Note:* 20 mg/100 ml = 340 µmol/ℓ. (Reproduced from Allen and Diamond (1958) with kind permission of authors and publishers)

to avoid unnecessary exchange transfusions. It is generally assumed that preterm infants and infants who have suffered from hypoxia, hypoglycaemia, septicaemia or other serious illness are at greater risk for the development of kernicterus. Although the above guidelines are considered safe, they are not based on sound scientific evidence and there is at present considerable debate regarding the pathogenesis of kernicterus and what constitutes an appropriate clinical response to a given serum bilirubin level in a specific infant.

Contraindications

A full exchange transfusion should not be done in hydropic infants or those who are severely anaemic (cord Hb <7.0 g/100 ml) with a central venous pressure greater than 12 cm H_2O. In such cases a partial (single volume) exchange should be done (*see* page 696).

Requirements

1. Blood: most blood banks now provide packed cells from citrate phosphate dextrose (CPD) blood, washed and reconstituted with fresh frozen plasma to a haematocrit of around 60 per cent. This preparation is less hyperosmolar than ACD blood and provides a lower acid and potassium load.
2. Whole concentrated or packed blood: if whole blood is provided some of the supernatant plasma should be removed before use and the blood should be preferably no more than 48 hours old, and certainly less than 5 days old.

3. Blood group: the blood should be cross-matched against the mother's serum and should be of the same ABO group as the infant, and Rhesus negative in all cases of Rhesus isoimmunization and all Rhesus negative infants requiring exchange transfusion for other reasons. In an emergency, O Rhesus negative blood can be used irrespective of the infant's ABO group provided that cross-matching is satisfactory.
4. Warming of the blood; the blood should be warmed during the exchange transfusion, using a commercial blood warmer or passed through a heating coil in a water bath at 37°C (98.6°F).
5. Volume of blood to be exchanged; in infants with hyperbilirubinaemia, normally a double volume (180 ml/kg) exchange should be carried out. Since an exchange transfusion is an exponential wash-out procedure, however, the first half of the exchange transfusion achieves most of the intended beneficial effects and in infants who do not tolerate the procedure well, a decision may have to be made to terminate the procedure after 85–100 ml/kg.

Preparation

1. Equipment; a complete list of the actual equipment is given in Appendix 22. It is important that the infant is nursed in a good light, preferably under a radiant overhead warmer and connected to cardiorespiratory monitor.
2. The infant's condition should be improved as much as possible before the exchange transfusion, particularly by correcting any blood gas abnormalities, and if it is anticipated that the infant will deteriorate with the handling required to carry out an exchange transfusion, serious thought should be given to prophylactic ventilation before the exchange transfusion. Feeds should be stopped 4 hours before the exchange and the stomach emptied by nasogastric aspiration before the transfusion begins.
3. Assistance; at least one assistant should be present to record the progress of the exchange and to confirm the cumulative blood volumes removed and transfused and to monitor the infant's response. Both operators should be aware of the 1–2 per cent chance of sudden unexpected cardiac arrest and have resuscitation equipment readily at hand.
4. Immobilization; the infant's limbs should be gently restrained to prevent dislodgement of the umbilical catheter.
5. Apparatus; the disposable exchange transfusion sets are safest and most convenient to use. A supply of heparinized saline should be available for rinsing out the tubing and syringes to prevent clotting (1 unit heparin/ml 0.9% NaCl).

Technique

Standard method

1. A piece of cord tape is loosely knotted around the base of the cord, and the umbilical cord divided about 2.5 cm (1 in) above its junction with the abdominal wall skin. A 5 or 8 FG catheter is connected to a three-way stopcock and a 10 ml syringe filled with heparinized saline and rinsed through to eliminate all air bubbles. The umbilical vein is identified and the catheter advanced a predetermined distance up the umbilical vein to bring the tip into the region of

the inferior vena cava above the diaphragm (*see Figure 87.2*). The actual position of the tip should be checked by X-ray or ultrasound. There should be a free flow of partly oxygenated blood through the catheter and when the catheter is found to be in a satisfactory position, it should be tied in, to prevent dislodgement. It is important to realize that with the tip of the catheter above the diaphragm, a sudden inspiratory effort by the infant will lead to sizeable venous air embolism if the catheter at any of its connections is permitted to be opened to atmospheric pressure. Central venous pressure may be measured using an umbilical vein catheter but this is not without risk of air embolism. Central venous pressure should be within 5–8 cm; if the pressure is higher than this a partial transfusion may be indicated.

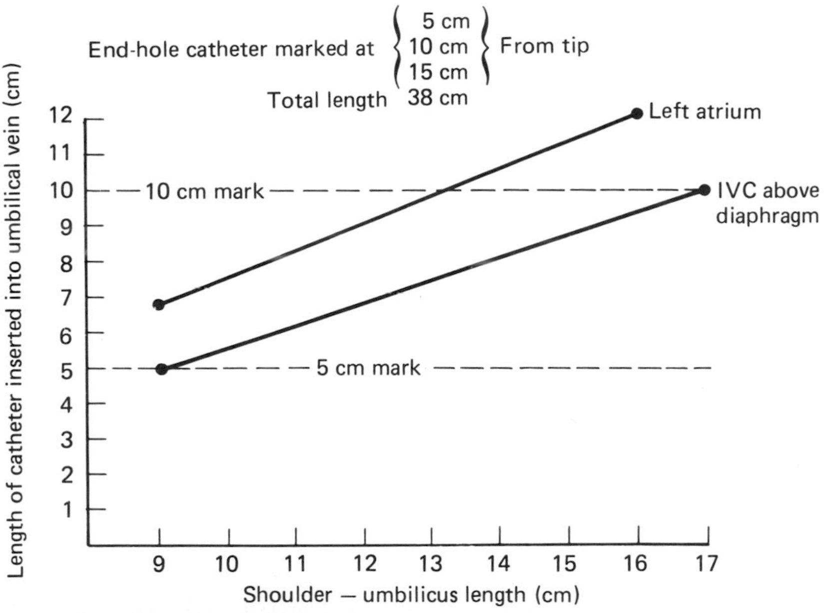

Figure 87.2 Umbilical vein catheterization. (Modified by M. A. Llewellyn from Dunn, in *Intensive Care of the Newly Born*. Swyer, p.188 (1975), by kind permission of publishers)

2. A 10 ml rather than a 20 ml syringe is preferable since the volume and pressure variation in the right atrium and the consequent fluctuations in the blood pressure are less. The use of the smaller syringe reduces the temptation to proceed too fast.
3. An initial blood sample should be retained for haemoglobin, bilirubin, and any other investigations that may be required, particularly if the reason for the severe jaundice is not yet known.
4. *Blood pH* – If washed, resuspended red cells made up with fresh frozen plasma is the blood source used for the exchange it is likely that no manipulation of pH will be required. However, if the initial pH is less than 7.2 the acidosis should be partly corrected by injection of 5 mmol sodium bicarbonate.
5. *Drugs* – Calcium gluconate is contraindicated as it is a potentially dangerous drug which has no lasting effect upon the infant's ionized calcium level. There is also no indication for digoxin, but frusemide may be used in hydropic infants or

those with a high CVP: dose 1 mg/kg IV. Infants receiving antibiotics should have the appropriate amounts of antibiotic added to the donor blood to produce the desired blood level in the baby, otherwise antibiotics will be washed out of the baby during the exchange transfusion.

6. *Duration of the procedure* – An exchange transfusion should not be completed in less than 1–1½ hours. A slow, gentle procedure which produces slower and less marked fluctuations in body chemistry will be better tolerated by an infant than a rapid procedure.
7. At the end of the transfusion, the umbilical vein catheter should be removed and the vein occluded by a ligature and purse-string suture around the base of the cord unless another transfusion is anticipated within the next 6 hours. The tip of the catheter should be sent for culture.

Difficulties in gaining central venous access for exchange transfusion

1. If there is difficulty in passing the catheter past the umbilical ring, this may be due to clots in the vein which may sometimes be sucked out by the syringe, on the end of the catheter. Difficulty may also be encountered owing to folding or narrowing of the vein; if this is so, the vein can usually be entered just before it passes upwards towards the liver. There are two approaches:
   (a) A vertical incision is made at 12 o'clock in the funnel of fibrous tissue at the base of the cord and the cut is extended upwards for 2–3 cm (about 1 in) into the skin of the abdomen. With gentle traction of the cord, the vein in its upward course usually becomes obvious. The vein is dissected free at its uppermost part and a 45° incision is made with fine-pointed scissors. A catheter can usually be passed upwards without any difficulty.
   (b) A crescentic incision is made about 1–2 cm (about ½ in) above the umbilicus and the underlying fascia is dissected until the vein is identified. This dissection is not easy since the peritoneum lies immediately beneath the vein and may be opened inadvertently. However, it can be sutured easily without appealing for surgical aid.
2. Use of the saphenous vein: this should be used only when all other approaches to the umbilical vessels have failed, or in the older child in whom the umbilical vessels are not available. A horizontal incision is made parallel to, but about 1 cm (½ in) below the inguinal fold medial to the femoral artery. The vein passes through the fascia at this point and joins the femoral vein. The saphenous vein is very small and a smaller than usual size of catheter may be required. The catheter should be passed up into the inferior vena cava in the usual way. Swelling of the leg is not uncommon after this procedure but appears to resolve without any evidence of permanent venous obstruction. The main danger of the saphenous vein approach is of uncontrollable venous oozing due to damage to the vein inside the fascia.

Exchange transfusion by the peripheral route

With this method, blood is withdrawn from an artery and returned to a major vein. The advantage of this procedure is that the umbilical vein is not used and that if blood is withdrawn from the artery at the same time as it is injected into the vein, there is no immediate circulating blood volume change and less fluctuation in central venous pressure and blood pressure. This may be of particular importance in low birth weight infants where blood pressure fluctuations are directly transmitted to the brain as fluctuations in intracranial pressure, which may be an important factor in the aetiology of intraventricular haemorrhage.

The arterial site for withdrawal may be the umbilical artery, if there is already umbilical arterial catheter *in situ* (*see* Chapter 93, page 728) or may be a radial or posterior tibial artery which may be cannulated using transillumination by someone experienced in this procedure. It is usually possible to insert a 21 or 22 FG Teflon venous catheter (Jelco or Abbocath) into a suitable vein on the back of the hand or into the long saphenous vein at the ankle. Withdrawals and infusions are carried out by two separate operators who synchronize their activities. The Arterial line should be rinsed with heparinized saline to prevent clotting. If venous and arterial access can be achieved, this technique can be an alternative to central exchange transfusion by the standard method and is more desirable than the alternative routes described above.

Care after exchange transfusion

1. Post-exchange levels of haemoglobin and bilirubin will indicate the effectiveness of the exchange transfusion but there is invariably a rebound rise at about 4 hours.
2. Hypoglycaemia is likely to occur in Rhesus infants (*see* page 460).
3. Repeat exchange transfusion may be required depending on the rate of rise of the serum bilirubin. In severely affected infants, obstructive jaundice may develop and the amount of conjugated bilirubin should be measured in addition to the total.
4. In cases of Rhesus isoimmunization follow-up should include weekly haemoglobin levels, and oral iron and folic acid from about 5 weeks of age onwards.

Late complications of exchange transfusion

1. *Sepsis* – This is more likely to occur as a result of prolonged retention of an umbilical catheter in the vein than from the exchange transfusion itself. Repeated exchanges increase the risk and some use prophylactic antibiotics for repeated exchange transfusions. Evidence of infection is usually seen 12–24 hours after the exchange transfusion.
2. *Portal thrombosis* – This may be a complication of septic thrombophlebitis of the portal vein, or it may occur without obvious infection. The infant has gross splenomegaly accompanied by prolonged obstructive jaundice and moderate hepatomegaly. It is usually advisable to treat with antibiotics because of the risk of an infective element. The involvement of exchange transfusion in the aetiology of necrotizing enterocolitis (*see* page 367) is debated but the two problems are frequently associated. The first sign is usually the passage of blood *per rectum*.

Partial exchange transfusion

Indications

1. *Hydrops;* in a severely ill infant, with chronic anaemia from any cause, with a high CVP.

2. Exchange transfusion for polycythaemia (*see* below).
3. Exchange transfusion for septicaemia.

Management

Hydropic and anaemic infants (see also page 700)

Concentrated or packed red cells should be used, of the same ABO group as the infant; Rhesus negative blood should be used in Rhesus isoimmunization, in Rhesus negative infants with other conditions, or in an extreme emergency after a rapid cross-match. If the CVP is greater than 12 cm the initial pressure should be recorded, and frusemide given IV or i.m. The transfusion is then started by the removal of 20 ml of blood and its replacement by 10 ml of donor blood. The venous pressure is measured again. A 10 ml deficit is left after each cycle and the CVP recorded until it is between 5 and 8 cm, by which time a cumulative deficit of 40–80 ml of blood will have been achieved. This procedure alleviates the infant's heart failure and raises the haemoglobin. The infant should be allowed to recover and conventional exchange transfusion is carried out later, based on the rate of bilirubin rise.

If the CVP is less than 5 cm the circulating volume should be expanded by incremental transfusion, taking 10 ml out and replacing with 20 ml donor blood. This is continued until the CVP is between 5 and 8 cm.

Polycythaemia (see below)

A dilutional exchange transfusion is carried out by replacing the infant's blood with plasma or dextran. The volume to be exchanged is between 15 and 25 ml/kg.

Septicaemia

There is inconclusive evidence that exchange transfusion may improve the survival rate in infants with fulminating septicaemia, presumably by removing endotoxin, replenishing opsonin and complement levels, and correcting coagulation abnormalities due to disseminated intravascular coagulation. Infants with severe respiratory problems may be benefited by the more favourable oxygen dissociation curve of adult haemoglobin compared with fetal haemoglobin. Under these circumstances a single volume exchange should be done using fresh whole blood, if possible. Consideration should also be given to 'topping up' the infant with fresh frozen plasma, platelets and perhaps white cells at the end of the exchange.

Polycythaemia

Polycythaemia (a venous PCV greater than 65 per cent) may be a serious problem due to the increase in the blood viscosity, when the packed cell volume rises above this value. Such infants appear cyanosed, and develop symptoms and disorders related to poor perfusion and cardiac decompensation; these include lethargy, irritability, seizures, poor perfusion, heart failure, poor renal output. At autopsy, such infants have been found to have sludging in the cerebral sinuses, and sinus thrombosis, and have an increased risk of necrotizing enterocolitis. Polycythaemia, thrombocytopenia, and hypoglycaemia tend to occur together, so that the infant with polycythaemia should be investigated for the other two disorders as soon as the need is recognized (Hathaway, 1983).

Recognition

Polycythaemia and hyperviscosity are most likely to occur in:

1. The infant of a diabetic mother.
2. SGA infant or post-mature infants.
3. In identical twins due to twin-to-twin transfusion.
4. Delayed cord clamping with the infant lower than the placenta may be a factor in causing polycythaemia.

A capillary PCV should be carried out in all infants at risk and if this is found to be greater than 65 per cent the infant must be given an adequate fluid intake to prevent dehydration and a further increase in PCV; a venous PCV should be determined and if this is greater than 65 per cent a dilutional exchange should be done (*see* above); this should be carried out before symptoms have developed. Recent studies underline the importance on behaviour and development in the first year of life of adequate treatment of polycythaemia (Black *et al.*, 1982; Goldberg *et al.*, 1982).

Religious objections to transfusion and refusal of consent

Depending on the unit, a formal, signed consent form may be required for exchange transfusion; at the least, verbal consent must be obtained and the indications for the exchange transfusion explained to the parents, emphasizing the fact that the procedure is less hazardous than the problem for which the procedure is to be carried out. On rare occasions this may be refused owing to the parent's religious beliefs. This situation can usually be foreseen and parental rights may have to be taken by the local Social Work department for the infant. This is enacted by obtaining a Place of Safety Order under the Children and Young Persons Act (1969), as for children who are neglected or injured by their parents. Under these circumstances it is usual practice to obtain a written statement in the infant's notes that the exchange transfusion is necessary and a life-saving procedure to be carried out as an emergency, signed by the consultant in charge of the patient's case and also by another consultant who has reviewed the patient and the situation. The hospital administration and possibly the doctor's defence association should also be consulted.

References

ALLEN, F. H. and DIAMOND, L. K. (1958) *Erythroblastosis Foetalis, Including Exchange Transfusion Technique*. Boston: Little, Brown

BLACK, V. D., LUBCHENKO, L. O., LUCKEY, D. W. *et al.* (1982) Developmental and neurological sequelae of neonatal hyperviscosity syndrome. *Pediatrics,* **69,** 426–431

GOLDBERG, K., WIRTH, F. H., HATHAWAY, W. E. *et al.* (1982) Neonatal hyperviscosity II: Effect of partial plasma exchange. *Pediatrics,* **69,** 419–425

HATHAWAY, W. E. (1983) Neonatal hyperviscosity. *Pediatrics,* **72,** 567–568

MAISELS, M. J. (1972) Bilirubin; on understanding and influencing its metabolism in the newborn infant. *Pediatric Clinics of North America,* **19,** 447

SWYER, P. R. (1975) *Intensive Care of the Newly Born,* pp. 147 and 188. Basle: S. Karger

Chapter 88

Neonatal hydrops

M. F. Whitfield

Hydrops fetalis exists when there is excess fluid subcutaneously, in the body cavities, and in the placenta. The ultrasound appearances *in utero* are characteristic and easily recognizable. The management of such a pregnancy and of the infant at delivery and during the first week of life, presents considerable problems. The mother should be transferred to the regional perinatal centre as soon as the diagnosis is suspected, and if an infant has to be transferred, the situation should be discussed both at the obstetric and neonatal level with the perinatal centre staff. Although in the past the majority of infants with hydrops were Rhesus isoimmunized, with effective Rhesus prevention programmes the majority of cases now are 'non-immune hydrops'. The differential diagnosis of hydrops is complex and if possible a diagnosis should be made before delivery.

Differential diagnosis (this does not include extreme rarities)

1. Anaemia; usually Rhesus isoimmunization or chronic fetomaternal haemorrhage, feto-fetal transfusion; in Oriental races, α-thalassaemia.
2. Cardiovascular – There may be an obstructive heart lesion or tachy- or brady-arrhythmias. Wolf–Parkinson–White syndrome is a common cause of tachyarrhythmias, and maternal systemic lupus should be considered if there is fetal heart block.
3. Intrauterine infection, commonly toxoplasmosis or cytomegalovirus.
4. Major pulmonary malformations.
5. Major renal malformations including renal vein thrombosis.
6. Multisystem abnormalities and syndromes including trisomy E, Turner's syndrome, achondroplasia, tuberose sclerosis, storage diseases.
7. Intrauterine intra-abdominal catastrophes including meconium peritonitis and volvulus.
8. Placental abnormalities including umbilical or chorionic vein thrombosis.

In addition to this differential diagnosis, in many cases the cause remains unknown. In practical terms, antenatal investigations include serological investigations to exclude congenital infection, haematological investigation of the mother to exclude Rhesus isoimmunization and chronic fetomaternal haemorrhage, fetal ECG and fetal ultrasound examination to assess fetal heart rhythm and the presence of major intracardiac defects. The possibility of digitalization of the mother, and hence the infant in fetal tachyarrhythmia should be considered. One unit of O Rhesus negative packed cells should be available at delivery where anaemia is suspected, along with exchange transfusion equipment. Equipment must also be available for emergency abdominal and chest paracentesis.

Recognition

The infant is obviously oedematous, may be clinically anaemic (but this is difficult to assess by inspection) and the abdomen is usually very protuberant. The severest cases have 'cauliflower' ears because of long-standing subcutaneous oedema.

Management

1. Full-scale resuscitation should be started as soon as the infant is delivered, including intubation and IPPV with 100% oxygen and heart rate monitoring (*see* page 614). A high inspiratory pressure is frequently required because of poor lung compliance (30–50 cm H_2O).
2. If the heart rate does not improve after 1 minute, emergency paracentesis of the abdomen in the right lower quadrant should be undertaken using a 20 ml syringe, three-way stopcock, and 18 gauge Teflon catheter (e.g. Abbocath or Jelco).
3. Bilateral chest paracentesis may also be required. Precautions should be taken not to cause pneumothorax. Ultrasound examination immediately before delivery may provide useful information about the presence and volume of fluid in both sides of the chest and the abdomen.
4. If the infant has Rhesus isoimmunization or anaemia from some other cause a cautious partial exchange with packed cells should be carried out with attention to the CVP (*see* page 696).
5. If there is a persisting tachyarrhythmia, emergency cardioversion may be required.
6. Failure to respond to the above management in the first half hour suggests that the infant may have hypoplastic lungs as a result of chronic pleural effusion *in utero*, or other intrinsic pulmonary disease.
7. The infant should be stabilized in an intensive care unit, with insertion of an umbilical arterial catheter, a chest X-ray, and the appropriate investigations initiated.
8. Respiratory management is usually difficult because of lung fluid and possible pulmonary hypoplasia.
9. Fluid intake should be conservative (40 ml/kg daily) usually 10% glucose, provided the blood glucose is maintained. No additional sodium should be given in the first few days, apart from sodium bicarbonate as required.
10. Frequent albumin infusions are of value in mobilizing tissue fluids.

Further reading

ETCHES, P. and LEMMONS, J. (1979) Non-immune hydrops fetalis: Report of 22 cases including 3 siblings. *Pediatrics,* **64,** 326–331

Chapter 89

Convulsions in the newborn*

M. F. Whitfield and J. A. Black

Recognition

Although convulsions in the newborn may be easy to recognize as classical tonic–clonic convulsions, or as Jacksonian fits starting in one limb and spreading to the rest of the body as a rhythmical jerking movement, more often the signs of a convulsion are subtle and difficult to recognize, particularly in the premature newborn, even by experienced medical or nursing staff. Signs which should suggest the possibility of convulsions are: cyanotic or apnoeic episodes, inexplicably fluctuating neurological signs, jerking eye movements, rhythmical blinking, rhythmical tongue protrusion, and lip smacking. It is often difficult to interpret these signs unless it is possible to observe the infant's behaviour when connected to an EEG machine. During a convulsion, the infant may or may not apparently lose consciousness, and there appears to be a continuum from normal behaviour with normal muscle tone to irritability and jitteriness, going on to rhythmical jerking in response to stimulation, eventually giving rise to convulsions without any initiating stimulus. The clinical localization of the seizure is of little prognostic value in anticipating ultimate outcome, or lateralization of possible neurological damage in later life.

It is important to recognize that in premature infants, uncoordinated movements, which are not convulsions involve jerking movements of one or more limbs, but these jerkings are not rhythmical or synchronized. Preterm infants also can be observed to have jerky eye movements during rapid eye movement sleep; premature infants are in this state for long periods.

Causes of convulsions

In the newborn, metabolic disturbances are more important than in older children both as primary initiators of convulsions, and as secondary effects of continued convulsions acting to prolong the convulsive state. Any infant suspected of having convulsions should therefore have blood glucose, serum calcium and magnesium and sodium levels measured.

* *See also* Chapter 28.

During the first 48 hours

1. Hypoxic ischaemic encephalopathy with cerebral oedema following severe perinatal asphyxia; the infant is abnormal from birth with abnormal neurological signs most evident as hypo- or hypertonia.
2. Mechanically difficult or precipitate delivery may cause venous sinus rupture, subarachnoid or subdural haemorrhage.
3. Hypoglycaemia in SGA infants, the smaller of twins, the infant of a diabetic mother. Hypoglycaemia may also occur in the asphyxiated infant.
4. Hypocalcaemia is likely to occur in sick, asphyxiated or premature infants, and in the baby of a diabetic mother, or may be due to maternal hyperparathyroidism or primary hyperparathyroidism in the infant.
5. Narcotic abstinence syndrome (*see* page 717).
6. Pyridoxine dependency is a rare cause of convulsions presenting during or after the first 48 hours. The fits are unresponsive to anticonvulsants but respond to pyridoxine. Pyridoxine should be given under EEG control (*see* page 715).
7. Early meningitis due to chorioamnionitis, usually associated with prolonged ruptured membranes.
8. Intrauterine infection with cytomegalovirus, toxoplasmosis or rubella.
9. Structural brain abnormalities.

3–4 days after delivery

1. In a small preterm infant particularly with hyaline membrane disease accompanied by pneumothorax, intraventricular haemorrhage with or without intracerebral extension is the most likely cause.
2. Hypocalcaemia and hypomagnesaemia in the infant of a diabetic mother.
3. Meningitis.
4. Structural brain abnormalities.
5. Inborn errors of metabolism (*see* Chapter 91).

4 days onwards

1. Meningitis.
2. Late hypocalcaemia in infants fed on unmodified cows' milk (this is now extremely rare with most currently available infant formulae).

Investigations

Lumbar puncture

Meningitis must be excluded in all infants having convulsions in the newborn period. The fluid may be blood-stained in meningitis or due to intracranial haemorrhage, and CSF protein and glucose should be measured in addition to Gram stain and culture. CSF and urine should be sent for the latex group B streptococcal antigen coagglutination test, if this is available, as it can provide an accurate diagnosis within hours, particularly in infants who have partially treated meningitis.

Biochemical screening

Blood glucose, serum calcium, magnesium and sodium should be measured. Dextrostix can be used as a quick screening procedure for hypoglycaemia but a formal blood glucose should be documented in all infants having convulsions.

Brain imaging

In preterm infants intraventricular haemorrhage and haemorrhagic infarction are readily identified by ultrasound sector-scanning through the anterior fontanelle. Seizures are unusual unless the haemorrhage is Papile Grade 3 or 4 on one side at least. In asphyxiated term infants, CT scan is the preferred technique and is most likely to show an abnormality at around 3–4 days of age. CT scanning is also useful for infants suspected of having a loculated intracranial haemorrhage. Radionuclide scanning may show parasagittal watershed lesions in asphyxiated term infants also, which may not be shown up by CT scanning. In the future nuclear magnetic resonance (NMR) scanning is likely to provide accurate anatomical location of lesions inadequately visualized by presently available techniques.

Exclusion of septicaemia

Consideration should be given to the possibility that the infant may have septicaemia as a cause of several metabolic upsets which have led to convulsions, without frank meningitis; a full infection screen may be indicated, followed by antibiotic treatment.

Continued fits resistant to anticonvulsants

The following additional investigations may be contemplated:

1. Injection of a test dosage of pyridoxine (100 mg IV), preferably under continuous EEG control, to exclude pyridoxine dependency (*see also* Chapter 91, page 715).
2. Blood and urine aminoacid determination and collection of urine for organic acids, and discussion with the laboratory about the advisability of doing a blood ammonia level (*see* pages 709–710).
3. Examination of blood and urine to exclude congenital infections.

Management

1. An adequate airway must be maintained by suction and positioning the baby in the semi-prone position and feeds should be temporarily stopped, as such infants are very likely to aspirate milk or secretions into the lungs. The baby should be given oxygen if cyanosed and blood gases monitored. If respiration is irregular and the baby's blood gas status is unsatisfactory the airway can be secured and the respiratory status improved by intubation and IPPV.
2. Metabolic defects such as hypocalcaemia, hypomagnesaemia, hypoglycaemia and hyponatraemia should be corrected.
3. Anticonvulsant therapy – Phenobarbitone (IV) is considered the anticonvulsant of first choice in the newborn period. A loading dose of 20 mg/kg is given in two

10 mg/kg aliquots over 5–10 minutes, separated by 20–30 minutes. If the infant is still convulsing after the first dose, the second dose should be given without the 20–30 minute delay. The maintenance dose is 3–4 mg/kg/24 hours in two divided doses, starting 12 hours after giving the loading dose. Adequacy of dosage and early recognition of overdosage should be monitored by blood levels. The therapeutic level is 20–30 μg/ml. If an adequate dose of phenobarbitone is unsuccessful in controlling convulsions, phenytoin should be added, using a loading dose of 20 mg/kg over 5–10 minutes, followed by maintenance of 3–4 mg/kg/24 hours in two divided doses, beginning 12 hours after the loading dose. The therapeutic blood level is around 15 μg/ml. If seizures continue despite adequate loading with phenytoin and phenobarbitone, continuous paraldehyde infusion intravenously may be added. Paraldehyde 5 ml is added to glucose 100 ml (5%) and the infusion is run at 1–4 ml/kg/hour.

4. Continuing seizures unresponsive to the above treatment may prove impossible to control. Reduction of cerebral oedema by mannitol (20%), in a dose of 1–2 g/kg IV over 45–90 min, preceded by a test dose of 1 ml/kg over 5 min IV may help. Another method of reducing intracranial pressure is deliberate hyperventilation down to PCO_2 levels below 35 mm Hg (4.7 kPa). The efficacy and long-term consequences of these procedures have not yet been adequately evaluated (*see also* Chapter 26, Raised intracranial pressure, and Chapter 71).
5. Seizures due to hypoxic ischaemic encephalopathy should be managed as above.
6. Hypoglycaemic convulsions (*see* page 460).
7. Hypocalcaemic convulsions (*see* page 134).
8. Meningitis (*see* page 335).
9. Intracranial haemorrhage (*see* page 628).

Further reading

FITZHARDINGE, P. M., FLODMARK, O., FITZ, C. R. and ASHBY, S. (1981) The prognostic value of computed tomography as an adjunct to assessment of the full term infant with post asphyxial encephalopathy. *Journal of Pediatrics,* **99,** 777–785

FITZHARDINGE, P. M., FLODMARK, O., FITZ, C. R. and ASHBY, S. (1982) The prognostic value of computed tomography of the brain in asphyxiated premature infants. *Journal of Pediatrics,* **100,** 476–481

PAPILE, L.-A., BURSTEIN, J., BURSTEIN, R. and KOFFLER, H. (1978) Incidence and evolution of subependymal and intraventricular hemorrhage; a study of infants with birth weights less than 1500 g. *Journal of Pediatrics,* **92,** 529–534

SWYER, P. R. (1975) *The Intensive Care of the Newly Born,* p. 152. Basle: S. Karger

Chapter 90

Infant of the diabetic mother

M. F. Whitfield

Pregnancy with diabetes constitutes a high-risk pregnancy and the infant of the diabetic mother (IDM) is at high risk, requiring special observation in the immediate neonatal period. The IDM is classically macrosomic and the birth of an infant of more than 4.5 kg suggests that the mother is pre-diabetic even though abnormal glucose tolerance may not have been documented before or during pregnancy. With careful pre-pregnant and antenatal management by a combined team of obstetric and diabetic specialists, a normally grown infant can be produced without any greater neonatal problems than normal term infants.

Recognition

Maternal history

A history of diabetes before the pregnancy, or abnormal glucose tolerance requiring treatment by diet or insulin during the pregnancy, must be recorded in the mother's records. Particular attention should be paid to the use of oral hypoglycaemic agents during pregnancy, as IDMs born to mothers receiving these drugs may develop severe hypoglycaemia lasting 4 or 5 days. For this reason, oral hypoglycaemics are not used during pregnancy. At delivery, the infant may be obviously macrosomic; or may be of normal appearance with weight appropriate for gestational age; or, particularly where there have been pregnancy complications or the mother has vascular complications of diabetes, the baby may be small for gestational age. This last group is probably at greatest risk of hypoglycaemia and neurological injury.

Macrosomia (greater than 4.5 kg at term)

There may or may not be any indication that the mother has diabetes but a macrosomic infant above the 90th percentile in weight for gestational age should be managed as an infant of a diabetic mother.

Possible problems in the IDM

1. Increased prematurity rate due to obstetric complications such as polyhydramnios, pregnancy induced hypertension, and abruption, all of which are more common in diabetic pregnancies.

2. Macrosomia: this increases the risk of delivery problems such as shoulder dystocia and asphyxia.
3. Hypoglycaemia; hyperinsulinaemia coupled with low glucagon and catecholamine levels induces reduced glucose production from the liver in the face of a high glucose utilization rate. Maintenance of the blood glucose is dependent on gluconeogenesis, which is diminished.
4. Respiratory distress syndrome:
   (a) There is an increased incidence of transient tachypnoea of the newborn.
   (b) Hyaline membrane disease is more frequent and more severe, due to a delay in the appearance of phosphatidyl glycerol (PG), one of the components of surfactant, even though the lecithin production may be adequate as reflected by a mature lecithin/sphingomyelin (L/S) ratio. Hyaline membrane disease may occur in a term infant who is an IDM.
5. Malformations. There is about a four times increase in major malformations, including vertebral and rib abnormalities, seen in its most severe form as the caudal deletion syndrome (sacral agenesis) which has a 600 times increased incidence over normals and is present in 1 per cent of IDMs. There is an increased incidence in neural tube defects and of congenital heart disease, transposition of the great vessels, ventricular septal defect, and coarctation of the aorta being the most common. Transient septal hypertrophy with ventricular outflow obstruction is a temporary echocardiogram finding in some IDMs.
6. Polycythaemia and hyperviscosity syndrome – Thirty four per cent of all IDMs have a PVC greater than 70 per cent in the first 8 hours, and this is frequently associated with thrombocytopenia and hypoglycaemia (*see* page 697).
7. Hypocalcaemia, hypomagnesaemia or both (*see* pages 133 and 138).
8. Jaundice (*see* page 682).
9. Renal vein thrombosis (*see also* pages 673 and 674). Renal vein thrombosis is common in IDMs, and presents with fever, vomiting, haematuria and proteinuria, and deterioration in renal function. Venous thrombosis may occur in other sites, e.g. adrenal and lung. It is not clear whether this is related to polycythaemia or has other causes.

Management

A watchful approach is adopted, looking for the problems outlined above. In the absence of asphyxia and respiratory problems maintenance of the blood glucose is the most pressing problem in the first few hours after delivery.

1. Early initiation of milk feeds within the first 2–3 hours. Use of normal baby formula will prevent hypoglycaemia in the majority of infants, tends to damp down insulin–glucose oscillations and favours a switchover to fat metabolism and gluconeogenesis. Feeds should be started at 60 ml/kg daily and increased to 150 ml/kg daily by the 4th day. There is little place for 10% glucose orally as it is slowly absorbed and delays gastric emptying.
2. The blood glucose should be monitored by formal blood measurements or a quick method such as Dextrostix using a glucometer, or Chemistrips or equivalent during the first 48 hours and should be monitored 1–2 hourly until feeding is well established. The aim is to maintain the blood glucose above 1.7 mmol/ℓ (>30 mg/100 ml).

3. If: (a) the infant develops signs of clinical hypoglycaemia or (b) the blood glucose level is less than 1.7 mmol/ℓ (<30 mg/100 ml) with or without symptoms, the blood glucose should be repeated and the infant started on 10% glucose 60 ml/kg daily (glucose 4 mg/kg/minute)* as a continuous infusion, in addition to continuation of oral milk feeds. Large intravenous boluses of glucose should be avoided. In a severely symptomatic hypoglycaemic infant, symptoms may be abolished by delivering around 3 ml/kg 10% glucose in addition to the calculated infusion rate during the first half hour of the infusion.
4. If the blood glucose is still low 1–1½ hours after commencing the infusion, the rate should be increased to 6 mg/kg/minute (90 ml/kg daily).
5. If the blood glucose continues to remain low, glucagon 1 mg daily should be given as a continuous infusion in addition to the current glucose infusion rate. The purpose of adding glucagon is not to stimulate glycogenolysis but to normalize the insulin/glucagon ratio to favour gluconeogenesis from glycerol, alanine and acetylCoA. After giving glucagon it is usually possible to reduce gradually the glucose infusion rate to 4 mg/kg/minute. Further reductions in the glucose infusion rate should not be made until the infant is tolerating 150 ml/kg daily of milk orally.
6. Other anticipated problems which occur should be managed as outlined in the appropriate chapters.

Further reading

DIGNAN, P. S. (1981) Teratogenic risk and counselling in diabetes. *Clinical Obstetrics and Gynecology,* **24,** 149–159

DAY, R. E. and INSLEY, J. (1976) Maternal diabetes mellitus and congenital malformation: survey of 205 cases. *Archives of Disease in Childhood,* **51,** 935–938

CUMMINS, M. and NORRISH, M. (1980) Follow-up of children of diabetic mothers. *Archives of Disease in Childhood,* **55,** 259–264

TSANG, R. C., BALLARD, J. and BROWN, C. (1981) The infant of the diabetic mother: Today and tomorrow. *Clinical Obstetrics and Gynecology,* **24,** 125–147

* 1 mg glucose is contained in 0.01 ml 10% glucose.

Chapter 91

Acute neonatal illness in inborn errors of metabolism

D. M. Danks

The diagnosis of an inborn error of metabolism (IEM) in an acutely ill newborn infant depends upon constant alertness to this possibility, correct interpretation of the clinical course of the illness, and ready availability of effective investigation. Every neonatal unit should know the nearest centre where specimens, and if necessary the infant, can be sent. Even the best laboratory must receive some guidance from the paediatrician about appropriate investigation, in the form of adequate clinical information.

The number of IEM known to be capable of causing death, or irreversible brain damage, in the newborn period has increased steadily over the last 25 years. Diagnosis of those conditions for which effective treatment is available must take special priority. However, correct diagnosis is important even when treatment cannot be offered because the parents can be warned of the risk of further affected children and because intrauterine diagnosis may be possible in future pregnancies.

It is therefore important that neonatal paediatricians should remember these conditions and know how to look for them in the appropriate patients.

Infants to investigate

1. Infants with any symptom or symptoms which could be caused by an IEM.
2. Sibs of an infant known to have had a specific IEM.
3. Sibs of infants which have died in the neonatal period without a satisfactory diagnosis or with symptoms which in retrospect suggest an IEM.
4. Infants discovered to have an IEM on routine screening.

Recognition

1. The symptoms of IEM are mainly non-specific and may equally be due to more common causes such as in birth trauma, hypoxia and infection. Suggestive symptoms are:
   Refusal of feeds, drowsiness, respiratory failure, jaundice, vomiting, diarrhoea, unconsciousness, convulsions, abnormal muscle tone, tachypnoea (metabolic acidosis), haemorrhagic tendency, pulmonary haemorrhage.

2. Development of symptoms after a period of normal performance lasting 12–72 hours is more characteristic than the symptoms themselves. The majority of the treatable IEM, and many of those that cannot be treated, have little effect upon the fetus because placental haemodialysis is generally very efficient. Once symptoms do develop they usually increase progressively in the absence of effective treatment. By contrast, many of the non-genetic causes of acute neonatal illness produce symptoms at or very soon after birth, and the progression of symptoms is not so relentless.
3. Symptoms are present at and before birth in a few IEM:
   (a) Severe hypotonia in non-ketotic hyperglycinaemia.
   (b) Pyridoxine-dependent convulsions which may start *in utero* but nevertheless have a good outcome with early treatment.
   (c) Some lysosomal storage diseases may cause hydrops fetalis.
4. Improvement with treatment involving stopping oral feeds may be the first clue.

Clinical improvement may follow treatment instituted for a quite different reason which happens to have a beneficial effect on the IEM. For instance, a very sick baby with probable septicaemia may be taken off oral feeds and given intravenous fluid and antibiotics. Dramatic improvement may occur and may be attributed to the antibiotics and not to the incidental withdrawal of galactose. Some patients with galactosaemia present in this manner and may be re-fed milk with serious consequences (Oberklaid, Danks and Davies, 1976).

Expertise in the diagnosis of these conditions must be centralized in a small number of specialized metabolic units. Otherwise no one will have the experience which is essential for the development of expertise. It is not just a matter of performing a number of laboratory tests. Correct interpretation of the results of these tests is vital. Specialized units need to be distributed within a country so that they are accessible to all patients. The initial tests must be performed on samples sent to a central laboratory where quick and efficient reporting of results is essential.

The following tests are now employed to detect unusual metabolites or unusual amounts of normal metabolites:

1. Colour reactions to recognize organic radicals; e.g. tests for ketone bodies, for ketoacids, for reducing substances, etc.
2. Rapid methods of screening for aminoacids in urine and serum by high voltage electrophoresis (HVE) and thin layer chromatography (TLC).
3. Gas-liquid chromatography (GLC) for identification of organic acids and of short-chain fatty acids (Goodman and Markey, 1981).
4. High performance liquid chromatography (HPLC) of CSF organic acids.
5. Quantitative determination of aminoacids in plasma or CSF.
6. Gas chromatography–mass spectrometry (GC-MS) is a method of identifying a compound which has been detected by GLC.

It has been usual to apply these techniques to urine and serum. Testing of CSF has proved valuable in our experience, allowing prompt diagnosis of glycine encephalopathy (non-ketotic hyperglycinaemia), of some other disorders of aminoacid neurotransmitters and of forms of lactic acidosis involving principally the brain.

Management

Emergency treatment in suspected IEM

A newborn baby with acute dangerous symptoms must be treated empirically while awaiting laboratory results, or when attempts to make a diagnosis have been unsuccessful. Since most of the relevant conditions are caused by defects in catabolic pathways it is essential to prevent a catabolic state and if possible to initiate anabolism. This is certainly possible in some of the known defects, e.g. hyperammonaemia, and it is reasonable to treat unknown defects on this assumption.

Empirical treatment with vitamins (*Table 91.1*)

Some of the acute IEM are vitamin responsive and there is some justification for blind use of massive doses of all water-soluble vitamins in the hope that the defect present may respond to one of them.

Table 91.1 Some of the IEM that may cause severe illness in the newborn period

Disease	*Methods of detection*	*Vitamin responsiveness in some cases*	*Inheritance*
Carbamyl phosphate synthetase deficiency	Blood ammonia	Nil	AR
Ornithine transcarbamylase deficiency	Blood ammonia	Nil	XL
Citrullinaemia	Blood ammonia HVE of urine or serum	Nil	AR
Other forms of hyperammonaemia	Blood ammonia HVE of urine or serum	Nil	AR
Propionic acidaemia	Metabolic acidosis GLC of urine	Nil	AR
Methylmalonic acidaemia	Metabolic acidosis GLC of urine	B_{12}	AR
Maple-syrup urine disease	Metabolic acidosis HVE of urine or serum GLC of urine	Thiamine*	AR
Isovaleric acidaemia	Metabolic acidosis GLC of urine	Nil	AR
Non-ketotic hyperglycinaemia	Clinical features HVE of urine and serum	Nil	AR
Galactosaemia	Clinical features Glycosuria	Nil	AR
Hereditary fructose intolerance	Clinical features Glycosuria	Nil	AR
Pyridoxine-dependent convulsions	Clinical features Therapeutic response	Pyridoxine	AR
Congenital lactic acidosis	Metabolic acidosis GLC of urine	Thiamine*	

* Noted only in mild cases presenting later in childhood.
XL = X-linked; AR = autosomal recessive; GLC = gas–liquid chromatography; HVE = high-voltage electrophoresis.

Exchange transfusion

Exchange transfusion and/or peritoneal dialysis can have both therapeutic and diagnostic value. Most of the diseases concerned produce their effects through accumulation of a circulating metabolite, and artificial removal of this metabolism may allow the baby to recover. Conversely a dramatic response to exchange transfusion or peritoneal dialysis may provide a clue to the existence of an IEM. It is even possible that these measures may allow a baby with an undiagnosed IEM to recover and that empirical dietary treatment may keep the baby alive in satisfactory condition.

Detailed management

Termination of catabolism

This requires a high calorie intake and subsequently the provision of exactly the amounts of aminoacids needed for growth.

The regimen suggested involves feeding glucose plus glucose polymer (Caloreen, Scientific Hospital Supplies*) orally or by intragastric tube to the maximum level of intestinal tolerance (generally a 5 per cent concentration of each) and/or feeding of a similar amount of glucose intravenously. If the glucose is given intravenously administration is monitored by repeated testing of urine for glucose and/or by intermittent measurement of blood glucose. If urine flow is adequate glucosuria will occur before dangerous levels of hyperglycaemia result. It is important to remember that hyperglycaemia can be dangerous through its osmotic effects.

It is very difficult to provide a sufficient caloric intake with glucose alone, and lipid must be added at a fairly early stage. We generally find that administration of lipid by the intragastric route is sufficient. We have used either medium chain triglyceride (MCT) oil or the more complex fats present in a commercially available powdered preparation which contains glucose, emulsified fat, minerals and vitamins (Nil Prote, *Mead Johnson*). MCT may cause transient urinary excretion of dicarboxylic acids (adipic, suberic and sebacic) in some babies. Alternatively intravenous lipids can be used.

Some forms of primary lactic acidosis (e.g. pyruvate dehydrogenase deficiency) are made worse by a high carbohydrate intake and improved by a high lipid, low carbohydrate regimen. These cases are very difficult to treat in a very ill newborn infant.

Introduction of protein

If the baby improves on this type of regimen it is important to introduce protein within 2 or 3 days to stimulate anabolism. The protein intake necessary to promote anabolism varies between 1 and 1.5 g/kg in different babies. This can be given as breast milk or as a humanized milk formula. There are some arguments for administering a mixture of essential aminoacids and excluding the non-essential ones and this argument is particularly strong in hyperammonaemia. The use of the keto derivatives of essential aminoacids may offer further advantage in hyperammonaemia. Their conversion to the corresponding aminoacids should utilize ammonia rather than liberate it.

* Scientific Hospital Supplies Ltd., 38 Queensland Street, Liverpool L7 3JG. (051 7088008).

Treatment of the infant diagnosed before symptoms

Finally, there are some circumstances in which it is possible to anticipate the birth of a baby with an IEM rather than having to treat a baby already very ill as a result of one of these conditions. This has been described elsewhere (Danks, 1974).

Specific diseases

Table 91.1 lists the more important IEM which can present with acute neonatal symptoms and the reader is referred to larger texts for descriptions of most of these (Raine, 1975; Galjaard, 1980; Stanbury *et al.*, 1983) and for details omitted from this brief description.

Galactosaemia

This is the most important IEM since it is one of the most easily treated and the diagnosis is simple; nevertheless, it is frequently forgotten, with tragic consequences (Oberklaid, Danks and Davies, 1976). Mass screening of newborn babies does not eliminate the clinical problem because *the illness can start before the test is done or before the result is returned.*

Recognition

Vomiting, jaundice, drowsiness, and convulsions are the most frequent symptoms. Onset is usually 24–28 hours after the start of milk feeding. Hepatomegaly is a constant finding and glycosuria (galactosuria) will be detected if the urine is tested with Clinitest (NOT dip tapes specific for glucose).

The illness may closely resemble septicaemia and in fact septicaemia commonly complicates the course of galactosaemia in the newborn period so that both dignoses are correct (galactosuria may be minimal, especially if oral feeds have been stopped).

Diagnosis

The assay of the red cell enzyme activity of galactose-l-phosphate uridyl transferase is now so simple that it should be applied in all patients with these symptoms. Misleading normal results may be obtained if the infant has been transfused.

Management

Exchange transfusion is valuable in critically ill patients with galactosaemia. A diet that excludes milk and milk products is then required.

Hereditary fructose intolerance

This condition is an exact parallel to galactosaemia and is equally easily treated. However, it is much less common.

Recognition

Symptoms are similar although even more acute. It may be excluded by showing that no fructose or sucrose has been ingested (e.g. in a fully breast fed infant). However, it is easy to overlook one sucrose-containing feed given during the night when the mother was asleep, or a dose of sweetened medicine. Delayed symptoms may occur when sucrose (or fructose) is given to an infant who has been exclusively breast fed for weeks or months.

Diagnosis

Demonstration of fructosuria (fructose gives a positive reaction to Clinitest but requires laboratory identification) and a dramatic improvement after dietary exclusion of sucrose (i.e. cane or beet sugar, 'ordinary sugar') will support the diagnosis.

Absolute proof requires assay of fructose-l-P aldolase in a liver biopsy, or fructose tolerance test. The former assay is not widely available and the tolerance test must be performed with care, because serious hypoglycaemia may occur.

Management

Strict exclusion of fructose and sucrose-containing feeds. Human milk and unaltered cows' milk do not contain either fructose or sucrose.

Hyperammonaemia

Defects of the first three steps of the urea cycle may cause very severe hyperammonaemia which may prove lethal in the first days after birth (Hsia, 1974).

Recognition

Carbamyl-phosphate synthetase deficiency, ornithine transcarbamylase (OTCase) deficiency, citrullinaemia, and severe argininosuccinic aciduria all cause similar symptoms of drowsiness, loss of consciousness, convulsions, hypotonia, and death. Breathlessness may also occur and sudden massive pulmonary haemorrhage has been described in several babies (Sheffield, *et al.*, 1976).

Diagnosis

Diagnosis rests upon blood ammonia estimation and HVE of urine aminoacids. Levels of ammonia in excess of 500 μmol/ℓ (normal 100 μmol/ℓ in the newborn) are usual in unconscious patients with these conditions. Citrullinaemia can be diagnosed by HVE on urine or serum, but the other two conditions show no characteristic findings though glutamine levels are usually elevated and changes secondary to liver damage may appear. OTCase deficiency is X-linked in inheritance and affected males generally die in the neonatal period; females possessing the gene can be quite severely affected, but more often are not; however, they may suffer quite severe transient symptoms in the newborn period. Impaired ability of a heterozygous mother to metabolize ammonia may compound the fetal metabolic problem.

Management

Peritoneal dialysis should be used immediately in any affected baby who is unconscious. Low protein diet or a diet based on essential aminoacids or keto derivatives of essential aminoacids may be used. The use of arginine to promote excretion of citrulline or argininosuccinate in blocks of the later steps in the cycle and of benzoate to remove ammonia by conjugation with glycine to form hippurate has improved the survival of these babies quite dramatically. However, some survivors have been severely damaged and good sense must be exercised in the application of these potent forms of therapy (Batshaw *et al.*, 1982; Msall *et al.*, 1984).

Congenital lactic acidosis

The distinction between this condition and the lactic acidosis which may occur in septicaemia or in cardiac disease may be impossible to determine in a baby who dies rapidly. If the patient recovers, secondary lactic acidosis will clear over about 48 hours after restoration of good tissue perfusion and oxygenation. Persistence suggests that the lactic acidosis is primary.

A number of different enzyme defects can cause primary lactic acidosis and several are susceptible to effective treatment. Fructose 1,6-diphosphatase deficiency causes lactic acidosis and hypoglycaemia and can be controlled by a low-protein, low-fructose diet. A thiamine-dependent defect of pyruvate carboxylase has been described but does not present so acutely. The basic defect remains unknown in some patients (Robinson, Taylor and Sherwood, 1980). In the majority of cases high fat low carbohydrate feeding is desirable, but very difficult to institute in the newborn period. The outcome of acute neonatal cases is rarely satisfactory.

Maple-syrup urine disease, propionic acidaemia, methylmalonic acidaemia, isovaleric acidaemia and multiple carboxylase deficiency

Recognition

All these diseases involve defects in the catabolism of the branched-chain aminoacids (leucine, isoleucine and valine) and all can cause acute neurological symptoms in the newborn period. Maple-syrup urine disease is easily diagnosed by elevation of all three aminoacids in the urine and by excretion of the three corresponding ketoacids (detected by GLC). Hyperglycinuria and hyperglycinaemia may occur in propionic acidaemia or methylmalonic acidaemia. The GLC pattern is the diagnostic test in these conditions and in isovaleric acidaemia. (Goodman and Markey, 1981). Staining of the region of the origin on the urine HVE with Fast Blue B provides a very sensitive method of detecting methylmalonic acid.

Management

A special diet is used in maple-syrup urine disease with restriction of the branched-chain aminoaicds. Low protein diet is the mainstay of treatment of the other three conditions. Fortunately vitamin-dependent forms exist, i.e. vitamin B_{12} dependent methylmalonic acidaemia and biotin-dependent multiple carboxylase deficiency.

Non-ketotic hyperglycinaemia (Glycine encephalopathy)

Recognition

This condition has a very characteristic clinical presentation with extreme hypotonia. Few other conditions cause such a rag-doll type of baby. Respiratory inadequacy develops and is the cause of death. Cerebral depression is severe.

The diagnosis is usually suggested by high levels of glycine in urine and serum, but it is the very high level of glycine in the CSF that is really diagnostic. A few babies have only a mild increase in urine glycine and near normal serum glycine. CSF glycine should be examined when a very floppy baby has moderate glycinuria.

Management

Strychnine specifically counteracts the inhibitory effect of excess glycine on spinal neurones and is tolerated in doses that would be lethal in adults. Benzoate can reduce plasma and CSF glycine to some degree. No good outcome has yet been reported in a severe case with neonatal onset of symptoms.

Pyridoxine dependent convulsions

This is generally regarded as a very rare condition causing convulsions from birth (or before) which are not influenced by anticonvulsants. Convulsions can start later, up to 6 or 8 weeks, and may be partially controlled by anticonvulsants. All babies with severe and persistent convulsions should be regarded as candidates for this diagnosis (Bankier, Turner and Hopkins, 1983). If convulsions are very frequent administration of pyridoxine IV 100 mg under EEG control is the best method of testing, remembering that control of convulsions may be delayed for an hour or two and that hypotonia and drowsiness may follow. If they are less frequent a trial of pyridoxine 50 mg twice daily for 1 or 2 weeks may be necessary.

References

BANKIER, A., TURNER, M. and HOPKINS, I. J. (1983) Pyridoxine dependent seizures – a wider clinical spectrum. *Archives of Disease in Childhood,* **58,** 415–418

BATSHAW, M. L., BRASILOW, S. and WABER, L. *et al.* (1982). Treatment of inborn errors of urea synthesis. Activation of alternative pathways of waste nitrogen synthesis and excretion. *New England Journal of Medicine,* **306,** 1387–1392

DANKS, D. M. (1974) Management of newborn babies in whom serious metabolic illness is anticipated. *Archives of Disease in Childhood,* **49,** 576–578

GALJAARD, H. (1980) *Genetic Metabolic Disease.* Amsterdam: Elsevier-North Holland

GOODMAN, S. I. and MARKEY, S. P. (1981) Diagnosis of organic acidaemias by gas chromatography – mass spectrometry. New York: Alan R. Liss

HSIA, Y. E. (1974) Inherited hyperammonemic syndromes. *Gastroenterology,* **67,** 347–374

MSALL, M., BATSHAW, M. L., SUSS, R., BRUSILOW, S. W. and MELLITS, E. D. (1984) Neurological outcome in children with inborn errors of urea synthesis – outcome of urea-cycle enzymopathies. *New England Journal of Medicine,* **310**, 1900–1505

OBERKLAID, F., DANKS, D. M. and DAVIES, H. E. (1976) Problems encountered in the diagnosis of galactosaemia. *Australian Paediatric Journal,* **12,** 14–18

RAINE, D. E. (ed.) (1975) *The Treatment of Inherited Metabolic Disease.* New York: Elsevier-North Holland

ROBINSON, B. N., TAYLOR, J. and SHERWOOD, W. G. (1980) The genetic heterogeneity of lactic acidosis: occurrence of recognisable inborn errors of metabolism in a paediatric population. *Paediatric Research,* **14,** 956–962

SHEFFIELD, L. J., DANKS, D. M., HAMMOND, J. W. and HOOGENNAD, N. H. (1976) Massive pulmonary haemorrhage as a presenting feature in congenital hyperammonemia. *Journal of Pediatrics,* **88,** 450–452

STANBURY, J. B. *et al.* (1983). *The Metabolic Basis of Inherited Disease* (5th edn.). New York: McCraw-Hill.

Chapter 92

Maternal drug dependence and the neonatal abstinence syndrome

M. F. Whitfield

An infant may develop symptoms of drug withdrawal after birth if the mother has been receiving prescribed or self-administered addictive or habit-forming drugs during pregnancy. Drugs capable of producing effects on the fetus, and subsequent withdrawal effects after birth are given in *Table 92.1*. It is worth noting that marijuana consumption does not appear to affect the fetus seriously but may have more subtle effects on fetal growth, similar to smoking; there is no evidence that LSD has a similar effect on the fetus although there is concern about the possible teratogenic effect of this drug in producing chromosomal abnormalities.

Table 92.1 Drugs potentially capable of producing withdrawal effects in the newborn

Opiates and opiate analogues:
Morphine
Heroin and related derivatives
Pethidine (Demerol, Meperidine)
Methadone (Physeptone)
Dihydrocodeine (DF 118)
Dipipanone/cyclizine combination (Diconal)
Barbiturates
Phenothiazines:
Chlorpromazine (Largactil) and related major tranquillizers
Prochlorperazine (Stemetil) and related antiemetics
Benzodiazepines:
Diazepam (Valium) and related minor tranquillizers and hypnotics
Alcohol

Maternal opiate addiction

Maternal opiate addiction is the most frequent cause of withdrawal effects in the newborn; but addicts frequently take mixtures of drugs deliberately or unwittingly because of adulteration of drugs by street dealers. In the first trimester of pregnancy, it is desirable to try to wean the mother from opiate addiction if possible, or therapeutic abortion may be contemplated. After the first trimester, abrupt reduction of opiate dosage may precipitate signs of withdrawal in the fetus, observable on real-time ultrasound examination, which may lead to fetal death. For this reason, many public health administrations provide a methadone maintenance programme for addicted mothers in which social work support is provided, and the mother is maintained on a regular dosage of methadone instead of an irregular dosage of street morphine of varying potency with or without additives. This clinic usually functions as an antenatal clinic in addition.

Recognition

Attempts must be made to get an accurate history of drug taking but it must be realized that the information obtained from the patient may not include all the important details. Examination of the mother's arms for injection sites and thrombophlebitis confirms the possibility that the baby may develop signs of withdrawal. Opiate withdrawal in the infant produces a defined syndrome ('neonatal abstinence syndrome', NAS) with wide-ranging symptomatology which is best assessed by serial objective observations recorded on a suitable chart (*Figure 92.1*) by nurses familiar with this problem. Symptoms usually develop between the 2nd and the 4th day but may occur on the 1st day of life or may take 2–3 weeks to develop.

Management

1. There is usually no problem at delivery unless the infant is asphyxiated and requires resuscitation. Naloxone (Narcan) is CONTRAINDICATED as it may provoke sudden severe withdrawal symptoms in the infant.
2. Blood (maternal and cord) should be collected at delivery and the infant's urine collected (preferably 60 ml or more) for toxicological analysis. It is important to include details from the history on the request form to aid the laboratory staff. (A negative result on blood, urine, or both does *not* indicate that the mother is not an addict.) Blood from the mother should also be sent for hepatitis screening.
3. The infant must be observed in a secure place by nurses with neonatal nursing expertise, for signs of withdrawal. The infant may be initially lethargic but may subsequently become agitated, irritable, and unconsolable, and may develop severe gastrointestinal symptoms or seizures.
4. Minimizing sensory input from bright lights, noise, and handling is important in controlling the severity of symptoms. Swaddling also helps to keep the infant settled.
5. The aim of treatment is to avoid the use of opiates by minimizing sensory input but if life-threatening symptoms occur, particularly diarrhoea and vomiting which may lead on to major fluid and electrolyte disturbances or seizures, it may not be possible to withhold opiates any longer. It is preferable to use a paediatric opium mixture made from tincture of opium diluted with distilled water to a morphine concentration of 0.4 mg/ml. The starting dose is around 0.2 ml per dose given 3–4 hourly for a 3 kg infant. Even a small dose of paediatric opium has a dramatic effect in abolishing symptoms. There are day-to-day fluctuations in symptoms which may require minor adjustments in the dosage, but over a period of weeks the intention is a gradual weaning from the drug. Downward reductions should not be made more frequently than every 48 hours; because of fluctuations in symptoms, this process may take several months.
6. The signs of NAS may mimic septicaemia, heart failure, gastroenteritis, or other neurological disorders. It is important to consider alternative diagnoses apart

Figure 92.1 Neonatal abstinence syndrome flowsheet

Date of beginning this page: ________________ 198__

Epoch From/To									
Convulsions, hyperreflexia									
Tremors, irritability									
Excessive cry									
Sucking									
Diarrhoea									
Skin abrasions (buttocks)									
Fast breathing									
Sneezing									
Yawning									
Diaphoresis									
Vomiting									
Weight									
Respiratory Rate									
Heart Rate									
Temperature									
Formula Intake (and type)									
Caloric Intake									
Medications									

GUIDE TO WITHDRAWAL SCORING

Convulsions, hyperreflexia 0–3
0. Normal
1. Increased reflexes
2. Markedly increased reflexes
3. Convulsions

Tremors, irritability 0–4
0. None
1. Minimally abnormal when handled
2. Marked when infant handled or touching crib
3. Marked when infant undisturbed
4. Continuously abnormal

Skin abrasions 0–4
0. None
1. Redness of knees and elbows
2. Breaking of the skin
3. #2 plus other abrasions
4. Increasing lesions daily

Fast breathing 0–1

Sneezing 0–1

Yawning 0–1

Excessive cry 0–2
0. Normal
1. High pitched
2. Continuous high pitched

Diarrhoea 0–2
0. Normal
1. More than average number of stools
2. Watery continuous diarrhoea

Sucking 0–4
0. Normal
1. Incoordinate
2. Weak
3. Stops early
4. Absent or almost

Diaphoresis 0–1

Vomiting 0–3
0. No vomiting
1. Occasional, without feeding
2. Occasional, any time
3. Frequent vomiting

from NAS in an infant who is known to have NAS, as it may have another significant disease in addition.
7. Infants with NAS have an abnormally high metabolic rate and may benefit from the use of hypercaloric feeds (81 kcal/100 ml; 339 kJ/100 ml) once they tolerate a normal infant formula. Weight gain is a sensitive indicator of the adequacy of control.
8. To be medically fit for discharge home, the infant must be gaining weight well on a standard formula (68 kcal/100 ml; 284 kJ/100 ml) and its behaviour must not be adversely affected by exposure to normal light, noise, and handling.
9. A mother, who is an addict, and her infant, pose a major social problem in which the interests of parents and infant must be considered; but the interests and safety of the infant must be considered paramount. Drug addicts are members of a sub-culture of society and are adept at manipulation of the situation and the professionals in what they perceive to be their own interests. The interests of the parent may directly conflict with those of the infant, particularly if the parents are not fully committed to rehabilitation and are intolerant of supportive supervision. Assessment of the social situation and parenting potential by social workers and medical and nursing staff should begin antenatally and continue during the baby's stay in the nursery. Before discharge decisions must be made about the most appropriate placement for the infant; home with the mother under supervision, fostering, or adoption. The social situation and parental attitudes may necessitate a Place of Safety Order to preserve the interests of the child.

Withdrawal effects of other drugs

Drugs other than opiates may be given to the mother and transient behaviour alterations in the newborn period may follow maternal ingestion of a wide range of drugs (*Table 92.1*). Symptoms can usually be controlled by phenobarbitone 10–15 mg then 2–5 mg/kg daily for maintenance with the intention of tailoring off the dosage over 1–2 weeks. The social connotations relating to drug addicts do not of course apply if the drugs have been prescribed for therapeutic reasons.

Acquired immune deficiency syndrome (AIDS)

Mothers who have used drugs intravenously are at risk for transmitting AIDS to the fetus or newborn infant (*see* page 659).

Further reading

COBRINIK, R. W., HOOD, R. T. and CHUSID, E. (1959) The effect of maternal narcotic addiction on the newborn infant. *Pediatrics,* **24,** 288–304

DESMOND, M. M., SCHWANECKE, R. P., WILSON, G. S., YASUNAGA, S. and BURGDORFF, I. (1972) Maternal barbiturate utilisation and neonatal withdrawal symptomatology. *Journal of Pediatrics,* **80,** 190–197

PIEROG, S., CHANDAVASU, O. and WEXLER, I. (1977) Withdrawal symptoms in infants with fetal alcohol syndrome. *Journal of Pediatrics,* **90,** 630–633

ROSEN, T. S. and JOHNSON, H. L. (1982) Children of methadone-maintained mothers; Follow-up to 18 months of age. *Journal of Pediatrics,* **101,** 192–196

TAMER, A., McKEY, R., ARIAS, D., WORLEY, L. and FOGEL, L. (1969) Phenothiazine-induced extrapyramidal dysfunction in the neonate. *Journal of Pediatrics,* **75,** 479–480

WEBSTER, P. A. C. (1973) Withdrawal symptoms in neonates associated with maternal antidepressant therapy. *Lancet,* **ii,** 318–319

Part XVII

Practical procedures

Chapter 93

Practical procedures

Andrew Boon, R. A. Minns, Ian Shellshear, Marian D. Smith

Introduction

Ian Shellshear

This section deals with procedures that involve penetration of the body tissues or cavities. Several points apply to all such procedures.

Preparation

For most procedures, local anaesthesia has little to offer, as it is painful and obscures landmarks. The exceptions occur with large instruments, e.g. trocar and cannula, or with prolonged manipulation. Overhead heaters should be used for any prolonged procedure in the neonate. Sedation beforehand is often of value, particularly in young children. Trimeprazine (0.9 mg/kg i.m. or 3–4 mg/kg orally) or diazepam (1 mg per year, orally or i.m.) are useful to calm the child. Ketamine may also be used.

Correct dosage

If drugs are to be inserted into a body cavity, it is the responsibility of the operator to ensure that he has the correct drug, the correct dose, and the correct route. Unlabelled syringes offered by an assistant should NEVER be accepted on the assumption that they are correct.

Comfort

Success is in proportion to the comfort of the operator. The operator should be sitting, and have an assistant, so that he is not attempting the procedure as well as restraining a patient.

Respiratory system

Ian Shellshear

1. Endotracheal intubation:
    (a) In the newborn (*see* page 619).
    (b) In the older child (*see* page 223).

2. Bag and mask ventilation in the newborn (*see* page 619).
3. Mouth-to-mouth ventilation in the newborn (*see* page 619).
4. Tracheostomy:
   (a) In the newborn (tetanus) (*see* page 330).
   (b) In the older child (*see* page 327).
5. Cricothyroid membrane puncture (*see* page 208).
6. Relief of pneumothorax
   (a) In the newborn (*see* pages 239 and 245).
   (b) In the older child (*see below*).
7. Aspiration of the chest:
   All procedures involving chest aspiration risk creating a pneumothorax and intrapulmonary haemorrhage. Local anaesthesia should be used. The chest should be examined clinically and X-rayed after the aspiration.

Indications

The diagnosis or treatment of intrapleural air, or effusion, pleural biopsy, or lung aspiration. The same approach is used for diagnostic procedures as for therapeutic ones.

Aspiration of air in pneumothorax

Equipment

Sterile procedure; needle and catheter, underwater drain and seal. In an emergency, intravenous cannulae may be used but these have the disadvantage of having a single-end hole and are too malleable. Suitable drainage catheters are of large bore, are stiff, and have a number of side holes.

Procedure

The needle should be inserted through the second intercostal space in the midclavicular line, or in the 2nd or 3rd space posteriorly, medial to the border of the scapula. The catheter is connected to the underwater drain. Suction pumps should be avoided, and should not be used if air is unable to escape when the pump is not in use. Water in the drainage tubing should rise and fall with respiration. Absence of this movement indicates a probable block.

Pleural effusion (pus, blood, chyle, etc.)

Equipment

Sterile procedure; 30 ml syringe, three-way valve, 22 × 1½ in needle. If a pleural biopsy is required a Franklin–Silverman or Abrams needle will be required.

Procedure

The needle is inserted in the lower chest where fluid has been demonstrated radiologically and at the highest space where the percussion note is still dull. This will usually be the lateral or posterior chest in the 6th–9th intercostal spaces. A three-way tap is inserted between the syringe and the needle so that large effusions can be aspirated slowly and expelled from a side-arm without disconnecting the needle. Fluid should be sent for culture (including tubercle bacilli), cell count, and cytology. If a pleural biopsy is required this should be done only when there is an effusion. An Abrams needle is safer than a Franklin–Silverman needle.

Complications

If fluid is aspirated too rapidly there may be a mediastinal shift which is usually indicated by a hoarse cough. The aspiration should be stopped temporarily. Pleural tears may be caused by inexperienced use of pleural biopsy needles.

Aspiration of the lung

Indication

When persistent consolidation is not responsive to normal therapy. The procedure is rarely indicated but may be necessary to establish a diagnosis, particularly if there is a possibility of pneumocystis infection.

Equipment

Sterile procedure; 22 gauge 2½ in needle, syringe, sterile normal saline.

Procedure

The aspiration procedure should be done as quickly as possible during one respiratory cycle. Good preparation including sedation is therefore essential. The needle is inserted in the area of lung thought to be suspicious radiologically. Sterile saline 1–2 ml is injected, provided aspiration has not drawn blood, and is then re-aspirated immediately. The needle is withdrawn and the aspiration fluid sent for culture, including tubercle bacilli. Special stains are necessary to demonstrate the presence of *Pneumocystis carinii.*

Cardiovascular system

Andrew Boon and Ian Shellshear

External cardiac massage

1. In the newborn (*see* page 619).
2. In the older child (*see* page 276).

Umbilical vein catheterization

See page 693.

Pericardial aspiration

See page 276.

Cardioversion

See page 270.

Capillary blood sampling in the newborn

Free-flowing capillary blood samples from a warmed extremity show a good correlation with arterial blood samples for pH and PCO_2. The PO_2 results from capillary blood underestimate the arterial PO_2 for values greater than 8 kPa (60 mm Hg).

Indications

Monitoring babies with *mild* hyaline membrane disease (idiopathic respiratory distress syndrome) (FiO_2 <0.3, 30 per cent), infants recovering from respiratory disease after removal of an arterial catheter, and babies with chronic lung disease.

Contraindications

Situations in which the $Pa0_2$ is likely to rise above 8 kPa (60 mm Hg), in particular in very preterm infants. Capillary blood gases are also inadequate if the FiO_2 is greater than 0.3 (30 per cent).

Procedure

If a baby is in an incubator and has good peripheral perfusion, warming of the heel is unnecessary. Otherwise the heel should be warmed for 3 minutes to 40°C (104°F) using a water bath at 38–40°C (100–104°F) or warm water compresses. The site should be cleaned with alcohol and a single puncture made on the medial or lateral aspect of the plantar surface of the heel. Blood is then collected into pre-heparinized glass capillary tubes.

Complications

Calcaneal osteochondritis and calcified heel nodules may result from heel punctures. Possible sources of error include inadequate warming of the heel, excessive squeezing of the heel leading to dilution of the capillary blood with interstitial fluid, and exposure of the blood to air bubbles during collection.

Arterial blood sampling in the newborn and in the older child

Intermittent arterial puncture

INDICATIONS

Arterial punctures have little or no place in the neonate as the disturbance of the infant makes interpretation of the results almost impossible. They may be helpful in the older child with respiratory insufficiency.

CONTRAINDICATIONS

In severe airway obstruction, an arterial puncture may produce rapid deterioration in the child's condition and is therefore best avoided. A severe coagulation disorder is an absolute contraindication.

PROCEDURE

The radial or brachial arteries are most commonly used for arterial punctures. The femoral artery should NOT be used in infants as thrombus formation could lead to the loss of a leg. Furthermore, it may be difficult to puncture the artery and not the vein.

The skin is first cleaned. Infiltration of the skin with lignocaine 1% may reduce crying and struggling and improve the validity of the PaO_2. A heparinized 2 ml syringe with a 23 gauge needle is suitable for most children. Care must be taken to eliminate air from the needle and syringe. The needle is inserted, bevel-up, at an angle of 45° to the skin, against the direction of arterial flow. *After sampling, continuous pressure must be applied to the artery for 5 minutes.*

COMPLICATIONS

Carpal tunnel syndrome has been described in a neonate after radial artery puncture. Median nerve damage has occurred with brachial artery sampling. Haematoma formation is common and often prevents further sampling from the artery.

Arterial cannulation (catheterization)

Arterial cannulation allows easy access for blood gas sampling without disturbing the patient. It also allows the continuous recording of arterial blood pressure.

INDICATIONS

In a neonate an FiO_2 of over 0.3 indicates the need for continuous arterial sampling. In older children arterial cannulation is an important adjunct to the intensive care of patients with severe cardiorespiratory problems. Umbilical artery catheterization also permits continuous monitoring of the PaO_2 using a catheter PO_2 electrode.

Peripheral arterial catherization

Catheters can be placed in the radial, brachial, posterior tibial, and dorsalis pedis arteries. The temporal artery should be avoided because of the risk of cerebral infarction (Simmons *et al.*, 1978).

Before cannulating the radial artery, the collateral circulation from the ulnar artery should be tested by squeezing blood out of the hand and observing whether the colour rapidly returns while the radial artery is occluded.

Peripheral arteries in neonates are best identified with the help of a cold light source.* The artery is cannulated with a fine Teflon catheter (e.g. 25 gauge Jelco) directing the catheter at an angle of 20° to the artery. Once in place, the catheter should be connected to extension tubing and a three-way tap. Continuous blood pressure monitoring is readily achieved using a peripheral arterial line.

COMPLICATIONS

Cerebral infarction is a well-recognized feature of temporal artery catherization. Loss of part of a limb and skin necrosis have been reported with peripheral arterial catheters.

* Obtainable from Bart & Stroud, Caxton Street, Anniesland, Glasgow G13 1HZ (Tel: 041 954 9601).

Umbilical arterial catheterization

Umbilical arteries are usually accessible for up to 4 days of age. The infant's femoral and dorsalis pedis pulses should be palpated and the buttocks and legs examined for bruising. The operator should then scrub and gown up; the umbilical stump and anterior abdominal wall are cleaned with an iodine/alcohol solution and then washed off with chlorhexidine in spirit. The abdomen is then draped with sterile towels. A sterile umbilical ligature is tied loosely around the umbilical stump. The cord is cut about 1–2 cm (½–¾ in) from the skin using a scalpel blade. Two thick-walled arteries and a thin-walled vein are identified. The lumen of one artery should be dilated very gently using iris forceps. A saline-filled catheter, attached to a three-way tap and syringe, is then inserted into the artery. A 5 FG catheter is suitable for babies over 1250 g. Babies of less than this weight usually require a 3.5 FG catheter. Obstruction may be encountered at the level of the abdominal wall and also where the internal iliac artery joins the aorta. Gentle pressure on the catheter usually overcomes this obstruction.

The catheter tip can be placed either in the 'high' position between T6 and T10 (just above the diaphragm; *Figure 93.1*), or in the 'low' position between L3 and L4. Providing the catheter is not used for fluid or drug administration, the 'low' position is probably preferable as it is below the renal and mesenteric arteries. Twice the distance from the umbilicus to the mid-inguinal point provides the distance of insertion for the low position.

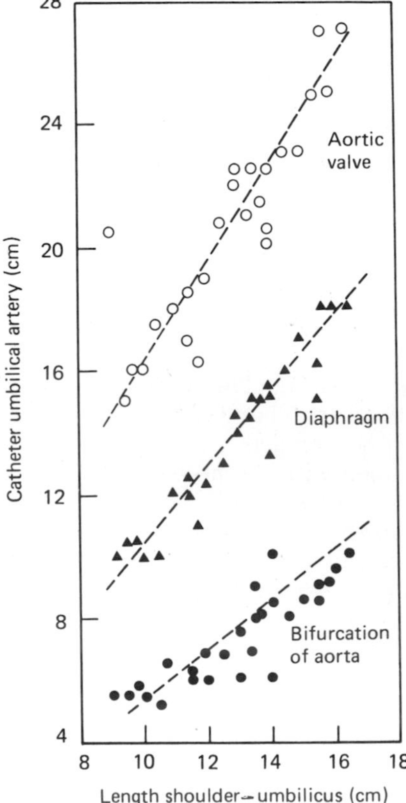

Figure 93.1 The relation between length of catheter inserted into the umbilical artery in order to reach the bifurcation of the aorta, the 'diaphragm', or the aortic valves, and the shoulder–umbilicus length of an infant. (Reproduced from Dunn (1966), with kind permission of authors and publishers.)

The catheter should be sutured in place and secured using a tape bridge. The femoral pulses should be palpated and the buttocks and legs inspected after catheter insertion. The position of the catheter should be checked radiographically or by ultrasound (Garg *et al.,* 1983).

COMPLICATIONS

Initially – Vasospasm leading to blanching of an extremity. The catheter should be removed at once.

Long term – Thrombosis and emboli, infection, haemorrhage, air embolism, necrotizing enterocolitis.

Venepuncture

Indications

To take blood for investigation, inject drugs, or place an intravenous line.

Blood specimens

THE OLDER CHILD

The procedure using the antecubital fossa is the same as for adults. An unhurried explanation should be given before approaching with a needle and syringe. Masks are frightening as well as unnecessary.

Equipment – A clean procedure; 5 or 10 ml syringe, 20–23 gauge 1 in needle and specimen containers.

Procedure – The venous return is obstructed by a cuff or an encircling hand. Care should be taken to have correct containers on hand as many laboratory procedures are rendered useless if the blood clots.

INFANTS

In small children, the external jugular vein is easier to use especially with a 21 or 23 butterfly needle (*see Figure 93.2*). The vein is superficial and should be punctured as it runs over the sternomastoid. Deep punctures risk striking the apex of the lung.

Other sites

Blood may also be taken from the dorsum of the hands or feet and from the scalp veins. Puncture of the femoral vein should be avoided as it risks spasm of the femoral artery and injury or infection of the hip joint, producing aseptic necrosis of the femoral head or a septic arthritis. If femoral vein puncture is necessary, the vein is found just medial to the artery and is best approached with the leg slightly flexed and abducted at the hips. In infants, the antecubital fossa is rarely considered, but the veins are often easily palpable, particularly in the preterm or small-for-dates infant with little subcutaneous fat. It is essential that the infant is firmly held on a firm surface at a convenient height for the operator. The arm is fully extended by placing a folded towel under the elbow. The assistant holds the infant's palm flat to restrain movement of pronation and supination. The upper arm is occluded by firm pressure sufficient to obstruct the venous return. If the arm is held too tightly arterial flow is obstructed and venous distension will be reduced.

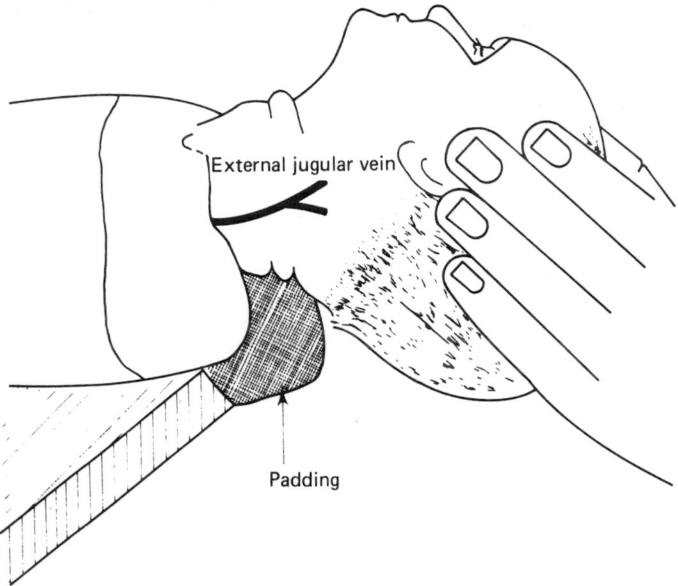

Figure 93.2 Venepuncture using the external jugular vein.

Administration of fluids

Umbilical artery

See page 728.

Umbilical vein

See page 693.

Exchange transfusion

See page 693.

Peritoneal dialysis and infusion

See page 434 (dialysis) and 739 (infusion).

Passage of nasogastric tube for oral rehydration

See page 736.

Intravascular infusions

Intravenous or intra-arterial lines should always have a paediatric chamber between the infusing solution and the patient to prevent accidental overload. Drip rates are best controlled by mechanical pumps, but if these are not available close supervision should be given. It should not be assumed that supervising staff know how to remove air from drip tubing, or other details of drip maintenance.

CATHETER SELECTION

Recent work on the irritant nature of catheters suggests a much lower incidence of thrombosis if Silastic rather than polyvinylchloride catheters are used. The Silastic catheters, however, have the disadvantage of being opaque and are less malleable.

Intravenous lines

INDICATIONS

To supply maintenance fluids, to replace lost fluids, to inject drugs or to insert monitoring devices. The site depends on these requirements and the age of the child. Butterfly needles are easiest to use and maintain in scalp veins. Silastic cannulae are easiest to maintain in other sites, but are more likely to produce long-term damage to the vein.

EQUIPMENT

Clean procedures; 21, 23 or 25 gauge butterfly needle or Silastic catheter; strips of plaster of Paris for scalp butterfly needles, non-irritant strips of surgical tape; cleansing solution; razor blade (to remove hair, for scalp veins); intravenous tubing and solution; microdrip chamber; infusion pump if available.

PROCEDURE

Scalp veins – The tubing should be primed with infusing fluid before beginning. The infant may be restrained by a sheet, and the hands restrained by tube gauze with one end placed over the wrists, and held by tape, and the other end tied to the cot sides. A rubber band is placed around the head to obstruct the veins. Alternatively the vein can be compressed with the finger. The frontal veins are particularly useful as the needle is less likely to be dislodged by movements of the head. The area is prepared with antiseptic. After insertion, needles are fixed either by plaster of Paris strips, or by surgical tape. Drip tubing should also be fixed at the side of the head so that an accidental sharp movement will not dislodge the needle. Accidental insertion of a needle into a scalp artery may cause distal skin necrosis. If this is suspected, the needle should be removed from the artery.

Even in the neonate the veins of the back of the hand, the antecubital fossa, or the ankle are available for cannulation, as for scalp veins. The essence of success is to have the vein stretched along its length to avoid sideways roll; e.g. for the neonate the back of the hand is easily accessible (*see Figure 93.3*).

FIXATION

Similar techniques can be used for older children. At 1–2 years of age, the subcutaneous veins are often hidden in fat. Short of a subclavian line, the veins on the palmar surface of the wrist, though small, can easily be found, and, with care, cannulated (21 or smaller Silastic catheter). The external jugular can be used if urgent fluids are required.

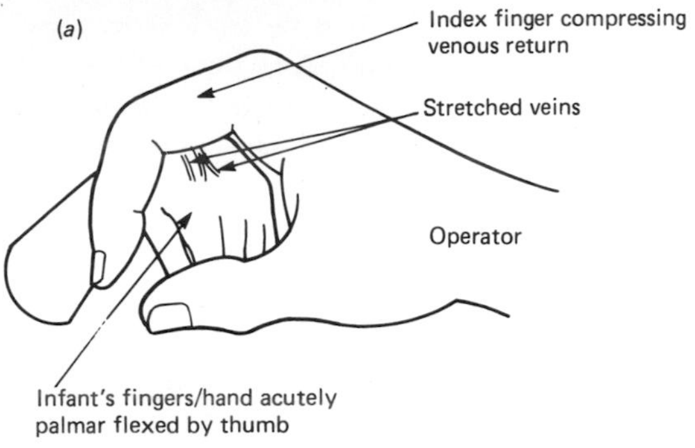

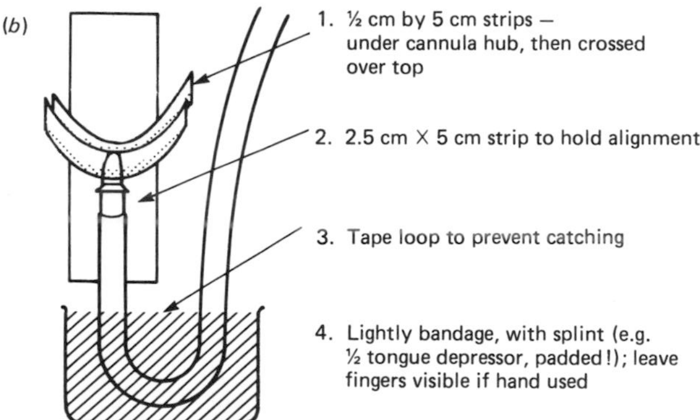

Figure 93.3 (*a*) Access to veins of dorsum of hand. (*b*) Fixation of needle in subcutaneous vein.

Intravenous cut-down

INDICATION

A cut-down to a vein may be necessary in an emergency, when peripheral veins are collapsed or cannot be found. The long saphenous vein is most easily approached but an arm vein gives the added advantage of being able to record central venous pressure (CVP).

EQUIPMENT

Sterile procedure; scalpel, two 10 cm (4 in) lengths of 00 catgut, 0000 catgut sutures, suture forceps, a pair of small scissors and three artery forceps. Local anaesthetic is required if the patient is conscious, preferably lignocaine 1% with adrenaline.

PROCEDURE (*FIGURE 93.4*)

The long saphenous vein is found most easily 1–2 cm (½–¾ in) in front of the medial malleolus of the ankle. A horizontal incision 2–3 cm (1 in) long is made in front of the medial malleolus. The subcutaneous tissues are opened longitudinally with a pair of artery forceps or blunt scissors until the vein is exposed. Two 00 catgut threads are passed under the vein. One thread is used to tie off the distal end of the vein and the other to stretch the upper part of the vein. With fine scissors, the vein is cut halfway through at 45° towards the groin. The plastic cannula (5or 8 FG) is inserted in the vein, care being taken not to strip the intima from the media. The upper thread is tied round the cannula and vein and the wound is sutured loosely.

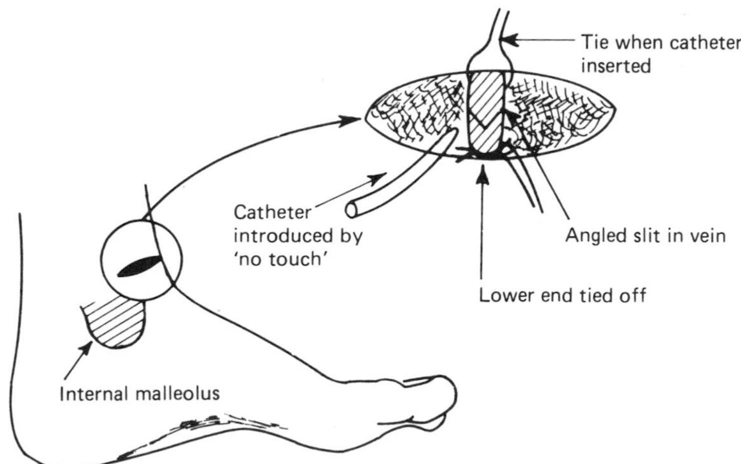

Figure 93.4 Cut-down to long saphenous vein.

A cut-down in the arm is made anterior to the medial epicondyle, or across the front of the antecubital fossa, and the vein is cannulated in the same way as the saphenous vein; the tip of the catheter should be in the superior vena cava or the right atrium and its position should be checked by X-ray.

For CVP monitoring a three-way tap is inserted in the line and connected to a section of vertical glass tubing with a scale attached, ranging from −10 cm to +15 cm H_2O (−7.7 to +11.5 mm Hg).

Zero is set at a level of the manubrium sterni, and for reading the CVP the glass manometer is first primed with infusing fluid to +15 cm H_2O (11.5 mm Hg). The manometer is then connected to the patient and the CVP read from the scale. If the equipment is working correctly, the top of the column of fluid in the manometer reflects the respiratory cycle. The normal CVP is between +5 and +10 cm H_2O (+3 to +7.7 mm Hg) water or saline. In an emergency, catheters may also be placed in other sites, using an intravenous needle and cannula. Possible sites are the right subclavian vein and the right internal jugular vein. The right subclavian vein is approached through the first intercostal space at the midclavicular point with the point of the needle aimed at the base of the sternal notch.

The internal jugular vein is approached between the two heads of the sternomastoid directed downwards and posteriorly. With both procedures there is a major risk of creating pneumothorax and of not being able to control bleeding on removal of the catheter. Introduction of infection or thrombosis of a major vein may occur and full aseptic technique should be used in the placement of catheters here.

Intravenous drugs (See also ***Appendix 11, Table 11.12)***

These may be injected into intravenous tubing or placed in the infusing chamber. It is important that the drug and the infusing solution are compatible (*see* Appendix 12). There should never be a toxic quantity of drug in the chamber at any time. Drugs which are locally toxic should never be injected into a line that is not running satisfactorily. This is particularly important with cytotoxic drugs, calcium gluconate, and hyperosmolar solutions. The sterile infusing solution should first be seen to run easily through the drip and then be used to clear the drip at the end of the drug injection. *See Tables 11.2* and *11.12* for use of intravenous antibiotics.

Gastrointestinal system

Oral rehydration solution for preparation at village level (*See also* Simmonds, Vaughan and Gunn, 1983)

Marian D. Smith

In many developing countries, packets of glucose–electrolyte are often not widely available, and a simple, easily understood pinch–scoop method of preparation is required.

Mothers are given instruction for the preparation and administration of the sugar (sucrose)–electrolyte solution in the home to any child with diarrhoea and vomiting. The following is demonstrated in under-5s clinics, by village health workers in homes, or broadcast over the local radio. The three-finger pinch of salt and the four-finger scoop of sugar are usually demonstrated or shown in pictures. For the technique of nasogastric feeding, *see* page 736.

Materials required

The only essential materials required are a clean, covered container in which to keep the solution, water, salt, sugar, a spoon and a standard sized measure. (In Nepal, for example, a local measure of one 'manna' is used, or three Nepali tea glasses, both of these amounts being roughly equivalent to 500 ml; an ordinary mug holds about 250 ml and an average sized teacup 150 ml.)

Preparation

The following details of preparation are given:

1. The hands should be washed with soap and water.
2. About 500 ml drinking water is boiled in a clean pot and allowed to cool. (If there is no fuel to boil the water, clean drinking water may be used; but boiled, cooled water is preferable.)
3. Two pinches of salt are added. The thumb, forefinger, and middle-finger are used to make the 'three-finger pinch of salt' (*Figure 93.5*). There is considerable variation in the amount of salt in a 'three-finger pinch' ranging from 0.5 to 2.0 g; with refined salt it is probably safe to assume that each pinch is 0.5–1.0 g, and for crude salt 1.5 g. Two pinches of refined salt to 500 ml of water would produce

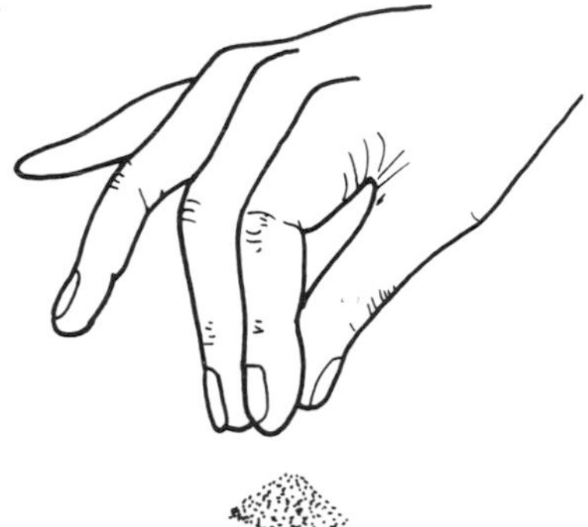

Figure 93.5 The 'three-fingers pinch' of salt. (Reproduced from Church (1972), with kind permission of authors and publishers.)

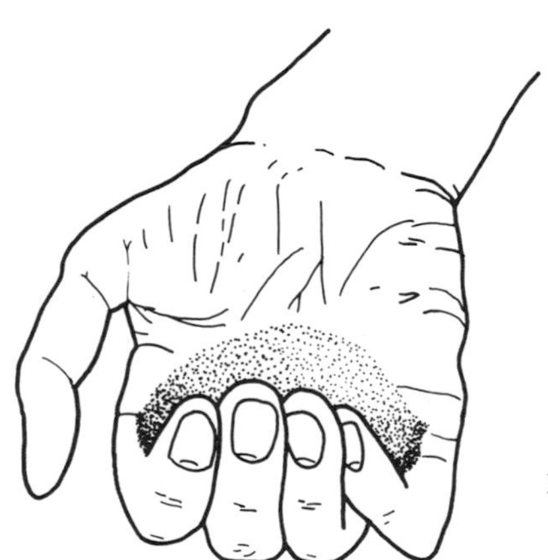

Figure 93.6 The 'four-fingers scoop' of sugar. (Reproduced from Church (1972), with kind permission of authors and publishers.)

a sodium content between 34 and 68 mmol/ℓ, more likely the higher figure. For crude salt the resulting sodium content for *1 pinch* of salt to 500 ml water would be 51 mmol/ℓ. The sucrose content of this mixture is 6 g/ℓ; a 'three-finger scoop' (15–20 g) may be better tolerated in the early stages (Morley, 1973). (*See also* Appendix 9 for comparison with other oral rehydration mixtures and Appendix 24 for domestic measurement of salt and sugar.)

4. A four-finger scoop of sugar is added. When the four fingers of the hand (but not the thumb) are curved, a scoop is formed (*Figure 93.6*). Sufficient sugar is taken to fill up the scoop and this is added to the water. An equal amount of brown sugar or honey may be used instead of sugar, if sugar is not available.
5. The mixture is then stirred with a clean spoon to completely dissolve the salt and sugar.
6. The mixture is stored in a clean, covered container to protect it from flies and dust. It is prepared fresh each day and never used when more than 24 hours old. After preparation, it should never be boiled again.

Instructions

The following details are given about administration and when to seek further medical advice (for alternative methods of measuring salt and sugar *see* Appendix 24):

1. The sucrose electrolyte solution must be given in proportion to the quantity of fluid lost through diarrhoea and vomiting. For a child below 2 years of age, half a cup or half a tea-glass of the mixture should be given for each stool or vomit. Older children should be given one full cup or tea-glass of the fluid for each stool or vomit.
2. Even though the child does not want to drink the mixture, it should be given slowly, a little at a time, several times an hour. It should not be stopped because the child vomits. After a vomit, wait a few minutes and then begin to feed it again. After two or three vomits, the vomiting stops and the child always retains more than he vomits.
3. Except where the diarrhoea is very severe, or there is frequent vomiting, it is important to continue to give the child food. Breast-feeding babies should continue to be breast fed. Older children can continue a usual diet except for very spicy foods. High potassium content foods should be given, e.g. bananas, oranges.
4. In any of the following situations, take the child to the nearest health-post or hospital:
   (a) When there are many, large fluid stools.
   (b) When there is blood in the stools.
   (c) When, for any reason, the child is unable to drink the sugar electrolyte solution.
   (d) When the urine becomes scanty.
   (e) When there is a high fever with the diarrhoea.
   (f) Where there is anything else unusual or worrying.

Nasogastric feeding

Christine E. Candy

Food, fluid and drugs are frequently given by nasogastric tube in children.

Indications

Many seriously ill children may require a nasogastric tube, such as the following:

1. Dehydrated infants (*see* Chapter 46).
2. Unconscious children:
   (a) Head injury.
   (b) CNS infections.
   (c) Diabetic coma.
   (d) Poisoning.
3. Before gut surgery.
4. Severe vomiting.

Technique of passing a nasogastric tube

1. Assemble the following equipment:
   (a) Nasogastric tube (narrow bore for conscious patients for comfort and less obstruction of nasal airway; wider bore if frequent aspiration required).

- (b) Lubricating fluid:
  - (i) KY Jelly (Johnson and Johnson).
  - (ii) Water, or ice.
  - (iii) Maternal saliva, if working under field conditions in developing countries.
- (c) Syringe.
  - (i) 20 or 50 ml.
  - (ii) This can be used subsequently as a funnel for administering feed.
- (d) Blue litmus paper, if available, to check that the end of the tube is in the stomach.
- (e) Adhesive tape to secure the tube beneath the nose and to the temple.
- (f) Stethoscope.
- (g) Fluid to be given.

2. Describe to the child's parents, if present, and the child if conscious, what you are going to do.
3. Put infants in supine position. Unconscious patients should be in the left lateral position, to avoid aspiration. Older children, if conscious, may prefer to sit, well supported.
4. Measure the approximate length from the child's anterior nostrils to the xiphisternum with the nasogastric tube, and mark the position on the tube. This will act as a guide to how far to insert the tube.
5. Clean around the anterior nostrils to remove mucus.
6. Lubricate the tip of tube and gently insert into the wider nostril.
7. Pass the tube slowly and smoothly along the floor of the nasal cavity:
   - (a) If child gags, stop and look with a spatula and a torch to see if tube is coiled in the oropharynx or mouth.
   - (b) If this is so, gently withdraw the tube and try again.
8. As the tube passes through the oropharynx, offer the conscious child a drink of water. This will aid the passage of the tube into the oesophagus and reduce discomfort.
9. If the child coughs, the tube is probably entering the trachea; withdraw gently and try again.
   Note: In the child with depressed consciousness, in whom the cough reflex may be depressed, it is important to watch for cyanosis and distress. These may be the only indication that the tube is entering the trachea.
10. Once the tube has been passed to the position previously marked on the tube, check once again for choking, restlessness, or cyanosis.
11. Secure the end of the tubing with adhesive tape beneath the child's nose and to the temple.
12. Open the spigot on the tube and aspirate, using the syringe.
13. Test the acidity of the aspirated fluid using blue litmus paper; if the colour changes to red, the end of the tube is in the stomach.
14. If litmus paper is unavailable, the aspiration of clear fluid containing mucus, or partially digested food, shows that the end of the tube is in the stomach (in intestinal obstruction, the fluid would be bile stained).
15. To test further for correct positioning of the tube, use the syringe to inject 5–10 ml/kg of air into the tube, while listening over the epigastrium with the stethoscope. A distinct 'gurgle' will be heard as air enters the stomach.
16. Once satisfied that the tube is in position, inject 5–10 ml of fluid, again noting any choking or cyanosis.

Nasogastric feeding

1. Where possible, fluid should be given by continuous infusion, using a pump or rate controller; a drip set and counting chamber can also be used.
2. Alternatively, fluid should be given in hourly boluses, using the syringe barrel to give small amounts. The syringe should be held vertically, approximately 30 cm (12 in) above the child's head, to produce a slow and gentle flow of the fluid.
3. When the feed is completed, spigot the tube, and record the amount of fluid given.
4. Before each subsequent feed (or 4 hourly in continuous feeding) the position of the nasogastric tube should be checked.
   (a) Look into the child's mouth to ensure that the tube is not coiled in the oropharynx.
   (b) Aspirate to check for 'pooling' of fluid in the stomach and test for acidity as above.
5. If the nasogastric feeding is continued, the following extra measures are required:
   (a) Daily cleansing of both nostrils with warm water, paying particular attention to nasal crusting around the tube.
   (b) Scrupulous oral hygiene is necessary; nasogastric feeding predisposes to stomatitis and parotitis if no oral fluids are taken. Cleansing with a solution of sodium bicarbonate 8.4% if available, or citrus fruit juice, can stimulate the flow of saliva and help to prevent these complications.
   (c) The skin beneath the adhesive tape quickly becomes sore if allowed to remain wet. Removal with plaster remover and gentle cleaning with water and thorough drying should be performed whenever the tape becomes damp. The site for securing the free end of the tape should be changed.
   (d) Infants should be encouraged to maintain their sucking reflex with a clean dummy or finger tip.

Stopping nasogastric feeding

1. If continuous nasogastric feeding has been used, this can be stopped by changing to hourly, then 2 hourly bolus feeds. Tube feeds are then alternated with oral feeds, during the day while tube feeds are continued at night. Tube feeds are then reduced progressively as oral feeds increase.
2. Severe loss of appetite and feeding problems may be encountered, after prolonged nasogastric feeding.

Removal of the nasogastric tube

1. Explain the procedure to the child.
2. Remove the adhesive tape with plaster remover.
3. Gently and smoothly withdraw the tube:
   (a) Older children may prefer to remove the tube themselves.
   (b) Rapid removal of the tube can stimulate the gag reflex and induce vomiting.
4. Offer the child a drink and gently cleanse the nostrils.

The use of nasogastric feeding in the dehydrated child (from King, King and Martodipoero, 1983) (*Table 93.1*)

Use the WHO oral rehydration mixture or a salt and sugar mixture (*see* page 405 or Appendix 9).
If the child is better after 12 hours, the drip can be slowed down. If he is not better, continue with the fluid at the same speed. Watch the eyes; swelling round the eyes indicates that too much fluid has been given or that it has been given too fast.

Table 93.1 Volumes of intragastric fluid in the first 12 hours

Weight of child (kg)	*No. of drops per minute*	(ml/hour)*
6	25	(75)
9	35	(100)
12	50	(150)

* The relationship between the number of drops per minute and the number of ml per hour depends upon the type of fluid given and even more importantly upon the type of drip chamber (*see* Appendix 24).

If the child vomits, slow the drip down to 20 drops per minute (60 ml/hour), or more slowly in a small child (<5 kg). Observe the child carefully, and take the drip down as soon as he can drink. If his dehydration gets worse despite intragastric fluid, he needs IV fluids. If the mother is present and there is no one else to look after the drip, show her how to regulate it and the level which it should reach in each hour.

Intraperitoneal fluids in dehydration

Marian D. Smith

In the developing world, intraperitoneal fluids can be used very successfully in the management of moderately dehydrated children. The technique is safe and simple and can be quickly mastered by paramedical staff.

Indications

Moderate dehydration, with any of the following:

1. No rapid improvement with oral therapy.
2. Persistent vomiting.
3. When the child appears too ill for complete reliance on oral fluids (e.g. when there is associated infection, respiratory or other).
4. In some field rehydration units where the duration of supervision may be limited to less than 6 hours in a day.
5. In some hospital situations where the skilled supervision of intravenous infusions is not available for the whole of the 24 hour period. Drips often stop, or run too quickly and overload the circulation.

Contraindications

Intraperitoneal fluids should not be given if there is abdominal distension or ascites, or severe skin sepsis. Its effect is not sufficiently rapid for a child who is more than moderately dehydrated. *Shocked children always require intravenous fluids.*

Apparatus required

Sterile fluid (0.45% NaCl in 2.5% or 5% glucose), drip stand, standard giving set with pinchcock and attached needle, antiseptic solution to clean the skin, adhesive tape.

Procedure

NaCl 0.45% in 2.5% or 5% glucose is normally used. Half-strength Darrow's solution (*see* Appendix 8) is also suitable. Sufficient to replace the child's estimated deficit can normally be given intraperitoneally (body weight in kg × 100 ml). The fluid should be warmed to *body heat* by standing in warm water.

The abdomen is first palpated to ensure that the liver, spleen, and bladder are not enlarged and at risk from the needle. The skin of the left iliac fossa is cleaned with antiseptic solution only, no anaesthetic is necessary. Mid-way between the umbilicus and the mid-inguinal point, a fold of skin is pinched up, and the needle inserted horizontally and subcutaneously through it. The pinchcock is opened fully, and the needle now turned vertically and pushed steadily into the peritoneal cavity. The pressure of fluid produced by fully opening the pinchcock, pushes any bowel away, and prevents damage by the needle.

After fixing the needle with adhesive tape, a volume of fluid sufficient to replace the calculated deficit can normally be given over about 30 minutes. The infant occasionally develops mild respiratory distress but this settles quickly as the fluid is usually absorbed rapidly over 6–8 hours.

After giving the necessary volume of fluid, the needle is removed and the entry site covered with adhesive tape only.

Additional fluids are offered orally to cover maintenance requirements. When intraperitoneal fluids are given as an out-patient, the child should be reviewed on the following day.

Complications

This procedure is extremely safe and effective. Complications are very rare. There is probably a very small risk of sepsis or damage to abdominal viscera.

Note: The same fluid, using the same apparatus, may also be given subcutaneously. This may be necessary where moderately dehydrated children have abdominal distension, or severe skin sepsis, or where the administering staff are *very* unskilled and poorly supervised. It is, however, slower and more painful than the preferred intraperitoneal route. Hyalase is expensive and unnecessary. The needle is inserted subcutaneously in the thigh or armpit. Fluid to replace the infant's estimated deficit can be given in several different sites over about 12 hours.

Peritoneal aspiration

Ian Shellshear

Indications

To determine the nature of unexplained intraperitoneal fluid or to relieve tense ascites.

Equipment

Sterile procedure; 20 ml syringe, 22 gauge 1½ in needle, trocar and cannula if indicated.

Procedure

If the effusion is large, it may be convenient to use a trocar and cannula under local anaesthetic, especially if large quantities of fluid are to be removed. Otherwise × 22 × 1½ in needle is inserted, with a 20 ml syringe attached, into either the right or left iliac fossa.

The fluid is aspirated and should be sent for cells, cytology and culture, including tubercle bacilli. For a trocar, a small incision is made in the skin under local anaesthetic. After completing the procedure, a butterfly tape or single suture is used to close the wound. Continuing leak of fluid may require careful re-suturing.

Complications

Particularly with trocar and cannula, there is a risk of puncture of the bowel.

Genitourinary system

Ian Shellshear

Aspiration of the bladder

Indication

Definitive diagnosis of a urinary-tract infection when bag urines have been equivocal, especially in the newborn.

Equipment

Aseptic procedure; 22 gauge 1½ in needle, 10 ml syringe, cleaning solution and swabs.

Procedure (Figure 93.7)

If there is time, liberal or extra fluids should be given 1–2 hours before the puncture. The direction of insertion of the needle varies with age, as the bladder is an abdominal organ in infancy and a pelvic organ in the older child. Rapid dart-like insertion of the needle greatly improves success. In a neonate, the needle is inserted 1 cm (½ in) above the symphysis pubis in the midline and directed 45° upwards. It is pushed in to a depth of 1–2.5 cm (½–1 in). In the older child, the needle is inserted just above the symphysis pubis inclined at 45° upwards towards the pelvis and pushed in for 4 cm (1½ in) before aspirating. If no urine is aspirated, the procedure should be delayed until the patient has had further fluids.

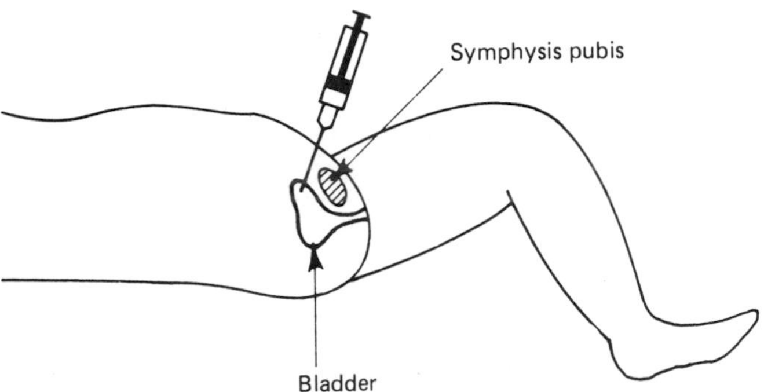

Figure 93.7 Bladder puncture.

Complications

There is often some haematuria afterwards but this should clear rapidly.

The bowel may be punctured and the urine contaminated with faeces. There is no danger to the child as the bowel appears to withstand this insult well, but the urine sample is useless.

Central nervous system

R. A. Minns

1. Monitoring of intracranial pressure (*see* pages 294–296).
2. Acute subdural haematoma: operative technique (*see* page 287).
3. Acute extradural haematoma; operative technique (*see* page 285).
4. Lumbar puncture.

Indications

Diagnostic:

1. Suspected meningitis.
2. First pyrexial convulsion under 3 years of age.
3. Suspected subarachnoid haemorrhage.
4. Suspected encephalitis.
5. Leukaemic meningitis.
6. Subacute sclerosing panencephalitis.
7. Guillain–Barré syndrome.
8. Myelography for spinal block.
9. Isotope encephalography and pneumo-encephalography.

Therapeutic:

10. Benign intracranial hypertension.
11. Subarachnoid haemorrhage.
12. Intrathecal steroids, antibiotics and anti-mitotics.
13. Neonatal intraventricular haemorrhage.
14. Spinal anaesthesia.

Preparation, equipment and method

1. Explanation and reassurance to the child and the parents about the procedure.
2. Sedate if necessary with diazepam.
3. Positioning the child on his side to open the lumbar interspinal spaces without lateral curvature or rotation of the spine. For right-handed doctors the patient is placed on his left side and with the help of an assistant the patient's back is arched and the knees are brought up to the chin, with the shoulders and pelvis in the same plane and vertical.
4. The skin is cleaned with betadine solution, merthiolate or other appropriate cleansing agent; it is important that the skin is dry before the procedure particularly if butterfly needles are to be used, or spinal needles without a stilette. The doctor scrubs up, and mask and gloves are put on. The infant or very small child may not necessarily be draped.
5. The landmark is a line drawn between the highest points of both iliac crests; this line crosses the spinal column at the L3–4 space. One space higher, L2–3, may be used after failure at the L3–4 space. It is not advisable to use higher spaces because of the risk of cord damage. The second and third fingers of the left hand are put on the adjacent L3 and L4 spines and the skin stretched gently between them.
6. A stiletted spinal needle is used 4–5 cm (1½–2 in) in length or a 21–23 gauge butterfly scalp vein needle for the newborn, or larger spinal needles for the older child. An acute-angled bevelled needle is better because it reduces the possibility of introducing skin into the subarachnoid space.
7. With most infants and young children local anaesthesia is not used as most doctors find it easier to perform the procedure carefully and quickly without it. Where lignocaine is used in the older child or adolescent, the infiltration is begun in the skin between the spine, and then on a line parallel to the slope of the vertebral spines in the direction of the umbilicus. The anaesthetic needle is left in position until anaesthesia occurs, as a guide for insertion of the spinal needle.
8. The needle is inserted with the bevel pointing laterally to separate rather than to cut any spinal roots. The needle is advanced through the ligamentum flavum where it is felt to 'give'; the same sensation occurs as it goes through the dura. The needle is advanced slowly, checking for any CSF flow by removing the stilette. Once the needle is fully advanced the stilette is removed and if no flow occurs the needle is rotated slightly in case a nerve root is obstructing it, and is again then advanced very slightly.
9. If CSF flows to the end of the needle this is suitable for measurement of the CSF pressure. The traditional open-ended manometric methods using a capillary tube column are less safe and of little value in children. It is important that the *CSF pressure is measured however,* and this is done using a non-displacement method by connecting up a strain gauge pressure transducer (attached to a 3-way tap to the end of the spinal needle) (Minns, 1984). This simple procedure requires inexpensive equipment which can be kept in the treatment room. The strain gauge transducer is calibrated before the procedure with a sphygmomanometer over a range of 0–50 mm Hg. The signal from the transducer is written out on a recorder. The transducer is sterilized in 'Cidex' solution and if it has a Luer connection is connected to a three-way tap. When the spinal needle stilette is removed and CSF has reached the proximal end of

the needle it is connected to the three-way tap. It is important that the CSF is in a continuous column from the patient's theca to the sensor of the diaphragm and that there are no air bubbles which falsify the recorded pressure. It is not essential that a chart recording is obtained, but it provides a permanent record of the measured pressure. The presence of a pulse wave verifies the position of the spinal needle and this is contributed to by the respiration. These oscillations may be damped when fine-bore spinal needles are used, but the mean CSF pressure will not be altered. A few minute's recording is obtained while the patient is permitted to relax a little, with reduced flexion, and with the head and neck in a neutral position and no abdominal compression. Over the next 3–4 minutes as the patient relaxes the pressure will drop to its true height, and where there is free communication of the CSF spaces, this reflects the intracranial pressure.

10. There are no routine indications for performing a lumbar puncture and a Queckenstedt's test. If a spinal block is known to exist or is suspected, one should proceed to myelography directly. The only situation where a Queckenstedt's test is justified is where at lumbar puncture a high CSF pressure is found, and after removal of a couple of drops of CSF the pressure falls markedly. One can then proceed to a Queckenstedt's test provided it is known that there is no disease above the level of the foramen magnum. With a complete spinal block, jugular venous compression causes no rise in the lumbar thecal pressure. Normally there is a rapid rise and fall of pressure. *In the presence of intracranial disease a Queckenstedt's test may induce tentorial or tonsillar herniation, with sudden death.* The test for the diagnosis of unilateral transverse sinus thrombosis, by failing to record a pressure rise on the side ipsilateral to the obstruction, is too rare to justify the Queckenstedt's test in any patient with intracranial pathology.
11. After the pressure record has been obtained the three-way tap is opened and the required volume of CSF drained, usually about 2 ml although all the required investigations can be performed on about 10 drops. Separate containers are used if the tap produces bloodstained fluid. Unless one is dealing with a known low pressure syndrome, or there is known to be purulent CSF, the spinal fluid should not be aspirated, and for low pressure syndromes the LP may be performed in the sitting position.

Absolute contraindications

1. *Intracranial space-occupying lesions,* such as tumours (in the cerebral hemisphere or posterior fossa), clot (such as extradural haematoma or a cystic external collection), cyst elsewhere in the intracranial cavity, or abscess.
2. *Hydrocephalus:*
   (a) Progressive, untreated, and moderately severe.
   (b) Non-communicating, with a potential compartment pressure difference.
   (c) Arnold–Chiari malformation.
3. *Evidence of coning or incipient herniation* – If coning is already present, there may be decerebrate or decorticate posturing (*see* page 293). If there is incipient herniation with pressure on the midbrain or the medullary region there will be a return of primitive reflexes, increasing coma, neck retraction, unequal pupils, and irregularities of pulse, blood pressure, and respiration.

The other clinical signs which might indicate intracranial space occupation or severe hydrocephalus may be quite diverse; certain combinations of local and general neurological signs constitute warning signs against lumbar puncture; for example, pyramidal and cerebellar signs with papilloedema; severe papilloedema alone with retinal haemorrhages; acute suture separation in a child of the toddler age or older; coma with papilloedema, or coma alone; where the cause of the coma is not known it would be unwise to puncture before a CT scan; focal neurological signs with papilloedema; *papilloedema is uncommon under the age of 5 years and there is no one single reliable sign of raised intracranial pressure in childhood.*

Complications and difficulties

1. The most serious complications is tonsillar or tentorial coning with a sudden collapse and cardiorespiratory arrest, when the lumbar puncture is done in the presence of one of the above contraindications. It may occur several hours after the lumbar puncture, owing to a persistent leak of CSF from the spinal theca. When it occurs while the needle is *in situ,* 1–2 ml of normal saline are injected back into the subarachnoid space and the child is inverted. In an infant with ventricles accessible via a patent fontanelle a ventricular puncture is performed and 10 ml of ventricular CSF removed. Resuscitative measures with intravenous mannitol, hyperventilation and immediate surgical decompression should be started immediately.
2. There are situations where it is essential to obtain CSF, in the presence of known raised intracranial pressure, by a 'careful LP'. The indications for the 'careful LP' include subarachnoid haemorrhage, meningitis with associated cerebritis and therefore oedema, tuberculous meningitis, and cryptococcal meningitis. Although lumbar punctures have been performed in tuberculous meningitis for many years, herniations were occasionally encountered, since nearly 90 per cent of tuberculous meningitis in childhood present with acute hydrocephalus. Where this is suspected, it is better to obtain an urgent CT scan to confirm the ventricular dilatation and to insert a ventricular reservoir, reduce the ventricular pressure by CSF removal, and obtain a cell count and bacteriological culture on the ventricular CSF. When the intracranial pressure is low, one may then safely proceed to a lumbar puncture for further cell count and identification of the tubercle bacillus. In such a situation spinal meningitis may occur without ventriculitis.

   The 'careful lumbar puncture' involves:
   (a) Cardiorespiratory resuscitation equipment close by.
   (b) Performing the lumbar puncture with a fine-bore needle.
   (c) Giving sedation for the procedure if one is likely to need it.
   (d) Having an intravenous infusion set up with mannitol ready to run in immediately, if necessary.
   (e) Having 2 ml of normal saline drawn up in a syringe ready to inject back into the spinal theca.

   A maximum of 10 drops of CSF is removed, two drops at a time and pressure measurement must only be done with the previously described non-displacement method.
3. The injudicious use of a Queckenstedt's test in patients with pathology above the foramen magnum may induce acute brain herniation, and similarly, removal of more than a few drops of CSF where the Queckenstedt's test is

positive, i.e. in a complete spinal block, may induce acute cord compression at the level of the block and result in a permanent paraplegia.

4. The introduction of infection into the CSF by lumbar puncture (i.e. meningitis) is an unusual complication but may occur when there is overlying infected skin such as in burns, or in septicaemia. The avoidance of the introduction of leukaemic cells into the subarachnoid space demands minimal trauma and struggling, and for most children this means a general anaesthetic or a dissociative anaesthetic such as ketamine.
5. In the absence of raised intracranial pressure, cardiorespiratory arrest may occur in young infants if there is cardiac or respiratory disease, such as respiratory distress syndrome, due to mechanical restriction of ventilation, from prolonged or restrictive positioning of the infant.
6. Transient low back pain and pain in the thigh.
7. Post-lumbar puncture (postural) headache. This occurs mainly in older children and may last for up to 3 days. It is probably due to leakage of CSF through the puncture site, and can be minimized if the patient remains lying flat after the procedure, and if a fine-bone needle is used. Analgesia may be required, and adequate fluid intake should be maintained.
8. A transient sixth nerve palsy, sometimes associated with headache and dizziness may occur a few days after lumbar puncture.
9. An intraspinal epidermoid tumour from introducing skin through a non-stiletted needle may occur years later.
10. Vertebral osteomyelitis is a rare complication from introduction of infection when the spinal needle pierces a vertebra.
11. Puncture of an intervertebral disc may cause acute localized pain lasting for several days.
12. Lumbar puncture performed early, in cases of meningitis, where the organism has not yet had time to excite a cellular response, may produce CSF free of cells; organisms may only be seen by careful scrutiny or cytocentrifuge techniques.
13. A traumatic tap may occur with blood in the CSF, if the needle punctures an epidural vein, or the intravertebral disc; traumatic haemorrhage may also result from piercing the epidural venous plexus on the posterior aspect of the vertebral body.

What to do with the CSF

1. Note the *appearance*. It should be 'gin clear', but may contain up to 350 red cells/mm^3 and yet still appear clear. With 500 red cells/mm^3 it will appear hazy or opalescent and with a greater number of red cells will be pink and then frankly bloodstained. Xanthochromia may result from neonatal hyperbilirubinaemia, previous traumatic tap, or intracranial haemorrhage. Cloudy CSF indicates a pleocytosis, probably due to meningitis; with more pus cells there is increasing turbidity.
2. The CSF is placed on a counting chamber and *cells are counted and identified*. There may be up to a few hundred red cells in the CSF of the newborn. If there was a traumatic tap, an attempt to estimate if there is an increased number of white cells, demands an idea of the peripheral red cell/white cell ratio and application of this ratio to the CSF; this ratio should hold true for the CSF is there is no meningeal inflammation. This usually means a correction factor, allowing 500–1000 red cells for each white blood cell seen. A similar correction

factor should be applied to the expected protein elevation in CSF contaminated by blood. Usually 1000 red cells/mm^3 equals 1 or 1.5 mg/100 ml.

A more accurate method of cell identification involves cytocentrifugation and a millipore filter, particularly where there is a mild CSF pleocytosis. This involves sedimentation in a cytospin machine, of the cellular elements in the CSF, onto a circumscribed area of a glass slide. This cellular deposit is then stained with standard May–Grunwald–Giemsa stain and is examined microscopically.

3. Bloody CSF may indicate a traumatic tap or an intracranial haemorrhage. Collection of CSF in three successive containers will clarify the position, as bloody CSF from trauma will clear in later containers; it may also clot in traumatic procedures, but will not clot with bloodstained CSF from an intracranial haemorrhage. Searching for crenated red cells is rarely useful but spectrophotometry after centrifugation may be helpful. Xanthochromia is due to the breakdown products of haemoglobin, which are protein-bound and consist of three groups of substances: (a) bilirubin and bilirubinoids, (b) methaemoglobin and methaemalbumin, and (c) oxyhaemoglobin. All of these have a characteristic absorption peak. They are not usually present in the CSF although in marked neonatal hyperbilirubinaemia, the CSF indirect bilirubin level correlates roughly with the serum indirect bilirubin; this CSF, however, contains no other pigments and no excess of cells.

   With bloody CSF due to either traumatic tap or intracranial haemorrhage both oxyhaemoglobin and methaemoglobin are present early, but in traumatic taps the xanthochromia usually disappears in 48 hours and specimens after this, show no oxyhaemoglobin. With bloody CSF due to subarachnoid haemorrhage, the xanthochromia appears within 8 hours, is at its maximum by 48 hours, the red cells disappear after 5–10 days, and the xanthochromia takes 10 days or more to disappear. Later CSF specimens after a subarachnoid haemorrhage reveal methaemoglobin with or without bilirubin.
4. The CSF is also sent for estimation of protein and sugar. The protein is mainly albumin and is increased in inflammatory conditions, in CSF blocks, and following bleeding into the CSF. The CSF protein is slightly less in ventricular fluid than in lumbar fluid, and is higher in full-term newborns than older children, and very much higher in preterm infants. In preterm babies of very low birth weight the protein level is 50–200 mg/100 ml. In the full-term newborn a level of 40–120 mg/100 ml may be expected, in infants, 20–80 mg/100 ml. and in the older child 15–45 mg/100 ml. The immunoglobin IG fraction may be elevated in multiple sclerosis and subacute sclerosing panencephalitis. The CSF glucose in the older child and adult is 40–60 per cent of the blood level, while in newborn it is 75–80 per cent of the blood glucose.
5. CSF is also sent for culture and sensitivities. Antibacterial titres for measles and immunofluorescent techniques to identify herpes simplex, haemophilus influenzae and tubercle bacilli may be required. Other investigations which may be indicated include creatine kinase, lactate, xanthine and hypoxanthine. Acid–base studies (in the newborn the CO_2 in the CSF is slightly higher than in the older child and the pH of the CSF is slightly lower compared with arterial blood). The CSF sodium is approximately that of serum, the chloride is slightly higher and the potassium slightly lower, but osmolality of CSF is approximately the same as serum (275–295 mosmol/kg). Lysosomal enzymes can now also be measured in the CSF, e.g. hexosaminidase A and B, α-mannosidase, α-fucosidase, β-glucuronidase, and acid phosphatase.

Subdural tap

Indications

Suspected subdural collections:

1. Haematoma.
2. Hygroma.
3. Effusions.

Procedure

1. The head is shaved in a 5 cm (2 in) radius around the fontanelle margins. A 3-minute Betadine scrub is used to prepare an aseptic surface. The skull is draped, leaving a window over the area.
2. The insertion point is the lateral angle of the fontanelle and the direction of needle is in the line of the coronal suture.
3. A 20 gauge 3–4 cm (1½ in) spinal needle without stilette is used with bevel uppermost, and introduced through the skin to immediately below the cranial bone at the edge of the fontanelle. The needle is then advanced and a 'popping' sensation is felt as it penetrates the dura. The needle base is secured by the operator's fingers close to the scalp, to avoid accidental movement. In the absence of a subdural collection, a dry tap results or produces no more than 1–2 ml of fluid. If more than 3 ml are obtained this indicates subdural fluid or effusion and the fluid is allowed to drain passively. When complete, slight rotation of the head or slight repositioning of the neede is made to ensure maximum drainage.
4. Penetration of the pia-arachnoid membranes may actually cause an effusion. However, this is not a disaster, as it means that the subdural space has been traversed, and therefore exclude a subdural collection; and any leakage of the CSF into the subdural space is quickly reabsorbed. Should traumatic fresh bleeding occur with the procedure, the needle is withdrawn and the site is compressed for 5 minutes. Repeated aspiration of large volumes may cause hypovolaemia and anaemia; blood transfusion may be required to rectify this. Gentle suction is sometimes necessary if the fluid is viscous, and drips very slowly.
5. While subdural collections may occasionally be missed with routine ultrasound, awareness of this possibility by the radiologist and the use of measures to detect sonic beams by a standoff jelly block, or an adapted probe with attached 2–3 mm water bath, lessens the risk of a false-negative scan. Similar difficulties may be experienced with CT scanning where bilateral isodense subdural haematomata may result in no shift of midline structures and no apparent abnormality of the scanning. While this is unusual, nevertheless a subdural tap is a simple procedure, and totally eliminates subdural collections except when they are loculated. Other false-negative taps include loculated subdural empyema, and acute subdural haemorrhage. In children acute subdural haemorrhage frequently starts as an acute subarachnoid haemorrhage which then moves over the surface of the brain in the subarachnoid space, by means of the CSF pump action of the surface vessel pulsations, towards the midline, where stasis results in alteration of arachnoid permeability and effusion of fluid into the subdural space.

6. It should be recognized that subdural effusions are frequently bilateral, and therefore, in most instances, both sides should be tapped.
7. In the absence of other methods of assessing the extent of the subdural collection, 5–10 ml of air can be injected after an adequate amount of fluid has been removed, and X-rays are then taken in the brow-up and brow-down positions.

Ventricular puncture

Indications

1. Acute hydrocephalus with evidence of raised intracranial pressure.
2. Ventriculography with myodil or water-soluble non-ionic contrast media, etc.
3. Sampling of ventricular CSF in ventriculitis.
4. Intraventricular antibiotic injection.
5. Closed ventricular drainage in head injury, for the relief of persistent raised pressure, etc.

Procedures

THROUGH THE ANTERIOR FONTANELLE

This is done without sedation in the infant:

1. The head is shaved in a 5 cm (2 in) radius around the fontanelle and the scalp prepared as before, for a sterile procedure.
2. The landmark for insertion is the outer lateral margin of the anterior fontanelle (or in a line drawn from the inner canthus of the eye to the coronal suture) depending on the size of the fontanelle.
3. A radio-opaque Teflon IV cannula (Angiocath) or a radio-opaque polyurethane IV catheter (Polycath) of 4–4½ cm (1¾ in) at least in length and of 20–23 gauge in diameter is used. A stiletted needle may be preferred. The normal ventricle will be reached at a depth of 4 cm in the newborn and 7 cm in the adult.
4. The cannula is inserted at an angle parallel to the falx and perpendicular to the base of the skull. Some operators prefer to angle the needle slightly anteriorly.
5. The stilette is withdrawn every 0.5 cm (¼ in) or so, to see if CSF flows, giving some indication of the thickness of the cortical mantle.
6. When the CSF is located, the ventricular pressure is measured by a non-displacement method as previously described for lumbar puncture, and the CSF is sampled or the required volume removed, as required to reduce the intracranial pressure to the normal range. If too great a volume of CSF is removed quickly, the brain hangs suspended, and the child becomes pale and sweaty, with a thready pulse. Air or normal saline may be reinjected, but with the foot of the bed elevated the symptoms usually subside quickly.

THROUGH BURR HOLES AT OTHER SITES

1. The position and angle of the cannula can be adjusted to penetrate the ventricle from most cranial sites, by imagining a line drawn from the nasion to the external occipital protuberance.

2. The needle or cannula is directed through the trephine towards this line, keeping the needle perpendicular to an anteroposterior tangent at the puncture site. This means that the ventricles can be located accurately from most sites on the cranium. The same guidelines can be used when puncturing the ventricle via the anterior fontanelle, and may be a more accurate way of locating normal or even small 'slit-like' ventricles from the fontanelle.

THROUGH THE FRONTAL BONE

By using a bone marrow needle puncture as described in the standard neurosurgical texts (Milhorat, 1977), and puncturing the ventricle through the frontal bone:

1. Locate a point a quarter of the distance over the surface of the skull, from the nasion to the external occipital protuberance, and then moving 2 cm (¾–1 in) from the midline, on the right hand side of the skull, the bone marrow puncture is made.
2. The catheter with guide wire stilette is directed to a point 1 cm (½ in) ipsilateral to the midline.
3. The anticipated ventricular depth with normal sized ventricles is no more than half the distance between the two external auditory meati.

Complications of ventricular puncture

1. If the CSF pressure is raised, porencephalic cysts may result, with focal epileptic activity later, or from leaking of CSF immediately after the procedure.
2. Intracranial bleeding.
3. Intracranial infection, such as ventriculitis.
4. Sudden release of intracranial pressure with peripheral circulatory collapse, or compartmental pressure changes with an *upward* cone.
5. Inadvertent penetration of intracranial structures due to misdirection of the cannula, for example the internal capsule, or puncture of the sagittal sinus.

C1–2 puncture

Indications

1. Any indication previously used for cisternal puncture. The C1–2 puncture is preferable not only because there is less discomfort but it is potentially a less dangerous procedure.
2. Myelography to determine the upper end of a spinal block from tumour or adhesive arachnoiditis.
3. Where CSF is required, to make a diagnosis of meningitis, and lumbar puncture is contraindicated; for example, in suspected epidural abscess, extensive spina bifida preventing a lumbar puncture, or a technically difficult lumbar puncture despite optimum positioning in the lateral recumbent manner or sitting position.
4. To introduce drugs above the level of an obstruction in the spinal theca, for example, steroids for spinal arachnoiditis.

Procedure

1. This should only be done by those with experience of it. The patient is conscious and the procedure is explained beforehand to the child and/or parent. An

assistant is required for the procedure which is an aseptic one, with the neck shaved to an area between the external occipital protuberance and the midcervical region.

2. Before the procedure, a lateral plain X-ray is taken of the craniovertebral junction, with the head extended.
3. Positioning of the patient is critical. The patient is placed prone with the head in the midline and chin resting on the bed. This causes hyperextension of the neck, and apart from the immobilization it affords, it also results in anterior bowing of the cervical cord with a resultant pool of CSF, which makes location of the subarachnoid space easier and provides a collecting gutter for contrast media, if the procedure is being used for radiology. If this is the case 10 ml of water-soluble non-ionic contrast is used and the pooling in the cervical region limits proximal flow.
4. The surface relations are an important guide to needle insertion. The mastoid process is identified clinically and radiologically and the position of the C1–2 space compared with the mastoid process is noted radiologically, and a similar distance is judged on the patient posterior to the process to insert the needle. One aims at the midpoint between C1 and C2 and posterior in the space.
5. A 22 gauge stiletted needle is used 8.5 cm (3½ in) in length in the adult, and 6 cm (2½ in) in the child. It is inserted some 5–6 cm (2–2½ in) in the adult and 2.5–3.5 cm (1–1½ in) in the child. It is inserted at right angles.
6. Should the cord be punctured, transient pain or paraesthesia may occur but invariably settle within 24–48 hours. It is unlikely that the vertebral artery will be punctured with these landmarks, as it ascends in the transverse processes and is only directed dorsally when proximal to C1, before entering the skull. The same mastoid process landmark is used when performing a vertebral angiogram. If a C1–2 puncture is performed and blood returns through the needle, it is withdrawn and will usually clot quite readily with surface pressure without a haematomyelia.

Cisternal puncture

Indications

The indications are the same as for C1–2 puncture, but cisternal puncture has been virtually superseded by C1–2 puncture which is less dangerous. Cisternal punctures are generally contraindicated with Arnold–Chiari malformation or with cerebellar herniation. There may still be a need for doing a cisternal puncture in rare instances and therefore the procedure is described.

Procedure

1. No sedation or premedication is required. The preparation of the skin with shaving, cleaning and antiseptic precautions are as previously described.
2. The position may be either in the lateral decubitus with the head flexed and with support, so that the cervical spine is horizontal, or with the infant in a sitting position, again with maximum flexion of the neck.
3. The first palpable cervical vertebra is the spinous process of C2, and if local anaesthetic is used it is injected subcutaneously in the midline, 1–2 cm (½ in) above this.

4. An imaginary line between the posterior superior borders of the mastoid processes will traverse the cisterna magna in the midline. A 20 gauge 5 cm (2 in) paediatric stiletted spinal needle is used for the older child, and is advanced through the skin 1–1½ cm (½ in) above the first palpable spinous process, in the direction of the nasion.
5. The needle is then further advanced in the midline. The first resistance that is felt is the atlanto-occipital ligament, this is then followed by a 'popping' sensation as the needle enters the cistern.
6. If the needle strikes bone, this is usually the occipital bone and the procedure then is to adopt a creeping manoeuvre, by gradual lowering the needle tip, until it passes just inferior to the occipital bone.
7. On removal of the stilette the CSF should drip out slowly. The needle is rotated fully if drugs are to be injected, to ensure that the needle tip is wholly within the cistern. In most cases radiological control is not necessary; however, screening may be helpful if difficulties are experienced at the first attempt. Gentle pressure is maintained for a few minutes after removal of the needle and the patient is nursed with slight head elevation for 25 minutes.

Complications and difficulties

The contraindications to this procedure are the Arnold–Chiari malformation, cerebellar herniation, raised intracranial pressure, mass lesions in the posterior fossa, and other contraindications as for lumbar puncture.

Complications

1. Puncture of the spinal cord.
   This may cause paraesthesia or hemi-distribution pain. Puncture of the spinal cord, while not advisable, does not necessarily carry any more morbidity than needle puncture through the cortex of the brain.
2. Puncture of the posterior inferior cerebellar artery, which may be variable in its position around the foramen magnum.
   This may give rise to an acute subarachnoid haemorrhage which ceases spontaneously, or persistent spasm which may cause coma and apnoea.

References

CHURCH, M. A. (1972) Fluids for the sick child; a method of teaching mothers. *Tropical Doctor,* **2,** 119–121

DUNN, P. M. (1966) Localization of the umbilical catheter by postmortem measurement. *Archives of Disease in Childhood,* **41,** 69–75

GARG, A. K., HOUSTON, A. B., LAING, J. M. and MacKENZIE, J. R. (1983) Positioning of umbilical arterial catheters with ultrasound. *Archives of Disease in Childhood,* **58,** 1017–1018

KING, M., KING, F. and MARTODIPOERO, S. (1983) *Primary Child Care; Book One; a Manual for Health Workers,* p. 122. Oxford: Oxford University Press

MILHORAT, T. H. (1977) *Pediatric Neurosurgery; Contemporary Neurology Series 16.* Philadelphia: F. A. Davis

MINNS, R. A. (1984) Intracranial pressure monitoring. *Archives of Disease in Childhood,* **59,** 486–488

MORLEY, D. (1973) *Paediatric Priorities in the Developing World,* p. 187. London: Butterworth

SIMMONDS, S., VAUGHAN, P. and GUNN, S. W. (ed.) (1983) *Refugee Community Health Care.* Oxford: Oxford University Press

SIMMONS, M. A., LEVINE, R. L., LUBCHENKO, L. O. and GUGGENHEIM, M. A. (1978) Warning: Serious sequelae of temporal artery catheterisation. *Journal of Pediatrics,* **92,** 284

Further reading

FLETCHER, M. A., MacDONALD, M. G. and AVERY, G. B. (eds.) (1983) *Atlas of Procedures in Neonatology.* Philadelphia: J. B. Lippincott

WALES, J. K. H., HALL, M. A. and WALTON, P. (1985) Neonatal infusion site complications. *British Journal of Parenteral Therapy,* **6,** 6–8

Part XVIII

Appendices

Appendix 1

Weight, height, and surface area

J. A. Black

Weight has the advantage that it can be easily and accurately measured, but as a basis for the calculation of water and energy requirements and drug dosage over the age range from infancy to adolescence it is unsatisfactory as it gives a considerable underestimate in infants.
For example:

> A 10 kg infant might be expected to require 1/7 of the dose of a drug appropriate for a 70 kg adult, but this would be quite inadequate. In practice the correct amount is approximately 1/4 of the adult dose. This fraction can be arrived at by dividing the surface area of the average adult (1.73 m^2) by the surface area of the child (for further details of this method of calculating drug dosage *see* Appendix 10). A similar calculation can be applied to water and energy requirements, or the desired result may be achieved by using one value per m^2 for the whole age range, excluding the neonatal period and preterm infants. Surface area is not a satisfactory basis calculation in these infants since there is a wide range of weights, it is difficult to measure length accurately, and the available data are unreliable for very small infants.

Drug dosage, fluid (or water) and energy requirements for neonatal and preterm infants are therefore calculated on a weight basis. Weight-based methods of calculation in older children are also available, using a series of different scales, according to age; these give values which are approximately the same as those arrived at by using surface area (*see* Appendix 10).

Difficulties in the use of weights

Circumstances that prevent the child from being weighed

These may arise because the child is too ill, is in a plaster cast or orthopaedic appliance, or because of refusal to be weighed. This difficulty may be overcome in a number of ways.

1. The parents may have recent records of the child's weight; but only written records should be accepted.
2. The probable weight can be obtained from any standard figures for weight-for-age (*Figure A1.3*); before doing this it is necessary to confirm that the child is of normal proportions and is neither wasted nor obese.

3. If the height can be measured, the probable weight can be read off a weight-for-height graph (*Figure A1.1*).
4. With small children a parent can be weighed alone, then again carrying the child.

Excessively fat children

For children above the 97th centile for weight, but of normal height, actual weight should not be used in a nomogram for arriving at the surface area, since fat is relatively inactive metabolically and does not influence water requirements. In such

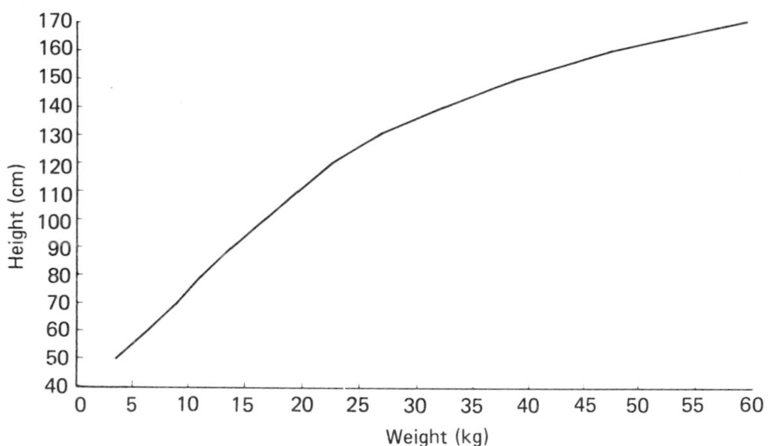

Figure A1.1 Weight-for-height. (Data from Tanner and Whitehouse charts using means of 50th centiles for boys and girls.)

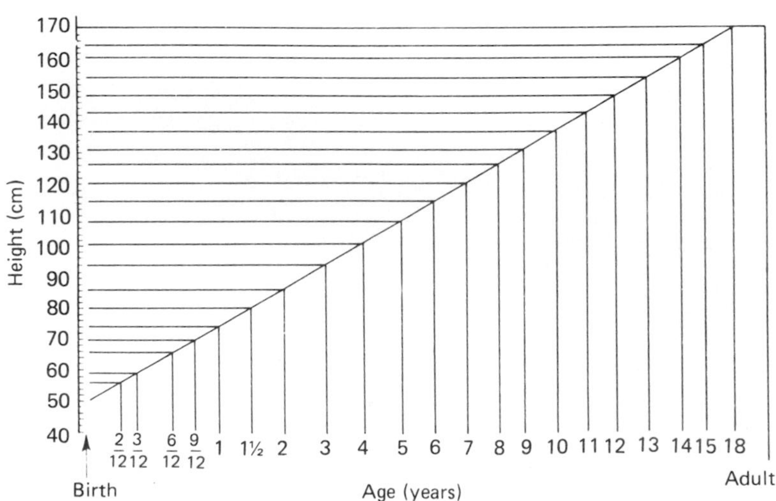

Figure A1.2 Height-for-age. 50th centiles means for boys and girls. (After Tanner, Whitehouse and Takaishi, 1966.)

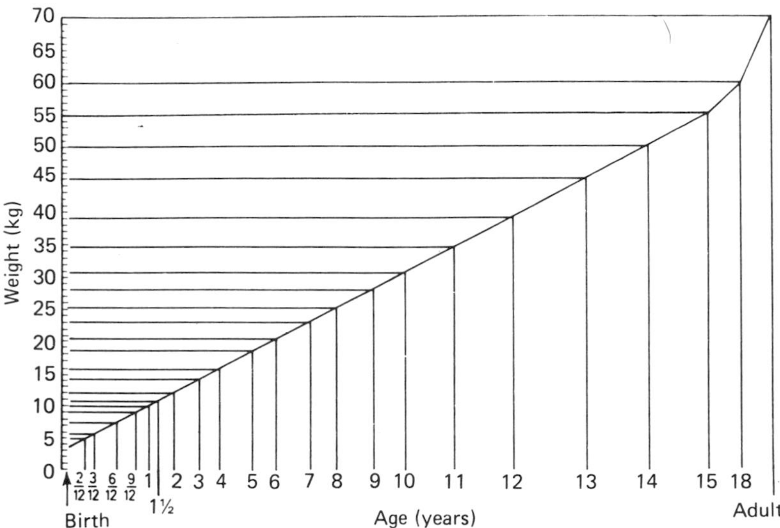

Figure A1.3 Weight-for-age. 50th centiles: means for boys and girls. (After Tanner, Whitehouse and Takaishi, 1966.)

circumstances the 'ideal' weight should be taken from a weight–height chart or from a standard centile chart, taking the same point on the chart for weight as is shown by plotting the height.

Determination of surface area

Both weight and height must be measured accurately, otherwise gross errors will occur. The standard nomograms can be used, provided that the child has normal body proportions. Many of the published nomograms have a very compressed scale and errors are common if they are used carelessley; those given in *Figures A1.5* and

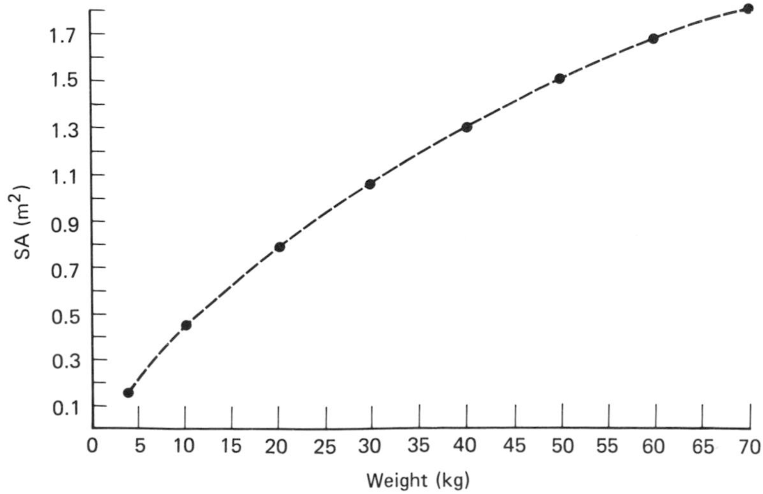

Figure A1.4 Surface area (SA)-for-weight for children of normal proportions.

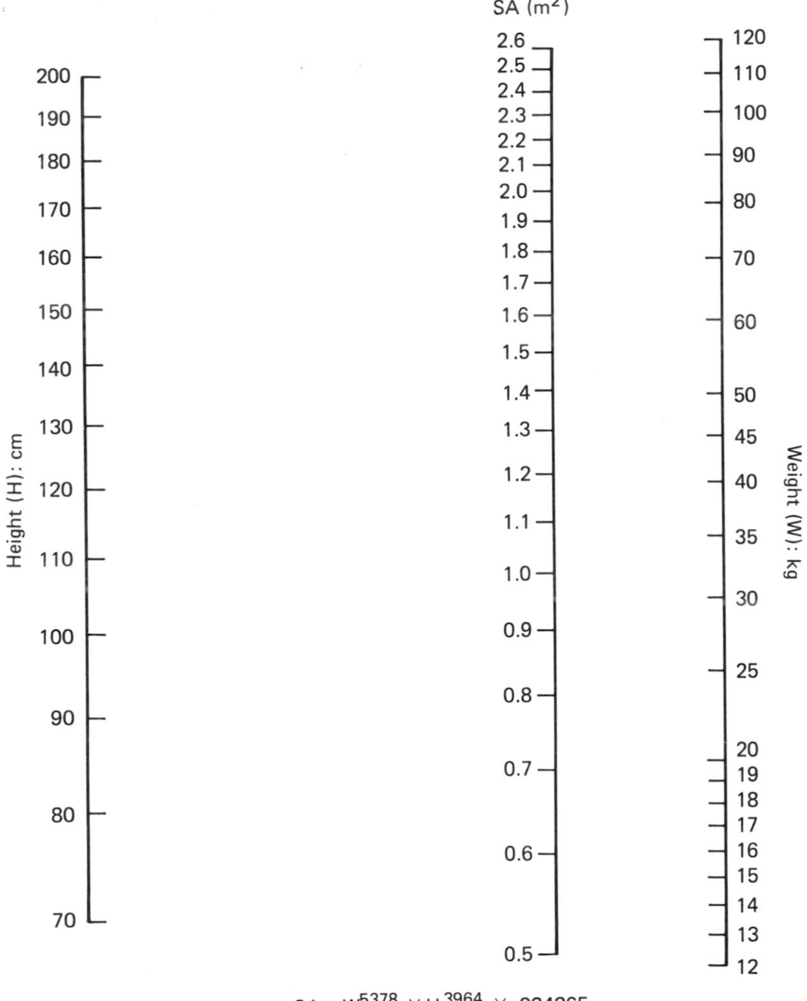

Figure A1.5 Nomogram showing the relationship between height, weight, and surface area in children and adults. To use the nomogram, a ruler is aligned with the height and weight on the two lateral axes. The point at which the centre line is intersected gives the corresponding value for surface area. (Reproduced from Haycock, Schwartz and Wisotsky (1978), with kind permission of authors and publishers.)

A1.6 appear to be the clearest and most accurate available. Alternatively, if only the weight is available, the surface area can be obtained from *Figure A1.4* provided the child is of normal weight for age. Surface area can be used, not only for calculating drug dosage, water, and energy requirements, but also for urine output (*see* Appendix 7). Apart from the nomogram, a number of formulae can be used to calculate surface area.

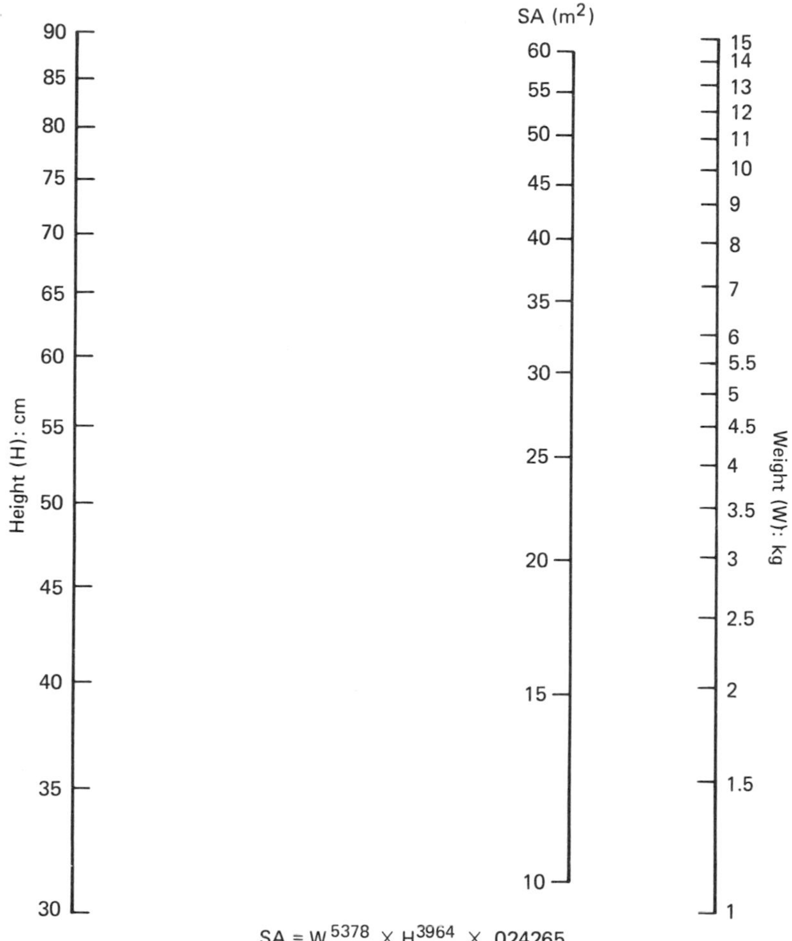

Figure A1.6 Nomogram showing the relationship between height, weight, and surface area in infants; use as for *Figure A1.5*. (Reproduced from Haycock, Schwartz and Wisotsky (1978), with kind permission of authors and publishers.)

1. Costeff's (1966) formula can be used, if only the weight is available.

$$SA(m^2) = \frac{4W + 7}{W + 90} \quad (W = \text{weight in kg})$$

2. An alternative method (Vaughan, 1983) of calculating surface area is:

Weight range (kg)	*Approximate SA*(m^2)
1–5	$0.05 \times W + 0.05$
6–10	$0.04 \times W + 0.10$
11–20	$0.03 \times W + 0.20$
21–40	$0.02 \times W + 0.40$

Over the extended range of 21–70 kg the formula $0.02 \times W + 0.40$ is reasonably accurate.

References

COSTEFF, H. (1966) A simple empirical formula for calculating approximate surface area in children. *Archives of Disease in Childhood,* **41,** 681–683

HAYCOCK, G. B., SCHWARTZ, G. J. and WISOTSKY, D. M. (1978) Geometric method for measuring body surface area; a weight–height formula validated for infants, children and adults. *Journal of Pediatrics,* **93,** 62–66

TANNER, J. M., WHITEHOUSE, R. H. and TAKAISHI, M. (1966) Standards from birth to maturity for height, weight, height velocity, weight velocity: British children. *Archives of Disease in Childhood,* **41,** 454–471

VAUGHAN, V. C. III (1983). In Behrman, R. E., Vaughan, V. C. (eds) *Nelson: Textbook of Pediatrics* (12th edn.), p. 26. Philadelphia: W. B. Saunders

Appendix 2

Energy requirements

J. A. Black

(For the requirements for the newborn and pre-term infants *see* Appendix 4). Metabolic requirements can be considered under three headings:

1. *Basal requirements* – As for the basal requirements for water (*see* Appendix 3), this is a physiological concept, and of no clinical significance.
2. *Requirements for normal activity* – It is necessary to know these figures in order to construct diets for diabetic children or for a nutritional survey.
3. Resting requirements (for patients on IV maintenance glucose–electrolyte solutions). Up to the age of 1 year, because of the relative inactivity of the infant, the energy requirements for normal activity and the IV glucose–electrolyte solutions are similar (*Figure A2.1*). The Surface Area method gives slightly lower figures.

Calculation of normal requirements

1. A commonly used method (*see also* page 453) is as follows, using an age-based formula: 1000 (+ 100 kcal for each year of age up to 18 years).
   Example:
   A 5-year-old boy would require:
   1000 + 500 = 1500 kcal
   (4200 + 2100 = 6300 kJ)*
   A table (*Table A2.1*) may be used, such as that given by Belton (1984), which gives slightly higher figures than the calculation in (1) above.

Calculation of resting maintenance requirements for on IV glucose–electrolyte solutions

(excluding the newborn and preterm infants, *see* Appendix 4)

1. Holliday and Segar (1957) suggest the following method:
   Up to 10 kg : 100 kcal/kg
   10–20 kg : 1000 + 50 kcal for each kg over 10 kg.
   20 kg and over : 1500 + 20 kcal for each kg over 20 kg.
   These weight-based values are given in graphic form in *Figure A2.1* for comparison with those in *Table A2.1* (normal activity) and those derived from surface area for IV glucose–electrolyte solutions.

* The 'calorie' of clinical medicine is actually a kilocalorie (kcal). 1 Cal = 4.2 kJ.

Table A2.1 Energy requirements for normal activity*

Age	Energy	
	per 24 hours (kcal/kJ)	*per kg per 24 hours* (kcal (kJ))
0–6 months	–	110 (460)
7 months–1 year	–	100 (420)
1–3 years	1200 (5040)	90 (380)
4–6 years	1600 (6700)	80 (340)
7–10 years	2100 (8800)	70 (300)
11–14 years (girls)	2500 (10500)	70 (300)
11–14 years (boys)	2750 (11500)	70 (300)
Adults	3000 (13600)	40–45 (170–190)

* *See also Figure A2.1* for these values compared with those for patients on IV glucose–electrolyte solutions. (Modified from Belton (1984).)

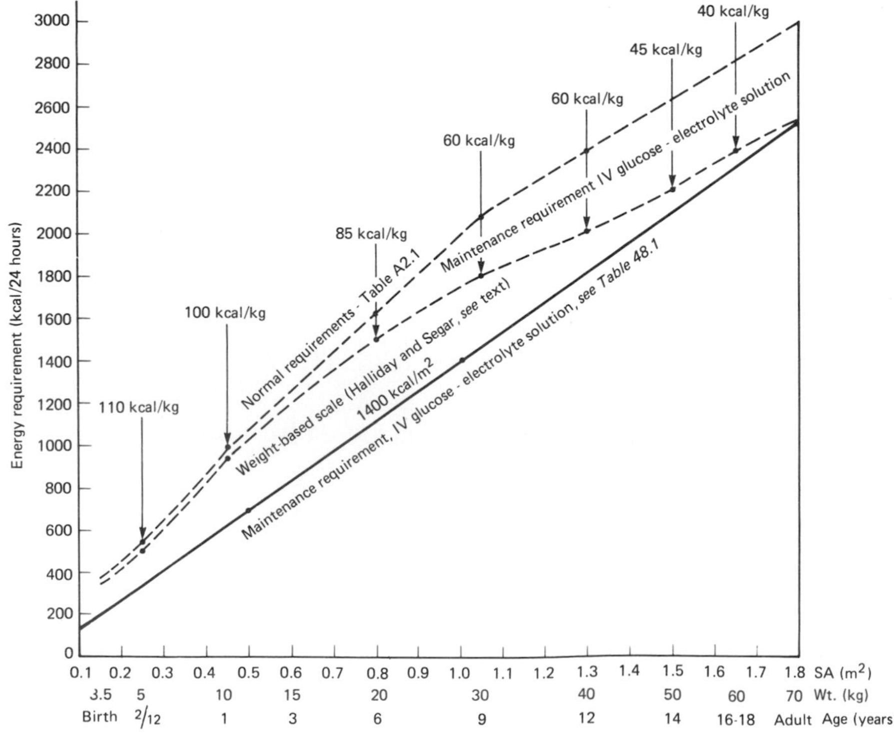

Figure A2.1 Energy requirements.

2. Surface area may be used as a reference; the usual value is 1400 kcal/m^2 (*see Table 48.1*). *Figure A2.1* shows that up to the age of 12 years the values obtained from the weight-based formula are slightly higher than those using surface area.

Factors that may alter energy requirements

Increased requirements

1. The energy requirement increases by 12 per cent for every rise in body temperature of 1°C (about 2°F).
2. In hypermetabolic states, such as thyrotoxicosis, salicylate poisoning, severe burns, and uncontrolled status epilepticus or tetanus, the energy requirements are increased by 25–75 per cent; in very extensive burns (>40 per cent of the body surface) the increased energy requirements may be as great as 100 per cent.

Decreased requirements

1. In hypothermia the energy requirement falls by 12 per cent for every fall of 1°C (about 2°F) of body temperature.
2. The energy requirement is presumably decreased in hypothyroidisis, but actual figures do not appear to be available.

References

BELTON, N. R. (1984) Biochemical and physiological tables and function tests. In Forfar J. O. and Arneil G. C. (eds.) *Textbook of Paediatrics* (3rd edn.), p. 1994. Edinburgh: Churchill-Livingstone

HOLLIDAY, M. A. and SEGAR, W. E. (1957) The maintenance need for water in parenteral fluid therapy. *Pediatrics,* **19,** 823–831

Appendix 3

Water and electrolyte requirements

(For requirements in the newborn and for low birth weight infants, *see* Appendix 4)

J. A. Black

Water requirements

Definitions

Water or fluid requirements

When calculating water requirements or measuring the intake of water, it should be assumed that all fluid consists solely of water.

Maintenance requirements

The term maintenance requirement implies that, excluding previous deficits, the requirement of water is that which equals the losses from all sources and at the same time provides for a urine flow which is sufficient to maintain homeostasis at different solute loads. However, 'maintenance' can be applied to three different situations:

1. *Basal maintenance requirement* – As for basal energy requirement, this is a physiological concept of no clinical importance.
2. *Normal maintenance requirement (Table A3.1 and Figure A3.1)* – This is the volume of water required to maintain homeostasis when the individual is undertaking normal physical activities on a normal diet, and there are no abnormal losses. Obviously this volume will vary with the age and size of the individual, the environmental temperature and humidity, the amount of physical activity, and the dietary intake of protein and salts (normally sodium and potassium salts).
   The normal maintenance requirement should not be confused with the *actual* intake, which, apart from the factors already mentioned, varies with the individual's personal habits, occupation and social customs. The volume of water actually drunk by active healthy individuals is usually much greater than the requirements for replacement of obligatory losses and for homeostasis.
3. *Resting maintenance requirements* – This is the volume of water required to maintain homeostasis on IV glucose–electrolyte fluids; that is, on a low solute load (this excludes total parenteral nutrition). This volume is therefore smaller than that required for the normal active person, as defined above. Resting maintenance can be calculated on the basis of weight or surface area (*Table A3.2, Figure A3.1*). Using the weight-based method, the values, up to the age of

Table A3.1 Normal water requirement according to age*

Age	*Daily requirement* (ml/kg)†
3 days	100–180
10 days	125–150
3 months	140–160
6 months	130–150
9 months	125–145
1 year	120–135
2 years	115–125
4 years	100–110
6 years	90–100
10 years	70–80
14 years	50–60
18 years	40–50

* Data, modified, from Documenta Geigy (1972) with permission of editors and publishers.
† These figures have been converted to ml daily using average weights for age, and incorporated into *Figure A3.1*.

See also Appendix 4.

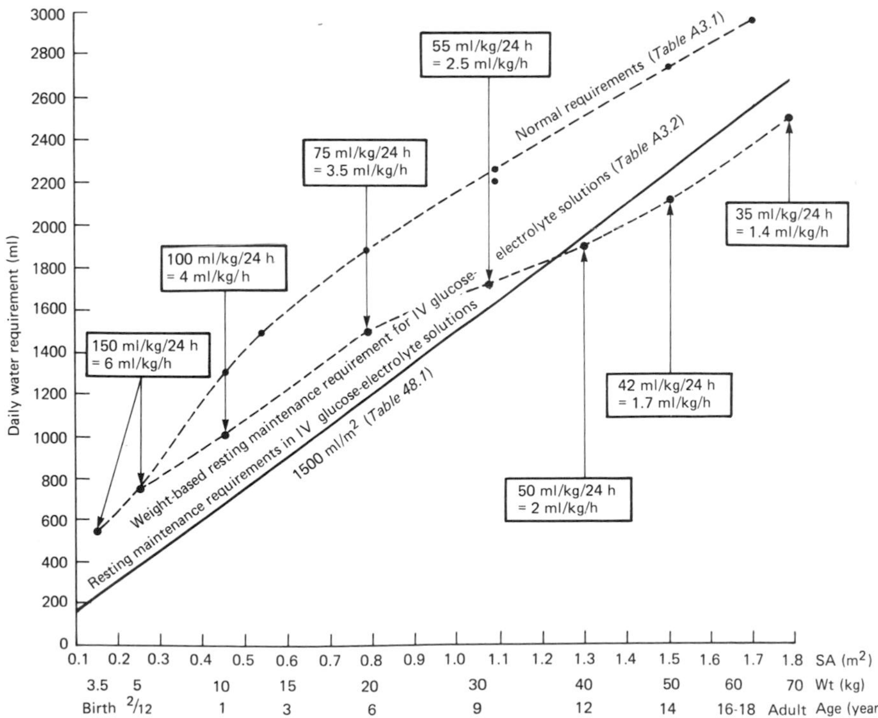

Figure A3.1 Maintenance requirements for water. For normal requirements *see Table A3.1;* for resting maintenance requirements *see also Table A3.2* and *Table 48.1*.

Table A3.2 Resting maintenance water requirements (*see also Table 48.1*, page 426)

Up to 10 kg	:	100 ml/kg
Over 10 kg	:	1000 ml + 50 ml for each additional kg up to 20 kg
Over 20 kg	:	1500 ml + 20 ml/kg for each additional kg over 20 kg

12 years, are about 30 per cent greater than those derived from surface area; after 12 years, they are about 12 per cent lower. As with energy, the normal and resting requirements for infants during the first year are similar.

In anuria the maintenance requirement is the volume of water required to replace losses through the skin and respiratory tract.

Factors that alter the maintenance water requirement

Age

The normal newborn infant during the first week of life, and the low birth weight infant need separate consideration (*see* Appendix 4).

Increased requirement

1. Raised environmental temperature; the water requirement is increased by 30 ml/kg for every rise of 1°C (about 2°F) above 30°C (80°F).
2. Raised body temperature, the water requirement increases by 12 per cent for every rise of 1°C (about 2°F) above 37°C (98°F).
3. Increased sweating.
4. Unusually low environmental humidity.
5. Exposure to radiant heat, as in phototherapy for neonatal jaundice (*see* page 686), or in using radiant heat shields for newborn or low birth weight infants; for either of these add 30 ml/kg/24 hours of water.
6. A sustained high respiration rate.
7. Polyuria due to renal disease, diabetes insipidus or to a high solute load, as in diabetic ketoacidosis and extensive burns; also, the polyuric phase following decompression of the obstructed renal tract (*see* page 776).
8. Continued losses from vomiting, gastric suction, fistulae, diarrhoea, and exudation and evaporative losses in extensive burns.

Reduced requirements

1. States of antidiuresis, which are usually transient; pain, trauma, operations, general anaesthesia, opioid drugs, cardiac failure, hepatic failure, head injury, bacterial meningitis, and other situations associated with the syndrome of inappropriate secretion of antidiuretic hormone (SIADH) (*see* page 124).
2. High environmental humidity.
3. Inspired air saturated with water vapour or containing aerosol droplets of water.
4. Anuria or oliguria due to renal disease (*see* Chapter 48).

Electrolyte requirements

1. *Short-term IV infusions* – For intravenous infusions lasting less than 48 hours, the maintenance requirements of sodium need only be considered (*see* Appendix 5).
2. *IV infusions lasting from 48 hours up to 5–7 days* – Potassium should also be added (*see* Appendix 5).
3. *IV infusions continued longer than 5–7 days* – Depending upon the circumstances total parenteral nutrition (TPN) or supplementary parenteral nutrition (SPN) is required, necessitating the calculation of the requirements of minerals, trace elements, vitamins, etc. (*see* Appendix 5).

Calculation of sodium and potassium requirements

Normally these are calculated on the basis of body weight; the requirements of chloride ion are covered by the fact that solutions are usually made up with sodium and potassium chloride.

Sodium: 2.0–3.0 mmol/kg (over 11 years or 35 kg, 1.5 mmol/kg).
Potassium : 2.0–3.0 mmol/kg (over 11 years or 35 kg, 1.5 mmol/kg).

Alternatively, sodium and potassium requirements may be based upon surface area, as 50 mmol/m^2 (Harris, 1972), or 75 mmol/m^2 if the higher requirement is used.

Factors that may alter electrolyte requirement

Increased requirement

SODIUM AND POTASSIUM

1. Continued loss by vomiting, gastric suction, fistulae, diarrhoea.
2. Renal disease with polyuria, as in acute tubular necrosis.
3. Polyuric phase following decompression of the obstructed renal tract.

SODIUM ONLY

1. Increased sweating.
2. Abnormally high sodium content of sweat, as in cystic fibrosis.
3. Renal sodium losing states (*see* Chapter 52, page 470).
4. Very low birth weight infants (*see* Appendix 4).

Decreased requirement

Postoperative sodium retention.

References

DOCUMENTA GEIGY (1972) Diem K., Lentner C. (eds) *Scientific Tables* (7th edn.). Basle: Ciba-Geigy
HARRIS, F. (1972) *Paediatric Fluid Therapy,* p. 144. Oxford: Blackwell Scientific Publications

Further reading

FINBERG, L., KRAVATH, R. E. and FLEISCHMAN, A. R. (1982) *Water and Electrolytes in Pediatrics.* Philadelphia: W. B. Saunders
WINTERS, R. (1982) *Principles of Pediatric Fluid Therapy* (2nd edn.). Boston: Little, Brown

Appendix 4

Energy, water, and electrolyte requirements of normal newborn and low birth weight infants

J. A. Black

Normal term infant (first week)

Only the requirements of the normal newborn during the first week are considered here; after the first week the calculations for infants in general apply. During the first week of life the newborn is physiologically adapted to receiving smaller amounts of energy and water than are required later, has ample supplies of glycogen and fat, and is well hydrated at birth. During this period of low intake, fat is metabolized to form water, and there may be, after an abnormal or hypoxic delivery, a short period of antidiuresis (Finberg, Kravath and Fleischman, 1982).

Energy (average intake)

Day 1 30 kcal/kg/24 hours (126 kJ/kg/24 hours).
Day 2 40–90 kcal/kg/24 hours (167–376 kJ/kg/24 hours).
Day 3 65–100 kcal/kg/24 hours (271–418 kJ/kg/24 hours).
Day 4 80–100 kcal/kg/24 hours (334–418 kJ/kg/24 hours).
Day 5 100–110 kcal/kg/24 hours (418–460 kJ/kg/24 hours).

Water

The water requirements during the first week are normally supplied from breast milk, or modified cows' milk formulae, with or without supplements of glucose water. The average requirements during the first week are shown in *Figure A4.1*.

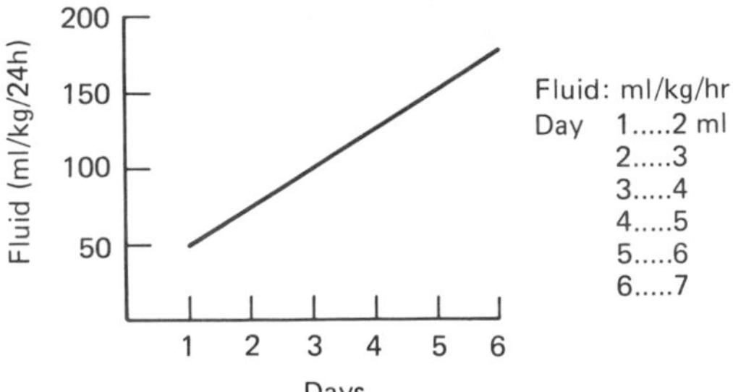

Figure A4.1 Water requirements in the first week of life. (Reproduced from Jones and Owen-Thomas (1971), with kind permission of authors and publishers.)

Electrolytes

The requirement for sodium and potassium during the first week of life appear to be met adequately by the intake of milk during this period.

Low birth weight (LBW) infants

Low birth weight infants differ from the normal newborn in having inadequate stores of glycogen and fat to cover a period of low energy intake. In addition, owing to their large surface area in relation to body weight, and their lack of subcutaneous fat, heat losses are very high. In very low birth weight infants (<1.5 kg), during the first week of life the skin is of a gelatinous consistency, causing large transcutaneous evaporative water losses, and heat loss. Even though these small infants really require large intakes of energy and water from birth it is usual to build up to their actual needs fairly slowly (*see* page 638) particularly if there are respiratory problems.

Energy

The energy requirement for the LBW infant is usually in the region of 120 kcal/kg/24 hours (502 kJ/kg/24 hours) though a greater intake may be required in infants of less than 1.5 kg.

Water

For infants of less than 2.5 kg, an intake of 180–200 ml/kg/24 hours is required, using the most appropriate route.

Electrolytes

Sodium

Though the conventional requirement of sodium of 2.0 mmol/kg/24 hours can be supplied by a volume of human milk (sodium 0.94 mmol/100 ml) or a low-sodium artificial milk (with the same content of sodium as human milk) of 200 ml/kg/24 hours these large intakes cannot always be achieved; but by using special premature infant formulae containing sodium 2.0 mmol/100 ml an adequate intake of sodium can be achieved with a small intake of milk. However Al-Dahhan *et al.* (1984) have shown that for infants on human milk or conventional artificial milks an increased weight gain (compared with controls) can be achieved and hyponatraemia can be avoided by supplementing sodium intake between 4 and 14 days of life up to a total of 5 mmol/kg/24 hours for infants of less than 31 weeks' gestation and to 4 mmol/kg/24 hours for those between 31 and 35 weeks' gestation.

Potassium

There is no evidence that the LBW infant requires more than the conventional 2 mmol/kg/24 hours, though the retention of potassium is of course greater where the infant is gaining weight rapidly (Al-Dahhan *et al.*, 1984).

References

AL-DAHHAN, J., HAYCOCK, G. B., NICHOL, B., CHANTLER, C. and STIMMLER, L. (1984) Sodium homeostasis in term and preterm infants. III. Effect of salt supplementation. *Archives of Disease in Childhood*, **59**, 945–950

FINBERG, L., KRAVATH, R. E. and FLEISCHMAN, A. R. (1982) *Water and Electrolytes in Pediatrics*, p. 222. Philadelphia: W. B. Saunders

JONES, R. S. and OWEN-THOMAS, J. B. (1971) *Care of the Critically Ill Child*, p. 288. London: Edward Arnold

Appendix 5

Intravenous maintenance fluids; surgery; total parenteral nutrition

(For low birth weight infants, including total parenteral nutrition, *see* Appendix 6).

J. A. Black, P. J. Milla and J. A. S. Dickson

As discussed in Appendices 2 and 3, the energy and water requirements for children on IV glucose–electrolyte solutions are lower than for normally active children. These requirements, and those for sodium and potassium, are summarized in *Table A5.1.* The requirements of the term newborn infant on IV fluids are given in *Table A5.2.* For total parenteral nutrition (*see* later), the water requirements are greater, owing to the higher solute load.

IV fluids: short-term maintenance (up to 48 hours)

In the absence of any known deficit of sodium, 0.18% NaCl in 4% glucose will cover the requirement of sodium. This solution is grossly deficient in energy but will suffice for a well-nourished child. This solution alone must NOT be used in

Table A5.1 Energy, water, sodium and potassium requirements for maintenance IV therapy with glucose–electrolyte solutions

Body weight (kg)	*Energy* (kcal/kg/24 hours (kJ/kg/24 hours))	*Water* (ml/kg/24 hours)	*Sodium* (mmol/kg/24 hours)	*Potassium* (mmol/kg/24 hours)
<10	110–75 (460–315)	150–100	2–3	2–3
10–20	100–65 (420–275)	100–75	2–3	2–3
>20	75–55 (315–230)	75–60	2–1.5	2–1.5

1. Use the higher figure for energy and water for the lower half of the weight range.
2. For sodium and potassium, use the lower figure for weights >35 kg.
3. For water requirements >25 kg use *Figure A3.1* or *Table A3.2*, and for energy requirements >50 kg use *Figure A2.1* or the method of calculation in Appendix 2, page 763.

Table A5.2 Water requirements of the term infant on IV fluids*

Day of life	*Volume* (ml/kg)
1	60
2	75
3	90
4 and 5	120
6	150
6+	150–200

* Tables A5.1 and A5.2 reproduced from C. A. Highes (1984), with kind permission of authors and publishers.

malnourished children who may have large deficits of potassium, magnesium and zinc (*see* Chapter 69). One litre of 0.18% NaCl in 4% glucose contains 31 mmol sodium and supplies 160 kcal (670 kJ) energy.

Example

A 10 kg child will require 100 ml water and 2–3 mmol sodium/kg/24 hours (1000 ml: 20–30 mmol). The sodium requirement will therefore be covered, but the energy requirement of 100 kcal/kg/24 hours (420 kJ/kg/24 hours; 1000 kcal, 4200 kJ) will not. The infusion rate will be 4 ml/kg/hour.

IV fluids: medium-term maintenance (48 hours up to 5–7 days)

For this period potassium *must* be given, to supply at least 1.5 mmol/kg/24 hours, though this is not the optimal requirement of 2–3 mmol/kg for small children.

0.18% NaCl in 4% glucose in the standard amounts will cover the requirement of sodium. The addition of one ampoule containing 0.15 g (2 mmol) potassium chloride to every 100 ml solution will produce a potassium concentration of 20 mmol/ℓ.

This solution is also deficient in energy and should only be used *alone* in well-nourished children, and is quite unsuitable for malnourished children who may require additional potassium and magnesium and zinc, and also 10% glucose to prevent hypoglycaemia (*see* Chapter 69).

Example

A 20 kg child will require:

Water: First 10 kg: 100 ml/kg = 1000 ml
Second 10 kg: 50 ml/kg = 500 ml
Total = 1500 ml, or 75 ml/kg/24 hours.

Sodium: Requirement is 2–3 mmol/kg/24 hours (40–60 mmol); 1500 ml of the solution supplies 46 mmol.

Potassium: Requirement is 2–3 mmol/kg/24 hours (40–60 mmol); 1500 ml of the solution supplies 30 mmol potassium which is slightly inadequate for small children (*see Table A5.1*).

Energy: Requirement is 65 kcal/24 hours (275 kJ/kg/24 hours) (1300 kcal, 5500 kJ), whereas 1500 ml of this solution supplies only 240 kcal (908 kJ).

IV fluids in surgery (*see* Appendix 6 for low birth weight infants)

Intraoperative requirements

The intraoperative need for fluid and electrolytes varies with the age of the child, the period of preoperative starvation, and the severity and duration of the operation. For operations lasting less than 1 hour, with a good prospect of resuming normal feeding within 4 hours, only the fluid required to give the anaesthetic need be given, and should not exceed 10 ml/kg/hour.

For longer operations it is usual to give 10 ml/kg/hour for the first hour, and in operations where there is much evaporative or other fluid loss, or a significant loss of extracellular fluid is expected, this rate should be continued. For other situations, the rate after the first hour should be reduced to 4 ml/kg/hour. In infants (under the age of 1 year), half-strength Hartmann's solution with 2.5% glucose (i.e. equal volumes of Hartmann's solution and 5% glucose) can be used. Blood loss of less than 10 per cent of the circulating volume does not need replacement. Losses in excess of this should be replaced totally and precisely, with an appropriate volume of blood to correct any anaemia and to cover anticipated postoperative losses. Other intraoperative losses should be replaced, taking into account the balance between the fluid, e.g. ascitic or within the lumen of the gut, and the general circulation.

The immediate postoperative period

During this time, depending upon the severity of the operation, there is a stage of antidiuresis and sodium retention. Large water loads with little or no sodium can cause hyponatraemic fits (water intoxication, *see* Chapter 11, page 124). 0.9% NaCl will not cause fits, but will be retained, causing tissues or pulmonary oedema, and will only be excreted later.

For children who will be able to return to a full oral intake after 48 hours, it is safest to give enough fluid and electrolytes to cover abnormal losses, and to meet obligatory urine output and insensible losses; this will require about 50–60 ml/kg/24 hours of 0.18% NaCl in 4% glucose.

In addition to the reduced urine output, postoperative catabolism releases intracellular potassium; therefore potassium should NOT be included in the maintenance fluid until at least 48 hours after the operation. Additional potassium may however be given (with careful monitoring of the serum potassium level) if there is clear evidence of potassium depletion (*see* Chapter 11, page 127), and the urinary output is at least 15 ml/kg/24 hours.

48 hours up to 5–7 days after operation

The schedule described previously under 'Medium-term Maintenance' can be used.

Obstructive uropathy and the effects of decompression

Obstruction of the renal tract impairs the following functions of the kidney:

1. Concentration.
2. Acidification.
3. Sodium reabsorption.

Severe renal damage leads to reduction of the glomerular filtration rate. Thus the child coming to surgery for relief of an obstruction is likely to suffer from metabolic acidosis and sodium loss, in addition to hyperkalaemia and raised serum urea and creatinine levels. Pre-operatively, correction of the sodium deficiency and acidosis is required. In severe renal failure, dialysis, either peritoneal or haemodialysis, is also necessary.

Postoperatively a considerable sodium losing diuresis is to be expected. The acute phase lasts about 24 hours. The urine output gradually returns to normal over the succeeding few days. During the diuresis the treatment is largely empirical. The circulation must be maintained by an intravenous infusion rate a little lower than the urine output. The electrolyte content of the infusion has to be assessed by measuring the serum and urinary electrolyte concentrations. When the serum potassium level falls to normal, potassium will also be required. Initially, sodium lactate 1/6 mol/ℓ is suitable, followed by Hartmann's solution (or lactate Ringer) made up with an equal volume of 5% glucose.

Total parenteral nutrition (For low birth weight infants, *see* Appendix 6)

Total parenteral nutrition (TPN) should be started in all children where it is expected that IV fluid will be required for longer than 7 days, or as soon as it becomes apparent that IV fluid will be required for longer than 7 days. It is essential, before starting TPN, that fluid, electrolyte, and acid–base balance are all normal, and that there is no septicaemia. Medical and nursing staff must be experienced in the management of TPN, and suitable micromethods for biochemical monitoring must be easily available.

Peripheral veins can be used if TPN is unlikely to be required for more than 2 weeks. For longer infusions a central venous catheter may be preferable, using a subcutaneous skin tunnel, with full surgical aseptic technique.

Solutions available for TPN (for full list of constituents and other properties *see* components of TPN Regimen below)

1. *Vamin-9-glucose* – This is an aminoacid mixture with 10% glucose, and sodium, potassium, calcium, magnesium and chloride. It supplies 650 kcal/ℓ (2700 kJ/ℓ).
2. *Glucose 15%* – 600 kcal/ℓ (2520 kJ/ℓ).

3. *Intralipid 20% (10% also available)* – This is a soya-bean oil emulsion stabilized with egg phospholipids and glycerol. The 20% preparation contains fat 20 g/100 ml, and 1 ℓ supplies 2000 kcal (8400 kJ). Dosage (*Tables A5.3* and *A5.4*) should be increased gradually up to the full dosage by the 5th day, with monitoring for lipaemia and measurement of serum triglyceride levels. Vitlipid, Diazemuls (emulsion of diazepam) and heparin can be added to Intralipid.
4. *Ped-El* – An electrolyte and trace element solution which is added to Vamin-9-glucose. This preparation is for use in infants of under 10 kg.
5. *Addamel* – This is an electrolyte–trace-element solution for use in children of over 10 kg body weight.
6. *Solivito* – A water-soluble vitamin preparation which is added to the glucose solution. It must be protected from light, using aluminium foil.
7. *Vitlipid infant* – A fat emulsion containing vitamins A, D_2 and K_1, which is added to Intralipid.
8. *Addiphos* – This contains potassium and sodium phosphate and can be added to Vamin or glucose solutions.

Table A5.3 TPN requirements for infants under 10 kg

Preparation	*Full dosage* (ml/kg/24 hours)
Vamin-9-Glucose	48
Glucose 15%	80
Intralipid 20%	20
Ped-El	5 (add to Vamin-9-Glucose)
Vitlipid Infant	1 (add to Intralipid)
Solivito	2 (add to 15% Glucose)
Total fluid intake	153 ml/kg/24 hours

Add also: calcium 1 mmol/kg/24 hours, magnesium 0.15 mmol/kg/24 hours, phosphate 0.5 mmol/kg/24 hours, copper 0.2 mmol/kg/24 hours, and zinc 2 mmol/kg/24 hours. These should be added to the glucose solution if Vamin and glucose are given by separate IV sets.

Table A5.4 TPN requirements for children over 10 kg

Preparation	*Full dosage* (ml/kg/24 hours)
Vamin-9-Glucose	30
Glucose 15%	30
Intralipid 20%	15
Addamel	0.2
Vitlipid Infant	4
Solvito	10
Total fluid intake	89 ml/kg/24 hours

Add calcium, magnesium, phsophate, copper and zinc, as in *Table A5.3*.

Apparatus (*Figure A5.1*)

Vamin-9-glucose plus Ped-El, and 15% glucose plus Solivito, can be given continuously over the 24 hours using separate intravenous sets, using a Y-connection, and a further Y-connection to join the aqueous (Vamin and glucose) lines to the lipid (Intralipid and Vitlipid) line. Intralipid is given continuously through a pump injector. Alternatively Vamin and Intralipid can be given together over 8 hours and the glucose and additives given over 16 hours. In some units, the Vamin and glucose are mixed in a single container and the quantities controlled by use of a microcomputer (MacMahon, 1984). A Millipore filter must be inserted in the aqueous line.

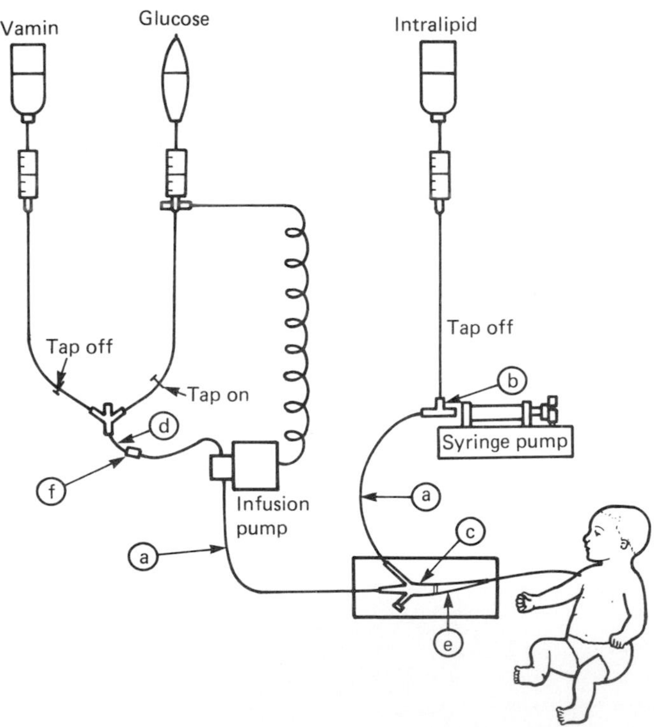

Figure A5.1 Arrangement of infusion pumps, giving sets and infusate. (*a*) Extension Set (S1028), Avon Medical Ltd., Redditch, UK. (*b*) Three-way stopcock (4011-3), Venflon, Viggo AB, Helsinborg S-252 27, Sweden. (*c*) Dual injection site (V5600), McGraw Laboratories, Irvine, California, USA. (*d*) L-S-Connector (409714/9), B Braun, Melsungen AG, West Germany. (*e*) Intravenous cannula (22 GA, 211473), Argyle Medicut, Sherwood Medical Industries, St Louis, Missouri 63101, USA. (*f*) Millipore filter. (After Candy (1980), with kind permission of author and publishers.)

Pharmacy

Solutions and giving sets should be changed every 24 hours. The solutions should be made up in the pharmacy under sterile conditions, using a laminar-flow hood, if this is available.

Dosage

One-third of the calculated amounts should be given on the first day, with the remainder of the daily requirements of fluid made up with 0.18% NaCl in 4% glucose. On days 2–4 two-thirds of the calculated amount is given, making up the fluid deficit, as before. The full regimen should be given on the 5th day.

Total fluid intake, 153 ml/kg/24 hours. Add also: calcium 1 mmol/kg/24 hours, magnesium 0.15 mmol/kg/24 hours, phosphate 0.5 mmol/kg/24 hours, copper 0.2 mmol/kg/24 hours, and zinc 2 μmol/kg/24 hours. These should be added to the glucose solution if Vamin and glucose are given by separate IV sets.

The total fluid and nutritional requirements for children of different ages are given in *Table A5.5;* for children over 10 kg, *pro rata* alterations should be made for the figures in *Table A5.4* to give the required total fluid per 24 hours.

Table A5.5 Daily intravenous nutritional requirements*

Age (years)	*Fluid* (ml/kg)	*Sodium* (mmol/kg)	*Potassium* (mmol/kg)	*Protein* (g/kg)	*Fat* (g/kg)	*Carbohydrate* (g/kg)	*Energy* (kcal/kg)
0–1	150	2.5	2.5	3.0–3.5	4	13	100–120
1–3	100	2.5	2.5	2.6–3.0	4	10	90–110
3–6	90	2.0	2.0	2.0	4	8	90–100
7–12	70	1.5	1.5	2.0	3	8	80
Adult	35	1.0	1.0	1.2	2	2	35

* Reproduced from Booth and Harrier (1982), with kind permission of authors and publishers.

Table A5.6 Biochemical monitoring

(a) During the first week of parenteral nutrition	
Daily	Twice weekly
Urea	Full blood count, including quantitative platelet count
Electrolytes	Bilirubin
Glucose	Alanine transaminase
Check plasma turbidity for Intralipid clearance	Calcium
Urinary glucose	Magnesium
	Phosphate
	Albumin
	Alkaline phosphatase
(b) After the first week of parenteral nutrition	
Alternate days	Weekly
Urea	Glucose
Electrolytes	Calcium
Check plasma for Intralipid clearance	Magnesium
Urinary glucose	Phosphate
	Albumin
	Bilirubin
	Alanine transaminase
	Alkaline phosphatase
	Copper
	Zn
	Full blood count including quantitative platelet count

* Reproduced from Booth and Harries (1982), with kind permission of authors and publishers.

Biochemical monitoring

This should be done according to the plan shown in *Table A5.6*. To avoid interference with the estimations by lipaemia, the Intralipid should be stopped for 4 hours before the blood samples are taken.

Complications (*Table A5.7*)

Most of the complications are avoidable, with scrupulous technique and good biochemical control.

Sepsis is the most serious complication (*Table A5.8*) and when it occurs, or is thought to be occurring, in a centrally placed catheter, it presents a difficult decision whether to remove the catheter. If other sites can be used, it is obviously better to re-site the catheter, but there may be occasions with no further sites available and no possibility of resuming enteral feeding, when it is better to attempt to overcome the infection with antibiotics while leaving the catheter *in situ*.

Table A5.7 Complications of TPN in childhood*

Infection	Hypo- and hyperglycaemia
Activation of infection	Trace element deficiency
Electrolyte disturbances	Hyperammonaemia
Hypophosphataemia	Hypo- and hypercalcaemia
Anaemia (investigational)	Essential fatty acid deficiency
Hypoxia	Hepatic dysfunction
Platelet and neutrophil dysfunction	(Cholestatic jaundice in infants)
Increased folic acid requirement	
Metabolic acidosis	

* Modified from Hughes (1984), with kind permission of authors and publishers.

Table A5.8 Features of catheter-related sepsis in parenterally fed infants*

Fever (or temperature instability)	Vomiting
Tachycardia	Irritability/lethargy
Local signs of infection	Tachypnoea/apnoea
Hepatosplenomegaly	Skin rash
Change in stool character	Abdominal distension
Thrombocytopenia	

* From Booth and Harries (1982), with kind permission of authors and publisher.

If any of the features shown in *Table A5.8* develop a full clinical examination should be made; this should include an examination of the retinae for 'candida spots'. The following investigations (Booth and Harries, 1982) should be performed:

1. Full blood count.
2. Blood culture (from a peripheral vein) for aerobes, anaerobes and candida.
3. Urine microscopy and culture.

4. Examination of the Gram stained buffy coat, using heparinized blood.
5. Culture of both male and female ends of the connection between giving set and the catheter.
6. Consider doing a lumbar puncture.

When an infant on TPN develops a fever but otherwise shows no clinical evidence of septicaemia, bacteriological investigations (as above) should be performed and, while awaiting the results, 0.18% NaCl in 4% glucose with additional potassium chloride should be substituted for TPN. If the child appears to have a septicaemia, or the culture results are positive, normally the catheter should be removed and antibiotics should be given through a peripheral vein. The factors governing the removal of a central catheter have already been discussed.

Components of TPN regimen:

All preparations are supplied by KabiVitrum, whose data sheets should be consulted for further information (KabiVitrum Ltd., KabiVitrum House, Riverside Way, Uxbridge, Middlesex (Tel: 0895 51144).

Vamin-9-glucose

In 1 ℓ:

L-alanine 3.0 g
L-arginine 3.3 g
L-aspartic acid 4.1 g
L-cysteine/cystine 1.4 g
L-glutamic acid 9.0 g
glycine 2.1 g
L-histidine 2.4 g
L-isoleucine 3.9 g
L-leucine 5.3 g
L-lysine 3.9 g
L-methionine 1.9 g
L-phenylalanine 5.5 g
L-proline 8.1 g
L-serine 7.5 g
L-threonine 3.0 g
L-tryptophan 1.0 g
L-tyrosine 0.5 g
L-valine 4.3 g
Glucose 100 g
Sodium 50 mmol
Potassium 20 mmol
Calcium 2.5 mmol
Magnesium 1.5 mmol
Chloride 5.5 mmol

pH 5.20
Osmolality 1350 mosmol/kg water
650 kcal/ℓ (2700 kJ/ℓ)
Bottles: 500 ml, 1000 ml

Glucose 15%

1 ℓ contains 150 g glucose (600 kcal, 2500 kJ)

Intralipid 20%

In 500 ml (as made up with water for injection):
Fractionated soya-bean oil 100 g
Fractionated egg phospholipids 6 g
Glycerol 11 g
pH 7.00
Osmolality 330 mosmol/kg water (plasma about 290 mosmol/kg water)
1 ℓ supplies 2000 kcal (8400 kJ)

Ped/El

Vials 20 ml.
In 1 ml:

Calcium 0.15 mmol	Copper 0.075 μmol
Magnesium 25 μmol	Fluoride 0.75 μmol
Ferric iron 0.5 μmol	Iodine 0.01 μmol
Zinc 0.15 μmol	Phosphate 75 μmol
Manganese 0.25 μmol	Chloride 0.35 mmol

This preparation does not cover sodium and potassium requirements. It should not be given undiluted. It contains sorbitol which is converted to fructose. pH 2.00.

Addamel

10 ml ampoules.
In 10 ml:

Calcium 5 mmol	Copper 5 μmol
Magnesium 1.5 mmol	Fluoride 50 μmol
Ferric iron 50 μmol	Iodine 1 μmol
Zinc 20 μmol	Chloride 13.3 mmol
Manganese 5 μmol	
pH 2.50	

Contains sorbitol (*see* Ped-El above)

Solivito

In one vial (to be dissolved in 10 ml of 5–20% glucose or water for injection):

B_1 (thiamine) 1.2 mg
B_2 (riboflavin) 1.8 mg
Nicotinic acid 10 mg
B_6 (pyridoxine) 2 mg
Pantothenic acid 10 mg
Biotin 0.3 mg
Folic acid 0.2 mg
B_{12} (cyanocobalamin) 2 μg
pH (reconstituted) 5.60

Vitlipid infant

10 ml ampoules.
In 1 ml:
Retinol palmitate (vitamin A) 100 μg (333 units).
Calciferol (D_2) 2.5 μg (100 units).
Phytomenadione (K_1) 50 mg.
Fractionated soya-bean oil 100 mg.
Fractionated egg phospholipids 12 mg.
Glycerol 22 mg.
Water to 1 ml.

Addiphos

20 ml vial.
In 20 ml:
Phosphate 40 mmol.
Potassium 30 mmol.
Sodium 30 mmol.

Not to be given undiluted or in the presence of renal or adrenal insufficiency.

References

BOOTH, I. W. and HARRIES, J. T. (1982) Parenteral nutrition in young children. *British Journal of Intravenous (now Parenteral) Therapy*, **3**, 31–48

CANDY, D. C. A. (1980) Parenteral nutrition in paediatric practice: a review. *Journal of Human Nutrition*, **34**, 287–296

HUGHES, C. A. (1984) In Insley J., Wood B. (eds) *Paediatric Vade-Mecum* (10th edn.). London: Lloyd-Luke (Medical Books)

MacMAHON, P. (1984) Prescribing and formulating neonatal intravenous feeding solutions by microcomputer. *Archives of Disease in Childhood*, **59**, 546–552

Further reading

FINBERG, L., KRAVATH, R. E. and FLEISCHMAN, A. R. (1982) *Water and Electrolytes in Pediatrics*. Philadelphia: W. B. Saunders

PANTER-BRICK, M. (1983) Principles of parenteral nutrition in infancy. In Peters J. L. (ed.) *A Manual of Central Venous Catheterization and Parenteral Nutrition*, pp. 231–240. Bristol: John Wright & Sons

WILKINSON, A. W. (1973) *Body Fluids in Surgery* (4th edn.) Edinburgh: Churchill-Livingstone

WINTERS, R. (1982) *Principles of Pediatric Fluid Therapy* (2nd edn.) Boston: Little Brown

Appendix 6

Feeding and intravenous nutrition (including total parenteral nutrition) and care during surgery of low birth weight infants

M. F. Whitfield

Enteral feeding (*see* also Chapter 74)

1. Human milk (per 100 ml: 71 kcal (298 kJ); protein 1.5 g; calcium 0.8 mmol; sodium 0.9 mmol). Human milk is the best food for term infants. Pooled, donated human milk (from mothers delivering at term), or their own mother's milk, is inadequate for very low birth weight premature infants, who require 180–200 ml/kg daily and supplementation with sodium (1 mmol/kg daily) and calcium (2 mmol/kg daily) to sustain adequate growth. (*See also* Appendix 4, page 771 for note on sodium supplementation.)
2. Infant formula (per 100 ml: 68 kcal (285 kJ); protein 2.3 g; calcium 1 mmol; sodium 0.9 mmol). Most standard infant formulae have a low sodium content, as in human milk, and therefore a large intake of 180 ml/kg daily or more and similar sodium and calcium supplementation is required to meet the needs of a very low birth weight infant.
3. Premature infant formula (per 100 ml: 81 kcal (340 kJ); protein 2.8 g; calcium 2 or more mmol; sodium 2 mmol). A number of such formulae have recently become available, designed for very low birth weight premature infants and appear to meet the nutritional needs, particularly in infants who cannot tolerate a high fluid load (e.g. infants with bronchopulmonary dysplasia).

Parenteral feeding

Glucose (10%) and electrolytes

(e.g., per 100 ml: sodium chloride 2 mmol; potassium chloride, 1.5 mmol; calcium gluconate 0.5 mmol).

This is the basic intravenous fluid for sick infants, to maintain fluid and electrolyte balance, with frequent appropriate adjustments to the electrolyte content. Five per cent glucose may have to be used if the blood glucose value rises consistently over 10 mmol/ℓ (180 mg/100 ml). 150 ml/kg daily of 10% glucose provides 61 kcal/kg daily (256 kJ/kg daily) which just covers basal energy requirements. Such a solution is satisfactory only for a short time (e.g. 5–7 days in infants previously in a good nutritional state, and 2–3 days in infants in a poor nutritional state or of extreme prematurity); 5% glucose at the same infusion rate leaves a major energy deficit.

Total parenteral nutrition (TPN)

For a full description of techniques, monitoring and complications of TPN, and for composition of the preparations mentioned below, *see* Appendix 5. The following are used to maintain adequate nutrition for periods of IV fluids longer than 5–7 days, or where it is obvious from the beginning that prolonged parenteral feeding is going to be required, or where the nutritional state is already very poor. (For dosage *see Table A6.1.*)

1. *Vamin-9-Glucose (Vamin-Glucose in North America)* – 35–40 ml/kg daily provides 2.1–2.4 g protein/kg daily. A newer preparation, Vaminolac (Neopham in North America) (Griffin and Gray, 1984; Meurling and Grotte, 1984) has a lower osmolality and a lower content of phenylalanine, serine, glutamic acid and proline; a higher content of leucine, lysine and alanine; and may prove superior to Vamin in meeting the aminoacid requirements of premature infants, by permitting the infusion of a higher 'protein' intake without major disturbance of the plasma aminoacid levels.
2. *Intralipid 20% (or 10%)* – The 10% preparation contains 10 g fat/100 ml and 100 kcal/100 ml) (420 kJ/100 ml, and the 20% preparation twice these amounts.
3. *Ped-El (electrolyte and trace element supplement)* – This is added to the Vamin-9-Glucose.
4. *Solivito (water-soluble vitamin preparation)* – This is added to the daily requirement of 10% glucose. This solution must be protected from light, using aluminium foil.
5. *Vitlipid Infant (fat emulsion containing vitamins A, D_2 and K_1)* – This preparation can only be added to Intralipid.

Risks and benefits of enteral and parenteral feeding in neonates and low birth weight infants

Enteral feeding

In all situations, enteral feeding – if it is tolerated, absorbed and supports a satisfactory rate of growth – is preferable to parenteral feeding.

Advantages of enteral feeding

1. Milk meets all the nutritional needs of the infant (except in some very low birth weight infants).
2. Use of the gastrointestinal tract is physiological and stimulates enterohormonal and digestive maturation.
3. Infection risk is low.
4. Enteral feeding is cheap.

Disadvantages of enteral feeding

1. Risks of regurgitation and pulmonary milk aspiration, delay in gastric emptying, exacerbation of respiratory distress and apnoeic attacks, inadequate peristalsis and constipation.
2. Malabsorption of fat due to functional bile salt deficiency in premature newborns, and of carbohydrate due to lack of adequate intestinal lactase; also glucose/galactose malabsorption.

3. Although the relationship of enteral feeding to necrotizing enterocolitis (NEC), is not fully understood, enteral feeding none the less appears to promote the disease process.
4. Enteral feeding is only possible if the gastrointestinal tract is intact and is functioning normally.

Alternative methods of enteral feeding

1. *Continuous nasogastric feeding* has been used to increase the amount of milk tolerated in the first weeks of life and to reduce the effects of feeding on respiratory mechanics; but the risk of feed aspiration remains. Some small infants who cannot tolerate intermittent feeding will tolerate slowly increasing continuous feeding. The potential advantages of continuous nasogastric feeding over conventional feeding have not been systematically evaluated in small infants.
2. *Transpyloric feeding (duodenal or jejunal),* using continuous milk infusion via a silicone rubber, preweighted tube (e.g. Vygon), has been used in small infants to establish early feeding, and combines the advantages of continuous nasogastric feeding with a (theoretically) reduced risk of feed aspiration. This technique has not been adequately evaluated in infants below 1000 g; tube dislodgement, malabsorption, and resultant poor growth appear to be the major disadvantages.

Parenteral feeding

Advantages

1. Absorption is certain because nutrients are delivered parenterally.
2. Integrity of the gastrointestinal tract and its absorptive function are not necessary.

Disadvantages and complications

1. Delivery of nutrients which are potentially toxic directly into the systemic circulation.
2. Risk of systemic infection at infusion sites.
3. Risk of infusion of nutrients at a faster rate than they can be assimilated, with resultant metabolic disorders (hyperammonaemia, hyperaminoacidaemia, lipaemia, hyperglycaemia).
4. Nutritional deficiencies due to relative lack of a particular nutrient in the solution. Requirements for many substances are not clearly established in the newborn, e.g. copper, zinc and other trace metals; carnitine; taurine (*see* page 787).
5. Cholestatic jaundice.
6. Investigational anaemia from repeated blood tests for TPN monitoring, and the risks of repeated transfusions (e.g. transfusion acquired cytomegalovirus infection).
7. Lack of stimulus to the gastrointestinal tract to mature functionally if feeding is withheld.
8. Expense.
9. Prescription errors.

Nutritional management in low birth weight infants

Appropriately grown infants of more than 1.5 kg (32 weeks' gestation or more), without respiratory problems

The majority of such infants manage on enteral feeding only, and rarely need intravenous fluids. Active sucking begins at around 33 or 34 weeks' gestation.

Plan – Initiate nasogastric feeding at 60 ml/kg daily on the first day, increasing slowly to 150 ml/kg daily by 5 days and then to 180–200 ml/kg daily by 14 days.

Appropriately grown infants of 1.25–1.5 kg (or 29–32 weeks' gestation), small for gestational age, or larger infant with respiratory problems

Such infants require intravenous fluids to maintain hydration and blood glucose until feeds can be established.

Plan – Initiate 10% glucose and electrolyte plus calcium infusion at 60 ml/kg daily (4 mg/kg/min of glucose) within the first hour of life. When there are bowel sounds and the baby has passed a stool (perhaps with the assistance of a glycerine suppository), start enteral feeding around the second to fourth day of life, as intermittent or continuous nasal, orogastric, or transpyloric feeding. Aim to reach 150 ml/kg daily by day 6 or 7 as tolerated, then increase slowly to 180–200 ml/kg daily or transfer to premature formula or breast milk with fortifier. Failure to start enteral feeding by the third or fourth day of life or to reach 150 ml/kg daily by day 6 or 7 because of feed intolerance, are indications for parenteral nutrition until full feeding can be established.

Appropriately grown or small for gestational age infant (500–1250 g; 24–28 weeks' gestation)

Such infants have very small nutritional reserves and usually take several weeks to get fully established on enteral feeding; the smallest infants are at special risk of feed intolerance, malabsorption, necrotizing enterocolitis, and frequently have severe respiratory and other complications. A period of TPN followed by Supplementary Parenteral Nutrition is required before feeding and growth are fully established.

Plan – Initiate IV fluids with 10% glucose and electrolytes. Do not add potassium for the first 24 hours. In well infants with bowel sounds, who have passed a stool, enteral feeding may be started in the first 3 days but must be increased very cautiously, as tolerated (e.g. 0.5–1.0 ml/kg per feed increase each day). By 3 days of life, TPN should be introduced and increased, as tolerated, to full dosage (*see Table A6.2*) then subsequently tailed off as milk intake becomes sufficient to meet the baby's needs.

Prolonged TPN (beyond 3 weeks) in such infants presents major technical problems. A central line may have to be used and should be inserted before suitable peripheral sites are exhausted. Nutritional deficiencies are likely to occur. Recent studies suggest that the trace element composition of the schedule given is inadequate for long-term use and will lead to zinc and copper deficiences. The zinc requirement for small, growing, premature infants, is around 6 mmol/kg daily (400 μg/kg daily) and the copper requirement is 0.6 mmol/kg daily (40 μg/kg daily) (Lockitch, *et al.*, 1983; Zlotkin and Buchanan, 1983), compared with zinc 0.6 mmol/kg daily and copper 0.3 mmol/kg daily supplied by the schedule. The requirements of taurine and carnitine which are not present in the currently used TPN solutions, are unknown but may be important.

Practical aspects of parenteral nutrition

For details of the apparatus required, *see Table A6.2* and *Appendix 5, Figure A5.1* (page 778). The final composition of the infusate at full dosage is given in *Table A6.3*.

1. Before starting TPN, correct fluid and electrolyte balance, acid–base status, check adequacy of urine output (>2 ml/kg/hour). Consider possible contraindications, particularly to the use of Intralipid (moderate to severe jaundice, septicaemia, thrombocytopenia, severe pulmonary disease), and review energy requirement for TPN.
2. Using *Table A6.1* calculate the 24-hour requirements of Vamin-9-Glucose and add Ped-El to the Vamin-9-Glucose bottle to supply 4 ml/kg daily of Ped-El with the daily allowance.
3. Calculate the 24-hour requirements of 10% glucose and sodium chloride, and add dipotassium hydrogen phosphate (1 mmol/kg daily) and Solivito (6.5 ml/kg daily) to the 10% glucose and sodium chloride mixture.
4. For details of procedure for setting up the aqueous lines, and diagrams, *see* Appendix 5, *Figure A5.1;* in some units the amounts of Vamin-9-Glucose and the 10% glucose mixture are combined in one container, sometimes with the aid of a microcomputer (MacMahon, 1984).
5. Calculate the 24-hour requirement of 20% Intralipid, and add 4 ml of Vitlipid Infant, and connect up as described in Appendix 5.
6. Monitoring of TPN: *see* Appendix 5, *Table A5.6.*
7. **The dosage may be increased progressively,** as in *Table A6.2* with due regard to the blood tests. The dosage of Intralipid can be increased by daily increments of 0.5 g/kg daily, up to a total of 3–4 g/kg daily.
8. *Biochemical complications:*
   (a) Many infants cannot tolerate large amounts of Intralipid without developing a significant lipaemia, and triglyceride levels should not be allowed to exceed 2.25 mmol/ℓ (200 mg/100 ml) because of the dangers of lipid deposition in the tissues. Plasma triglycerides should be measured daily for the first week, and then twice weekly.
   (b) Sudden intolerance of glucose or fat is usually a sign of septicaemia, the most likely source being the infusion site. If this occurs, the fat infusion should be stopped, and the rate of glucose infusion should be halved until blood glucose results are available. Investigations for infection should be started and then appropriate antibiotics given.
   (c) Blood ammonia levels should be measured in small infants on prolonged TPN who become inexplicably unwell, having first excluded septicaemia, acid–base and electrolyte disturbances and any other of the commoner complications (*see* Appendix 5, *Tables A5.7* and *A5.8).*

Surgery in term and low birth weight infants

Term neonates and low birth weight infants requiring major surgery for gastrointestinal abnormalities may require TPN if enteral feeding has to be stopped for more than 5–7 days. Term infants in the first week of life requiring IV fluids need one third of their normal requirements on the first day of life, and two thirds on the third day, and their normal requirement by the sixth to seventh day (*see* schedule in Appendix 5, *Table A5.2*).

Table A6.1 Schedule for introduction of total parenteral nutrition (TPN) in neonates and infants; and resultant nutritional intake

Day of TPN	*Nutrient solution* (ml/kg daily)			*Infused intake/kg body weight/daily*					
	*Vamin-9-Glucose**	*Intralipid 20%†*	*10% Glucose + NaCl* 2 mmol/100 ml‡	*Total fluid* (ml)	*Total calories* (kcal)§	*Protein equivalent* (g)	*Fat* (g)	*Na* (mmol)	*K* (mmol)
0 (Glucose and electrolytes only)	0	0	150	150	62	0	0	3.0	2.3
1	12	5	133	150	73	0.7	1	3.3	2.2
2–4	25	10	115	150	83	1.5	2	3.4	2.5
5 onwards (full dosage)	40	15–20	95–90	150	95–102	2.4	3–4	3.6–3.7	2.8

* Add Pel-El 4 ml/kg daily.
† Add 4 ml Vitlipid Infant (Dose of Intralipid increased as permitted by triglyceride monitoring. (*See* text)).
‡ When using 10% glucose and electrolytes only, add potassium chloride 1.5 mmol/100 ml and calcium gluconate 0.5 mmol/100 ml. When using TPN add dipotassium hydrogen phosphate (1 mmol/kg) and Solvito 6.5 ml/kg.
§ 1 kcal = 4.2 kJ.
Total fluid intake may be increased by increasing 10% glucose intake in infants who will tolerate the glucose and fluid load. Gastrointestinal losses can be compensated for by increasing the volume of 10% glucose and adding extra potassium chloride or providing a separate gastrointestinal replacement solution which can be connected to the burette.

Table A6.2 Equipment for total parenteral nutrition in infants

Solutions

Vamin-9-glucose 100 ml bottle
10% glucose 500 ml bag
20% Intralipid 100 ml bottle
Ped-El 20 ml vial
Solivito ampoule (to be reconstituted with the addition of 5 ml 10% glucose)
Vitlipid Infant 10 ml vial
30% (hypertonic) sodium chloride (5 mmol/ml)
Di-potassium hydrogen phosphate (1 mmol/ml)

Disposable infusion equipment
(See also Appendix 5, Figure A5.1)

Travenol Paediatric TPN Set
An alternative is a standard paediatric giving set with a 100 or 120 ml burette, the additional bottle being connected to the burette using an adult giving set inserted through the rubber injection port in the Burette, using a 21 gauge needle)
Millipore filter
Luer Y-connector
30–50 ml syringe to fit syringe pump (*see* below)
Narrow bore anaesthetic extension tubing (e.g. Travenol)

Infusion pumps

Volumetric infusion pump which can deliver accurately 2–20 ml/h (e.g. Ivac cassette-type infusion pump).
Syringe pump capable of delivering 0.1–4 ml/h (many commercially available, e.g. Sage, Vickers)

Preoperative

Preoperative nutritional status appears to be an important determinant of postoperative morbidity in infants; patients in poor nutritional condition in whom non-urgent surgery is planned benefit from several days of preoperative TPN. TPN should be stopped on the day of the operation and replaced by 10% glucose and electrolytes to permit effective and prompt adjustments of fluid and electrolyte status.

Postoperative

First 48 hours

Fluid intake should be reduced by about 30% (to 90–100 ml/kg daily) of 10% glucose and electrolytes. Electrolyte additions should be adjusted in accordance with postoperative electrolytes and urine output, and potassium should not be added in the first 24 hours postoperatively because of potassium release from tissue catabolism and low urinary output due to postoperative antidiuresis. Glucose 5% may be required if there is glucose intolerance.

After 48 hours

Fluid intake should be increased once the urine output has improved (2 ml/kg/hour or more), TPN should be started in infants in poor nutritional status in whom successful enteral feeding is not anticipated in the next few days (by 5–7 days postoperatively).

Table A6.3 Total parenteral nutrition infusate composition (per kg daily) (full dosage: day 5 onwards)

Carbohydrate and fat		*Vitamins*	
Glucose	13.0 g	Thiamine	0.12 mg
Soya bean oil	4.0 g*	Riboflavin	0.18 mg
Egg lecithin	0.24 g*	Nicotinamide	1 mg
Glycerol	0.5 g	Biotin	0.03 mg
		Pyridoxine	0.2 mg
Amino acids		Pantothenic acid	1 mg
L-Alanine	120 mg	Ascorbic acid	3 mg
L-Arginine	132 mg	Folic acid	0.02 mg
L-Aspartic acid	164 mg	Vitamin B_{12}	0.2 μg
L-Cysteine/Cystine	56 mg	Vitamin A	400 μg
Glycine	84 mg	Calciferol (D_2)	400 U
L-Histidine	96 mg	Vitamin K_1	200μg
L-Isoleucine	156 mg		
L-Leucine	212 mg	*Minerals*	
L-Lysine	156 mg	Sodium	3.6 mmol
L-Methionine	76 mg	Potassium	2.8 mmol
L-Phenylalanine	220 mg	Calcium	0.7 mmol
L-Proline	324 mg	Magnesium	0.16 mmol
L-Serine	300 mg	Chloride	4.1 mmol
L-Threonine	120 mg	Phosphate	1.4 mmol
L-Tryptophan	40 mg	Iron	2.0 mmol
L-Tyrosine	20 mg	Zinc	0.6 mmol
L-Valine	172 mg	Manganese	1.0 mmol
Glucose	360 mg	Copper	0.3 mmol
		Fluoride	3.0 mmol
		Iodine	0.04 mmol
Water to	150 ml		

* 50% of esterified fatty acids derived from linoleic acid.

References

GRIFFIN, E. and GRAY, P. (1984) A study evaluating the metabolism of Vaminolac in the sick preterm infant. *Acta Chirurgica Scandinavica,* **Suppl. 517,** 89–102

MacMAHON, P. (1984) Prescribing and formulating neonatal intravenous feeding solutions by microcomputer. *Archives of Disease in Childhood,* **59,** 548–552

MEURLING, S. and GROTTE, G. (1984) Total parenteral nutrition in pediatric surgery using a new aminoacid solution (Vaminolac). *Acta Chirurgica Scandinavica,* **Suppl. 517,** 79–88

LOCKITCH, G., GODOLPHIN, W. and PENDRAY, M. *et al.* (1983) Serum zinc, copper, retinol binding protein, prealbumin and caeruloplasmin concentrations in infants receiving intravenous zinc and copper supplementation. *Journal of Pediatrics,* **102,** 304–308

ZLOTKIN, S. and BUCHANAN, B. (1983) Meeting zinc and copper intake requirements in the parenterally fed pre-term and full term infant. *Journal of Pediatrics,* **103,** 441–446

Further reading

DEAR, P. R. F. (1984) Nutritional problems in the newborn. *Hospital Update,* **10,** 915–927

HEIRD, W., McMILLAN, R. and WINTERS, R. (1976) In Fisher J. E. (Ed.). Total parenteral nutrition of the pediatric patient. *Total Parenteral Nutrition,* pp. 253–283. Boston: Little Brown

KANAREK, D., WILLIAMS, P. and CURRAN, J. (1982) Total parenteral nutrition in infants and children. *Advances in Pediatrics,* **29,** 151–181

WINTERS, R. and HASSELMEYER, E. (eds.) (1974). *Intravenous Nutrition of the High Risk Infant.* New York: Wiley

Appendix 7

Urine output in acute disease

J. A. Black

Although much information can be obtained from random samples of urine, measurement of the volume passed in timed periods is of much greater value. Catheterization should be reserved for children with actual or suspected renal failure, or in whom spontaneous micturition has not occurred in spite of a full bladder, or when rupture of the bladder or clot retention is suspected. Catheterization in children should be done with gentleness and great care to avoid infection.

The information which can be obtained from measurement of the urine output is as follows:

1. In resuscitation from states of shock or dehydration:
   (a) Has an adequate flow of over 0.5 ml/kg/hour or over 12.5 ml/m^2/hour been established within 4 hours of starting IV fluids?
   (b) If the urine flow is below that expected, the reason may be:
   Inadequate resuscitation or rehydration.
   Impending renal 'shut-down'.
   Persisting antidiuresis.
   Extravasation of urine (rupture of bladder or kidney).
   Bilateral obstruction to the renal tract (calculi or uric acid nephropathy).
   (c) If the bladder is distended but there is no spontaneous micturition the following should be considered:
   Blocked catheter.
   Clot retention.
   Spinal injury.
2. In cardiac conditions. An inadequate urine flow may be due to shock or more commonly to cardiac failure with fluid retention.
3. In the polyuric phase of acute tubular necrosis. The rate of flow is very high in spite of clinical dehydration.

Standards of reference

The urine flow can be based upon the body weight or surface area but the same calculations cannot be used throughout the age range from infancy to adolescence. It is therefore necessary to establish standards of reference at different ages based upon surface area and per kg body weight. Surface area is an unsatisfactory basis for the low birth infants, and under the age of 1 year a different basis for surface area calculations must be used (*Figure A7.1*).

Definitions

Normal output (*Figure A7.1, Table A7.1*)

This is the urinary output in a healthy individual on a diet appropriate for age. There are very large individual variations, depending upon the type of diet (amount of water and solutes), environmental temperature and humidity, muscular activity and personal habits (e.g. amount of fluid taken with meals). The values used here are the best available from the literature (Lafourcade and Gorin, 1962; Rubin, 1969) and are intended to represent average values at certain ages, without any statistical validity. It is to be expected that variations above and below these values will be of the order of about 50 per cent.

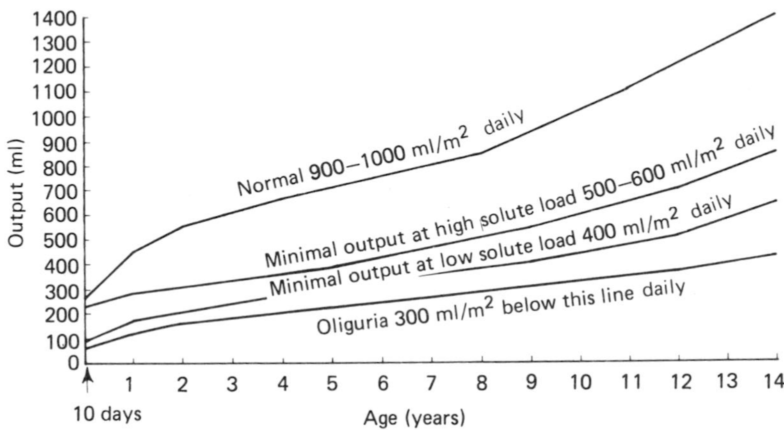

Figure A7.1 Urine output by surface area. (*See also Tables A7.1–A7.4.*)

Table A7.1 Normal urine output*

Age	*ml/24 h*	*ml/h*	*ml/kg/24 h*	*ml/kg/h*	*ml/m²/24 h*	*ml/m²/h*
10 days†	250	10	70	2.5	1250	50
2 months	450	18	90	3.5	1800	75
1 year	500	20	50	2.0		
2 years	550	22	40	1.7		
4 years	650	27	40	1.7		
7 years	750	30	40	1.7	900–1000	37–40
11 years	1100	45	35	1.4		
14 years	1200	50	35	1.4		
Adult	1500	60	20	0.8		

* Midpoint figures for the ranges of age and output are given from Lafourcase and Gorin (1962) and Rubin (1969). Variations will be ±50 per cent of the figures given.

† Output during the first 10 days depends upon the ability or desire of the infant to feed, also upon the type of milk (solute load). Thomson (1944) gives the following range for breast-fed infants. Day 1: 0–68, 2: 0–82, 3: 0–96, 4: 5–180, 6– 42–268, 8: 59–330, 10: 106–320.

Obligatory urine output (*Figure A7.1, Tables A7.2 and A7.3*)

This is the minimum urine flow which is required to excrete the solute load (that proportion of solutes which is available for excretion by the kidney) in order to maintain the electrolyte content and acid–base state of the ECF within normal

Table A7.2 Minimal urine volumes for high solute load during resuscitation (Burns) (After Muir and Barclay, 1974)

Age	*ml/24 h*	*ml/h*	*ml/kg/24 h*	*ml/kg/h*	*ml/m²/24 h*	*ml/m²/h*
10 days	240	10	70	3.0	1200	50
2 months	240	10	50	2.0	900	37.5
1 year	290	12	30	1.2	600	25
2 years	310	13	24	1.0	600	25
4 years	360	15	21	0.9	500	20
7 years	430	18	20	0.8	500	20
11 years	625	26	19	0.8	500	20
14 years	840	35	19	0.8	500	20
Adult	840	35	12	0.5	480	20

Table A7.3 Minimal urine volumes for low solute load (maintenance IV glucose–electrolyte solutions); based on 400 ml/m²/24 hours (West, 1975) except uner 1 year where the figures are ⅖ of the normal rate per m² as given in *Table A7.1*)

Age	*ml/24 h*	*ml/h*	*ml/kg/24 h*	*ml/kg/h*	*ml/m²/24 h*	*ml/m²/h*
10 days	100	4.0	28	1.2	500	20
2 months	180	7.5	36	1.5	720	30
1 year	180	7.5	18	0.75		
2 years	220	9.0	17	0.7		
4 years	280	12.0	16	0.65		
7 years	335	14.0	15	0.6	400	17
11 years	400	18.0	13	0.55		
14 years	550	20.0	12	0.5		
Adult	700	30.0	10	0.4		

limits. The higher the solute load the larger the obligatory urine volume and therefore the higher the water requirement.

Obligatory urine volume is high in:

1. Tissue catabolism (e.g. severe burns).
2. Increased production of solutes and acid metabolities (e.g. diabetic ketoacidosis).
3. Ingestion of abnormal solutes which are mainly or exclusively excreted through the kidney (e.g. salicylate poisoning).

Obligatory urine volume is low in:

1. Maintenance IV fluids using glucose–electrolyte solution of low sodium content such as NaCl 0.18% in 4% glucose.
2. Starvation in the absence of catabolism.

Therefore it is not possible to give one obligatory urine flow for all situations, but figures are given for minimal flow rates under the following conditions:

1. High solute load (*Table A7.2*) (Muir and Barclay, 1974).
2. Low solute load (*Table A7.3*) (West, 1975).

In practice the solute load will be excreted without difficulty if the urine osmolality is maintained between 250 mosmol/kg (specific gravity 1008) and 450 mosmol/kg (specific gravity 1014).

Oliguria

When the urine flow is less than 1/4 to 1/3 of the expected normal (i.e. <0.5 ml/kg/hour or <12.5 ml/m^2/hour) oliguria is present (*see Figure A7.1* and *Table A7.4* for actual values at different ages).

Oliguria in the absence of obstruction or extravasation may be:

1. The physiological response of the normal kidney to dehydration, shock, hypotension, reduced blood flow, antidiuresis, or adrenocortical insufficiency.
2. The pathological response (renal 'shut-down') of a kidney damaged by ischaemia, haemoglobinuria, myoglobinuria, or poisons.

Table A7.4 Oliguria: based on 300 ml/m^2/24 hours except under 1 year (where the figures are approximately one-third of normal values as given in *Table A7.1*)

Age	*ml/24 h*	*ml/h*	*ml/kg/24 h*	*ml/kg/h*	*ml/m^2/24 h*	*ml/m^2/h*
10 days	80	3.5	25	1.0	400	16.5
2 months	140	6.0	28	1.25	600	25.0
1 year	140	6.0	14	0.6		
2 years	160	6.5	12	0.5		
4 years	210	8.5	12	0.5		
7 years	250	10.0	11	0.45	300	12.5
11 years	330	13.5	10	0.4		
14 years	420	17	9.5	0.4		
Adult	500	20	7.0	0.3		

Physiological oliguria cannot always be distinguished from pathological oliguria on the basis of urine flow alone, but examination of the urine (osmolality, specific gravity, urea or sodium content) in relation to the clinical state or plasma urea and electrolytes (*see* page 429) will usually distinguish between the two situations, as will the response to a controlled increase in the rate of infused fluids or the giving of a potent diuretic such as IV frusemide (*see* page 111).

It should be emphasized that extreme oliguria, whether physiological or pathological, will result in a rising blood urea, a metabolic acidosis and also electrolyte disorders in certain situations.

Polyuria and diuresis

The distinction between polyuria and diuresis is somewhat arbitrary; polyuria is generally used to describe a continued state of high urine flow (e.g. uncontrolled diabetes), and a diuresis to describe a transient increase in urine flow, usually as a result of treatment. In either case the urine flow exceeds the normal value for age.

Polyuria (or diuresis) may be due to:

1. The physiological reaction of the normal kidney to an increased intake of water or solutes, a diuretic drug, or absence of antidiuretic hormone (diabetes insipidus).
2. The pathological reaction of a damaged kidney in chronic renal disease, or acute tubular necrosis (inability of the renal tubules to modify the glomerular filtrate).
3. Decompression of an obstructed renal tract (*see* page 776).

Special situations

Burns

There is usually shock with diminished ECF during the first 48–72 hours. Antidiuresis may also be present but this is usually overcome by the high solute infusions used in most resuscitation regimens. In extensive burns there is a danger of toxic damage to the kidneys by free haemoglobin or myoglobin. In most schemes of resuscitation minimal hourly flow-rates are suggested, depending upon the type of fluids used. The antidiuretic effect is usually seen only in small painful burns or scalds in which excessive drinking of water or low-solute fluids may cause water intoxication. After initial resuscitation has been completed a higher urine flow (up to 800–900 ml/m^2/24 hours or equivalent rates per hour, or on a body weight basis) can be safely maintained provided there is no evidence or risk of pulmonary oedema.

References

LAFOURCADE, J. and GORIN, R. (1962) *Les Spoliations Hydro-Salines du Nourrisson et leur Traitment,* p. 64. Paris: G. Doin et Compagnie

MUIR, I. F. K. and BARCLAY, T. L. (1974) *Burns and their Treatment.* 2nd edn., p. 33; London: Lloyd Luke

RUBIN, M. I. (1969) In Nelson W. E., Vaughan V. C., McKay R. J. (eds), *Textbook of Pediatrics* (9th edn.), p. 1106. Philadelphia: W. B. Saunders*

THOMSON, J. (1944) Observation on the urine of the new-born infant. *Archives of Disease in Childhood,* **19,** 169–177

WEST, C. D. (1975) In Shirkey H. C. (ed.) *Pediatric Therapy* (5th edn.) p. 280. St. Louis: C. V. Mosby

* Similar figures are given by:

BELTON, N. R. (1984) In Forfar J. O., Arneil, G. C. (eds) *Textbook of Paediatrics* (3rd edn.) p. 1985. Edinburgh: Churchill-Livingstone

Composition of preparations and solutions used in intravenous infusions

J. A. Black

Table A8.1 Composition of preparations and solutions commonly used in intravenous infusions

Name	*Electrolyte content* (mmol/litre)				*pH**	*Glucose* (g/ℓ)†	kcal (kJ/ℓ)‡	*Remarks*
	Na^+	*K^+*	*Cl^-*	*HCO_3^- or equivalent*				
Sodium chloride 0.18% in 4% glucose	30		30		3.5–4.3	40	150 (628)	Maintenance solution short term
Sodium chloride 0.45% in 2.5% glucose	77		77		3.5–4.3	25	94 (397)	
Sodium chloride 0.9%	150		150		5.7–6.9			
Sodium chloride 0.9% in 5% glucose	154		154		3.5–4.3	50	188 (785)	
Sodium chloride 0.18%, potassium chloride 0.15% in 4% glucose	30	20	50			40	150 (628)	Maintenance solution medium term
Darrow's solution	121	35	103	53 (lactate)	6.7–7.1			
Dacca solution	133	14	99	48		0	0	Cholera (Chapter 63)
Compound sodium lactate§ (Hartmann's solution)	131	5	111	29 (lactate)				With Ca 2 mmol/ℓ
Plasma–protein fraction (PPF)	140–160	<2	100–120	15 (citrate)				400 ml contains 17–19 g protein, replaces freeze dried pooled plasma
Fresh frozen plasma (FPP)	138–148							
Plasma from whole stored (ACD) blood, PCV 60% (citrated plasma)	150 at 0 days 148 at 7 days	3–4 at 0 days 12 at 7 days	55	103	6.9–7.0 at 0 days 6.8 at 7 days			Expiry time 21 days. Each 495 ml contains 1.7 g sodium citrate and 0.6 g citric acid

Table A8.1 Continued

Name	*Electrolyte content* (mmol/litre)				*pH**	*Glucose* (g/ℓ)†	kcal (kJ/ℓ)‡	*Remarks*
	Na^+	K^+	Cl^-	HCO_3^- *or equivalent*				
Salt-poor albumin								25 g contains ≯17 mmol sodium and ≯1.2 mmol potassium
Whole blood, packed red cells	138–148							
Dextran 40 10% (molecular weight 40 000)								Available in 5% glucose or 0.9% sodium chloride
Dextran 70 6% (molecular weight 70 000)								Available in 5% glucose or 0.9% sodium chloride
Dextran 110 6% (molecular weight 110 000)								Available in 5% glucose or 0.9% sodium chloride
Hydroxyethyl starch in 0.9% NaCl	140–150		140–150					
Sodium bicarbonate 8.4% (1 ml = 1 mmol)	1000			1000				Store at −10 to −25°C. Rapid injection may be harmful. Dilute with 5% glucose
Sodium bicarbonate 4.2% (2 ml = 1 mmol)	500			500				Store at −2 to −25°C
Sodium chloride 5%	855		855					
Sodium chloride 1.8%	308		308					
Sodium lactate M/6 (1.85%)	167			167 (lactate)				Avoid rapid infusion

Potassium chloride 0.15% in 5% glucose		20	20		50	188 (785)	Avoid rapid infusion
Potassium chloride 0.3% in 5% glucose		40	40		50	188 (785)	Avoid rapid infusion
Glucose 10%				3.7–4.2	100	375 (1570)	Avoid rapid infusion
Ammonium chloride M/6			167				Avoid rapid infusion
Miscellaneous							
Intralipid 10%						1100 (4200)	Total parenteral nutrition
Intralipid 20%						2200 (8400)	Total parenteral nutrition
Vamin glucose	50	20	55	5.2	100	650 (2730) including 450 (1890) from glucose	Magnesium 1.5 mmol/ℓ and calcium 2.5 mmol/ℓ
Lignocaine 0.1% in 5% glucose					50	188 (785)	Cardiac arrhythmias (*see* page 269)
Lignocaine 0.2% in 5% glucose					50	188 (785)	

* Values for pH from Harris F. (1972). *Paediatric Fluid Therapy* p. 141. Oxford, Blackwell.
† For consistency 'glucose' is used instead of 'dextrose', though bottles are often labelled in terms of dextrose content.
‡ The clinical 'Calorie'.
§ Almost identical with Lactate Ringer (Na^+ 130 mmol/ℓ; K^+ 4 mmol/ℓ; Cl^- 100 mmol/ℓ; lactate 28 mmol/ℓ; Ca^{2+} 3 mmol/ℓ).
NOTE: IV solutions containing fructose or sorbitol should NOT be used, since they can produce fatal hypoglycaemia, with hepatic and renal damage in undiagnosed cases of fructose intolerance (*see* page 712 and Schulte M. J. and Lenz W. (1977) *Lancet* **ii**: 188) and a metabolic acidosis in the newborn.

Appendix 9

Composition of commonly used milks and oral electrolyte solutions

J. A. Black and J. A. Walker-Smith

Table A9.1 Composition of commonly used milks and oral electrolyte solutions

Name	*Electrolyte content* (mmol/ℓ)				*Carbohydrate* (g/100 ml (mmol/ℓ))	*Osmolality* (mosmol/kg)	*Remarks*
	Na^+	K^+	Cl^-	HCO_3^- *or equivalent*			
Human milk	6	15	12	9	7.0 (lactose) (211)	264	
Cows' milk (unmodified)	22	36	28	30	4.5 (lactose) (137)	281–301	
WHO oral rehydraton solution (ORS)	90	20	80	30	2.0 (glucose) (110) (if sucrose is used make up with 4 g/100 ml)	331	Sodium chloride 3.5 g, sodium bicarbonate 2.5 g, potassium chloride 1.5 g, glucose 20 g (sucrose 40 g), water 1 ℓ
Sodium chloride and glucose oral powder compound (BP); also Dioralyte (Armour)	35	20	37	18	4.0 (glucose) (222	310	B.P. preparation: 1 powder (22 g) into 500 ml water or 8 g into 200 ml water. Dioralyte 1 sachet (8 g) in 200 ml water

Dextrolyte (Cow & Gate)	35	13.4	30.5	17.7 (lactate)	3.6 (glucose) (200)	297	Oral solution: no reconstitution required (100 ml)
Rehidrat (Searle)	50	20	50	20	1.6 (glucose) (91) 3.2 (sucrose) (94) 0.3 (fructose)	331	1 sachet into 500 ml water
Alhydrate (Nestlé)	60	20	60	18 (citrate)	6.0 (maltodextrin) (–) 2.0 (sucrose) (110)	<300	1 sachet into 500 ml water
Simple salt and sugar solution	55	–	55	–	3.0 (sucrose) (80)	190	½ level teaspoon salt and 5 level teaspoons sugar in 750 ml water (*see* page 407)
Alternative salt and sugar solution	34–68	–	36–68	–	6.0 (sucrose) (160)		For further details of method *see* p. 734
Oral solution for burns	133	–	85	48	0		*See* page 31

Note: for domestic methods of measuring salt and sugar *see* Appendix 24.

Appendix 10

Drug dosage: general principles

J. A. Black

Use of surface area for the calculation of drug dosage in children

There are two methods of using surface area for calculating drug dosage, etc.:

1. Then the adult dose is known, and the child's dose is to be calculated. Assuming the adult has a surface area of 1.73 m^2, the child's dose will be:

   $$\frac{\text{adult dose} \times \text{child's surface area}}{1.73}$$

   For less accurate purposes the fraction or percentage of adult dose can be read off a figure relating surface area at different weights (and ages) to the percentage of the adult dose required.
2. A standard dose can be used throughout childhood (except the neonatal period) giving the dose in kg/m^2, ml/m^2, etc. This of course can be calculated from a known adult dose simply by dividing the adult dose by 1.73.

For ordinary purposes the dosage scales given in *A Paediatric Vade-Mecum* (Insley and Wood, 1984) (*see* Appendix 11) are satisfactory and are given in the following form:

1. First year: dose based upon body weight, from birth to 2 weeks, then from 2 weeks to 1 year.
2. At ages 1 year and 7 years the dosage is based upon surface area:
   At 1 year the dose of 1/4 adult dose.
   At 7 years the dose is 1/2 adult dose.

Intermediate doses can be arrived at by extrapolation, from *Figure A10.1* or from *Table A10.1.*

Difficulties in paediatric dosage

1. Many doses after the age of 1 year in this book, are, for ease of calculation, based upon body weight. It is important that unless there is some very good reason, *the maximum adult dose should be not exceeded,* so that no child should normally receive more than four times the dose at 1 year.
2. When the dose must be very accurately calculated (as in cytotoxic drugs) the initial scale should be based upon the dose/m^2, and the actual surface area of the child should be accurately determined, using a nomogram or formula.

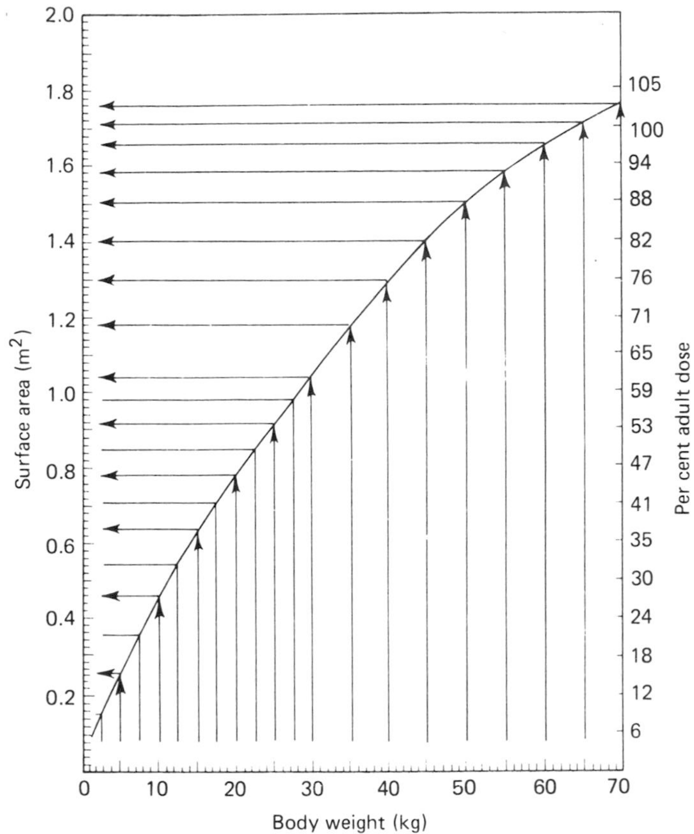

Figure A10.1 Relation between body weight, surface area and adult dosage. (Reproduced from Talbot, Richie and Crawford (1959), with kind permission of authors and publishers.)

Table A10.1 Simplified scheme for drug dosage based on surface area

Age	*Average weight* (kg)	*Surface area* (m^2)	*Fraction of adult dose*
Birth	3–3.5	0.2	⅛
4 months	6	0.3	⅙
1 year	10	0.45	¼
2 years	13	0.58	⅓
7 years	25	0.9	½
12 years	40	1.3	¾
14 years	50	1.5	9/10
14 years +	65+	1.7	Adult

3. When a child has abnormal proportions the surface area should be used rather than the age or weight.
4. Fat children: *see* page 758.
5. In renal insufficiency, the dosage of certain drugs, particularly the aminoglycoside antibiotics (streptomycin, kanamycin, gentamicin, tobramycin, amikacin) and the polymyxins (Colistin) should be reduced or the intervals between doses should be increased, published data should be consulted or the maker's literature, and serum levels should be measured at frequent intervals if this is practicable (*see* also Appendix 13).

References

INSLEY, J. and WOOD, B. (eds) (1984) *A Paediatric Vade-Mecum* (10th edn.) London: Lloyd Luke Medical Books

TALBOT, N. B., RICHIE, R. H. and CRAWFORD, J. D. (1959) *Metabolic Homeostasis*. Harvard University Press

Appendix 11

Doses of drugs

J. A. Black

The drugs listed below are mainly those mentioned in the text, but some other widely used drugs have also been included.

Names – These are the British Approved Names, as used in the *British National Formulary* (1985); American official names where they differ, are given in brackets preceded by 'US'. Proprietary names are given in italics and are used either because they have gained widespread acceptance, or when it is helpful to refer to a specific preparation, as in intravenous preparations (*see Table A11.12*).

Strength of formulations – The strength of tablets, solutions, and other preparations, and information on IV injections and infusions are those given in the *British National Formulary* and in the *ABPI Data Sheet Compendium* (1984). Strength and formulations may be different in other countries. No compound preparations are given nor with a few exceptions are special formulations such as slow release tablets.

Dosage – In general the dosage scales are those given in *'A Paediatric Vade-mecum* (Insley and Wood, 1984). Unless otherwise indicated the quantity given is for a single dose. Drugs mentioned in the tables, which can be given intravenously are shown in *Table A11.12. ('Intravenous additives')*. When the dosage or method of administration is complicated or related to one specific condition, reference is made to the instructions given in the text. Page references also indicate a discussion in the text on the usage of the drug, and its more important indications.

Contraindications – Where special care is required in administration, or because of dangerous side-effects, these are indicated. Where a drug is not normally given in a particular age group, this is shown by a – in the relevant column; a stronger prohibition is indicated by 'Avoid'. Routes which are not recommended are shown in brackets.

Special groups of drugs – The following drugs or therapeutic agents are given in separate Tables:

Some commonly used drugs, *Table A11.1.*
Antibacterial agents, *Table A11.2.*
Antituberculous agents: *Table A11.3.*
Antiviral agents: *Table A11.4.*
Antifungal agents: *Table A11.5.*
Antiprotozoal agents: *Table A11.6.*
Anthelminthic agents: *Table A11.7.*

Glucocorticoids and corticotrophins: *Table A11.8.*
Mineralocorticoids and anabolic steroids: *Table A11.9.*
Characteristics of glucocorticoids: *Table A11.10.*
Vaccines, immune globulins and antisera: *Table A11.11.*
Intravenous additives: *Table A11.12.*
Intrathecal antibacterial agents: *Table A11.13.*
Leukaemia: for information on drugs used in the treatment of leukaemia in children, and their dosage, *see* Chapter 54 pages 489–493.

References

ASSOCIATION OF THE BRITISH PHARMACEUTICAL INDUSTRIES (ABPI) (1984) *Data Sheet Compendium 1984–5.* London: Datapharm Publications

BRITISH NATIONAL FORMULARY No. 9 (1985). London: The British Medical Association and the Pharmaceutical Society of Great Britain

INSLEY, J. and WOOD, B. (1984) *A Paediatric Vade-Mecum* (10th edn.) London: Lloyd Luke Medical Books

Table A11.1 Some commonly used drugs. Drugs referred to in the text are given below, with the more important page refverences. Some commonly used drugs not referred to in the text are also included. Single doses are given unless otherwise indicated

Name and formulations	*Routes*	*Doses per 24 hours*	*0–2/52*	*2/52–1 year*	*1 year*	*7 years*	*14 years to adult*	*Remarks*
Acetazolamide Caps (slow release) 500 mg Tab. 250 mg Powder (oral use) Sodium parenteral Vial 500 mg	Oral: IV	Once	–	–	125 mg	250 mg	500 mg	Raised Intracranial Pressure, page 296
Acetylcysteine Amp. (200 mg/ml) 10 ml	IV infusion*		Paracetamol poisoning (*see* page 66 for dosage)					
Adrenaline (US epinephrine) 1:1000 (0.1%; 1 mg/ml) Amps. 0.5, 1 ml Disp. syringe 0.5, 1 ml	S.C. i.m.	Single dose repeated as required	0.1 ml/kg (0.1 mg/kg)	0.1 ml/kg (0.1 mg/kg)	0.12 ml (0.12 mg)	0.25 ml (0.25 mg)	0.5 ml (0.5 mg)	Standard dosage; see also page 114 for Anaphylactic shock and page 559 for anaphylaxis after antivenom
	IV Intracardiac	Single dose, normally	1–2 ml (1–2 mg)	1–2 ml (1–2 mg)	1–2 ml (1–2 mg)	7 ml (7 mg)	10 ml (10 mg)	Cardiac arrest; *Table 2.1* page 6 for intermediate doses
Adrenaline 1:10 000 (0.01%, 0.1 mg, 100 μg/ml) Disp. syringe (300 μg) 3 ml	IV continuous infusion*		Shock (page 108) and *Table 10.2* (page 106) for dosage					
	IV injection	Once	1–3 ml (100–300 μg)	1–3 ml (100–300 μg)	1–3 ml (100–300 μg)	1–3 ml (100–300 μg)	1–3 ml (100–300 μg)	Cardiac arrest or extreme bradycardia (alternative scheme) page 6

Table A11.1 continues

Table A11.1 continued

Name and formulations	*Routes*	*Doses per 24 hours*	*0–2/52*	*2/52–1 year*	*1 year*	*7 years*	*14 years to adult*	*Remarks*
Alcuronium Amp. (5 mg/ml) 2 ml	IV i.m.	Single doses repeated as required	Neonatal period 1.25 mg (1250 μg)	Neonatal period 1.25 mg (1250 μg)	125–200 μg/kg, then ⅓ of initial dose	125–200 μg/kg, then ⅓ of initial dose	125–200 μg/kg, then ⅓ of initial dose	Tetanus in Childhood, page 328, Neonatal Tetanus, page 330)
Alfacalcidol (1α-hydroxycholecalciferol) Caps. 250 ng, 1 μg Drops 5 μg/ml; 250 ng/drop	Oral	Once	Neonatal hypocalcaemia (page 135) for dosage					
Alprostadil (Prostaglandin E_1) Amp. (500 mg/ml) 1 ml, in alcohol, for dilution	IV infusion*		Ductus dependent cardiac lesions (page 266)					See manufacturer's data sheet (Prostin VR, Upjohn) for further details of administration
Aluminium hydroxide Mixture (gel) 4% w/w in water	Oral	3–4	1–2 ml/kg/24 hours	1–2 ml/kg/24 hours	1–2 ml/kg/24 hours	1–2 ml/kg/24 hours	5 ml	Hyperphosphataemia in Acute Renal Failure, page 433
Amiloride Tab. 5 mg	Oral	1–2	0.2 mg/kg, with another diuretic	0.2 mg/kg, with another diuretic	0.2 mg/kg, with another diuretic	0.2 mg/kg, with another diuretic	0.2 mg/kg, with another diuretic Max. dose 20 mg	Diuretic in Cardiac Failure, page 264
Aminocaproic acid (EACA) Powder: Sachet 3 g Syrup: 1.5 g/5 ml	Oral	4–6	–	100 mg/kg	1.5 g	3 g	6 g	Dental bleeding, page 163

Aminophylline Tab. 100 mg Amp. (25 mg/ml), 2 ml, 10 ml; (250 mg/ml) 2 ml Slow-release tablet (Paediatric 100, 225 mg. (Phyllocontin Continus)	Oral	2 (dosage for Phyllocontin S/R tabs)	–	–	–	100 mg daily up to 225 mg twice daily	225 mg twice daily, up to 450 mg twice daily	Dosage for asthma
	IV over 30 min	Once (25 mg/ml strength)	–	0.5 ml (12.5 mg)	1 ml (25 mg)	7 ml (175 mg)	10 ml (250 mg)	Acute asthmatic Attack, Status Asthmaticus, or Anaphylaxis with bronchial spasm, *Table 2.3*, page 8
	IV infusion	As required	Acute asthmatic attack (page 234) for method and dosage					
	IV	3	Neonatal period Loading dose 6 mg/kg/24 hours, then 4 mg/kg/24 hours in divided doses	Neonatal period Loading dose 6 mg/kg/24 hours, then 4 mg/kg/24 hours in divided doses	–	–	–	Apnoeic attacks in Newborn, page 253, and page 642. *Monitor blood levels*
Ascorbic acid Tabs. 25 up to 500 mg Amp. 100, 500 mg	Oral: IV	3–4	300–400 mg/24 hours	300–400 mg/24 hours	300–400 mg/24 hours	300–400 mg/24 hours	300–400 mg/24 hours	Methaemoglobinaem-ia, page 666
Atropine Tab. 0.6 mg Amp. 0.4 mg/ml, 1 ml; 0.6 mg/ml, 1 ml; 0.8 mg/ml, 1 ml; 1.0 mg/ml, 0.5 ml; 1.2 mg/ml, 1 ml; 1.25 mg/ml, 1 ml	Oral S.C. i.m.	Once	0.15 mg/kg	0.15 mg/kg	0.15 mg	0.3 mg	0.6 mg	Routine pre-medication; Emergency pre-medication page 188
	IV	Once	0.1 mg	0.1 mg	0.2 mg	0.4 mg	0.5–0.6 mg	Bradycardia in Cardiorespiratory Collapse, *Table 2.2* page 7

Table A11.1 continues

Table A11.1 continued

Name and formulations	*Routes*	*Doses per 24 hours*	*0–2/52*	*2/52–1 year*	*1 year*	*7 years*	*14 years to adult*	*Remarks*
A, vitamin	*See* Retinol acetate and palmitate							
BAL (British Anti-Lewisite)	*See* Dimercaprol							
B_1, vitamin	*See* Thiamine							
B_6, vitamin	*See* Pyridoxine							
C, vitamin	*See* Ascorbic acid							
Caffeine citrate	Oral	Apnoeic attacks in the newborn (page 253) for dosage						
Calciferol Tab. 10 000 units (250 μg) Solution, 3 000 units (75 μg)/ml	Oral	Once	Neonatal period 1000 units (25 μg)	Neonatal period 1000 units (25 μg)				Neonatal Hypocalcaemia page 135
Calcitonin (*see also* Salcatonin) Vial, 160 units with gelatine diluent	S.C. i.m.	3–4	–	4–8 units/kg/24 hours according to clinical and biochemical response	4–8 units/kg/24 hours according to clinical and biochemical response	4–8 units/kg/24 hours according to clinical and biochemical response	4–8 units/kg/24 hours according to clinical and biochemical response	Acute hypercalcaemia page 137
Calcitriol (1α, 25-hydroxycholecalciferol) Cap. 250 ng	Oral	Once	Neonatal hypocalcaemia (page 135) for dosage					

Calcium chloride 10% solution	IV slow infusion	Once	0.1–0.2 ml/kg (10–20 mg/kg)	0.1–0.2 ml/kg (10–20 mg/kg)	0.1–0.2 ml/kg (10–20 mg/kg)	0.1–0.2 ml/kg (10–20 mg/kg)	0.1–0.2 ml/kg (10–20 mg/kg)	Hypocalcaemia in Shock, page 105
	(Oral)		Oral route not recommended; use alternative preparations					
Calcium glubionate with calcium galactogluconate (*Calcium Sandoz*) Syrup 325 mg (8.1 mmol) calcium per 15 ml Amp. 93 mg (2.32 mmol) calcium per 10 ml: 10 ml	Oral	Six, with feeds	5 ml	–	–	–	–	Neonatal
	IV (slow, over 5–10 mins)* i.m.	Once or on alternate days	–	2.5–5.0 ml IV or (i.m.)	2.5–5.0 ml IV or (i.m.)	2.5–5.0 ml IV or (i.m.)	2.5–5.0 ml IV or (i.m.)	Hypoglycaemia, page 105
Calcium gluconate Amp. (10%), 5, 10 ml, 1 g contains 2.25 mmol calcium. Use amp. for oral treatment	Oral	4	–	100 mg/kg	1 g	2 g	4 g	Standard dosage, Hypocalcaemia
	IV (slow, over 5–10 mins)*	1–2	–	0.3 ml/kg (30 mg/kg) of 10% solution diluted to 2.5%	0.3 ml/kg (30 mg/kg) of 10% solution diluted to 2.5%	0.3 ml/kg (30 mg/kg) of 10% solution diluted to 2.5%	Max. dose 10 ml of 2.5% solution	Also *Table 2.1* page 6 for dosage scale in Cardiorespiratory Collapse
	IV (slow, over 5–10 mins)*	Once repeated if required	–	0.5–1.0 ml/kg (50–100 mg/kg)	0.5–1.0 ml/kg (50–100 mg/kg)	0.5–1.0 ml/kg (50–100 mg/kg)	0.5–1.0 ml/kg (50–100 mg/kg)	Hypocalcaemia in Shock, page 105. Neonatal Hypocalcaemia page 136 and Acute Hyperkalaemia pages 132 and 433
Calcium lactate 6% suspension	Oral	Up to 4	5 ml	5 ml	10–30 ml	10–30 ml	20–60 ml	Neonatal Hypocalcaemia page 135

Table A11.1 continues

Table A11.1 continued

Name and formulations	*Routes*	*Doses per 24 hours*	*0–2/52*	*2/52–1 year*	*1 year*	*7 years*	*14 years to adult*	*Remarks*
Calcium Resonium Powder 300 g	Oral, gastric tube Enema	Up to 3	–	–	1 g/kg	1 g/kg	1 g/kg	Acute Hyperkalaemia, pages 132 and 433
Carbamazepine Tab. 100, 200, 400 mg Syrup, 100 mg/5 ml	Oral	2–3	–	10–20 mg/kg	100 mg	200 mg	400 mg	Anticonvulsant dosage
Carbimazole Tab. 5 mg	Oral	3		Over 1 month 0.25 mg/kg	2.5 mg	5 mg	10 mg	Standard dosage for thyrotoxicosis
	Oral	3–6	Neonatal period 1 mg/kg/24 hours in divided doses	Neonatal period 1 mg/kg/24 hours in divided doses				Neonatal Thyrotoxicosis page 479
Charcoal, activated. Powder 50 g bottle Effervescent granules, 5 g sachet	Oral or gastric tube	Every 2 hours, as indicated	–	5–10 g	5–10 g	5–10 g	Over 10 years 50 g	Antidote in Acute Poisoning pages 55–64
Chloral hydrate Caps. 500 mg Mixture 500 mg/5 ml Paediatric Elixir 200 mg/5 ml	Oral	Once	–	30–50 mg/kg	30–50 mg/kg	600 mg–1.0 g	1.5–3.0 g	Single dose at night, page 82
	Oral	3	–	30 mg/kg	300 mg	600 mg	1.0 g	For repeated doses only: *See also* Dichloralphenazone and Triclofos
Chlorothiazide Tab. 500 mg	Oral	2	–	25 mg/kg Increase to 40–50 mg/kg if [illegible]	25 mg/kg Increase to 40–50 mg/kg if [illegible]	25 mg/kg Increase to 40–50 mg/kg if [illegible]	0.5–1.0 g	Diuretic in Cardiac Failure, page 264

Chlorpheniramine Tab. 4 mg Elixir (2 mg/5 ml) Amp. (10 mg/ml) 1 ml	Oral	3–4	–	–	1 mg	2 mg	4 mg	Dose may be doubled
	IV	Once	–	0.25 mg/kg	2.5 mg	5 mg	10 mg	Anaphylactic Shock, page 114
Chlorpromazine Tab. 10, 25, 50, 100 mg Elixir 25 mg/5 ml Amp. (25 mg/ml) 1, 2 ml	Oral	3	–	–	–	–	75–100 mg	Anorexia Nervosa, page 522
	Oral, nasogastric tube i.m.	Tetanus in Childhood (page 327), Neonatal Tetanus with IPPV (page 330) without IPPV (page 332), for dosage						
	Oral i.m.	3–4	–	1 mg/kg	10 mg	25 mg	50 mg	Sedative or antiemetic effect
Cimetidine Tab. 200, 400 mg Syrup 200 mg/ml Amp. (100 mg/ml) 2 ml	Oral	4	–	5–10 mg/kg	5–10 mg/kg	5–10 mg/kg	200 mg	Standard dosage for reduction of gastric acidity
	IV over 2 hours	4–6	–	2 mg/kg in 5% glucose	2 mg/kg in 5% glucose	2 mg/kg in 5% glucose	2 mg/kg in 5% glucose	Bleeding Peptic Ulcer, page 390
	or slow infusion*	4	–	10 mg/kg in 5% glucose or 0.9% NaCl	10 mg/kg in 5% glucose or 0.9% NaCl	10 mg/kg in 5% glucose or 0.9% NaCl	10 mg/kg in 5% glucose or 0.9% NaCl	Gastrointestinal Bleeding in Acute Liver Failure, page 414
Clonazepam Tab. 0.5, 2 mg Amp. (1 mg/ml), 1 ml with 1 ml water for injection	Oral	2	–	0.5 mg	1 mg	2 mg	4 mg	Anticonvulsant dosage
	IV slow over 1 min*	Dose and rate according to response	–	0.5 mg in 0.5 ml water	0.5 mg in 0.5 ml water	0.5 mg in 0.5 ml water	0.5 mg in 0.5 ml water	Status epilepticus, page 309
	IV slow infusion*	Dose and rate according to response	–	3 mg in 250 ml 0.9% NaCl or 5% glucose	3 mg in 250 ml 0.9% NaCl or 5% glucose	3 mg in 250 ml 0.9% NaCl or 5% glucose	3 mg in 250 ml 0.9% NaCl or 5% glucose	Status epilepticus, page 309

Table A11.1 continues

Table A11.1 continued

Name and formulations	*Routes*	*Doses per 24 hours*	*0–2/52*	*2/52–1 year*	*1 year*	*7 years*	*14 years to adult*	*Remarks*
Cyclizine Tab. 50 mg Amp. (50 mg/5 ml) 1 ml	Oral	Up to 3	–	–	–	25 mg	Above 10 years 25–50 mg	Travel Sickness, page 80
	IV i.m.	Up to 3	–	–	–	–	Above 10 years 50 mg	Travel Sickness, page 80
DDAVP				*See* Desmopressin				
D_2, vitamin				*See* Calciferol				
Dantrolene Vial, 20 mg, powder for reconstitution	IV		Malignant hyperpyrexia (page 184) for dosage					
Dapsone Tab. 50, 100 mg	Oral	Once	–	–	100–200 mg *daily*	100–200 mg *daily*	100–200 mg *daily*	Dermatitis Herpetiformis, page 512
Desferrioxamine Vial 500 mg, powder for reconstitution	i.m. (S.C.) IV slow infusion*		Acute iron poisoning (page 68) for dosage					
Desmopressin	Nasal	1–2	–	–	5–10 μg	5–10 μg 10–20 μg	Diabetes insipidus	
	i.m. IV	Once	–	–	400 ng	400 ng	1–4 μg	Dental bleeding, page 163
Diazepam Tab. 2.5, 10 mg Elixir, 2 mg/5 ml Amp. (5 mg/ml) 2, 4 ml Amp. Emulsion	Oral	3	–	–	–	–	2–5 mg	School Phobia, page 253
	Oral, nasogastric tube	6	Neonatal period 2 mg	Neonatal period 2 mg	–	–	–	Neonatal tetanus with IPPV page 331, without IPPV

	Oral i.m.	Once	–	–	1 mg per year of age	1 mg per year of age	1 mg per year of age	Sedation for Practical Procedures, page 723
	IV i.m.		Posthypoxic convulsions (Table 2.2) for dosage scale					Emergency Intubation, page 228
	IV	Once	–	0.05 mg/kg	0.05 mg/kg	0.05 mg/kg	0.05 mg/kg	
	IV over 2–3 min IV infusion*	As required	–	0.25 mg/kg	2.5 mg (1–6 years)	5 mg (7–12 years)	10 mg (12 years on)	Status Epilepticus, page 308
Diazoxide Tab. 50 mg Amp. (15 mg/ml) 20 ml	Oral	2–3	–	5–25 mg/kg per 24 hours	5–25 mg/kg per 24 hours	5–25 mg/kg per 24 hours	100 mg	Hypoglycaemia, page 467
	IV	Up to 4	–	1.5–5.0 mg/kg	1.5–5.0 mg/kg	1.5–5.0 mg/kg	300 mg	Hypertensive Crises, *Table 48.4*, page 431
Dichloralphenazone (*Welldorm*) Tab. 50 mg Elixir 225 mg/5 ml	Oral	Once, for hypnotic effect	–	30–50 mg/kg	30–50 mg/kg	650 mg	1.3 g	Sedative, page 82
Digoxin Tab. 0.0625 mg (62.5 μg), 0.125 mg (125 μg), 0.25 mg (250 μg)	Oral i.m.		Digitalizing dose at various body weights (page 265) Digitalizing dose in protein–energy malnutrition (page 605)					
Paediatric Elixir 0.05 mg/ml (50 μg/ml) Amp. (250 μg/ml) 2 ml	IV slow*							
Dimercaprol Amp. (50 mg/ml) 2 ml	i.m.	6	–	4 mg/kg	4 mg/kg	4 mg/kg	4 mg/kg	Acute Lead Poisoning, page 357
Diphenoxylate			No longer recommended; use loperamide					

Table A11.1 continues

Table A11.1 continued

Name and formulations	*Routes*	*Doses per 24 hours*	*0–2/52*	*2/52–1 year*	*1 year*	*7 years*	*14 years to adult*	*Remarks*
Dipotassium hydrogen phosphate	IV over 4–6 hours		5–10 mg/kg of phosphorus (0.15–0.33 mmol/kg)	5–10 mg/kg of phosphorus (0.15–0.33 mmol/kg)	5–10 mg/kg of phosphorus (0.15–0.33 mmol/kg)	5–10 mg/kg of phosphorus (0.15–0.33 mmol/kg)	5–10 mg/kg of phosphorus (0.15–0.33 mmol/kg)	Hypophospataemia in Shock, page 105. Substitute Disodium hydrogen phosphate in hyperkalaemia, page 105; *see* also Tables A5.3 and A5.4, page 777)
Disodium hydrogen phosphate	IV over 4–6 hours		5–10 mg/kg of phosphorus	5–10 mg/kg of phosphorus	5–10 mg/kg of phosphorus	5–10 mg/kg of phosphorus	5–10 mg/kg of phosphorus	Use in hypophosphataemia in shock, in presence of hyperkalaemia; *see* also Tables A5.3 and A5.4, page 777)
Dobutamine Vial 250 mg, for reconstitution	IV infusion*	Shock (page 107) and *Table 10.2* (page 106), and *Table 2.2* (page 17) for rate of infusion and dosage scale						
Dopamine Amp. or syringe (40 mg/ml). 5 ml, for dilution Amp. (160 mg/ml), 5 ml, for dilution	IV infusion*	As above						*See* also Septic Shock in Mengitis
Doxapram Amp. (20 mg/ml) 5 ml. Bottle for infusion (2 mg/ml) in 5% glucose, 500 ml	IV	Post-anaesthetic respiratory depression, *Table 2.1* for dosage scale (page 6)						
Edrophonium Amp. (10 mg/ml) 1 ml	IV i.m.	Once	0.5–1.0 mg (test dose only)	0.5–1.0 mg (test dose only)	0.5–1.0 mg (test dose only)	0.5–1.0 mg (test dose only)	0.5–1.0 mg (test dose only)	Myasthenia Gravis, page 225

EDTA				*See* Sodium Calciumedetate				
Epoprostenol (prostacylin, prostaglandin I_2) Vial, 500 µg with 50 ml diluent	IV infusion continuous*			Shock (pages 106 and 109)				
Epsi-amino-caproic acid (EACA)				*See* Aminocaproic acid				
Felypressin				*See* Prilocaine with Felypressin				
Folic acid Tab. 0.1 mg (100 µg), 5 mg	Oral	Once	–	0.25 mg/kg	2.5 mg	5 mg	10 mg	Folic acid deficiency
Frusemide (US Furosemide) Tabs. 20, 40, 50 mg	Oral	Once or alternate days	1–4 mg/kg	1–4 mg/kg	20 mg	40 mg	40–80 mg	Acute hypercalcaemia (IV also) page 137
Paediatric liquid 1 mg/ml for reconstitution in water.	I.V. i.m.	1–2 1–2	1–5 mg/kg 1–2 mg/kg	1–5 mg/kg 1–2 mg/kg	1–5 mg/kg 1–2 mg/kg	5–10 mg 5–10 mg	10–20 mg 5–10 mg	Diuretic in cardiac failure page 264
Amp. (10 mg/ml) 2, 5, 25 ml	IV infusion*							Also, Pulmonary Oedema (page 267) or Renal Shutdown (IV), *Table 2.3*, page 8; in Burns, page 38; Oedema in Protein–Energy Malnutrition, page 605; Renal Failure in Shock, page 111; Exchange Transfusion, page 694

Table A11.1 continues

Table A11.1 continued

Name and formulations	*Routes*	*Doses per 24 hours*	*0–2/52*	*2/52–1 year*	*1 year*	*7 years*	*14 years to adult*	*Remarks*
Glucagon Vial, 1 mg (1 unit), 10 mg (10 units) with diluent	S.C. i.m. IV	Once but repeat after 20 min if required	0.5–1.0 mg (0.5–1.0 units)	0.5–1.0 mg (0.5–1.0 units)	0.5–1.0 mg (0.5–1.0 units)	0.5–1.0 mg (0.5–1.0 units)	0.5–1.0 mg (0.5–1.0 units)	Hypoglycaemia page 467, also hypoglycaemia in diabetes, page 456
Glycerol	Oral	Up to 6	1 g/kg	1 g/kg	1 g/kg	1 g/kg	1 g/kg	Benign Intracranial Hypertension page 299 and Coma, page 314
Glyceryl trinitrate Tab. 300 µg (0.3 mg), 500 µg (0.5 mg), 600 µg (0.6 mg).	Sublingually	Once, or repeat if required	–	–	0.4 mg with Vasopressin	0.4 mg with Vasopressin	0.4 mg with Vasopressin	Portal Hypertension page 419
Amp. 500 µg/ml (5 mg/ml), 10 ml	IV infusion*							Left ventricular failure
Glypressin					*See* Terlipressin			
Heparin Amp/Vial (1000 units/ml) 5 ml, (5000 units)/ml 5 ml	IV infusion*	Continuous	25 units/kg *per hour*	25 units/kg *per hour*	25 units/kg *per hour*	25 units/kg *per hour*	25 units/kg *per hour*	Disseminated Intravascular Coagulation, page 498: also Exchange Transfusion, page 693
	IV injection	4–6	100 units/kg *per dose*	100 units/kg *per dose*	100 units/kg *per dose*	100 units/kg *per dose*	100 units/kg *per dose*	

Hydrazaline (US Hydrallazine) Tab. 25, 50 mg Amp. (powder for reconstitution) 20 mg	(Oral)		–					
	i.m.	Effect lasts a few hours; repeat if required	–	0.15 mg–0.5 mg/kg	0.15 mg–0.5 mg/kg	0.15 mg–0.5 mg/kg	0.15 mg–0.5 mg/kg Max. dose per 24 hours, 200 mg	Shock, page 109; Hypertensive Crises, page 431
	IV	Effect lasts a few mins; repeat if required	–	0.15 mg–0.5 mg/kg	0.15 mg–0.5 mg/kg	0.15 mg–0.5 mg/kg	0.15 mg–0.5 mg/kg Max. dose per 24 hours, 200 mg	Shock, page 109; Hypertensive Crises, page 431
	IV infusion*							
Hyoscine (scopolomine) Tab. 0.3, 0.6 mg Amp. 0.4 mg, 1 ml; 0.6 mg, 1 ml	Oral s.c.	Once	–	0.15 mg/kg	0.15 mg	0.3 mg	0.6 mg	Travel Sickness, page 80
Imipramine Tab. 10, 25 mg Syrup, 25 mg/5 ml	Oral	3	–	–	–	10 mg	25 mg	For antidepressin effect, dose may be doubled, page 525
	Oral	Once at night	–	–	–	10–25 mg, up to 50–75 mg	10–25 mg, up to 50–75 mg	Nocturnal Enuresis
Indomethacin Caps. 25, 50 mg Suspension, 25 mg/5 ml	(Oral) IV	Persistent Patent Ductus (page 262) for dosage and method						
Insulin	s.c. i.m. IV infusion*	Diabetes Mellitus						Also Shock, page 105 and Contraindication in hypernatraemia, page 410

Table A11.1 continues

Table A11.1 continued

Name and formulations	*Routes*	*Doses per 24 hours*	*0–2/52*	*2/52–1 year*	*1 year*	*7 years*	*14 years to adult*	*Remarks*
Iodine, aqueous solution (Lugol's Iodine or solution) (Iodine 5%, potassium iodide 10%, in water). Total Iodide content 130 mg/ml	Oral	3	1 drop	–	–	–	–	Neonatal Thyrotoxicosis, page 479
Ipecacuanha Emetic Mixture, Paediatric Total alkaloids, as emetine 14 mg/10 ml	Oral	1 or 2	–	6 months–1 year 15 ml	15 ml	Up to 4 years 15 ml Over 4 years 30 ml	30 ml	Emetic in Acute Poisoning, page 163; and *Table 8.6*
Isoprenaline (US Isoproterenol) 1:1000 (0.1%, 1 mg/ml) Amp. 0.2 mg (200 μg/ml, 1, 5 ml); 1 mg/ml, 2 ml	IV bolus or infusion*	For dosage and method of administration *see* Cardiorespiratory arrest or persistent bradycardia (*Table 2.2*, page 7), also Shock (page 108 and *Table 10.5*, page 106)						
	IV	Once	–	–	1–2 μg/kg	1–2 μg/kg	1–2 μg/kg	Stokes–Adams attacks, page 271
	IV infusion*	As required	–	–	0.075 μg/kg *per min*	0.075 μg/kg *per min*	0.075 μg/kg *per min*	Stokes–Adams attacks, page 271
Isosorbide Tab 20, 40 mg	Oral	2–3	8 g/kg *per 24 hours*	8 g/kg *per 24 hours*	8 g/kg *per 24 hours*	8 g/kg *per 24 hours*	8 g/kg *per 24 hours*	Hydrocephalus, page 298
K_1, vitamin				*See* Phytomenadione				
Labetalol Tab. 100, 200, 400 mg Amp. (5 mg/ml) 20 ml	(Oral) IV infusion*	As required	–	1–3 mg/kg *per hour*	1–3 mg/kg *per hour*	1–3 mg/kg *per hour*	Max. dose 120 mg/*hour*	Hypertensive Crises, page 431; and *Table 48.4*

Lactulose (Duphalac) Syrup 3.35 g/ml	Oral	2	–	2.5 ml	5 ml	10 ml	15 ml	Acute Liver Failure, page 413
Lignocaine (US Lidocaine) 0.1% (1 mg/ml), 500 ml, 1 ℓ containers in 5% glucose. 0.2% (2 mg/ml), 500 ml, 1 ℓ containers in 5% glucose. Syringe, 100 mg (20 mg/ml) 5 ml. IV infusion (200 mg/ml), 5, 10 ml syringes	IV	Once	–	1 mg/kg for ventricular extrasystoles or ventricular tachycardia	1 mg/kg for ventricular extrasystoles or ventricular tachycardia	1 mg/kg for ventricular extrasystoles or ventricular tachycardia	1 mg/kg for ventricular extrasystoles or ventricular tachycardia	Arrhythmias, *Table 2.2* page 7 for dosage scale; also page 272
	IV infusion*	As required	–	1 mg/kg/*hour* for recurring tachycardia	1 mg/kg/*hour* for recurring tachycardia	1 mg/kg/*hour* for recurring tachycardia	1 mg/kg/*hour* for recurring tachycardia	Arrhythmias, *Table 2.2* page 7 for dosage scale; also page 272
Liothyronine (tri-iodothyronine) Tab. 20 µg Amp. (20 µg) powder, with glucose, for reconstitution	Oral IV	Alternate days	Neonatal period 20 µg/m^2 *per 24 hours*	Neonatal period 20 µg/m^2 *per 24 hours*				Hypothyroidism in Newborn, acute complications page 478
Loperamide Caps. 2 mg Syrup 1 mg/5 ml	Oral	4	–	–	–	4–8 years 1 mg	9–12 years 2 mg Adult 4 mg initially	Diarrhoea, *see* page 397
Lugol's iodine				*See* Iodine, aqueous solution				
Magnesium hydroxide (Milk of Magnesia) 8% suspension; 6.8 mmol/5 ml	Oral	Up to 3–4	–	1–2 ml	5 ml	10 ml	15 ml Adult dose 3–6 g *per 24 hours*	Start oral treatment after i.m. treatment for 3–4 days. Magnesium depletion in Protein–Energy Malnutrition, page 604

Table A11.1 continues

Table A11.1 continued

Name and formulations	*Routes*	*Doses per 24 hours*	*0–2/52*	*2/52–1 year*	*1 year*	*7 years*	*14 years to adult*	*Remarks*
Magnesium sulphate 50% (2 mmol/ml)	i.m. (deep)	Once	–	0.3 mmol/kg (0.15 ml/kg) once, then half dose for 3–4 days	0.3 mmol/kg (0.15 ml/kg) once, then half dose for 3–4 days	0.3 mmol/kg (0.15 ml/kg) once, then half dose for 3–4 days	0.3 mmol/kg (0.15 ml/kg) once, then half dose for 3–4 days	Magnesium depletion in Protein–Energy Malnutrition, page 604
	i.m. (deep)	Once	–	0.1 mmol/kg (0.05 ml/kg)	0.1 mmol/kg (0.05 ml/kg)	0.1 mmol/kg (0.05 ml/kg)	0.1 mmol/kg (0.05 ml/kg)	Hypomagnesaemia in Shock, page 105
Magnesium sulphate 25% or 12.5% (1 or 0.5 mmol/ml)	Oral (non-urgent symptoms)	3–4	0.5–1.0 mmol/kg (0.25–0.5 ml/kg) 50% solution to be diluted	0.5–1.0 mmol/kg (0.25–0.5 ml/kg) 50% solution to be diluted	–	–	–	Neonatal Hypocalcaemia and Hypomagnesaemia, pages 135–139
Magnesium sulphate 50% (2 mmol/ml); dilute to 25% or 12.5% for small infants	i.m. (deep) (acute symptoms)	2	0.2–0.5 mmol/kg (0.1–0.25 ml/kg) 50% solution to be diluted	0.2–0.5 mmol/kg (0.1–0.25 ml/kg) 50% solution to be diluted	–	–	–	Neonatal Hypocalcaemia and Hypomagnesaemia, pages 000–000
Magnesium sulphate 1% (0.04 mmol/ml)	IV ($\ngtr$1 ml/min; very acute symptoms)	Once	0.5–1.25 mmol (12–30 ml) NOT PER KG	0.5–1.25 mmol (12–30 ml) NOT PER KG	–	–	–	Neonatal Hypocalcaemia and Hypomagnesaemia, page 138

Mannitol 10%, 500 ml; 15%, 500 ml; 20%, 200, 250, 500 ml	IV	Once or slow infusion*				Dosage scale *Table 2.3*, page 9. Raised Intracranial Pressure, management, page 296; also Raised ICP in Head Injury, page 290; in Acute Liver Failure, page 415. Neonatal Convulsions, page 704. Pulmonary Oedema, Haemoglobinuria in Burns, pages 36 and 38
Metaraminol Amp. (10 mg/ml) 1 ml	(S.C.) (i.m.) IV infusion*	Acute hypotension in cardiorespiratory collapse, dosage scale (*Table 2.3*, page 9)				
Methionine Tab. 250 mg	Oral	6	Paracetamol poisoning (page 67) for dosage			
Methoxamine Amp. (20 mg/ml) 1 ml	(i.m.) IV slow infusion*	Cardiorespiratory collapse, dosage scale (*Table 2.3*, page 9)				
Methylene Blue 1% solution	IV	Once or more as required	1–2 mg/kg (0.1–0.2 ml/kg)	1–2 mg/kg (0.1–0.2 ml/kg)	1–2 mg/kg (0.1–0.2 ml/kg)	Methaemoglobinaemia, page 666

Table A11.1 continues

Table A11.1 continued

Name and formulations	*Routes*	*Doses per 24 hours*	*0–2/52*	*2/52–1 year*	*1 year*	*7 years*	*14 years to adult*	*Remarks*
Morphine Amp. (10, 15, 20, 30 mg/ml) 1, 2 ml	i.m.	1–3	Avoid if possible, respiratory depression (0.15 mg/kg)	Avoid if possible, respiratory depression (0.2 mg/kg)	2 mg	4 mg	8–16 mg	Dosage scale for general use
	i.m.	Once repeat as required	–	–	0.2 mg/kg	0.2 mg/kg	0.2 mg/kg Max. dose 5–10 mg	Pulmonary Oedema, page 267
	i.m.	6	–	–	0.2 mg/kg	0.2 mg/kg	0.2 mg/kg Max. dose 5–10 mg	Acute Liver Failure, page 417
	IV	Once, repeat if required	–	–	0.1–0.2 mg/kg	0.1–0.2 mg/kg	0.1–0.2 mg/kg Max. dose 10–20 mg	Burns, page 29, Venomous Bites and Stings, page 564
	IV infusion over 30 min	2–3	–	–	1 mg/kg	1 mg/kg	1 mg/kg	Tetanus in Childhood, page 328
Nalorphine	Not recommended; use naloxone							
Naloxone *Adult* Amp. (0.4 mg/ml, 400 µg/ml) 1 ml *Neonatal* Amp. (0.02 mg/ml, 20 µg/ml) 2 ml	IV or infusion*	As required, can be repeated after 2–3 min	Term infant 0.04 mg (2 ml); <2.5 kg 0.02 mg (1 ml)				Drug depression in newborn, page 617	Drug depression in newborn, page 617
	IV or infusion*	As above	–	0.2 mg	0.2 mg	0.2 mg	0.2 mg	Opioid Poisoning, page 69
	i.m.	As above	–	0.06 mg/kg	0.06 mg/kg	0.06 mg/kg	0.06 mg/kg	Opioid Poisoning; less effective than IV, page 69

Neostigmine Tab. 15 mg Amp. (0.5 mg/ml, 500 µg/ml) 1 ml; 2.5 mg/ml, 1 ml	(Oral) i.m. IV	Once	0.06 mg/kg (60 µg/kg)	0.06 mg/kg (60 µg/kg)	0.625 mg (625 µg)	1.25 mg	2.5 mg	Myasthenia gravis; atropine usually given first, page 225
Nikethamide Amp. (250 mg/ml), 2, 5 ml	IV	Once	Respiratory arrest when intubation is not possible (*Table 2.1*, page 6) for dosage scale					
Nitrazepam Tab. 5, 10 mg Caps. 5 mg Suspension (2.5 mg/5 ml)	Oral	1–2	–	0.25 mg/kg	2.5 mg	5 mg	10 mg	Anticonvulsant dose
Nitroprusside			*See* Sodium Nitroprusside					
Nitroglycerine			*See* Glyceryl Trinitrate					
Opium tincture (Morphine 1%, 10 mg/ml)	Oral	Maternal Drug Dependence and the Neonatal Abstinence Syndrome *see* page 717 for dosage						
Pancuronium Amp. (2 mg/ml) 2 ml	i.m. IV	Once	0.1 mg/kg (single dose)					Diaphragmatic Hernia page 635
Paracetamol Tab. 500 mg Syrup or suspension 120 mg/5 ml	Oral	4–6	–	12 mg/kg	120–140 mg	250–500 mg	1 g	

Table A11.1 continues

Table A11.1 continued

Name and formulations	*Routes*	*Doses per 24 hours*	*0–2/52*	*2/52–1 year*	*1 year*	*7 years*	*14 years to adult*	*Remarks*
Paraldehyde Amp. 5, 10 ml	i.m. (deep)	Once repeated if required	–	–	1.0–1.5 ml	1–5 years 3 ml 6–10 years 8 ml	10 ml	Status Epilepticus page 309; dosage scale, *Table 2.3* page 9
	IV infusion*	According to response	Neonatal convulsions (page 704) for dosage	Neonatal convulsions (page 704) for dosage				
Penicillamine Tab. 50, 125, 250 mg	Oral	4	–	–	–	5 mg/kg	5 mg/kg Max. dose 2 g/*24 hours*	Acute Lead Poisoning, page 357
Pentobarbitone (US Pentobarbital) Caps. 100 mg	Oral IV	For dosage in raised intracranial pressure *see* Chapter 26, page 296						
(Nembutal)	(Oral)							
Pethidine (US Meperidine) Tab. 25, 50 mg Amp. (50 mg/ml) 1, 2 ml	i.m. IV	Once	Avoid if possible: respiratory depression	Avoid if possible: respiratory depression	0.2 mg/kg	0.2 mg/kg	0.2 mg/kg Max. dose IV 25 mg	Intubation, page 228; Venomous Bites and Stings, page 564
Phenelzine Tab. 15 mg	Oral	3–4	–	–	–	–	15 mg	Antidepressant; *Note*, Dietary precautions for monoamine oxidase inhibitors, page 525

Phenobarbitone (US Phenobarbital) Tab. 15, 30, 60, 100 mg Elixir 30 mg/10 ml Amp. (200 mg/ml), 1 ml and water for injection	Oral i.m. IV	Once Once	6 mg/kg 10 mg/kg Danger: transient respiratory depression	6 mg/kg 10 mg/kg Danger: transient respiratory depression	30–60 mg 10 mg/kg Danger: transient respiratory depression	60–90 mg 10 mg/kg Danger: transient respiratory depression	60–90 mg 8 mg/kg Max. dose 50–200 mg	Anticonvulsant dose. For other indications see Drowning, page 47; Tetanus, page 327; Acute Liver Failure, page 417; Meningitis, page 339; Neonatal Convulsions, page 703; Maternal Drug Dependence, page 719
Phentolamine Amp. (10 mg/ml) 1, 5 ml	IV infusion*	According to response	–	–	–	–	–	Shock, page 110 for dosage
Phenytoin (US Diphenylhydantoin) Tab. 25, 50, 100 mg Parenteral injection (50 mg/ml) in water for injection, 5 ml	Oral IV slow* (i.m.)	2 According to response	– Neonatal period Convulsions (page 704) for dosage	– Neonatal period Convulsions (page 704) for dosage	5 mg/kg –	2.5 mg/kg –	2.5 mg/kg Max. dose 150–300 mg –	Anticonvulsant dose
Phosphate	*See* dipotassium hydrogen and disodium hydrogen phosphate							
Physostigmine salicylate	IV infusion	According to response	–	–	–	0.5–1.0 mg/kg *per hour*	0.5–1.0 mg/kg *per hour*	Tricyclic antidepressant poisoning, page 68

Table A11.1 continues

Table A11.1 continued

Name and formulations	*Routes*	*Doses per 24 hours*	*0–2/52*	*2/52–1 year*	*1 year*	*7 years*	*14 years to adult*	*Remarks*
Phytomenadione (US Phytodiadone) Tab. 10 mg Amp. (2 mg/ml) 0.5 ml (10 mg/ml) 1 ml	Oral i.m.	Once repeated if required	0.3 mg/kg	0.3 mg/kg	3 mg	5 mg	10 mg	
	IV	Once repeated if required	1 mg (IV)	–	–	–	–	Acute Neonatal Bleeding, IV dosage required, page 678
Practolol (US Practol) Amp. (2 mg/ml) 5 ml	IV	Repeated as required	–	–	–	0.5 mg	0.5 mg	Tricyclic antidepressant poisoning, page 68
Prilocaine, with Felypressin	Locally	As required	Dental bleeding (page 162)					
Prochlorperazine Tab. 5, 25 mg Syrup 5 mg/5 ml Amp. (12.5 mg/ml) 1, 2 ml	Oral	3	–	1.25–2.5 mg	5 mg	5–10 mg	5–10 mg	Antiemetic effect
	i.m. (deep)	Once or up to 3	–	–	3.125–6.25 mg	3.125–6.25 mg	12.5 mg	Antiemetic during cytotoxic treatment
Promethazine Tab. 10, 25 mg Elixir 5 mg/5 ml Amp. (25 mg/ml) 1, 2 ml	Oral	3	–	1.5 mg/kg	15 mg	25 mg	25–50 mg	Antihistamine effect
	IV slow (i.m. deep)	Once	–	0.5 mg/kg	5 mg	5 mg	7–14 years 10–25 mg >14 years 25–50 mg	Anaphylactic Shock, page 114
Propranolol Tab. 10, 40, 80, 160 mg Amp. (1 mg/ml) 1 ml	Oral	3	–	–	1–2 mg/kg	1–2 mg/kg	1–2 mg/kg Max. dose 40 mg	Cyanotic attacks, page 269; Paroxysmal supraventricular tachycardia, page 270

	IV infusion over 1 hour*	As required	–	–	–	2 mg *over 1 hour*	2 mg *over 1 hour*	*Table 2.2*, page 7 for dosage scale over larger age range. Theophylline poisoning, page 71
Propylthiouracil Tab. 50 mg	Oral	3–6	Neonatal thyrotoxicosis 1 mg/kg/*24 hours*	Neonatal thyrotoxicosis 1 mg/kg/*24 hours*	–		300–450 mg/*24 hours*	Neonatal Thyrotoxicosis, page 479
Prostacyclin (Prostaglandin I_2)					*See* Epoprostenol			
Prostaglandin E_1					*See* Alprostadil			
Protamine Amp. (10 mg/ml), 5, 10 ml	IV slow*	As required	1 mg (0.1 ml) for each 100 units of Heparin up to max. of 50 mg (5 ml)	1 mg (0.1 ml) for each 100 units of Heparin up to max. of 50 mg (5 ml)	1 mg (0.1 ml) for each 100 units of Heparin up to max. of 50 mg (5 ml)	1 mg (0.1 ml) for each 100 units of Heparin up to max. of 50 mg (5 ml)	1 mg (0.1 ml) for each 100 units of Heparin up to max. of 50 mg (5 ml)	Neutralizes effect of heparin
Pyridostigmine Tab. 60 mg Amp. (1 mg/ml) 1 ml	Oral	6	Neonatal period 5–10 mg	Neonatal period 5–10 mg Up to 1 year 10 mg initially	10 mg initially	10 mg initially	0.3–1.2 g/*24 hours*	Myasthenia gravis, page 225
	S.C. i.m. IV	6	Neonatal period 200–400 μg	Neonatal period 200–400 μg Up to one year 0.25–1.0 mg initially	0.25–1.0 mg initially	0.25–1.0 mg initially	2–5 mg/*24 hours*	Myasthenia gravis, page 225

Table A11.1 continues

Table A11.1 continued

Name and formulations	*Routes*	*Doses per 24 hours*	*0–2/52*	*2/52–1 year*	*1 year*	*7 years*	*14 years to adult*	*Remarks*
Pyridoxine Tabs. 10, 20, 50 mg	Oral	1–2	25 mg/24 *hours*	25 mg/24 *hours*	25 mg/24 *hours*	25 mg/24 *hours*	25 mg/24 *hours*	To accompany antituberculous treatment with isoniazid, page 344
	IV	Once	Neonatal period 100 mg with EEG control	Neonatal period 100 mg with EEG control				Neonatal Pyridoxine Dependent Fits, page 715
Resin, Resonium				*See* Calcium Resonium				
Retinol acetate Tab 50 000 units (16 000 μg)	Oral		Vitamin A deficiency and Xerophthalmia (page 148) for dosage					
Retinol palmitate Amp. (300 000 units, 100 000 μg/ml) 1 ml	i.m. (deep)		Vitamin A deficiency and Xerophthalmia (page 148) for dosage					
Salbutamol Tab. 2, 4 mg Elixir 2 mg/5 ml Amp. (50 μg/ml), 5 ml; (0.5 mg/ml. 500 μg/ml) 1 ml.	Oral	3–4	–	0.1 mg/kg	1 mg	2 mg	4 mg	Asthma, standard dose
	Nebulized	6–12						Aerosol solution for acute asthma
For IV infusion: Amp. (1 mg/ml) 5 ml, for dilution before use For aerosol solution 5 mg/ml diluted with 0.9% NaCl	IV infusion*							Can also be given by inhalation with metered dose, *Rotacaps*; s.c., i.m., slow IV injection or continuous IV infusion

Salcatonin (*see also* calcitonin) Amp. (100 units/ml) 1 ml; (200 units/ml) 2 ml	s.c. i.m.	3–4	–	Up to 8 units/kg per dose; adjust later dosage according to clinical and biochemical response	Up to 8 units/kg per dose; adjust later dosage according to clinical and biochemical response	Up to 8 units/kg per dose; adjust later dosage according to clinical and biochemical response	Up to 8 units/kg per dose; adjust later dosage according to clinical and biochemical response	Acute Hypercalcaemia, page 137
Sodium bicarbonate 8.4% (1 mmol/ml) Other strengths available	IV		Metabolic acidosis (calculation and dosage, page 119)					Also Cardiorespiratory Arrest, *Table 2.1* for dosage scale, page 6; and Resuscitation of the Newborn, page 615
Sodium calciumedetate Amp. (200 mg/ml) 5 ml	i.m. IV infusion*		Acute Lead Poisoning (page 357) for dosage					
Sodium iodide	IV infusion	As required	Neonatal period 1–2 g/*24 hours*	Neonatal period 1–2 g/*24 hours*	–	–	–	Thyrotoxic Crises, page 480
Sodium nitroprusside Amp. 50 mg, powder for reconstitution with solvent	IV infusion*	As required	–	–				Shock, page 109 and *Table 10.5* page 106. Acute Hypertension in renal failure, page 431
Somatostatin	IV infusion	As required	–	–	250–500 µg/*hour*	250–500 µg/*hour*	250–500 µg/*hour*	Bleeding in Portal Hypertension, page 419
Spironolactone Tab. 25, 50, 100 mg	Oral	2	–	1.2 mg/kg	12.5 mg	25 mg	50 mg	Diuretic: standard dosage

Table A11.1 continues

Table A11.1 continued

Name and formulations	*Routes*	*Doses per 24 hours*	*0–2/52*	*2/52–1 year*	*1 year*	*7 years*	*14 years to adult*	*Remarks*
Sulphapyridine Tab. 0.5 g	Oral	4	–	–	1–2 g/24 *hours*	1–2 g/24 *hours*	1–2 g/24 *hours*	Dermatitis Herpetiformis, page 512
Terlipressin (*Glypressin*) Vial, 1 mg, with diluent	IV infusion*	As required	–	–				Bleeding in Portal Hypertension (page 419) for dosage
Theophylline Tab. 100, 125 mg Elixir 60 mg/5 ml	Oral		Neonatal period 4 mg/kg/24 *hours*	Neonatal period 4 mg/kg/24 *hours*				Apnoeic attacks in Newborn, page 253
Thiamine Tab. 3, 10, 25, 50, 100, 300 mg Amp. (25 mg/ml) 1 ml; (100 mg/ml) 1 ml	i.m. IV	Once	25 mg	25 mg	–	–	–	Infantile Beri-beri, page 275
Thiopentone sodium Injection 2.5%; Amp. 500 mg; Vial, 2.5 g (powder) Injection 5%; Amp. 500 mg, 1 g; Vial, 5 g (powder)	IV	For dosage in raised intracranial pressure, *see* Chapter 26, page 296						

Thyroxine (US Levothyroxine) Tab. 25, 50, 100 μg	Oral	Once	Neonatal period 100 μg/m² or 10 μg/kg/ *24 hours*	Neonatal period 100 μg/m² or 10 μg/kg/ *24 hours* Up to 1 year 12.5 μg	25 μg	50 μg	100 μg	Hypothyroidism in Newborn, page 478
Tolazoline Vial 25 mg/ml (*Priscoline* Ciba US)	IV bolus, then infusion	As required	Persistent fetal circulation (pages 251 for dosage)					
Tranexamic acid Tab. 500 mg Syrup 500 mg/5 ml Amp. (100 mg/ml) 5 ml	Oral	3	30 mg/kg	30 mg	30 mg	30 mg	30 mg Max. dose 1–1.5 g	Dental Bleeding, page 163
	IV slow, over 10 min	3–4	15 mg/kg	15 mg/kg	15 mg/kg	15 mg/kg	15 mg/kg Max. dose 1 g	Dental Bleeding, page 163
Triclofos Elixir 500 mg/5 ml	Oral	Once, as sedative	–	30–50 mg/kg	30–50 mg/kg	600 mg	Max. dose 1–2 g	Sedative at Night, page 82
Trimeprazine Tab. 10 mg Syrup 7.5 mg/5 ml Syrup (strong) 30 mg/5 ml	Oral	Once	–	–	3–4 mg/kg	3–4 mg/kg	Max. dose 100 mg	Sedative before Practical Procedures page 723
	i.m.	Once	–	–	0.9 mg/kg	0.9 mg/kg		
L-Tri-iodothyronine			*See* Liothyronine					
Vasopressin (*Pitressin*) Amp. (20 units/ml) 1 ml	IV*	As required	–	–				Bleeding in Portal Hypertension (page 419) for dosage and method

Table A11.1 continues

Table A11.1 continued

Name and formulations	*Routes*	*Doses per 24 hours*	*0–2/52*	*2/52–1 year*	*1 year*	*7 years*	*14 years to adult*	*Remarks*
Verapamil Tab. 40, 80, 120, 160 mg Amp. (2.5 mg/ml) 2 ml	IV slow, over 10 min*	As required	Paroxysmal Supraventricular Tachycardia (page 270) for dosage and method					
Vitamin A			*See* Retinol acetate and palmitate					
Vitamin B_1			*See* Thiamine					
Vitamin B_6			*See* Pyridoxine					
Vitamin C			*See* Ascorbic Acid					
Vitamin D_2			*See* Calciferol					
Vitamin K_1			*See* Phytomenadione					
Vitamin multiple (Solivito) Vial for injection	*See* Appendix 5, *Tables A5.4* and page 782 for composition and dosage							
Zinc sulphate Caps. 320 mg Tab. (effervescent) 200 mg (45 mg zinc)	Oral	1–3	10 mg/kg/*24 hours*	10 mg/kg/*24 hours*	10 mg/kg/*24 hours*	200 or 220 mg once, up to 3 times *per 24 hours*	200 or 220 mg once, up to 3 times *per 24 hours*	Acrodermatitis Enteropathica and iatrogenic zinc deficiency, page 515. For dosage in nutritional zinc deficiency see page 604.

* See *Table A11.12* for details of IV injections and infusions.

Table A11.2 Antibacterial agents. Conditions requiring special regimens or dosage scales are indicated, or a page reference to the text is given. In calculating doses on a 'per kg' basis, the dose should NOT normally exceed the maximum adult dose. For details of IV infusions, *see Table A11.12*. Intrathecal doses are given in *Table A11.13*

Name and formulations	*Routes*	*Doses per 24 hours*	*0–2/52*	*2/52–1 year*	*1 year*	*7 years*	*14 years to adult*	*Remarks*
Amoxycillin Caps. 250, 500 mg Tab. 125 mg Syrup 125 mg/5 ml 250 mg/5 ml Vial 250, 500 mg	Oral	3	62.5 mg	62.5 mg	125 mg	250 mg	500 mg	
	Oral	3	100 mg/kg/ *24 hours*	100 mg/kg/ *24 hours*	100 mg/kg/ *24 hours*	100 mg/kg/ *24 hours*	100 mg/kg/ *24 hours*	Typhoid, page 584; use parenteral routes if necessary
	i.m.	3	50–100 mg/ *kg/24 hours*	50–100 mg/ *kg/24 hours*	50–100 mg/ *kg/24 hours*	50–100 mg/ *kg/24 hours*	500 mg	
	IV (injection or infusion*)	4	50–100 mg/ *kg/24 hours*	50–100 mg/ *kg/24 hours*	50–100 mg/ *kg/24 hours*	50–100 mg/ *kg/24 hours*	1 g	
Ampicillin Caps. 250, 500 mg Tab 125 mg Syrup 125 mg/5 ml 250 mg/5 ml, 250 mg/5ml Vial 250, 500 mg	Oral (i.m.)	4	–	62.5 mg	125 mg	250 mg	500 mg	
	IV (injection or infusion*)	4–6	Neonatal period Chapter 77 and *Table 77.2* page 662	Over 1 month 125 mg	250 mg	250 mg	500 mg	Neonatal meningitis: 200 mg/kg/24 hours i.m. or IV with chloramphenicol page 338. meningitis: 300 mg/kg/ 24 hours i.m. or IV with chloramphenicol, page 342

Table A11.2 continues

Table A11.2 continued

Name and formulations	*Routes*	*Doses per 24 hours*	*0–2/52*	*2/52–1 year*	*1 year*	*7 years*	*14 years to adult*	*Remarks*
Benzylpenicillin Vial 300, 600 mg, 3, 6 g	i.m.	4	Neonatal period Chapter 77 and *Table 77.2*, page 662	Over 1 month 15 mg/kg	150 mg	300 mg	600 mg	1 mg = 10 000 units
	IV infusion*			Over 1 month 25–50 mg/kg	25–50 mg/kg	25–50 mg/kg	25–50 mg/kg	Severe infections, use bolus injection over 5 min; Neonatal Meningitis, page 338; Meningitis, page 343
Carbenicillin Vial, 1, 5 g Infusion set 5 g	i.m.	4	Neonatal period 100 mg/kg IV, 2–3 doses per 24 hours	50 mg/kg	50 mg/kg	500 mg	2 g	
	Slow infusion*	4–6		Over 1 month 250–400 mg/kg/24 *hours*	250–400 mg/kg/24 *hours*	5 g	IV for severe infections	
Cefotaxime Vial, 500 mg, 1, 2 g	i.m. IV*	2–4	Neonatal period Chapter 77 and *Table 77.2* page 662	Over 1 month 100–150 mg/kg/24 *hours*	100–150 mg/kg/24 *hours*	100–150 mg/kg/24 *hours*		Neonatal Meningitis, page 338. Reduce dose in severe renal impairment
	IV infusion*			*See Table A11.2*				

Cefoxitin Vial 1, 2 g	i.m. IV slow*	3–4	–	>3 months 80–60 mg/ kg/*24 hours*	80–60 mg/ kg/*24 hours*	80–60 mg/ kg/*24 hours*	1–2 g (single dose)	Reduce dose in renal impairment
	IV infusion*			*See Table A11.2*				
Cefuroxime Vial 250, 750 mg, 1.5 g	i.m. IV*	3	Neonatal period 30 mg/kg in 2–3 doses *per 24 hours*	30 mg/kg	250 mg/kg	500 mg/kg	1 g	Reduce dose in renal impairment
	IV infusion*	3–4		30–100 mg/ kg/*24 hours*	30–100 mg/ kg/*24 hours*	30–100 mg/ kg/*24 hours*	1.5 g	
Cephalexin Caps. 250, 500 mg Mixture 125 mg/5 ml Paediatric drops 125 mg/ 1.25 ml	Oral	4	12 mg/kg	12 mg/kg	125 mg	250 mg	500 mg	
Cephazolin Vial 500 mg, 1 g	i.m. IV*	2–4	–	25 mg/kg	250 mg	500 mg	1 g	Renal dose in renal impairment
	IV infusion*			*See Table A11.2*				
Chloramphenicol Caps. 250 mg Suspension 125 mg/5 ml Vial 300 mg, 1, 1.2 g	Oral	4	Neonatal period Chapter 77 and *Table 77.2*, page 662	12.5 mg/kg	12.5 mg/kg	250 mg	500 mg	Neonatal Meningitis, Meningitis, pages 342–343. Typhoid, page 584
	IV infusion*	3		25 mg	25 mg	25 mg/kg	25 mg/kg	
Clindamycin Caps. 75, 150 mg Paediatric suspension 75 mg/5 ml Amp. (150 mg/ml) 2 ml, 4 ml	Oral	3–4	–	31.5 mg	75 mg	150 mg	300 mg	Side effect, pseudo-membranous colitis
	IV infusion*	4	–	5–10 mg/kg	5–10 mg/kg	5–10 mg/kg	300–600 mg	

Table A11.2 continues

Table A11.2 continued

Name and formulations	*Routes*	*Doses per 24 hours*	*0–2/52*	*2/52–1 year*	*1 year*	*7 years*	*14 years to adult*	*Remarks*
Cloxacillin Caps. 250, 500 mg Syrup 125 mg/5 ml Vial 250, 500 mg, 1 g	Oral i.m. IV infusion*	4–6	Neonatal period Chapter 77 and *Table 77.2*, page 662					Meningitis, page 343; *flucloxacillin* better absorbed *orally*
Co-trimoxazole Tab. 480, 960 mg Paediatric tab. 120 mg Mixture 480 mg/5 ml Paediatric Mixture 240 mg/5 ml Amp. (320 mg/ml) 3 ml (i.m.) Amp. (96 mg/ml) 5 ml (IV infusion for dilution)	Oral	2	Avoid	6 weeks to 5 months 120 mg	6 months to 5 years 240 mg	6–12 years 480 mg	960 mg	Dosage in terms of number of mg sulphamethoxazole plus trimethoprim (5:1 ratio). i.m. not advised under 6 years. Reduce dose in renal impairment
	i.m. IV infusion*	2	Avoid	120 mg	240 mg	480 mg	960 mg	
Doxycyline Tab. 100 mg Caps. 100 mg Syrup 50 mg/5 ml	Oral						200 mg on first day then 100 mg daily	Cholera, page 581, otherwise avoid in children under 12 years
Erythromycin Caps. 250 mg Tab. 250, 500 mg Mixture, 125 mg/5 ml, 250 mg/5 ml, 500 mg/5 ml Vial 1 g (IV)	Oral	4	12.5 mg/kg	12.5 mg/kg	125 mg	250 mg	500 mg	Mycoplasma Pneumonia, page 237. Chlamydia Conjunctivitis, page 652. If i.m. usage unavoidable obtain special i.m. preparation
	(i.m.)	3	2.5 mg/kg	2.5 mg/kg	25 mg	50 mg	100 mg	
	IV slow*	4	8–12 mg/kg	8–12 mg/kg	8–12 mg/kg	300 mg	300–600 mg	
	IV infusion*							

Flucloxacillin Caps. 250, 500 mg Syrup 125 mg/5 ml, 250 mg/5 ml Vial 250, 500 mg	Oral i.m. IV slow* IV infusion*	4 4 4	Neonatal period 30 mg/kg i.m. or IV	62.5 mg 62.5 mg 62.5 mg	62.5 mg 62.5 mg 62.5 mg	125 mg 125–250 mg 125–250 mg	250 mg 250–500 mg 250–500 mg	
Fusidic acid (*Fucidin*)				*See* Sodium fusidate				
Gentamicin Amp. (40 mg/ml) 1, 2 ml Syringe (80 mg/ml) 1.5 ml Paediatric injection (5 mg/ml) 2 ml. (10 mg/ml) 2 ml Vial 1 g	i.m. IV bolus*	3	Neonatal period Chapter 77 and *Table 77.0*, page 662	2 mg/kg *8 hourly*	2 mg/kg *8 hourly*	2 mg/kg *8 hourly*	2–5 mg/kg *8 hourly*	Infection in leukaemia, page 492. Reduce dose in renal impairment
Kanamycin Amp. (250 mg/ml) 4 ml Vial 1 g Caps. 250 mg	i.m. IV infusion*	2–3	Neonatal period Chapter 77 and *Table 77.2*, page 662	15 mg/kg/ *24 hours*	15 mg/kg/ *24 hours*	15 mg/kg/ *24 hours*	15 mg/kg/ *24 hours*	Meningitis, page 339. Reduce dose in renal impairment
Latamoxef (*Moxalactam*) Vials, 500 mg, 1, 2 g	i.m. (deep) IV IV infusion*	2, 3 in severe infections	0–1 week 25 mg/kg *12 hourly* –	1–4 weeks 25 mg/kg *12 hourly*	50 mg/kg *12 hourly*	50 mg/kg *12 hourly*	0.25–3 up to 4 g *8 hourly*	Meningitis, page 338. Reduce dose in renal impairment
Methicillin Vial 1 g	i.m. IV slow*	4–6	50 mg/kg i.m. in single dose per 24 hours	62.5 mg	125 mg	250 mg	1 g	Meningitis, page 338

Table A11.2 continues

Table A11.2 continued

Name and formulations	*Routes*	*Doses per 24 hours*	*0–2/52*	*2/52–1 year*	*1 year*	*7 years*	*14 years to adult*	*Remarks*
Metronidazole Tab. 200, 400 mg Suspension 200 mg/5 ml	Oral	3	7–8 mg/kg *12 hourly*	7–8 mg/kg	7–8 mg/kg	7–8 mg/kg	400 mg	Neonatal Anaerobic Meningitis, page 339. Neonatal Trypanosomiasis (Chagas' Disease), page 657. Amoebiasis, page 585. Necrotizing Enterocolitis, page 368
Amp. (5 mg/ml) 20, 100 ml Also available in sterile mini packs (*Zadstat*)	IV infusion*	3	7–8 mg/kg *12 hourly*	7–8 mg/kg	7–8 mg/kg	7–8 mg/kg	500 mg	
Mezlocillin Vial 500 mg, 1, 2 g Infusion vial 5 g	i.m. IV	3–4	75–100 mg/kg/*24 hours*	75–100 mg/kg/*24 hours*	75–100 mg/kg/*24 hours*	75–100 mg/kg/*24 hours*	0.5–2 g 2 g IV	Infection in Leukaemia, page 492. Increase interval between doses in renal impairment
	IV infusion*			*See Table A11.12*				
Moxalactam				*See* Latamoxef				
Nalidixic acid Tab. 500 mg Mixture 300 mg/5 ml	Oral	4	Avoid	25 mg/kg	250 mg	500 mg	1 g	Urinary tract infection
Neomycin Tab. 500 mg Elixir 100 mg/5 ml	Oral	4	12 mg/kg	12 mg/kg	125 mg	250 mg	500 mg	Acute Liver Failure, page 413. Not absorbed from gastrointestinal tract

Netilmycin Amp. (10 mg/ml) 1.5 ml, (50 mg/ml) 1 ml, (100 mg/ml) 1.5 ml	i.m. IV IV infusion*	2–3	0–1 week 3 mg/kg *12 hourly*	1 week–1 year 2.5–3 mg/kg *8 hourly*	2–2.5 mg/kg *8 hourly*	2–2.5 mg/kg *8 hourly*	4–6 mg/kg/*24 hours* 7.5 mg/kg/*24 hours* in severe infections	Neonatal Meningitis, page 337. Reduce dose in renal impairment
Penicillin G				*See* Benzylpenicillin				
Pencilillin, prolonged action (*Triplopen*) 1 vial contain benzylpenicillin 300 mg, procaine penicillin 250 mg, benethamine penicillin 475 mg	i.m. (deep)	Every 2–3 days	¼ vial every 2–3 days	¼ vial every 2–3 days	¼ vial every 2–3 days	½ vial every 2–3 days	1 vial every 2–3 days	
Phenoxymethyl penicillin (Penicillin V) Tab. 125, 250, 300 mg Caps. 250 mg Elixir 62.5 mg, 125 mg, 250 mg/5 ml	Oral	4	62.5 mg	62.5 mg	125 mg	250 mg	500 mg	
Piperacillin Vial 1, 2 g Infusion unit, 4 g with 50 ml water for injection	i.m. IV slow* IV infusion*	2–4	100–150 mg/kg/*24 hours* (200–300 mg/kg/*24 hours* in severe infections)	100–150 mg/kg/*24 hours* (200–300 mg/kg/*24 hours* in severe infections)	100–150 mg/kg/*24 hours* (200–300 mg/kg/*24 hours* in severe infections)	100–150 mg/kg/*24 hours* (200–300 mg/kg/*24 hours* in severe infections)	100–150 mg/kg/*24 hours* (200–300 mg/kg/*24 hours* in severe infections)	Infections in Leukaemia, page 492. Increase interval between doses in renal impairment

Table A11.2 continues

Table A11.2 continued

Name and formulations	*Routes*	*Doses per 24 hours*	*0–2/52*	*2/52–1 year*	*1 year*	*7 years*	*14 years to adult*	*Remarks*
Rifampicin Caps. 150, 300 mg Mixture 100 mg/5 ml (Vial 300 mg)	Oral	2	–	20 mg/kg/24 hours for 4 days	20 mg/kg/24 hours for 4 days	20 mg/kg/24 hours for 4 days	20 mg/kg/24 hours for 4 days	Caution with liver impairment. Prophylaxis against Meningococcal and *H. influenzae* Meningitis, page 343.
	IV infusion*							Antituberculous treatment, page 344
Sodium fusidate Tab. 250 mg Suspension 250 mg/5 ml (= sodium fusidate 175 mg) Vial (= 500 mg sodium fusidate)	Oral	4	–	12.5 mg/kg	12.5 mg/kg	250 mg	500 mg	
	IV infusion*	3	6–7 mg/kg	6–7 mg/kg	6–7 mg/kg	6–7 mg/kg	500 mg	
Tetracycline Caps. 250 mg Tab. 250 mg Syrup 125 mg/5 ml Vial 100 mg (i.m.) Vial 250 mg (IV)	Oral	4	Avoid	Avoid	Cholera only 50 mg/kg/24 *hours*	Cholera only 50 mg/kg/24 *hours*	Cholera 250–500 mg	Avoid under the age of 12 years unless for Cholera, page 581
	i.m.	2–3	Avoid	Avoid		Cholera only 50 mg/kg/24 *hours*	100 mg	
	IV infusion*	2	Avoid	Avoid		Cholera only 50 mg/kg/24 *hours*	500 mg	

Tobramycin Vial (10 mg/ml) 2 ml, (40 mg/ml) 1, 2 ml	i.m. IV*	3	Neonatal period Chapter 77 and *Table 77.2*, page 662	Over 1 month 2–2.5 mg/kg	2–2.5 mg/kg	3–5 mg/kg	3–5 mg/kg	Reduce dose in renal impairment
	IV infusion*			*See Table A11.2*				
Trimethoprim Tab. 100, 200, 300 mg Mixture 50 mg/5 ml Amp. (10 mg/ml) 5 ml	Oral	2	–	4 mg/kg	50 mg	100 mg	200 mg	Contraindicated in severe renal failure
	IV slow* IV infusion*	2	–	6–9 mg/kg/*24 hours 8 or 12 hourly*	6–9 mg/kg/*24 hours 8 or 12 hourly*	6–9 mg/kg/*24 hours 8 or 12 hourly*	150–250 mg	
Vancomycin Powder (oral) 10 g bottle Vial 500 mg	(Oral) IV infusion*	4 2 4	Neonatal period Chapter 77 and *Table 77.0*, page 662	Neonatal period Chapter 77 and *Table 77.0*, page 662	Over 1 month 40 mg/kg/*24 hours*	40 mg/kg/*24 hours*	125 mg 1 g *12 hourly* 500 mg *6 hourly*	Drug of choice in antibiotic-associated pseudomembranous colitis

* *See Table A11.12* for details of IV injections and infusions.

Table A11.3 Antituberculous agents

Name	*Routes*	*Doses per 24 hours*	*0–2/ weeks*	*2 weeks – 1 year*	*1 year*	*7 years*	*Over 14 years*	*Remarks*
Ethambutol Tab. 100, 200, 400 mg	Oral	Once	–	15 mg/kg	15 mg/kg	15 mg/kg	15 mg/kg	Tuberculous Meningitis, page 344; *see also* Amoebic Meningencephalitis, page 344. Add pyridoxine 25 mg daily when using isoniazid
Isoniazid (INA, INAH) Tab. 50, 100 mg Elixir 50 mg/5 ml Amp. (25 mg/ml) 2 ml	Oral i.m.	Once	–	10 mg/kg	10 mg/kg	10 mg/kg	300 mg or 1 g twice weekly	
Rifampicin Caps. 150, 300 mg Mixture 100 mg/5 ml Vial 300 mg	Oral IV infusion*	Once 3	– –	20 mg/kg ⅓ above doses *8 hourly*	20 mg/kg ⅓ above doses *8 hourly*	20 mg/kg ⅓ above doses *8 hourly*	450–600 mg ⅓ above doses *8 hourly*	Reduce dose of rifampicin to 8 mg/kg/*24 hours* in hepatic impairment
Streptomycin Vial 1 g	i.m.	Once	Avoid	20 mg/kg	20 mg/kg	20 mg/kg	1 g	
Thiacetazone Tab. 50 mg (with 133 mg isoniazid, combined tablet)	Oral	Once	25 mg	25 mg	50 mg	100 mg	150 mg	Use with isoniazid when low cost is important (Simmonds, Vaughan and Gunn, 1983; King, King and Martodipoero, 1983); add pyridoxine 25 mg daily when using isoniazid

* *See Table A11.12* for details of IV infusion.

King M., King F., Martodipoero S. (1983). *Primary Child Care, Book One*. Oxford: Oxford Medical Publications.
Simmonds S., Vaughan P., Gunn S. W. (1983). *Refugee Community Health Care*, p. 218. Oxford: Oxford University Press.

Table A11.4 Antiviral agents

Name	*Routes*	*Doses per 24 hours*	*0–2 weeks*	*2 weeks – 1 year*	*1 year*	*7 years*	*Over 14 years*	*Remarks*
Acyclovir Tab. 200 mg Vial 250 mg	Oral	5	–	120 mg/m^2/ dose	120 mg/m^2/ dose	120 mg/m^2/ dose	200 mg	Varicella or Herpes Zoster in Leukaemia, page 492.
	IV infusion*	3	Neonatal period 10 mg/kg/ *24 hours*	5 mg/kg/ 24 hours 50 mg/m^2/ dose	5 mg/kg/ 24 hours 50 mg/m^2/ dose	5 mg/kg/ 24 hours 50 mg/m^2/ dose	5 mg/kg/ 24 hours 50 mg/m^2/ dose	Herpes Virus Encephalitis, page 347. Disseminated Neonatal Herpes Infection, page 653
Idoxuridine Eye drops 0.1% Ointment 0.5%	Locally	Drops every hour by day; every 2 hours at night; Ointment every 4 hours						Herpetic Corneal ulceration, page 150
Vidarabine Vial (200 mg/ml) 5 ml	IV infusion*	Over 24 hours	Neonatal period 30 mg/kg/ *24 hours*	10 mg/kg/ *24 hours*	10 mg/kg/ *24 hours*	10 mg/kg/ *24 hours*	10 mg/kg/ *24 hours*	Disseminated Neonatal Herpes Infection, page 653

* For details of IV infusion *see Table A11.12*

Table A11.5 Antifungal agents

Name	*Routes*	*Doses per 24 hours*	*0–2 weeks*	*2 weeks – 1 year*	*1 year*	*7 years*	*Over 14 years*	*Remarks*
Amphotericin Tab. 100 mg Lozenges 10 mg Suspension 100 mg/ml Vial 50 mg	Oral	4	–	5 mg/kg	50 mg	100 mg	200 mg	Oral moniliasis
	IV infusion*	4	–	–	300 μg/kg/ *24 hours*	300 μg/kg/ *24 hours*	250 μg/kg/ *24 hours*. Max. dose 1.0–1.5 mg/ kg/*24 hours*	Cryptococcal Meningitis, page 344
Flucytosine Tab. 500 mg IV infusion bottle (10 mg/ml) 250 ml	Oral IV infusion*	4	–	50 mg/kg *12 hourly*	150 mg/kg/ *24 hours*	150 mg/kg/ *24 hours*	150 mg/kg/ *24 hours*	Cryptococcal Meningitis, page 344 Reduce dose in renal impairment
Griseofulvin Tab. 125, 500 mg Suspension 125 mg/5 ml	Oral	2	–	5 mg/kg	5 mg/kg	5 mg/kg	250–500 mg or 500 mg– 1 g once	Dermatophyte infections of skin, nails or scalp
Ketoconazole Tab. 200 mg Suspension 100 mg/5 ml	Oral	Once	–	3 mg/kg	3 mg/kg	3 mg/kg	200 mg Max. dose 400 mg	Dermatophyte infections, systemic fungal infections, candidiasis
Miconazole Tab. 250 mg Oral gel 25 mg/ml Amp. (10 mg/ml) 20 ml	Oral	4	62.5 mg *12 hourly*	62.5 mg *12 hourly*	125 mg *12 hourly*	125 mg *6 hourly*	250 mg *6 hourly*	As for ketoconazole, *see also* Amoebic Meningencephalitis, combined treatment, and page 344
	IV infusion*	3	–	12–15 mg/ kg	12–15 mg/ kg	12–15 mg/ kg	600 mg	
Nystatin Tab. 500 000 units Suspension 100 000 units/ ml	Oral		Oral moniliasis, 100 000 units on the tongue after each feed					Oral, oesophageal or intestinal candidiasis

* *See Table A11.12* for details of IV injections and infusions.

Table A11.6 Antiprotozoal agents

Name	*Routes*	*Doses per 24 hours*	*0–2 weeks*	*2 weeks – 1 year*	*1 year*	*7 years*	*Over 14 years*	*Remarks*
Amodiaquine Tab. 200 mg				Malaria (page 571) for dosage				
Amphotericin Tab. 100 mg Lozenge 10 mg Suspension 100 mg/ml Vial 50 mg	Oral IV infusion*	4 4	– –	5 mg/kg –	50 mg 300 μg/kg/ *24 hours*	100 mg 300 μg/kg/ *24 hours*	200 mg 250 μg/ *24 hours*; Max. dose 1.0–1.5 mg/kg/*24 hours*	Amoebic Meningoencephalitis, as part of combined treatment, page 344
Chloroquine Tab. 200, 250 mg Syrup 68 mg/5 ml, 80 mg/5 ml Amp. (40 mg/ml) 5 ml	i.m. IV			Malaria (page 571) for dosage				
Co-trimoxazole Tab. 480, 960 mg Paediatric tab. 120 mg Mixture 480 mg/5 ml Paediatric mixture 240 mg/5 ml Amp. (320 mg/ml) 3 ml (i.m.) Amp. (96 mg/ml) 5 ml, IV infusion for dilution	Oral (i.m.) IV infusion*	2 2	Avoid Avoid if possible	6 weeks–5 months 120 mg –	6 months–5 years 240 mg 240 mg	6–12 years 480 mg 480 mg	960 mg 960 mg	*Dosage as sulphamethoxozole plus trimethoprim.* Pneumocystis infection in Leukaemia, page 492. Avoid i.m. under the age of 6 years if possible

Table A11.6 continues

Table A11.6 continued

Name	*Routes*	*Doses per 24 hours*	*0–2 weeks*	*2 weeks – 1 year*	*1 year*	*7 years*	*Over 14 years*	*Remarks*
Erythromycin Caps. 250 mg Tab. 250, 500 mg Mixture 125 mg/5 ml, 250 mg/5 ml, 500 mg/5 ml Vial 1 g (I.V.)	Oral (i.m.) IV infusion*			*Table A11.2* for dosage				Mycoplasma pneumonia, page 237
Metronidazole Tab. 200, 400 mg Suspension 300 mg/5 ml Amp. (5 mg/ml) 20, 100 ml	Oral	3	16 mg/kg	16 mg/kg	16 mg/kg	16 mg/kg	800 mg	Amoebiasis 5 day course, page 585; Giardiasis 3 day course
	Oral IV infusion*	3	Neonatal period 6 mg/kg *for 1 month*					Neonatal Trypanosomiasis (Chagas' disease) with nifurtimox, page 651
Miconazole Tab. 250 mg Oral gel 25 mg/ml Syrup (10 mg/ml) 20 ml Amp. (10 mg/ml) 20 ml	Oral	4	6.25 mg *12 hourly*	6.25 mg *12 hourly*	125 mg *12 hourly*	125 mg	217 mg	Amoebic Meningoencephalitis, combined treatment, page 344
	IV infusion*	3	–	12–15 mg/kg	12–15 mg/kg	12–15 mg/kg	600 mg	
Nifurtimox (*Lampit*, Bayer)	Oral	4	Neonatal period 25 mg/kg/*24 hours* for 15 days then 15 mg/kg/*24 hours* for 75–120 days (initially 5–7 mg/kg/*24 hours*)					Neonatal Trypanosomiasis (Chagas' disease) with metronidazole, page 651

Pyrimethamine Tab. 25 mg	Oral	Once	Neonatal period 2 mg/kg for 1 day then 1 mg/kg for 30 days	6.25 mg	6.25 mg	12.5 mg	25 mg	Neonatal Toxoplasmosis with sulphadiazine, page 651. Add folinic acid
Quinine bisulphate (as salt) Tab. 125. 200. 300 mg Quinine hydrochloride Tab. 300 mg Quinine dihydrochloride Tab. 300 mg Amp. 300, 500 mg Quinine sulphate Tab. 125, 200, 300 mg	Oral i.m. IV IV infusion*			Malaria (page 572) for dosage				
Rifampicin Caps. 150, 300 mg Mixture 100 mg/5 ml Vial 300 mg	Oral	Once	–	Up to 15–20 mg/kg	Up to 15–20 mg/kg	Up to 15–20 mg/kg	450–600 mg	Amoebic Meningoencephalitis as part of combined treatment, page 341. Reduce dose in hepatic impairment to ≯8 mg/kg/*24 hours*
	IV infusion*	3	–	⅓ above doses given *8 hourly*	⅓ above doses given *8 hourly*	⅓ above doses given *8 hourly*	⅓ above doses given *8 hourly*	
Sulphadiazine Tabs. 0.5 g Injection (250 mg/ml) 4 ml	Oral (IV infusion*)	4	Neonatal period 37.5 mg/kg for 30 days					Neonatal Toxoplasmosis with pyrimethamine, page 651. Add folinic acid
Tinidazole Tab. 500 mg IV infusion (2 mg/ml) 400, 800 ml bottle	Oral	Once	–	60 mg/kg	60 mg/kg	60 mg/kg	2 g initially then 1 g	Amoebiasis 3 day course, page 585
	IV infusion*	Once					800 mg	

* *See Table A11.12* for details of IV infusion.

Table A11.7 Anthelminthic agents

Name	*Routes*	*Doses per 24 hours*	*0–2 weeks*	*2 weeks – 1 year*	*1 year*	*7 years*	*Over 14 years*	*Remarks*
Bephenium Sachet 2.5 g (as hydroxynaphthoate)	Oral	Once	–	2.5 g	2.5 g	5 g	5 g	Hookworm (Ankylostoma and Necator). Roundworm (Ascaris)
				Give on empty stomach, no food for 1 hour after dose				
Mebendazole Tab. 100 mg Suspension 100 mg/5 ml	Oral	2	–	–	–	2 years to adult 100 mg: 3 day course	2 years to adult 100 mg: 3 day course	Hookworm, roundworm, theadworm (Enterobius), whipworm (Trichuris)
Niclosamide Tabs 500 mg (can be chewed)	Oral	Once	–	–	500 mg	1 g	2 g (Two doses of 1 g separated by 1 hour; followed by purgative after 2 hours)	Tapeworm (Taenia). Dwarf tapeworm (*Hymenolepis nana*), stated dose on first day, half stated dose for the next six days
Piperazine Tab. 500 mg Elixir 750 mg/5 ml Doses as equivalent of piperazine hydrate	Oral	Once	–	50 mg/kg	750 mg	1.5 g	2 g	Threadworm: stated dose for 7 days. Roundworm: twice stated dose once in the morning (*see also* Chapter 42, page 384)
Thiabendazole Tab. 500 mg (can be chewed)	Oral	2–3	–	25 mg/kg	25 mg/kg	25 mg/kg	1.5 g	Hookworm and roundworm: treat for 2–3 days. Threadworm treat for 1 day repeat in 7 days. Whipworm and Strongyloides treat for 2–3 days

Table A11.8 Glucocortoids and corticotrophins

Name	*Routes*	*Doses per 24 hours*	*0–2 weeks*	*2 weeks – 1 year*	*1 year*	*7 years*	*Over 14 years*	*Remarks*
ACTH (adrenocorticotrophin)				*See* corticotrophin and tetracosactrin				
Beclomethasone								
Inhalers 50 µg/metered inhalation; 250 µg/ metered inhalation	Metered inhalation	2–4	–	–	–	50 µg	100 µg	Asthma use 50 µg/ dose inhaler
Rotacaps, 100, 200 µg	Inhaler (*Rotacaps*)	2–4	–	–	–	100 µg	200 µg	Use *Rotacaps*, 100 or 200 µg
Suspension for nebulization (50 µg/ml) 10 ml	Nebulized suspension	2–4	–	–	–	100 µg; max. dose 1 g/*24 hours*	100 µg; max. dose 1 g/*24 hours*	Use suspension 50 µg/ ml
Corticotrophin gel Vial (20 units/ml) 5 ml; (40 units/ml) 1, 2, 5 ml; (80 units/ml) 5 ml	S.C. i.m.	Once	–	1 unit/kg	10 units	20 units	40 units	Long-acting preparation; use only for test of adrenal function; page 472
Cortisone acetate Tab. 5, 25 mg Vial (aqueous suspension) (25 mg/ml) 10 ml	Oral (i.m.)			Dose depends upon indications				Adrenal insufficiency. *Absorption from i.m. injection is slower than by oral route*. For rapid effect use hydrocortisone IV

Table A11.8 continues

Table A11.8 continued

Name	*Routes*	*Doses per 24 hours*	*0–2 weeks*	*2 weeks – 1 year*	*1 year*	*7 years*	*Over 14 years*	*Remarks*
Dexamethasone Tab. 0.5 mg (500 μg), 2 mg Amp. (3.33 mg dexamethasone ≡ 4 mg dexamethasone phosphate/ml) 1, 2 ml; dexamethasone phosphate (20 mg/ml) 5 ml	Oral	2	Dose depends upon indications					Adrenal hyperplasia, page 471. Inflammatory and allergic conditions
	i.m. IV slow IV infusion*	4–6	0.1 mg/kg IV immediately, then 0.05 mg/kg *6 hourly*	0.1 mg/kg IV immediately, then 0.05 mg/kg *6 hourly*	0.1 mg/kg IV immediately, then 0.05 mg/kg *6 hourly*	0.1 mg/kg IV immediately, then 0.05 mg/kg *6 hourly*	0.1 mg/kg IV immediately, then 0.05 mg/kg *6 hourly*	Cerebral oedema, page 296.
Hydrocortisone Tab. 10, 20 mg Vials (hydrocortisone sodium succinate) 100, 500 mg Amp. (hydrocortisone phosphate 100 mg/ml) 1, 5 ml	Oral		20–30 mg/*24 hours* in 2–3 divided doses	20–30 mg/*24 hours* in 2–3 divided doses	20–30 mg/*24 hours* in 2–3 divided doses	20–30 mg/*24 hours* in 2–3 divided doses	20–30 mg/*24 hours* in 2–3 divided doses	Adrenal suppression in adrenal hyperplasia, page 472.
	i.m. IV slow IV infusion*		50–100 mg repeated *6 hourly* if required	50–100 mg repeated *6 hourly* if required	50–100 mg repeated *6 hourly* if required	50–100 mg repeated *6 hourly* if required	50–100 mg repeated *6 hourly* if required	Acute adrenal insufficiency, page 472.
Methylprednisolone Tab. 2, 4, 16 mg Vials 40, 125, 500 mg 2 g (with solvent)	Oral	4					4 mg	Anti-inflammatory effect
	i.m. IV slow IV infusion*		15–30 mg/kg	15–30 mg/kg	15–30 mg/kg	15–30 mg/kg	15–30 mg/kg	Adjust intervals according to response; sometimes used in severe shock

Prednisolone Tab. 1, 5, 25 mg Vial (prednisolone sodium phosphate, 16 mg/ml) 2 ml Vial (Prednisolone acetate 25 mg/ml) 5 ml	Oral	3	Up to 10 mg each dose	Up to 10 mg each dose	Up to 10 mg each dose	Up to 10 mg each dose	Up to 10 mg each dose	Adrenal hyperplasia, page 472
	i.m. IV IV infusion*		4–60 mg/ *24 hours* each dose, as divided doses	4–60 mg/ *24 hours* each dose, as divided doses	4–60 mg/ *24 hours* each dose, as divided doses	4–60 mg/ *24 hours* each dose, as divided doses	4–60 mg/ *24 hours* each dose, as divided doses	Suppression of inflammatory and allergic conditions
	i.m. (phosphate only)	1–2 times per week	25–100 mg each dose	25–100 mg each dose	25–100 mg each dose	25–100 mg each dose	25–100 mg each dose	Suppression of inflammatory and allergic conditions
Prednisone		Avoid, since activity depends upon conversion to prednisolone; conversion impaired in liver damage						
Tetracosactrin (*Synacthen*) Amp. (250 µg/ml) 1 ml Depot: Amp. (1 mg/ml) 1, 2 ml	i.m.	6–8	250 µg each dose	250 µg each dose	250 µg each dose	250 µg each dose	250 µg each dose	250 µg equals approx. 25 units.
	IV infusion*	4	250 µg in 500 ml over 6 hours	250 µg in 500 ml over 6 hours	250 µg in 500 ml over 6 hours	250 µg in 500 ml over 6 hours	250 µg in 500 ml over 6 hours	Therapeutic use: adjust dose according to response. For diagnostic test use 250 µg once only
	i.m. (depot)	Twice weekly or once daily for 3 days	250 µg (0.25 mg)	250 µg (0.25 mg)	250 µg (0.25 mg)	0.25–0.5 mg	0.5–1.0 mg	Depot; long acting preparation; use twice weekly except in acute conditions when it is given once daily for the first 3 days
Triamcinolone Tabs. 2, 4, 16 mg Vials 40, 125, 500 mg. 1 g (with solvent)	Oral	2	–				12 mg each dose	Avoid in chronic conditions, danger of proximal myopathy
	i.m. (deep)	Repeat according to response	–	–	–	–	40 mg each dose. Max. single dose 100 mg	

* For details of IV injections and infusions *see Table A11.12*.

Table A11.9 Mineralocorticoids and anabolic steroids

Name	*Routes*	*Doses per 24 hours*	*0–2 weeks*	*2 weeks – 1 year*	*1 year*	*7 years*	*Over 14 years*	*Remarks*
Deoxycortone pivalate Amp. (25 mg/ml) 1 ml (aqueous suspension)	i.m.	Once every 2–4 weeks	50–100 mg each dose	50–100 mg each dose	50–100 mg each dose	50–100 mg each dose	50–100 mg each dose	Mineralocorticoid replacement in adrenal insufficiency, page 473
Fludrocortisone Tab. 0.1 mg (100 μg)	Oral	Once	5 μg/kg	5 μg/kg	0.05 mg (50 μg)	0.1 mg	0.2 mg	Mineralocorticoid replacement in adrenal insufficiency and salt-losing adrenal hyperplasia, page 472
				ANABOLIC STEROIDS				
Nandrolone Syringe or amp. (25 mg/ml) 1 ml; (50 mg/ml) 1 ml; (100 mg/ml) 1 ml (oily preparations)	i.m. (deep)	Once every 3 weeks	–	–	–	–	Adolescents 12.5–25 mg	Anorexia Nervosa, page 522

Table A11.10 Characteristics of glucocorticoids

Name	*Anti-inflammatory equivalent dose** (mg)	*Mineralocorticoid activity†‡*	*Time to achieve maximal plasma cortisol level†*			*Biological half-life†*
			Oral	*i.m.*	*I.V.*	
Betamethasone	0.75	Negligible	–	–	–	
Cortisone acetate	25	20 mg	2 hours	20–24 hours	–	30 minutes
Dexamethasone	0.75§	Negligible	–	–	–	200 minutes
Hydrocortisone sodium succinate	20	20 mg	1–2 hours	½–1 hour	Immediate	90 minutes
Methylprednisolone	4	–	–	–	–	–
Prednisolone	5	20 mg				200 minutes
Triamcinolone	4	–	–	–	–	–

* Data from *British National Formulary* (1985). No. 9, p. 236. London: British Medical Association and the Pharmaceutical Society of Great Britain.
† Data from Conte F. A., Grumbach M. M. (1973). In Pascoe D. J., Grossman M. (ed.) Endocrine Emergencies. *In Pediatric Emergencies*, p. 223. Philadelphia: J. B. Lipincott.
‡ Expressed as equivalents to DOCA in mg; 2.5 mg DOCA ≡ 0.1 mg fludrocortisone.
§ For adrenal suppression in adrenal hyperplasia the dose ratio between dexamethasone and cortisone appears to be between 1 in 80 and 1 in 200.

Table A11.11 Vaccines, immune globulins and antisera

Name	*Routes*	*Dose*	*Remarks*
Diphtheria antitoxin	i.m. IV	Chapter 20 (pages 212–213) for dosage and precautions	
Hepatitis A	i.m.	Use normal standard immunoglobulin (*see* below) 0.02–0.02 ml/kg gives protection for 3 months	At-risk groups
Hepatitis B immune globulin	i.m.	Neonatal dosage: 0.5 ml (200 i.u., 200 mg) at birth (with vaccine)	Newborn at risk for hepatitis B, *see* page 654, also for other at risk groups
Hepatitis B vaccine		Neonatal dosage: 0.5 ml (10 μg at birth (with immune globulin) and again (vaccine only) one and 6 months later. Age 6 months–10 years 0.5 ml; adult 1 ml, 3 doses, 1 and 6 months after the first dose	
Measles immune globulin	i.m.	0.25 ml/kg on two consecutive days	Measles contacts in leukaemia (or other conditions with depressed immunity), page 492
Rabies antiserum	i.m. and locally	For heterologous serum 40 i.u.; for human serum 20 i.u. Half dose infiltrated locally, and half i.m.	Chapter 68 (page 599) for details of procedures, types of vaccine, dosage and where products can be obtained
Rabies vaccine	s.c. deep	Chapter 68	Chapter 68
Snake and other bite antivenoms		Chapter 61 (pages 559–566) for details and dosage	
Tetanus antitoxin (Human tetanus immune globulin, HTIG)	i.m.	500 units at all ages including newborn	Chapter 33, page 327 for dosage of horse antitetanus serum (ATS)
Varicella (Zoster immune globulin, ZIG)	i.m.	250–750 mg at all ages	Varicella or herpes zoster contacts in Leukaemia (or other conditions with depressed immunity), page 492

Table A11.12 Intravenous additives (page references are for dosage or method of administration); volumes as for adults unless stated otherwise*

Name	*Method†*	*Intravenous infusion fluids*	*Stability: precautions*	*Remarks*
Acetylcysteine *Parvolex*	C	5% glucose	Acetylcysteine is not compatible with rubber and metals, especially iron, copper and nickel. Use silicon rubber or plastics	*See* page 67 for details of dose and rate
Acyclovir *Zovirax IV*	I	0.9% NaCl, 0.9% NaCl in 5% glucose, Hartmann's solution. See page 845 for details of dosage	Reconstitute immediately before used. Discard turbid solutions	Dilute to concentration of 250 mg in at least 50 ml. Give over 1 hour.
Adrenaline	C			Page 807 for details of dosage
Alprostadil *Prostin VR*	C	5% glucose, 0.9% NaCl	Infusion pump recommended. Prepare fresh solution every 24 hours. Do not refrigerate.	*See* manufacturer's data sheet for details of administration (Prostin VR, Upjohn), page 266
Aminophylline	C	5% glucose, 0.9% NaCl, Hartmann's solution		Page 809 for details of dosage
Amoxycillin *Amoxil*	(C)	Continuous infusion not advised		
	I	5% glucose, 0.9% NaCl	Use reconstituted solutions without delay	100 ml of diluted solution over 30–60 minutes
	D	5% glucose, 0.9% NaCl, Ringer's solution. Sodium lactate ⅙ M. Hartmann's solution		Direct injection over 3–4 minutes, page 835
Amphotericin sodium deoxycholate complex *Fungizone*	C	5% glucose: recommended dilution 0.1 mg/ml	Protect infusion from light	Dissolve thoroughly at reconstitution stage. Dilute in large volume of infusion. pH must not be <4.2. Infuse over 6 hours, pages 846 and 847

Table A11.12 continues

Table A11.12 continued

Name	*Method†*	*Intravenous infusion fluids*	*Stability: precautions*	*Remarks*
Ampicillin *Penbritin*	(C)	Continuous infusion not recommended		
	I	5% glucose, 0.9% NaCl	Use reconstituted solution without delay	Use 100 ml of diluted solution over 30–60 minutes, page 835
	D	As for Amoxycillin, above		
Azlocillin sodium *Securopen* (5 g)	I	5% or 10% glucose, 0.9% NaCl, Ringer's solution, 5% fructose. Use a 10% solution of the drug	10% solution stable at room temperature for 6 hours	Intermittent infusion for doses over 2 g; give over 20–30 minutes, page 836
Benzylpenicillin sodium *Crystapen*	(C)	Continuous infusion not recommended		
	I	5% glucose, 0.9% NaCl	Use immediately after preparation	100 ml over 30–60 minutes
Calcium glubionate with calcium galactogluconate *Calcium-Sandoz*; Calcium gluconate 10%	C	5% glucose, 0.9% NaCl		Avoid solutions containing bicarbonates, phosphates and sulphates. Also given by slow injection, page 811
Carbenicillin sodium *Pyopen*	I	5% glucose; water for injection. Add 20 ml of diluent to 5 mg vial. Shake vigorously and dilute to 100–150 ml	Store dry powder at 5°C. Use solution within 30 minutes of preparation	100–150 ml over 30–40 minutes. page 811
Cefotaxime sodium *Claforan*	I	5% glucose, 0.9% NaCl, Hartmann's solution; water for injection	Stable as diluted solution for 24 hours	40–100 ml over 20–60 minutes. Intermittent infusions every 12 hours, or 6–8 hours in severe infections. Page 836
Cefoxitin sodium *Mefoxin*	(C)	Continuous infusion not recommended		
	I.D.	5% or 10% glucose, 0.9% NaCl, sodium lactate ⅙ M	Store in dry state below 30°C. Reconstituted solutions stable for 24 hours at room temperature	By direct injection, give over 3–5 minutes. Intermittent infusions every 8 hours. Page 837

Cefuroxime sodium *Zinacef*	I.D.	5% glucose, 0.9% NaCl, Hartmann's solution. Dissolve 1.5 g in 50 ml diluent	Reconstituted solution stable for 24 hours at room temperature	Give in 50–100 ml over 30 minutes. Page 837
Cephazolin sodium *Kefzol*	(C)	Continuous infusion not recommended		
	I.D.	5% or 10% glucose, 0.9% NaCl, Hartmann's solution, water for injection. Dilute 500 mg or 1 g in 50–100 ml		Direct injection over 3–5 minutes. Intermittent doses every 8–12 hour. Page 837
Chloramphenicol sodium succinate *Kemicetine*	I.D.	5% glucose, 0.9% NaCl	Reject cloudy solutions	Infuse over 30–60 minutes; by direct injection over 3–4 minutes. Page 837
Chloroquine sulphate *Nivaquine*			*See* under Malaria, page 571	
Cimetidine *Tagamet*	C.I.	5% glucose, 0.9% NaCl		For intermittent infusion, give in 250 ml over 2 hours, page 813
Clindamycin phosphate *Dalacin*	C.I.	5% glucose, 0.9% NaCl	Dilute to 300 mg in 50 ml or more of fluid *Dose* (mg) / *Diluent* (ml) / *Time* (min) 300 mg / 50 ml / 10 min 600 mg / 100 ml / 30 min 900 mg / 150 ml / 40 min 1200 mg / 200 ml / 45 min Not more than 1200 mg over 60 min	Give by continuous infusion or over 10–60 minutes. Do not use bolus injections. Page 837
Clonazepam *Rivotril*	I	5% or 10% glucose, 0.9% NaCl		250 ml for intermittent infusion. Page 813

Table A11.12 continues

Table A11.12 continued

Name	*Method†*	*Intravenous infusion fluids*	*Stability: precautions*	*Remarks*
Cloxacillin sodium *Orbenin*	(C)	Continuous infusion not recommended		
	I	5% glucose, 0.9% NaCl	Use within 30 minutes of preparation	100 ml over 30–60 minutes, page 838
	D	As for Amoxycillin, above		
Co-trimoxazole *Bactrim for infusion*	C	5% or 10% glucose, 0.9% NaCl, Ringer's or Hartmann's solutions, Fructose 5%. Dextrans 40 or 70	Dilute immediately before use. Solution faintly yellow. Shake well after dilution; reject turbid solutions	Ampoule has pH of about 10.0 infuse over 90 minutes, page 838
Septrin for infusion	C	As above, but exclude Hartmann's solution		Page 491
Cyclophosphamide *Endoxana*	I.D.	Water for injection		For intermittent infusion, use 50–100 ml given over 5–15 minutes. Maximum time for completion of injection is 30 minutes. Direct injection over 1–2 minutes
Cytarabine *Alexan, Cytosar*	C.I.D.	5% glucose, 0.9% NaCl	Check container for haze or precipitate during administration	*See* data sheets from Upjohn (Cytostat) and Pfizer (Alexan) for methods of administration, page 491
Desferrioxamine mesylate *Desferal*	C.I.	5% glucose, 0.9% NaCl	Infusion pump recommended for continuous infusion	Page 491
Dexamethasone sodium phosphate *Decadron*	C.I.D.	5% glucose, 0.9% NaCl		Maximal effects with injections every 3–4 hours or continuous infusion. Dosage adjusted according to effect, page 852
Oradexon	C.I.D.	5% or 10% glucose, 0.9% NaCl, Ringer's or Hartmann's solutions, ⅙M. sodium lactate		

Diazepam *Diazemuls*	C	5% or 10% glucose	Diazepam is absorbed to some extent by plastic of giving set	
	D	5% or 10% glucose, 0.9% NaCl		Dilute to maximum concentration of 200 mg in 500 ml. Administration should be completed within 6 hours
Stesolid	C	5% glucose, 0.9% NaCl		Dilute to concentration of $\not>$10 mg in 200 ml
Valium	C	5% glucose, 0.9% NaCl		Dilute to concentration of $\not>$40 mg in 500 ml. Complete administration within 6 hours. *See also* page 814
Digoxin *Lanoxin*	C	5% glucose, 0.9% NaCl		To be given slowly, page 815
Dipotassium hydrogen phosphate Disodium hydrogen phosphate	I	*See Tables A5.3* and *A5.4* for details, also page 105		Infuse over 4–6 hours
Dobutamine hydrochloride *Dobutrex*	I	5% glucose, 0.9% NaCl, sodium lactate ⅙ M	Diluted solutions should be used within 24 hours	250–500 ml for infusion, pages 17, 106 and 107
Dopamine hydrochloride *Intropin*	C	5% glucose, 0.9% NaCl, Hartmann's solution, ⅙ M sodium lactate	Discard discoloured solutions. Infusion pump recommended	Dilute to 1.6 mg/ml. Incompatible with bicarbonate or other alkaline solutions, pages 17, 106 and 107
Doxorubicin hydrochloride *Adriamycin*	D	5% glucose, 0.9% NaCl		Page 491
Epoprostenol *Cyclo-Prostin, Flolan*	*C*	*See page 817* for details of administration		

Table A11.12 continues

Table A11.12 continued

Name	*Method†*	*Intravenous infusion fluids*	*Stability: precautions*	*Remarks*
Erythromycin lactobionate *Erythrocin*	C.I.	5% glucose, 0.9% NaCl, Hartmann's solution. 6 ml diluent added to 300 mg vial to make stock solution	Reconstituted solution stable for 2 weeks at 4°C	Dilute to 1 mg/ml for continuous infusion, and 1–5 mg/ml for intermittent infusion. Adjust glucose solution to pH >5.5 using sodium bicarbonate, page 838
Flucloxacillin sodium *Floxapen*	(C)	Continuous infusion not recommended		
	I	5% glucose, 0.9% NaCl	Use within 30 minutes of preparation	100 ml over 30–60 minutes, page 839
	D	As for amoxycillin, above		
Flucytosine *Alcobon*	I		Use special giving set, with filter	Infuse over 20–40 minutes, page 846
Frusemide (sodium salt) *Dryptal, Lasix*	I.C.	0.9% NaCl, Ringer's solution		Infusion pH must be >5.5, *glucose solutions unsuitable*. Infusion can be given over 1 hour, page 817
Fusidic acid		*See* sodium fusidate		
Gentamicin sulphate *Cidomycin* *Garamycin* *Genticin*	I.D.	5% glucose, 0.9% NaCl	Incompatible in mixed solutions with penicillins, cephalosporins, erythromycin, heparin, and sodium bicarbonate	For intermittent infusion give in 50–100 ml over 20–120 minutes. Direct injection over 2–3 minutes is preferred I.V. route, page 839
Glyceryl trinitrate *Tridil*	C	5% glucose, 0.9% NaCl	Syringe pump recommended. Solution is stable for 24 hours at room temperature in glass or other recommended containers (*see* next column)	For Tridil dilute to a concentration of 400 μg/ml. Incompatible with polyvinyl chloride containers (Viaflex, Steriflex). Use glass or polyethylene containers, page 818

Heparin sodium	C	5% glucose, 0.9% NaCl. Heparin loses potency in contact with solutions of pH <6.0 and should only be added to 5% glucose immediately before use.	Heparin in aqueous solution is incompatible with antibiotics, antihistamines, phenothiazines, narcotic analgesics, hydrocortisone and hyaluronidase	Use infusion pump, page 818
Hydralazine hydrochloride *Apresoline*	C	0.9% NaCl, Ringer's solution. *Do not use glucose solutions*	Reconstituted solutions should be used immediately	Infuse volume, 500 ml. Page 819
Hydrocortisone sodium phosphate *Efcortesol*	C.I.D.	5% glucose, 0.9% NaCl		Direct injections should be given over at least one minute. The effect of an intravenous injection lasts for 8 hours, page 852
Hydrocortisone sodium succinate *Efcortelan Soluble* *Solucortef*	C.I.D.	5% glucose, 0.9% NaCl		Direct injections should be given over at least one minute. The effect of an intravenous injection lasts for 8 hours, page 852
Insulin	C	0.9% NaCl, Hartmann's solution	Most infusion pumps can be used but roller (peristaltic) pumps are not suitable for Actrapid MC, due to the risk of precipitation	Adsorbed to some extent by plastics of infusion set, page 819
Isoprenaline hydrochloride *Saventrine IV*	C	5% glucose, 0.9% NaCl		Must be given in large volume. Minimum volume 500 ml, with pH <5.0, page 820
Kanamycin sulphate *Kannasyn* *Kantrex*	I	5% glucose, 0.9% NaCl. Use concentration of 2.5 mg/ml	IV route only to be used when injection is not practicable	To be given slowly; for adult, 80–90 drops per minute, with proportionate rates for children. Normally IV administration divided into 2 or 3 doses per 24 hours
Labetalol hydrochloride *Trandate*	I	5% glucose, 0.9% NaCl in 5% glucose		Dilute to 1 mg/ml. Give in 200 ml. Adjust rate with in-line burette; rate according to effect

Table A11.12 continues

Table A11.12 continued

Name	*Method*†	*Intravenous infusion fluids*	*Stability: precautions*	*Remarks*
Latamoxef sodium *Moxalactam*	I.D.	5% glucose, 0.9% NaCl, Hartmann's solution, sodium lactate ⅙ M; water for injection		Direct I.V. doses normally given every 12 hours, page 839
Lignocaine hydrochloride *Xylocard* 20% preferably use 0.1 and 0.2% in glucose	C	5% glucose, 0.9% NaCl, Ringer's solution, Dextrans. Use 1 g Xylocard syringe added to 500 ml diluent		Dilute to large volume: use concentration of 0.2% ready prepared solution when available. Different formulations available for bolus injection. For adults use an injection rate of 1–2 ml/min of the 0.2% solution, page 821
Magnesium sulphate 1% (0.4 mmol/ml)		*See Table A11.1*, page 822		
Mannitol	I.D.	Dilute with 5% glucose or any of the commonly used electrolyte solutions. *Do not add to a blood transfusion*	If crystals are present, either (1) heat water bath to 80°C; remove from heat and immerse ampoule for 15–20 min or (2) autoclave for 20 minutes at 15 psi. As soon as cool enough to handle, shake gently. Do not use an ampoule containing crystals	Usage depends upon indications; *see* page 823
Metaraminol tartrate *Aramine*	C.D.	5% glucose, 0.9% NaCl, Ringer's or Hartmann's solutions, Dextran 70. Normally, dilute 15–100 mg in 500 ml diluent		Direct injection only in grave emergencies. For infusion, use a volume of 500 ml, and adjust rate to maintain desired blood pressure, page 9

Methicillin sodium *Celbenin*	(C) Continuous infusion not recommended			
	I	5% glucose, 0.9% NaCl	Use solution within 30 minutes of preparation	100 ml, over 30–60 minutes, page 839
	D	As for Amoxycillin, above		
Methoxamine *Vasoxine*	I	For details of administration, *see* page 823		
Methylprednisolone sodium succinate *Solu-Medrone*	C.I.D.	5% glucose, 0.9% NaCl	Prepared solutions should be used within 48 hours	High dosage should be given over 10–20 minutes, page 852
Metronidazole *Flagyl* *Zadstat*	I	5% glucose, 0.9% NaCl. *Zadstat* available in sterile minipack	Protect from direct sunlight. Discard solutions which are not clear	Adult dose should be given in 100 ml at 5 ml/hour, page 840
Mezlocillin sodium *Baypen*	I	5% or 10% glucose, 0.9% NaCl, Ringer's solution, fructose 5%. Water for injection	Use freshly prepared diluted solutions	50 ml given over 15–20 minutes, page 840
Miconazole *Daktarin*	C.I.	5% glucose, 0.9% NaCl		Minimum period of infusion 30 minutes. For intermittent infusion use 250–500 ml, pages 846 and 848
Naloxone *Narcan*	C	5% glucose, 0.9% NaCl		Dilute to concentration of 4 μg/ml, page 824
Netilmycin sulphate *Netillin*	I.D.	5% or 10% glucose, 0.9% NaCl		For intermittent infusion use 50–200 ml over 30–120 minutes, page 841

Table A11.12 continues

Table A11.12 continued

Name	*Method†*	*Intravenous infusion fluids*	*Stability: precautions*	*Remarks*
Noradrenaline strong solution *Levophed* (2 mg per ml)	C	5% glucose, 0.9% NaCl in 5% glucose	Brown solutions should be discarded	Give in large volume. pH must be <6.0. Dosage adjusted according to response
Paraldehyde Amp 5, 10 ml	I.D.	0.9% NaCl	Inject slowly; use glass or opaque plastic syringe	Dilute with several times volume of 0.9% NaCl, page 826
Phentolamine mesylate *Rogitine*	I	5% glucose, 0.9% NaCl		For diagnosis, give over 10 minutes; for treatment give over 180 minutes, page 110
Phenytoin *Epanutin parenteral* (Ready mixed solution)	D	–		Slow injection; for adults ≯50 mg/minute, page 827
Piperacillin sodium *Pipril*	I.D.	5% glucose, 0.9% NaCl, Hartmann's solution, water for injection, Dextrans	Diluted solutions are stable for 24 hours at room temperature and 48 hours at 4°C	Use 50 ml over 20–40 minutes. Direct injection over 3–5 minutes, using 5 ml water for injection to each 1 g of piperacillin, page 841
Potassium chloride	C	5% glucose, 0.9% NaCl		Give in large volume. Mix thoroughly to avoid 'layering' especially in non-rigid containers. Use ready prepared solutions when possible, pages 129–130
Prednisolone sodium phosphate *Codelsol*	C.I.D.	5% glucose, 0.9% NaCl	If added to an infusion solution, use within 24 hours	page 853
Propranolol hydrochloride *Inderal*	D	5% glucose, 0.9% NaCl, 5% glucose in 0.9% NaCl	Use ECG control during injection	page 828

Protamine	D	None required		Slow injection over 10 minutes, page 829
Quinine dihydrochloride	C	0.9% NaCl	*See also* Malaria (Chapter 62) for further details of dosage and administration	To be given over 4 hours: rate 50 mg/minute. For infusion dilute in up to 200 ml of 0.9% NaCl, with a concentration of quinine 0.5–1.0 mg/ml
	D	Water for injection, 10 times original volume		*Inject over at least 3 minutes*
Rifampicin *Rimactane infusion*	I	5% glucose, Hartmann's solution		600 mg in 500 ml diluent. Give over 2–3 hours, pages 842, 844 and 849
Salbutamol sulphate *Ventolin for IV infusion*	C	5% glucose, 0.9% NaCl		Use volume of 500 ml, containing 10 μg/ml. Different formulations available for bolus injections, page 831
Sodium calciumedetate *Ledclair*	C	5% glucose, 0.9% NaCl		Dilute to concentration of >3%. Suggested volume 250–500 ml given over 1 hour, page 831
Sodium fusidate (diethanolamine salt) *Fucidin*	C	5% glucose, 0.9% NaCl, 20% fructose	Diluted solution should be used within 24 hours	Reconstitute with buffer solution provided and dilute to maximum equivalent to sodium fusidate 1 mg/ml; give over 6 hours, page 842
Sodium nitroprusside *Nipride*	C	*5% glucose only*	Prepared solution should be used within 4 hours. Protect from light	Use volume 500–1000 ml. Reconstitute with diluent provided. Complete administration within 4 hours, page 831
Solivito (multiple vitamin preparation)	C	*See* Appendix 5, *Tables A5.4* and page 782 for details and method of administration		

Table A11.12 continues

Table A11.12 continued

Name	*Method†*	*Intravenous infusion fluids*	*Stability: precautions*	*Remarks*
Sulphadiazine sodium	C	0.9% NaCl, water for injection		Use 500 ml. Ampoule solution has pH of >10.0, page 849
Terlipressin *Glypressin*	I.D.	For details of administration *see* page 832		
Tetracosactrin *Synacthen*	C	5% glucose, 0.9% NaCl		Use 500 ml, given over 6 hours, page 853
Tetracycline hydrochloride *Achromycin intravenous*	C	5% glucose, 0.9% NaCl, Hartmann's solution		Minimum volume 100 ml. Give over ≯8 hours, page 842
Thiopentone sodium *Intraval sodium*	C.D.	0.9% NaCl	Check container for haze and precipitate before giving	Page 832
Tinidazole *Fusigyn*	I	5% glucose, 0.9% NaCl		800 mg to be given over at least 30 minutes; rates pro rata for other doses. Page 849
Tobramycin sulphate *Nebcin*	I.D.	5% glucose, 0.9% NaCl		For intermittent infusion use 100–150 ml, given over 20–60 minutes, page 843
Trimethoprim lactate *Monotrim*	C.D.	As for Syraprim (below), also 0.9% NaCl, Hartmann's solution, Dextrans 40 or 70 in NaCl		1–2 mg/kg/hour constant I.V.
Syraprim	I.D.	5% glucose, ⅙ M sodium lactate, 5% fructose		Consult data sheets (Wellcome)

Vancomycin hydrochloride *Vancocin*	(C)	Continuous infusion not recommended		Page 843
	I	5% glucose, 0.9% NaCl		Use 100–200 ml given over 20–30 minutes, every 6 hours
Vasopressin synthetic *Pitressin*	I	5% glucose		Use concentration of 20 units/ml, given over 15 minutes, page 833
Verapamil hydrochloride *Cordilox*	C	5% glucose, 0.9% NaCl, fructose solutions		Page 834
Vidarabine *Vira-A*	C	5% glucose, 0.9% NaCl in 5% glucose, Hartmann's solution. Dilute 1 ml of microcrystalline solution in 500 ml to produce strength of 0.4 mg/ml	With good aseptic technique a week's supply can be prepared at one time. Store at room temperature, *not* in refrigerator	Limited solubility in infusion fluids. Give in large volume over 12–24 hours, page 845
Vinblastine sulphate *Velbe*	D	0.9% NaCl, water for injection		*See* data sheet (Lilly)
Vincristine sulphate *Oncovin*	D	0.9% NaCl, water for injection		Reconstitute with diluent provided. *See* data sheet (Lilly) and page 491
Vitamins *Solivito*	I	5% or 10% glucose. Water for injection	Use within 24 hours of dilution	500–1000 ml given over 2–3 hours, page 782

* Data from *British National Formulary* (1985). No. 9, pp. 420–434. London: British Medical Association and the Pharmaceutical Society of Great Britain; and from *ABPI* (Association of the British Pharmaceutical Industries) *Data Shet Compendium 1984–85*, London: Datapharm Publications Limited. For further details consult these publications or the manufacturers data sheets. Proprietary names are shown in italics.

† C = Continuous infusion; I = intermittent infusion; D = direct injection into drip tubing. Method not advised in parentheses.

Table A11.13 Intrathecal preparations of antibiotics currently available

Antibiotic	*Birth to 1 year*	*Other ages*
Ampicillin	5 mg	10 mg
Carbenicillin	10 mg	Up to 2 years: 10 mg 2–12 years: 20 mg Over 12 years: 40 mg
Chloramphenicol	1–2 mg	5–10 mg
Cloxacillin	5 mg	10 mg
Colistin	0.2 mg	Adult 2–5 mg
Gentamicin	1 mg	Adult up to 8 mg
Kanamycin	2 mg	Adult 10 mg
Benzylpenicillin	6.0 mg (10 000 units)	6–12 mg (10 000 – 20 000 units)
Streptomycin	1.0 mg/kg	Up to 50 mg

Appendix 12

Drug interactions

J. A. Black

The interactions of different combinations of drugs are extremely complex. If any doubt, consult the hospital pharmacist as well as the manufacturer's drug literature; or the manufacturer's medical department should be consulted direct.

In Britain information on drug interactions is available in any of the following publications:

British National Formulary, published by the British Medical Association and the Pharmaceutical Society of Great Britain.

Monthly Index of Medical Specialities, (MIMS), Medical Publications Ltd., London.

Drug Interaction Guide, Abbot Laboratories Ltd., Queenborough, Kent, England.

Association of the British Pharmaceutical Industries (ABPI) Data Sheet Compendium 1984–5 (and subsequent years). London, Datapharm Publications.

Clinical and Resuscitative Data by R. P. H. Dunnill and B. E. Crawley, Oxford (1977), Blackwell Scientific Publications.

Intravenous drug interactions

IV drugs can be given in a number of different ways.

Direct injection

The following drugs are particularly dangerous if injected rapidly (i.e. in <3 minutes) IV:

Aminophylline
Calcium gluconate
Chloroquine
Digoxin
Magnesium salts
Potassium salts
Practolol
Quinine
Sodium bicarbonate

Potassium salts should NEVER be injected directly IV.

Drugs added to an IV line

1. Avoid mixing drugs in an infusion: only one drug should be given at one time.
2. No drugs of any sort should be added to bottles containing:

Blood	Parenteral lipid preparations
Plasma	(Vitlipid may be added to
Plasma protein fraction	Intralipid, *see* page 782)
Parenteral amino acid	Mannitol
preparations	Sodium bicarbonate solutions

3. The following drugs should NEVER be mixed with any other drugs in an infusion:

Amphotericin	Magnesium sulphate
Barbiturates	Mannitol
Calcium gluconate	Phenothiazines (e.g. chlorpromazine)
Diazepam	Sodium bicarbonate
Frusemide	Sulphonamides
Heparin	Vitamin B complex
	± vitamin C

Methods of administration into an IV line

There are three alternative methods:

1. Injection into the tubing followed by flushing through with infusion fluid. *Usual duration of injection:* 3–4 minutes.
2. Addition of the drug to the drip chamber, which may contain 30–100 ml fluid. *Usual duration:* 30–40 minutes.
3. Addition to the bottle of infusion fluid: this normally involves a slow infusion over 4–6 hours and can only be used when the added drug is exceptionally stable under these conditions (room temperature, and in the presence of the infusion fluid) and in which a peak plasma level is not required.

For antibiotics, methods (1) or (2) are nearly always used.

When giving more than one drug in an IV infusion always check compatibilities. Always discard any IV solution of a drug which is discoloured, or opaque, when it should be colourless or clear. If in doubt about the best route of administration and compatibility with the infusion fluid:

1. Check the manufacturer's instruction insert. *Or*
2. Check with the hospital pharmacist. *Or*
3. Check with the manufacturer by telephone.

Appendix 13

Drug prescribing in renal failure

The data given below are for general guidance on the use of drugs in renal failure. In some situations blood levels will need to be estimated. For further information, the *British National Formulary,* or the manufacturers themselves, should be consulted.

The following text, figures and tables are reproduced by permission of the authors and publishers of *Safer Prescribing; a Guide to Some Problems in the Use of Drugs* (Linda Beeley (1983) (3rd Edn.), pp. 33–43. Oxford: Blackwell Scientific Publications).

The following topics are covered:

1. Drugs requiring dose reduction in renal failure.
2. Drugs to avoid in renal failure.
3. Other drugs that may be harmful to patients in renal failure.
4. Drugs that are ineffective or less effective in renal failure.

Drugs requiring dose reduction in renal failure

Drugs eliminated entirely or partly by renal excretion accumulate in renal failure and smaller doses must be used.
The extent of dose reduction depends on:

1. Whether the drug is eliminated entirely by excretion or is partly metabolized.
2. The toxicity of the drug, and if this is related to the amount of drug present in the body. A smaller dose will result in toxic amounts in renal failure than if renal function is normal.
3. The safety margin (therapeutic ratio) of the drug.

Increased sensitivity to some drugs occurs in renal failure for reasons other than impaired excretion and this may necessitate dose reduction.

In the following table drugs are classified into three groups according to the severity of renal failure. In each group the drugs are classified by body system and listed alphabetically. Renal function is expressed in terms of glomerular filtration rate and serum creatinine level but is should be remembered that the latter is only a rough guide to renal function as it depends also on age, weight and sex. In particular it may be normal in elderly patients despite the fact that glomerular filtration rate falls with increasing age. The dose of drugs in group 3 should be reduced in all patients over 60 whatever the value of the serum creatinine.

Glomerular filtration rate can be estimated from serum creatinine, weight, age and sex, using a nomogram (*Figure A13.1*).

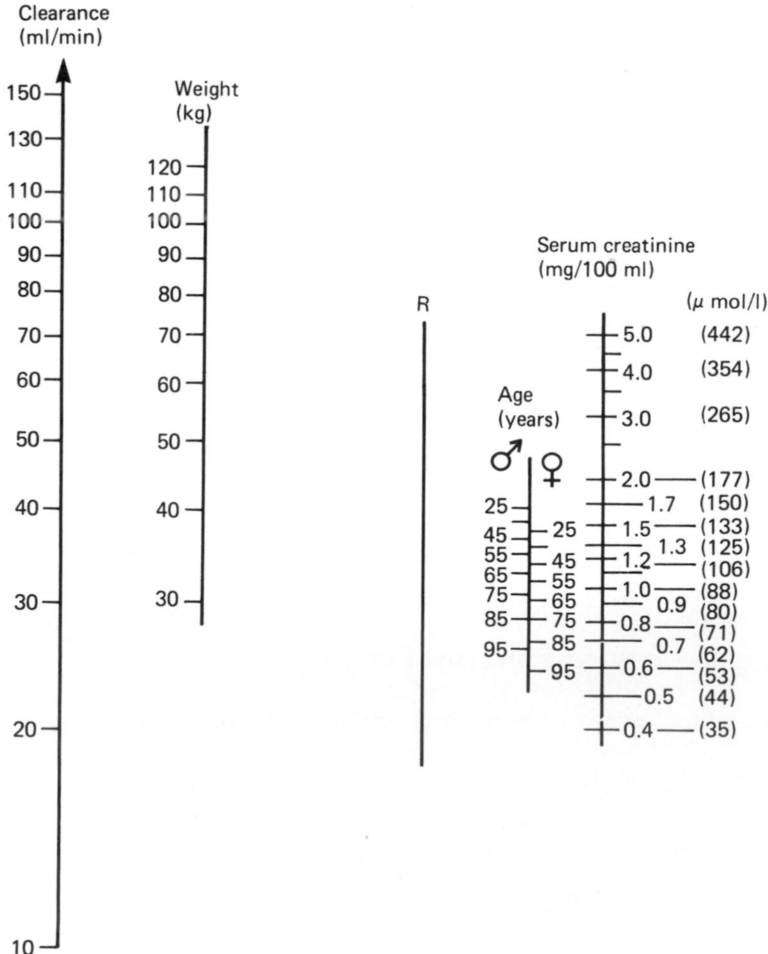

Figure A13.1 Nomogram for rapid evaluation of endogenous creatinine clearance. With a ruler, join weight to age. Keep ruler at crossing point of line marked R. Then move the right-hand side of the ruler to the appropriate serum creatinine value and read the patient's clearance from the left-hand side of the nomogram.

DRUG	UNWANTED EFFECTS

GROUP 1 Dose reduction necessary only in severe renal failure (GFR <10 ml/min, serum creatinine >700 μmol/ℓ).

DRUG	UNWANTED EFFECTS
Gastrointestinal system	
Metoclopramide	Increased risk of extrapyramidal reactions.
Sulphasalazine	Metabolites accumulate and may produce toxicity (blood dyscrasias, rashes).
Cardiovascular system	
Beta-adrenoceptor antagonists: acebutolol, metoprolol, propranolol	Increased hypotensive effect, bradycardia. May reduce renal blood flow and adversely affect renal function.
Diazoxide	Increased hypotensive effect of IV injection.
Hydralazine	Increased hypotensive effect. Possibly increased risk of SLE syndrome.
Methyldopa	Increased hypotensive effect.
Prazosin	Increased hypotensive effect. Postural hypotension.
Nervous system	
Amylobarbitone	Increased sedation due to accumulation of active metabolite.
Lorazepam	May accumulate with regular therapy.
Phenobarbitone	Increased sedation.
Phenothiazines e.g. chlorpromazine, prochlorperazine, trifluoperazine	Increased incidence of extrapyramidal side effects.
Primidone	Increased sedation.
Thiopentone	Increased sensitivity, probably due to reduced protein binding.
Drugs used in infections	
Amoxycillin Ampicillin	Rashes.
Benzylpenicillin	Neurotoxicity with high doses; bleeding diathesis.
Cephalexin	
Cefotaxime	
Cotrimoxazole	Rashes and blood dyscrasias. Increase in serum creatinine may occur.
Erythromycin	Ototoxicity.
Isoniazid	Peripheral neuropathy (more likely in slow acetylators).
Lincomycin	
Metronidazole	Neurotoxicity. Bone marrow depression.

DRUG	UNWANTED EFFECTS
Mezlocillin	Neurotoxicity possible with high doses.
Piperazine	Increased risk of neurotoxicity.
Sulphonamides	Metabolites accumulates and may produce toxicity (blood dyscrasias, rashes). Crystalluria. Ensure high fluid intake.
Trimethoprim	Avoid sulphadiazine.
Immunosuppressants	
Azathioprine	Bone marrow suppression.

GROUP 2 Dose reduction necessary when GFR 25 ml/min or less (serum creatinine >250 μmol/ℓ).

Gastrointestinal system	
Cimetidine	Confusional states. Transient deterioration in renal function may occur.
Cardiovascular system	
Beta-adrenoceptor antagonists: atenolol, pindolol, sotalol	Increased hypotensive effect, bradycardia. May reduce renal blood flow and adversely affect renal function.
nadolol	As above but does not reduce renal blood flow.
Clofibrate	Myopathy. Avoid in severe renal failure.
Sodium nitroprusside	Thiocyanate accumulates. Avoid prolonged use.
Nervous system	
Alcuronium Pancuronium Tubocurarine	Prolonged neuromuscular block.
Drugs used in infections	
Aminoglycosides: amikacin, gentamicin, kanamycin, streptomycin, tobramycin	Nephrotoxicity, ototoxicity, neuro-muscular block.
Azlocillin	
Carbenicillin, Ticarcillin	Neurotoxicity. Bleeding diathesis.
Cefsulodin	
Piperacillin	

DRUG	UNWANTED EFFECTS
Malignant disease and immunosuppressants	
Bleomycin Cyclophosphamide Melphalan Mercaptopurine Procarbazine Thioguanine	Bone marrow suppression.
Drugs used in arthritis	
Allopurinol	Rashes.
Sulindac (*see also* group 4)	

GROUP 3 Dose reduction necessary even with mild degrees of renal failure (GFR <50 ml/min. Serum creatinine >150 μmol/ℓ); and in all patients over 60.

DRUG	UNWANTED EFFECTS
Cardiovascular system	
Captopril	Increased risk of hyperkalaemia.
Disopyramide	Anticholinergic effects – dry mouth, blurred vision, urine retention. Myocardial depression, arrhythmias.
Digoxin, medigoxin	Nausea, confusional states, visual symptoms, arrhythmias.
Procainamide	CNS toxicity. Avoid if possible.
Nervous system	
Baclofen	Sedation. Muscle hypotonia.
Lithium	Nausea and vomiting. CNS toxicity. Avoid in severe renal failure.
Nomifensine	Sleep disturbance, restlessness. Avoid if serum creatinine greater than 250 μmol/ℓ.
Drugs used in infections	
Acyclovir	
Capreomycin	Neurotoxicity, ototoxicity, neuromuscular block.
Cefamandole Cefoxitin Cefuroxime Cephazolin Cephradine Ciclacillin Colistin, polymixin B	Nephrotoxicity, neurotoxicity, neuromuscular block
Flucytosine	Bone marrow suppression. Hepatotoxicity.
Ethambutol	Optic nerve toxicity.
Vancomycin	Ototoxicity.

DRUG	UNWANTED EFFECTS
Endocrine system	
Propylthiouracil	
Cytotoxic and immunosuppressant drugs	
Methotrexate	Bone marrow suppression. Nephrotoxicity. Avoid in severe renal failure.
Drugs used in arthritis	
Azapropazone (*see also* group 4)	
Chloroquine	Accumulation occurs during prolonged therapy. Avoid in severe renal failure.
Diflunisal (*see also* group 4)	

Drugs to avoid altogether in renal failure

DRUG	UNWANTED EFFECTS
Gastrointestinal system	
Magnesium salts, e.g. magnesium trisilicate magnesium sulphate	Magnesium toxicity may occur in severe renal failure.
Cardiovascular system	
Bethanidine, debrisoquine, guanethidine	Reduce renal blood flow. Severe postural hypotension common.
Ethacrynic acid	Deafness may follow IV injection in severe renal failure.
Nervous system	
Amantadine	Confusion, agitation, hallucinations.
Dextropropoxyphene (Distalgesic)	Increased CNS toxicity due to accumulation of metabolites. Avoid in severe renal failure.
Gallamine	Prolonged neuromuscular block.
Pethidine	Increased CNS toxicity due to accumulation of metabolites.
Sulthiame	Produces a metabolic acidosis.
Drugs used in infections	
Amphotericin	Nephrotoxic. Use only if there is no alternative.
Bacampicillin	Potentially toxic products of hydrolysis of the ester may accumulate. Avoid in severe renal failure.
Cephaloridine Cephalothin	Nephrotoxic – especially if renal function already impaired.
Chloramphenicol	Increased risk of bone barrow suppression. Use only if there is no alternative.
Cinoxacin	Nausea, rashes.
Nalidixic acid	Nausea, rashes, photosensitivity.

DRUG	UNWANTED EFFECTS
Neomycin	Ototoxicity, nephrotoxicity, neuromuscular block.
Nitrofurantoin	Neurotoxicity. Nausea.
Pivampicillin	*See* bacampillin.
Talampicillin	*See* bacampicillin.
Tetracyclines (except doxycycline and minocycline)	Anorexia, nausea, vomiting. Increase in blood urea. Further deterioration in renal function.
Endocrine system	
Chlopropamide	Prolonged hypoglycaemia.
Metformin phenformin	Lactic acidosis.
Malignant disease	
Cisplatin	Nephrotoxicity. Avoid in severe renal failure.
Drugs used in arthritis	
Anti-inflammatory analgesics all – indomethacin, naproxen, etc.	May cause fluid retention and deterioration in renal function. Avoid in severe renal failure.
Aspirin	As above; and increased risk of gastro-intestinal bleeding.
Gold salts	Nephrotoxicity
Penicillamine	Nephrotoxicity. Avoid if possible, or reduce dose.
Miscellaneous	
Acetazolamide	Produces a metabolic acidosis.
Phenazopyridine	Methaemoglobinaemia. Haemolytic anaemia. Crystalluria.

Other drugs that may be harmful to patients with renal failure

Preparations containing large amounts of sodium, e.g. Sandocal – 6 mmol/tablet Magnesium trisilicate mixture – 6 mmol/10 ml. Gaviscon – 6 mmol/10 ml. Carbenicillin – 5.4 mmol/g Sodium polystyrene sulphonate (Resonium A) – 67 mmol/15 g	May produce sodium overload and heart failure. Avoid, or allow for in patients on restricted salt intake.

DRUG	UNWANTED EFFECTS
Drugs producing fluid retention, e.g. anti-inflammatory analgesics. carbenoxolone. oestrogens	Use alternative if possible. Avoid in severe renal failure.
Potassium-sparing diuretics Potassium supplements Salt substitutes (contain potassium salts)	Risk of hyperkalaemia. Serum potassium does not usually rise spontaneously until GFR <5 ml/min. but inability to excrete a potassium load occurs earlier.
Corticosteroids, ACTH	Increase blood urea by inhibiting protein synthesis.
Drugs producing nausea, e.g. narcotic analgesics, many oral antibiotics	Nausea and vomiting may cause dehydration with deterioration in renal function.
Antidiabetic drugs	In severe renal failure insulin requirements fall and the compensatory response to hypoglycaemia is impaired. Insulin dependent diabetics usually need a smaller dose, and there is an increased risk of prolonged hypoglycaemia with oral hypoglycaemic drugs. Tolbutamide is the safest sulphonylurea as it is inactivated by metabolism and is short acting, but the dose should be reduced. Metformin and phenformin should be avoided because they can produce lactic acidosis.
Hypnotics, sedatives, tranquilisers	Increased 'cerebral sensitivity' and increased incidence of CNS side effects. May require smaller doses.
Vitamin A – present in many multivitamin preparations	Increases the already raised serum Vitamin A concentration in patients with chronic renal failure. Hypervitaminosis A may contribute to hypercalcaemia, possibly by an osteolytic effect.

Drugs that are ineffective or less effective in renal failure

DRUG	COMMENTS
Diuretics	Thiazides (except metolazone) ineffective when GFR <20 ml/min. (Serum creatinine >300 μmol/ℓ.) Frusemide and bumetanide are effective down to GFR of 3 ml/min. but large doses are often needed.
Antihypertensive drugs	Salt and water retention produce resistance. Dialysis or large doses of frusemide may restore sensitivity.
Uricosuric drugs	Ineffective. Use allopurinol instead.

DRUG	UNWANTED EFFECTS
Drugs used to treat urinary tract infections	Problem of achieving adequate urine concentrations without systemic toxicity.
Nitrofurantoin	Avoid – urine concentration inadequate and high risk of peripheral neuropathy.
Nalidixic acid	Adequate urine concentrations can be achieved only by increasing the dose. Toxicity may occur. Avoid.
Sulphonamides	Sulphadimidine and sulphamethoxazole achieve adequate urine concentrations but metabolites accumulate in severe renal failure and may produce toxicity.
Trimethoprim (cotrimoxazole)	Good urine concentrations even in severe renal failure but reduce dose to avoid toxicity.
Ampicillin Amoxycillin	Good urine concentrations with little toxicity unless GFR <10 ml/min. (Serum creatinine >700 µmol/ℓ.)
Cephalexin	Urine concentrations adequate at GFR down to approx. 3 ml/min. Risk of toxicity probably small (but N.B. some cephalosporins are nephrotoxic).
Hexamine mandelate Hexamine hippurate	Avoid. Ineffective when GFR <25 ml/min.

Further reading

BRITISH NATIONAL FORMULARY (1986) No. 11 (and in subsequent issues). Prescribing in renal impairment, pp. 11–17. London: British Medical Association and the Pharmaceutical Society of Great Britain

SHARPSTONE, P. (1977) Prescribing for patients with renal failure. *British Medical Journal,* **ii,** 36–37

Appendix 14

Prescribing in pregnancy

Data in *Table A14.1* are reproduced by permission of the authors and publishers of the *British National Formulary* No. 11 (1986), pp. 17–21. London, British Medical Association and The Pharmaceutical Society of Great Britain.

Drugs can have harmful effects on the fetus at any time during pregnancy. During the *first trimester* they may produce congenital malformations (teratogenesis), and the period of greatest risk is from the third to the eleventh week of pregnancy. Few drugs have been shown conclusively to be teratogenic in man but no drug is safe beyond all doubt in early pregnancy. During the *second and third trimester* drugs may affect the growth and functional development of the fetus or have toxic effects on fetal tissues; and drugs given shortly before term or during labour may have adverse effects on the neonate after delivery.

Drugs should be prescribed in pregnancy only if the expected benefit to the mother is thought to be greater than the risk to the fetus, and all drugs should be avoided if possible during the first trimester. Drugs that have been extensively used in pregnancy and appear to be usually safe should be prescribed in preference to new or untried drugs; and the smallest effective dose should be used.

The Table below lists drugs which may have harmful effects in pregnancy and indicates the trimester in which these effects occur.

Experience with many drugs in pregnancy is limited. The Table is based on human data and *animal* toxicological studies have been excluded. Information on animal studies has been included for some newer drugs when its omission might be misleading. However, it should be noted that the absence of a drug from the list does not imply safety.

Table A14.1 Drugs to be avoided or used with caution in pregnancy

Drugs	*Trimester of risk*	*Adverse effects*
1. Gastrointestinal system		
Chenodeoxycholic acid	1, 2, 3	Theoretical risk of effects on fetal metabolism
Stimulant laxatives	1, 2, 3	Best avoided during pregnancy as they may increase uterine activity in susceptible patients
Sulphasalazine	3	Theoretical risk of neonatal haemolysis and of kernicterus in jaundiced neonates

Drugs	*Trimester of risk*	*Adverse effects*
2. *Cardiovascular system*		
2.2 Diuretics	3	Reduce plasma volume and placental perfusion and should not be used to treat hypertension in pregnancy
Thiazides	3	May cause neonatal thrombocytopenia
2.3 Antiarrhythmic drugs		
Amiodarone	2,3	Releases iodine with possible risk of neonatal goitre. Use only if no effective alternative
Flecainide, Tocainide		Manufacturer advises toxicity in *animal* studies
2.4 Beta-adrenoceptor blocking drugs	3	Neonatal hypoglycaemia and bradycardia. The risk is greater in women with severe hypertension
2.5 Antihypertensive drugs		
Bethanidine, Debrisoquine, Guanethidine	3	Postural hypotension and reduced uteroplacental perfusion. Should not be used to treat hypertension in pregnancy
Captopril, Enalapril	1,2,3	May adversely affect fetal and neonatal blood pressure control, and manufacturers advise toxicity in *animal* studies
Diazoxide	2, 3	Prolonged use may produce alopecia and impaired glucose tolerance in the neonate. Inhibits uterine activity during labour
Reserpine	3	Neonatal bradycardia, drowsiness, and nasal stuffiness
2.6 Vasodilators		
Nifedipinc, Verapamil	3	Calcium-channel blockers may inhibit labour
Diltiazen		As for above; manufacturers advise toxicity in *animal* studies
2.7 Vasoconstrictors		
Metaraminol, Noradrenaline, etc.	1, 2, 3	Avoid – may reduce placental perfusion
2.8 Anticoagulants		
Heparin	1, 2, 3	Osteoporosis has been reported after prolonged use
Oral anticoagulants	1, 2, 3	Congenital malformations. Fetal and neonatal haemorrhage. Subcutaneous heparin should be substituted in the last few weeks of pregnancy in deep-vein thrombosis
2.10 Fibrinolytic drugs		
Streptokinase, Urokinase	1, 2, 3	Possibility of premature separation of placenta in first 18 weeks. Theoretical possibility of fetal haemorrhage throughout pregnancy. Avoid postpartum use – maternal haemorrhage

Drugs	*Trimester of risk*	*Adverse effects*
2.11 Antifibrinolytic drugs		
Aminocaproic acid	1, 2, 3	Avoid – may increase the risk of thrombosis
2.12 Drugs used in hyperlipidaemia		
Clofibrate, Probucol	1, 2, 3	Avoid – theoretical possibility of interference with embryonic growth and development due to anticholesterol effect
3. Respiratory system		
Aminophylline	3	Neonatal irritability and apnoea have been reported
Astemizole		Manufacturer advises toxicity in *animal* studies
Iodides (in preparations for cough)	2, 3	Neonatal goitre and hypothyroidism
Selective beta-adrenoceptor stimulants (such as salbutamol)	3	Large parenteral doses given for asthma at term could delay the onset of labour
4. Central nervous system		
4.1 Hypnotics and sedatives	3	Depress neonatal respiration
Alcohol	1, 2	Teratogenic and may cause growth retardation
	3	Withdrawal syndrome may occur in babies of alcoholic mothers
Barbiturates	3	Withdrawal effects in neonate
Benzodiazepines	3	Neonatal drowsiness, hypotonia, and withdrawal symptoms. Avoid large doses and regular use. Oxazepam and temazepam may be safer than longer-acting benzodiazepines
4.2 Antipsychotic drugs		
Lithium salts	1, 2, 3	Congenital malformations. Neonatal goitre has been reported. Lithium toxicity (hypotonia and cyanosis) in the neonate if maternal therapy poorly controlled. Maternal dose requirement increased during pregnancy
Phenothiazine derivatives	3	Extrapyramidal effects in neonate occasionally reported
4.3 Antidepressants		
Tricyclic antidepressants	3	Tachycardia, irritability, muscle spasms, and convulsions in the neonate reported occasionally
4.7 Analgesics, Anti-inflammatory analgesics		
Aspirin	3	Impaired platelet function and risk of haemorrhage. Kernicterus in jaundiced neonates. With regular use of high doses, closure of fetal ductus arteriosus *in utero* and possibly persistent pulmonary hypertension of the newborn. Delayed onset and increased duration of labour with increased blood loss. Avoid if possible in last week of pregnancy

Drugs	Trimester of risk	Adverse effects
Indomethacin, Naproxen, etc.	3	With regular use closure of fetal ductus arteriosus *in utero* and possibly persistent pulmonary hypertension of the newborn. Delayed onset and increased duration of labour
Narcotic analgesics Dextropropoxyphene, Diamorphine, Pentazocine, etc.	3	Depress neonatal respiration. Withdrawal effects in neonates of dependent mothers. Gastric stasis and risk of inhalation pneumonia in mother during labour
Antimigraine drugs		
Ergotamine	1, 2, 3	Oxytocic effects on the pregnant uterus
4.8 Antiepileptics		Benefit of treatment outweighs risk to the fetus
Ethosuxamide	1	May possibly be teratogenic
Phenytoin, Phenobarbitone	1, 3	Congenital malformations. Neonatal bleeding tendency – prophylactic vitamin K_1 should be given. Caution in interpreting maternal plasma phenytoin concentrations which may be reduced without a fall in the effective (free) phenytoin concentration
Sodium valproate	1	Increased risk of neural tube defects reported
5. *Infections*		
5.1 Antibacterial drugs		
Aminoglycosides	2, 3	Auditory or vestibular nerve damage. Risk greatest with streptomycin and kanamycin, probably small with gentamicin and tobramycin
Chloramphenicol	3	Neonatal grey syndrome
Dapsone	3	Neonatal haemolysis and methaemoglobulinaemia
Rifampicin	3	Risk of neonatal bleeding may be increased
Sulphonamides (and co-trimoxazole)	3	Neonatal haemolysis and methaemoglobulinaemia. Increased risk of kernicterus in jaundiced neonates
Tetracyclines	2, 3	Dental discoloration. Maternal hepatotoxicity with large parenteral doses
Trimethoprim (and co-trimoxazole)	1	Possible teratogenic risk (folate antagonist)
5.2 Antifungals		
Flucytosine	1	Possible teratogenic risk
5.4 Antimalarials	1, 3	Benefit of prophylaxis and treatment in malaria
Primaquine	3	Neonatal haemolysis and methaemoglobulinaemia
Pyrimethamine	1	Possible teratogenic risk (folate antagonist)
Quinine	1	High doses are teratogenic

Drugs	*Trimester of risk*	*Adverse effects*
5.5 Anthelminthics		
Mebendazole		Manufacturer advises toxicity in *animal* studies
6. Endocrine system		
6.1 Oral hypoglycaemic drugs		
Sulphonylureas	3	Neonatal hypoglycaemia. Insulin is normally substituted in all diabetics. If oral drugs are used therapy should be stopped at least 2 days before delivery
6.2 Antithyroid drugs Carbamizole, Iodine, Propylthiouracil	2, 3	Neonatal goitre and hypothyroidism
Radioactive iodine	1, 2, 3	Permanent hypothyroidism – avoid
6.3 Corticosteroids	2, 3	High doses (>10 mg prednisolone daily) may produce fetal and neonatal adrenal suppression. Corticosteroid cover will be required by the mother during labour
6.4 Sex hormones		
Androgens, Oestrogens, Progestogens (high doses)	1, 2, 3	Virilization of female fetus
Progestogens used to prevent abortion	1	May possibly be teratogenic
Stilboestrol	1	High doses associated with vaginal carcinoma in female offspring
6.7 Other endocrine drugs		
Danazol	1, 2, 3	Has weak androgenic effects and virilization of female fetus has been reported
Trilostane	1, 2, 3	Interferes with placental sex hormone production
7. Obstetrics, gynaecology, and urinary-tract disorders		
Oral contraceptives	1	May possibly be a small risk of congenital malformations
8. Malignant disease and immunosuppression		
Cytotoxic drugs		
Alkylating drugs. Methotrexate	1	Teratogenic – high risk
Others	1	Teratogenic – lower risk
Immunosuppressants		
Azathioprine	1	The risk of teratogenicity appears to be small
9. Nutrition and blood		
Vitamin A	1	Excessive doses may possibly be teratogenic
Vitamin K		
Menadiol sodium diphosphate	3	Neonatal haemolysis. Increased risk of kernicterus in jaundiced neonates

Drugs	*Trimester of risk*	*Adverse effects*
10. Musculoskeletal and joint diseases		
Gold (sodium aurothiomalate)	1, 2, 3	No good evidence of harm but avoid if possible
Penicillamine	1, 2, 3	Fetal abnormalities have been reported rarely. Avoid if possible
13. Skin		
Etretinate	1, 2, 3	Teratogenic. Effective contraception must be continued for one year after stopping treatment
Isotretinoin	1, 2, 3	Teratogenic. Causes serious CNS malformations. Effective contraception must be continued for at least 4 weeks after stopping treatment
Podophyllum resin	1, 2, 3	Avoid application to large areas or in the treatment of anogenital warts. Neonatal death and teratogenesis have been reported
Povidone-iodine	2, 3	Sufficient iodine may be absorbed to affect the fetal thyroid
14. Vaccines		
Live vaccines	1	Theoretical risk of congenital malformations
15. Anaesthesia		
Inhalational and intravenous anaesthetics	3	Depress neonatal respiration
Local anaesthetics	3	With large doses, neonatal respiratory depression, hypotonia, and bradycardia after paracervical or epidural block
Prilocaine, Procaine	3	Neonatal methaemoglobinaemia
Neostigmine, Pyridostigmine etc.	3	Neonatal myasthenia with large doses
Treatment of alcoholism		
Disulfiram	1	The high levels of acetaldehyde which occur in the presence of alcohol may be teratogenic

Appendix 15

Prescribing during breast feeding

Data in *Tables A15.1–A15.3* are reproduced by permission of the authors and publishers of the *British National Formulary* No. 11 (1986), pp. 22–25. London, British Medical Association and the Pharmaceutical Society of Greaty Britain.

Administration of some drugs to nursing mothers may cause toxicity in the infant, for example diazepam, barbiturates, and ergotamine (*Table A15.1*), whereas administration of other drugs, for example digoxin, has little effect on the neonate (*Table A15.2*). For many drugs there is insufficient information available and it is advisable to administer only essential drugs to the mother during breast feeding.

Toxicity to the infant can occur if the drug enters the milk in pharmacologically significant quantities. Milk concentrations of some drugs, for example iodides, may exceed those in the maternal plasma and cause toxicity to the infant but not the mother. Some drugs inhibit the infant's sucking reflex, for example phenobarbitone, or inhibit lactation, for example, bromocriptine and oestrogens. Drugs may, at least theoretically, cause hypersensitivity in the infant even when concentrations are too low for a pharmacological effect.

Table A15.1 lists drugs that should be used with caution or which are contraindicated in breast feeding for the reasons given above.

Table A15.2 lists drugs that, on present evidence, may be given to the mother during breast feeding, because they are excreted in milk in amounts which are too small to be harmful to the infant.

Table A 15.3 lists drugs that are not known to be harmful to the infant although they are present in milk in significant amounts.

These tables should be used only as a guide because of the inadequacy of currently available information on drugs in breast milk and absence from the tables does not imply safety.

Table 15.1 Drugs to be avoided or used with caution in breast-feeding

Drugs	*Comments*
1. Gastrointestinal system	
Atropine	May possibly have anticholinergic effects in infants
Laxatives	
Anthraquinones	Avoid; large doses may cause increased gastric motility and diarrhoea, particularly cascara and danthron
Phenolphthalein	Avoid; increased gastric motility, diarrhoea and possibly rashes
Sulphasalazine – *see* 5 (sulphonamides)	

Drugs	*Comments*
2. *Cardiovascular system*	
Amiodatone	Avoid. Present in milk in significant amounts. Theoretical risk from release of iodine – *see* 6.2
Beta-adrenoceptor blocking drugs	Monitor infant; possible toxicity due to beta-blockade but amount of most beta-blockers excreted in milk is too small to affect infant
Oral anticoagulants	Risk of haemorrhage; increased by vitamin-K deficiency. Warfarin appears safe but some authorities consider breast feeding is contraindicated during therapy. Phenindione should be avoided
3. *Respiratory system*	
Aminophylline	Irritability in infant has been reported
Clemastine	Drowsiness in infant has been reported
Cough mixtures containing iodides – *see* 6.2	Use alternative cough mixtures
Ephedrine, Pseudoephedrine	Irritability and disturbed sleep reported with ephedrine. Significant amounts of pseudoephedrine in milk
4. *Central nervous system*	
4.1 Hypnotics and sedatives	
Alcohol	Large amounts may affect infant
Barbiturates	Avoid if possible (*see also* 4.8 – phenobarbitone). Large doses may produce drowsiness
Benzodiazepines	Avoid repeated doses; lethargy and weight loss may occur in infant
Bromide salts	Avoid; sedation and rash in infant
Chloral hydrate, dichloralphenazone	Sedation in infant
Meprobamate	Concentration in milk may exceed maternal plasma concentrations fourfold and may cause drowsiness in infant
4.2 Antipsychotic drugs	
Haloperidol	Amount excreted in milk probably too small to be harmful
Lithium salts	Monitor infant for possible intoxication; low incidence of adverse effects but increased by continuous ingestion. Good control of maternal plasma concentrations minimises the risk
Phenothiazine derivatives	As for haloperidol, but drowsiness has been reported with chlorpromazine
4.7 Analgesics	
Diamorphine, Morphine	Therapeutic doses are unlikely to affect infant. Withdrawal symptoms occur in infants of dependent mothers. Breast feeding is no longer considered best method of treating dependence in offspring of dependent mothers and should be stopped
Methadone	Withdrawal symptoms in infant; breast feeding permissible during maintenance dosage
Antimigraine drugs	
Ergotamine	Avoid where possible; ergotism may occur in infant. Repeated doses may inhibit lactation

Drugs	*Comments*
4.8 Antiepileptics	
Phenobarbitone, Primidone	Avoid when possible, drowsiness may occur but risk probably small. One case of methaemoglobinaemia reported with phenobarbitone and phenytoin
5. *Infections*	
Chloramphenicol	Stop breast feeding: may cause bone-marrow toxicity in infant. Concentration in milk usually insufficient to cause grey syndrome
Dapsone	Haemolytic anaemia. Risk to infant very small
Isoniazid	Monitor infant for possible toxicity; theoretical risk of convulsions and neuropathy. Prophylactic pyridoxine advisable in mother and infant
Metronidazole	May give a bitter taste to the milk
Nalidixic acid	Risk to infant very small but one case of haemolytic anaemia reported
Sulphonamides and co-trimoxazole	Monitor infant, especially in first few weeks of life. Small risk of kernicterus in jaundiced infants and, in G6PD-deficient infants, haemolytic anaemia, particularly with long-acting sulphonamides
Tetracyclines	Some authorities recommend avoidance but absorption and therefore discoloration of teeth in infant probably prevented by chelation with calcium in milk
6. *Endocrine system*	
6.1 Antidiabetic drugs	
Oral hypoglycaemic drugs	Caution: theoretical possibility of hypoglycaemia in infant
6.2 Antithyroid drugs	
Carbimazole	Stop breast feeding; danger of neonatal hypothyroidism or goitre
Iodine	Iodine appears to be concentrated in the milk
Propylthiouracil	Monitor infant's thyroid status but amounts in milk probably too small to affect infant
Radioactive iodine	Breast feeding contraindicated after therapeutic doses. With diagnostic doses withhold breast feeding for at least 24 hours
6.2 Thyroid hormones	
Liothyronine, Thyroxine	May interfere with neonatal screening for hypothyroidism
6.3 Corticosteroids	Continuous therapy with high doses (>10 mg prednisolone daily) could possibly affect the infant's adrenal function – monitor carefully
6.4 Sex hormones	High doses of oestrogens, progestogens, and androgens suppress lactation – see also 7
Androgens	Avoid breast feeding; may cause masculinization in the female infant or precocious development in the male infant
Cyproterone	Caution; possibility of anti-androgen effects in neonate
6.7 Other endocrine drugs	
Bromocriptine	Suppresses lactation

Drugs	Comments
7. Obstetrics, gynaecology, and urinary-tract disorders	
Oestrogen/progestogen contraceptives	Usually have little effect on milk flow. In some women, usually when lactation is not well established, suppression of milk flow may occur. Progestogen-only contraceptives do not appear to adversely affect established milk flow but may alter milk composition
Povidone-iodine	Iodine absorbed from vaginal preparations is concentrated in milk. Avoid
8. Malignant disease and immunosuppression	
Cytotoxics and immunosuppressants	Discontinue breast feeding
Cyclosporin	Caution – excreted in milk
9. Nutrition and blood	
Calciferol (vitamin D)	Caution with high doses; may cause hypercalcaemia in infant
Thiamine	Severely thiamine-deficient mothers should avoid breast feeding as the toxic methylglyoxal is excreted in milk
Vitamin A	Theoretical risk of toxicity in infants of mothers taking large doses
10. Musculoskeletal and joint diseases	
Carisprodol	Concentrated in milk. No adverse effects reported but best avoided
Colchicine	Caution because of its cytotoxicity
Gold (sodium aurothiomalate)	Caution – excreted in milk. Theoretical possibility of rashes and idiosyncratic reactions
Phenylbutazone	Caution, theoretical possibility of blood dyscrasias in infant but amounts excreted in milk are very small
Salicylates	Occasional doses are safe (preferably taken after feeding) but caution with continuous therapy, as rashes and hypoprothrombinaemia (with inadequate neonatal vitamin K stores) may occur in infant
11. Skin	
Idoxyuridine	May make milk taste unpleasant

Table A15.2 Drugs present in milk in amounts too small to be harmful. The list of drugs given below is not comprehensive and is based on current information concerning the use of these drugs in therapeutic dosage

Acetazolamide	Flupenthixol	Nomifensine
Antidepressants, tricyclic	Frusemide	Phenytoin
Azathioprine	Heparin	Pirenzepine
Baclofen	Hyoscine	Piroxicam
Captopril	Ibuprofen	Procainamide
Chlormethiazole	Insulin	Pyrazinamide
Codeine	Labetalol	Pyridostigmine
Corticotrophin	Loprazolam	Rifampicin
Cycloserine	Mebeverine	Sodium valproate
Dextropropoxyphene	Mefenamic acid	Suprofen
Diclofenac	Methyldopa	Terbutaline
Digoxin	Metoclopramide	Thiazide diuretics
Dispyramide	Mexiletine	Tolmetin
Domperidone	Mianserin	Verapamil
Ethambutol	Naproxen	Warfarin (*see also* Table 1)
Fenbufen	Nitrazepam	

Table A15.3 Drugs present in milk in significant amounts but not known to be harmful. The list of drugs given below is not comprehensive and is based on current information concerning the use of these drugs in therapeutic dosage

Antihistamines	Ethosuximide	Quinidine
Cimetidine	Hydroxychloroquine	Ranitidine
Diltiazem	Mioxidil	Spironolactone
Erythromycin	Paracetamol	Trimethoprim
Ethamsylate	Pyrimethamine	

Appendix 16

Other drug effects

Information on the following can be obtained from *Pediatric Therapy* (1980). (6th edn.) Editor H. C. Shirkey, St. Louis, C. V. Mosby Company.

1. Modification of laboratory tests caused by drugs, pp. 151–160 (T. C. Cashman).
2. Drugs that discolour the faeces* and the urine*, pp. 163–166 (H. C. Shirkey).

Also, *Interpretation of Pediatric Tests* (1983), J. Wallach, pp. 147–148 (urine) and 645–646 (faeces). Boston and Toronto, Little Brown and Company.

* Rifampicin may give a reddish colour to faeces, saliva, sputum, sweat, tears, soft contact lenses and urine.

Appendix 17

Normal blood pressure

J. A. Black

The data for normal blood pressure have been taken from different sources, using different methods of measurement. It is important, when using these figures, to employ the same methods and cuff sizes as those used by the authors (*Table A17.1*).

Table A17.1 Appropriate cuff size according to age

Cuff name	*Range of dimensions of bladder* (cm)	
	Width	*Length*
Newborn	2.5–4.0	5.0–10.0
Infant	6.0–8.0	12.0–13.5
Child	9.0–10.0	17.0–22.5
Adult	12.0–13.0	22.0–23.5
Large adult arm	15.5	30.0

Data from Recommendations of the Task Force on Blood Pressure Control in Children (1977), with kind permission of the Publishers and the National High Blood Pressure Education Program, Bethedsa, Maryland.

Table A17.2 Average systolic, diastolic and mean aortic blood pressures during the first twelve hours of life in normal newborn infants grouped according to birth weight*

Birth weight (g)	*Hour:*	*1*	*2*	*3*	*4*	*5*	*6*	*7*	*8*	*9*	*10*	*11*	*12*
1001–2000	Systolic	49	49	51	52	53	52	52	52	51	51	49	50
	Diastolic	26	27	28	29	31	31	31	31	31	30	29	30
	Mean	35	36	37	39	40	40	39	39	38	37	37	38
2001–3000	Systolic	59	57	60	60	61	58	64	60	63	61	60	59
	Diastolic	32	32	32	32	33	34	37	34	38	35	35	35
	Mean	43	41	43	43	44	43	45	43	44	44	43	42
Over 3000	Systolic	70	67	65	65	66	66	67	67	68	70	66	66
	Diastolic	44	41	39	41	40	41	41	41	44	43	41	41
	Mean	53	51	50	50	51	50	50	51	53	54	51	50

* From Kitterman, Phibbs and Tooley (1969).

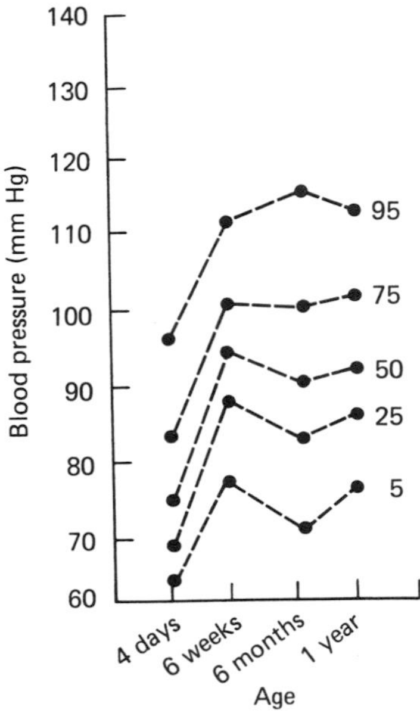

Figure A17.1 Percentiles of blood pressure in infants awake (both sexes pooled) at age 4 days to 1 year. (Reproduced from de Swiet, Fayers and Shinebourne (1980), with kind permission of authors and publishers.)

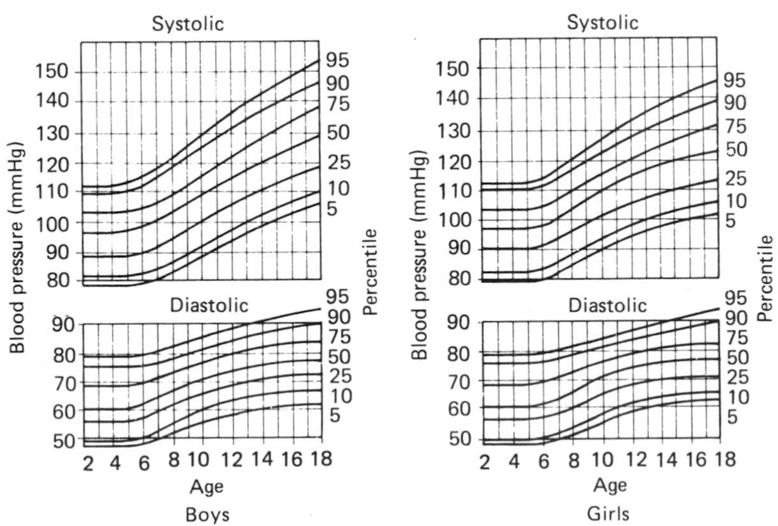

Figure A17.2 Percentiles of blood pressure measurement in boys and girls (right arm, seated). (Reproduced from Recommendations of the Task Force on Blood Pressure Control in Children (1977), with kind permission of the publishers and the National High Blood Pressure Education Program, Bethesda, Md., USA.)

Table 17.2 gives systolic and diastolic *aortic* pressures during the first 12 hours of life, using an umbilical arterial catheter, and a pressure transducer and electronic recorder. Readings were made when the infant was quiet. The value in *Figure 17.1* from the age of 4 days up to 1 year, were measured when the infants were awake and quiet, using a Doppler ultrasound system and a random zero-reading sphygmomanometer reading to the nearest 2 mm Hg. *Figure 17.2* shows the data from the ages of 2–18 years, using standard sphygmomanometer cuffs (*see Table 17.1*), taking the diastolic pressure as the fourth Korotkoff sound (muffling of sound).

References

de SWIET, M., FAYERS, P. and SHINEBOURNE, E. A. (1980) Systolic blood pressure in a population of infants in the first year of life; the Brompton Study. *Pediatrics,* **65,** 1028–1035

KITTERMAN, J. A., PHIBBS, R. H. and TOOLEY, W. H. (1969) Aortic blood pressure in infants during the first 12 hours of life. *Pediatrics,* **44,** 959–968

Recommendations of the task force on blood pressure control in children (1977). *Pediatrics,* **59,** 797–820

Appendix 18

Chemical tests

J. A. Black

Fantus' test for chloride in urine

(*See* Heat Illnesses, Heat Cramps (Chapter 60, page 546)
10 drops of urine are placed in a wide-mouthed test tube and 1 drop of 20% potassium chromate is added. A 2.9% solution of silver nitrate is added drop by drop until the colour changes from yellow to brown.

The number of drops added is approximately equal to the concentration of chloride in the urine expressed as g/ℓ sodium chloride (1 g NaCl is the equivalent of 17 mmol).

It is important that distilled water is used in the preparation of the solutions and for cleaning the test tube. The same dropper should be used both for urine and for silver nitrate solutions and rinsed with distilled water after delivering the urine.

Test for verdoglobin in urine (verdoglobinuria)

This test is used to detect the green pigment verdoglobin which is excreted in the urine in severe infections with *Pseudomonas aeruginosa,* as may occur in severe burns (*see* Chapter 5, page 38):

> 'Equal volumes of urine and glacial acetic acid are mixed in one tube, urine and water in the second and urine and ammonium hydroxide in the third. The three tubes are examined with ultraviolet light in the dark. Verdoglobin is present if an olive fluorescence appears in each, although the alkaline tube may be a chalky-blue. This reaction should not be confused with the yellow–green fluorescence of fluorescein, which may occur in urinary infections due to Pseudomonads.'
>
> (Monafo, 1971)

Test for paraquat poisoning (*See* Chapter 8, page 76)

> 'An indication to prognosis can be derived from a relatively simple test on the urine. This test relies on the reduction of paraquat to a blue free radical by alkaline sodium dithionite. The reagent must be freshly prepared by adding 10 ml sodium hydroxide (1 mol/ℓ) to 100 mg pure sodium dithionite. Aqueous paraquat

standards are prepared containing 1.0, 5.0, and 10.0 mg/ℓ (μg/ml) of paraquat ion and 2 ml aliquots of the sodium dithionite reagent are added to 10 ml volumes of the test samples and paraquat standards. Quantitation is by visual inspection and the test is sensitive to 1.0 mg/ℓ (μg/ml) in clear urine. Since diquat is reduced to a green free radical, a green to blue coloration indicates Weedol ingestion.

'If no colour change occurs (that is, the result is negative) it can be assumed that no significant quantity of paraquat is being excreted and accordingly that no toxic amount has been absorbed. Active treatment can then be withheld. On the other hand a colour change to some shade of green or blue, while being no absolute criterion, certainly points towards an unfavourable outcome.'

(Goulding *et al.*, 1976)

APT's test for distinguishing between fetal and maternal haemoglobin (*See* Chapter 43, pages 386 and 676)

Soak the blood-stained material in water or mix with some of the stool, until a pink colour is obtained. Filter or centrifuge to obtain a clear solution. Add one part of 10% sodium hydroxide (NaOH) and wait for 1–2 minutes. An unchanged pink colour indicates fetal blood, and a yellow–brown colour indicates maternal blood. If in doubt, do control tests using blood of known origin.

References

GOULDING, R., VOLANS, G. N., CROME, P. and WIDDOP, B. (1976) Paraquat poisoning. *British Medical Journal,* **i,** 42

MONAFO, W. W. (1971) *The Treatment of Burns,* p. 213. St. Louis: Warren Green II

Appendix 19

Temperature conversions

Table A19.1 Temperature conversions

°F	*°C*	*°C*	*°F*
76	24.4	24	75.2
78	25.6	25	77.0
80	26.7	26	78.8
82	27.8	27	80.6
84	28.9	28	82.4
		29	84.2
86	30.0	30	86.0
88	31.1	31	87.8
90	32.2	32	89.6
92	33.3	33	91.4
94	34.4	34	93.2
		35	95.0
96	35.6	36	96.8
98	36.7	37	98.6
99	37.3		
100	37.8	38	100.4
102	38.9	39	102.2
104	40.0	40	104.0

Intermediate values

°C	0.1	0.2	0.3	0.4	0.5	0.6	0.7	0.8	0.9
°F	0.18	0.36	0.54	0.72	0.90	1.08	1.26	1.44	1.62

Appendix 20

Système international (SI) units: conversions

In view of the gradual acceptance of SI units, both 'old' and SI units have been given wherever possible, except for values used in pharmacology or toxicology where the use of a system based upon chemically active units has no special advantage.

Multiples of SI units

The prefixes most likely to be encountered in clinical medicine are listed in *Table A20.1*.

Table A20.1

Factor	*Name*	*Symbol*	*Factor*	*Name*	*Symbol*
10^6	Mega	M	10^{-1}	deci	d
10^3	Kilo	k	10^{-2}	centi	c
10^2	hecto	h	10^{-3}	milli	m
10^1	deca	da	10^{-6}	micro	μ
			10^{-9}	nano	n

Units not previously in use

Pressure:	kilopascal (kPa). 7.5 mm Hg = 1.0 kPa (Torr is sometimes used for mm Hg)
Energy (nutrition):	joules (J). 1 kilocalorie ('Calorie' in clinical medicine) = 4.2 kilojoules (kJ)

Conversions that require no calculation

Bicarbonate, Chloride, Potassium, Sodium: mEq/litre = mmol/litre

Conversion to and from SI units (*Figures A20.1–A20.7*)

The following conversion scales are reproduced, by kind permission of authors and publishers, from *Clinical Chemistry; Conversion Scales for SI Units,* (1975) by A. M. Bold and P. Wilding, Oxford; Blackwell Scientific Publications (the normal adult ranges have not been included here).

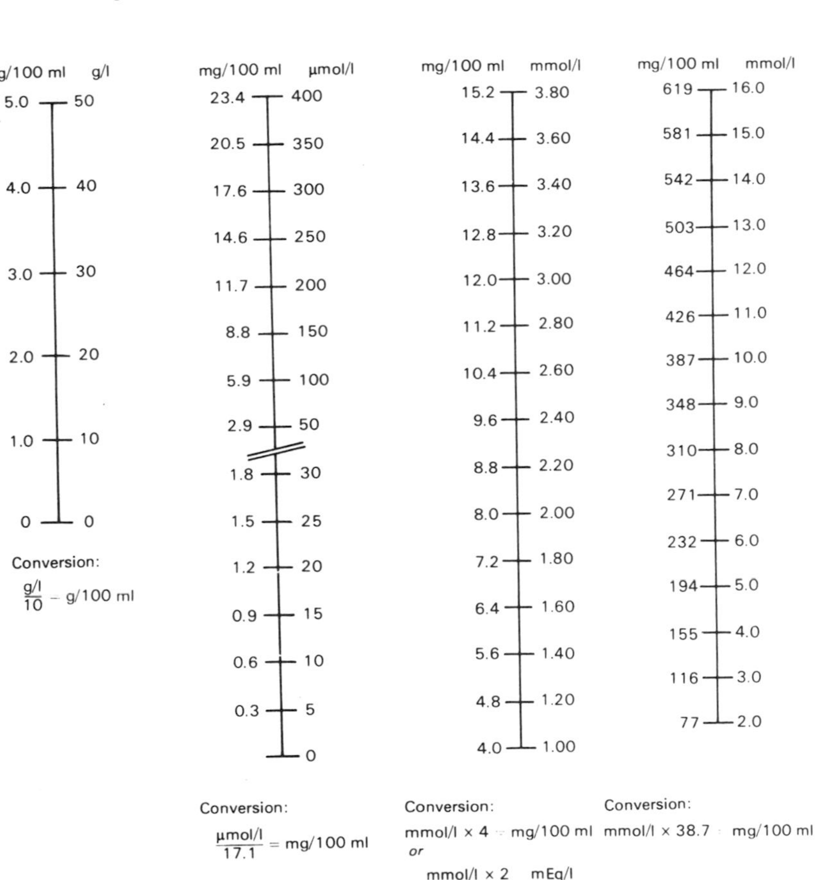

Figure A20.1 SI unit conversions; serum albumin, serume bilirubin, serum calcium and serum cholesterol.

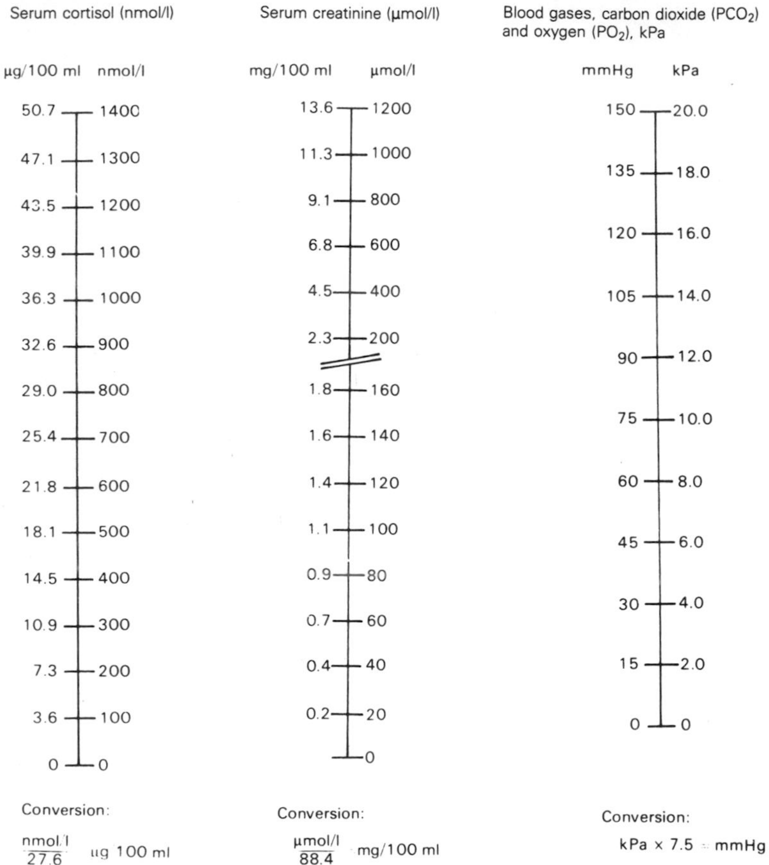

Figure A20.2 SI unit conversions: serum cortisol, serum creatinine, blood gases, carbon dioxide ($PC0_2$) and oxygen ($P0_2$).

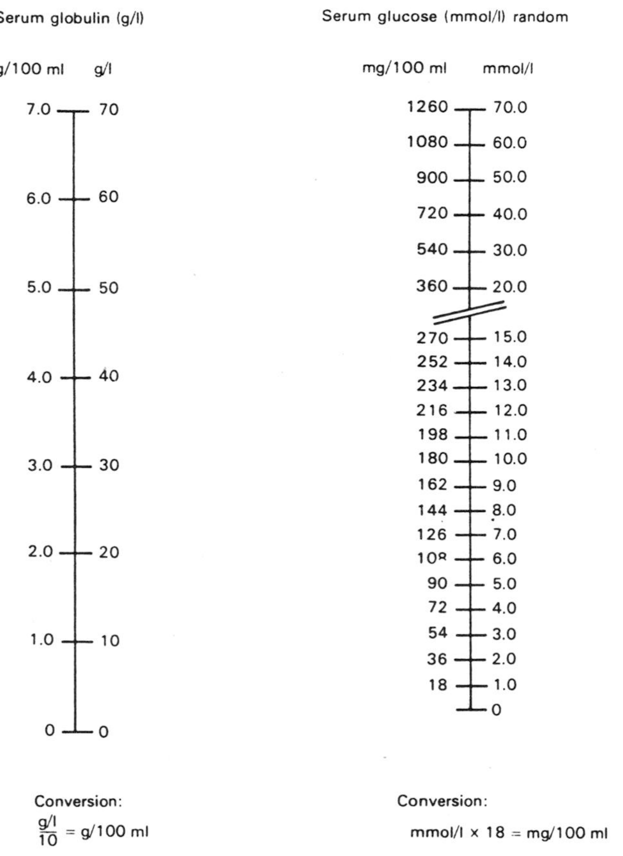

Figure A20.3 SI unit conversions: serum globulin and serum glucose.

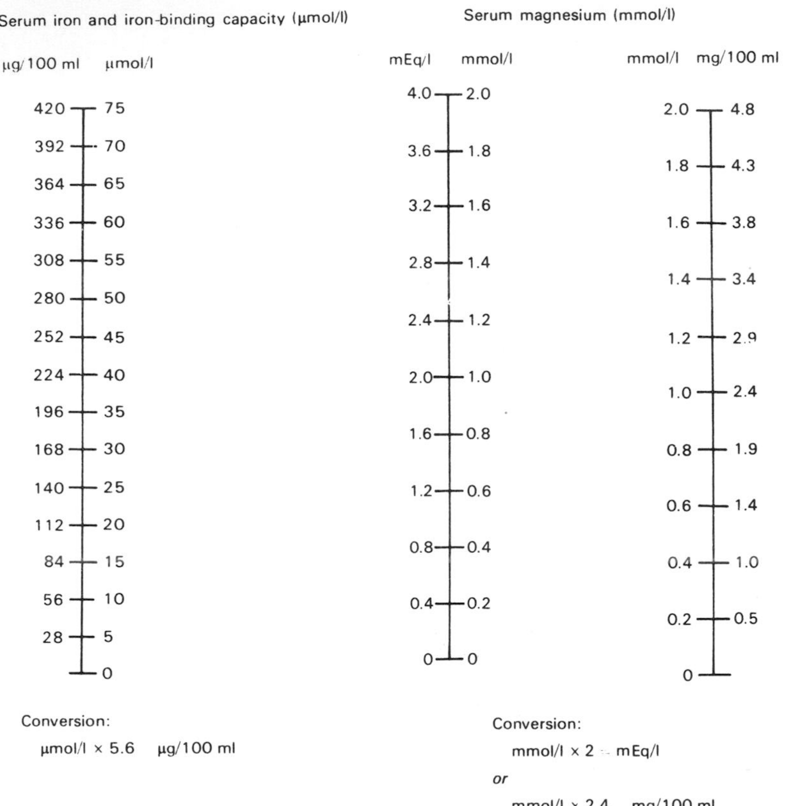

Figure A20.4 SI unit conversions: serum iron and iron-binding capacity, serum magnesium.

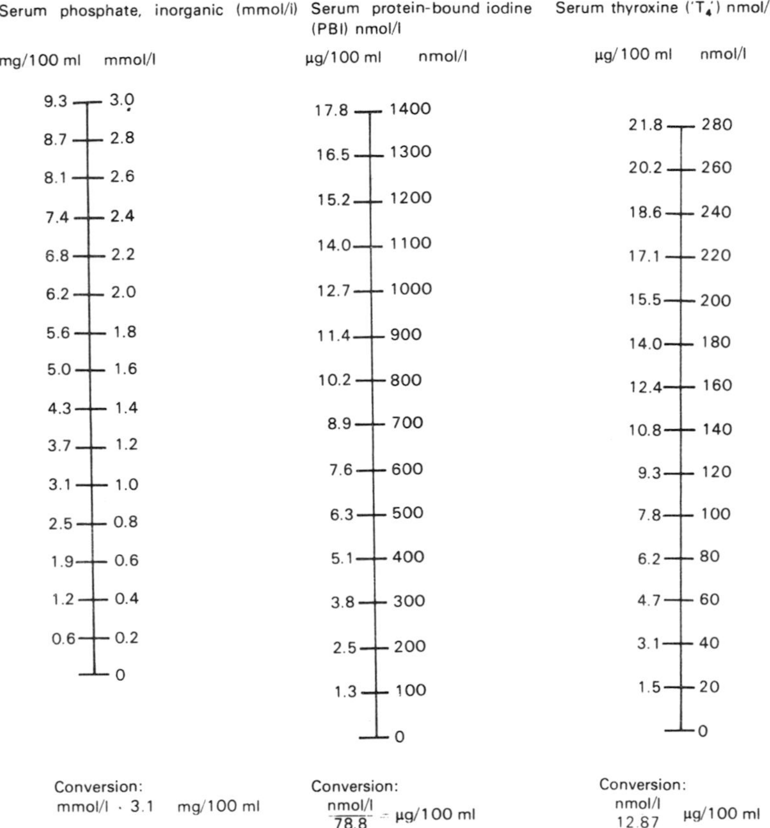

Figure A20.5 SI unit conversions: serum phosphate (inorganic), serum protein-bound iodine (PBI), serum thyroxine (T_4).

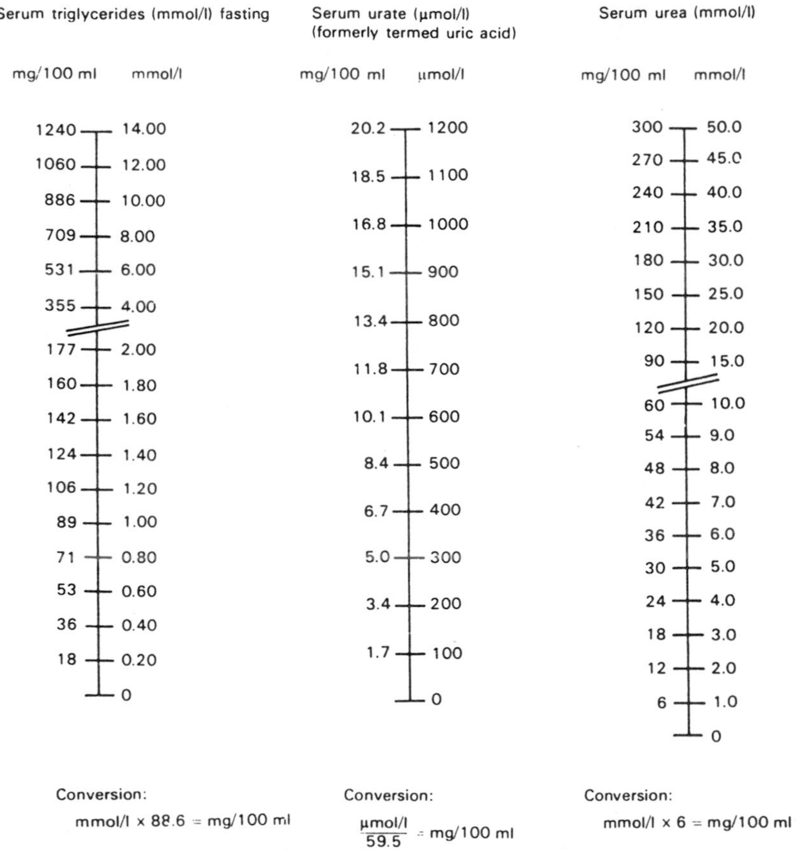

Figure A20.6 SI unit conversions: serum triglycerides (fasting), serum urate (formerly termed 'uric acid'), serum urea.

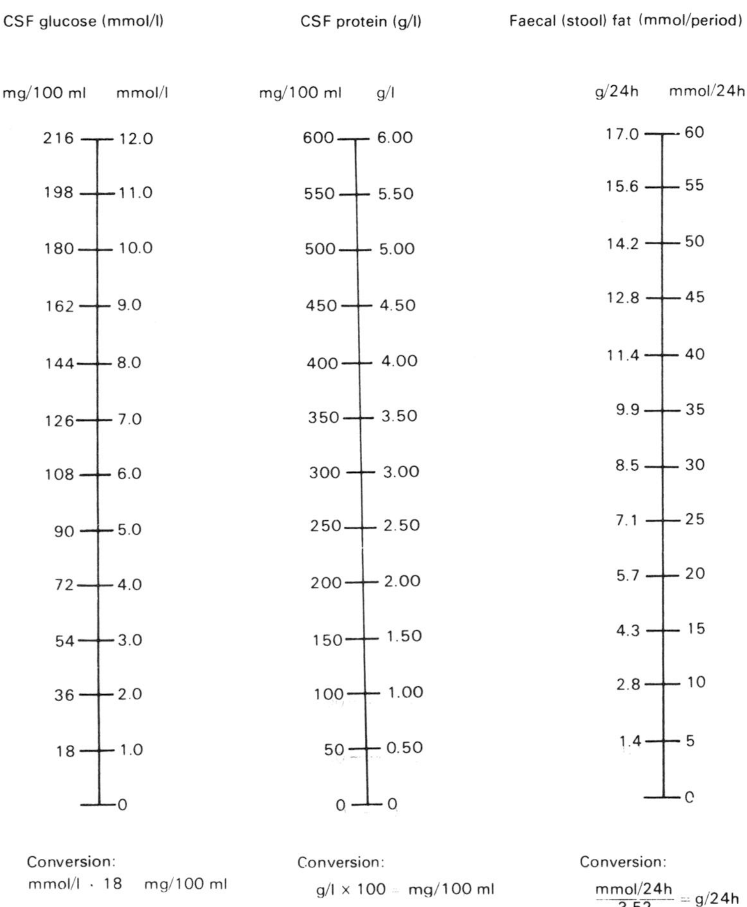

Figure A20.7 SI unit conversion: CSF glucose, CSF protein, faecal (stool) fat.

Appendix 21

Equipment for resuscitation of the newborn (*See also* Chapter 71)

M. F. Whitfield

1. *Resuscitation trolley providing:*
   (a) Facilities for O_2 IPPV by mask or endotracheal tube with a pressure-limiting blow-off valve designed to limit pressure in the circuit to 30 cm H_2O.
   (b) Suction.
   (c) Stop clock.
   (d) Sloping surface on which to place baby with head-down tilt.
   (e) Overhead heater.
2. *Mucus extractors.*
3. *Suction catheters*
   (e.g. Argyle 5, 8 and 10).
4. *Infant bag and mask* of the reinflating type which can be connected to the oxygen line, e.g. Laerdal bag.
5. *Infant laryngoscope* with blades for the premature, and spare batteries and bulbs.
6. *Infant orotracheal tubes* e.g. Warnes 8, 10, 12 and 14 Portex resuscitation sets 2.0, 2.5, 3.0 mm and open angle connector (Cobb) to fit these tubes. (The Portex resuscitation set contains an endotracheal tube with open right angle connector and a suction catheter which passes through the constricted portion of the tube.)
7. *Oral (Guedel) airways* size 0 and 00.
8. *Paediatric McGill forceps* (small size) and endotracheal tube introducer.
9. *Towels.*
10. *Drugs.*
    10% glucose: 10 ml ampoules.
    Sodium bicarbonate: 8.4% 10 ml ampoules or 5%.
    Naloxone (Narcan Neonatal): 2 ml ampoules (0.02 mg/ml).
    Adrenaline 1:1000: 1 ml ampoules.
    Vitamin K_1 (phytomenadione): 0.5 ml ampoules (1 mg per 0.5 ml).
11. *Syringes:* 1 ml, 2 ml, 5 ml, 10 ml, 20 ml.
    Needles: 21, 23 and 25.
    Butterfly needles: 23 and 25.
    Alcohol swabs.
    Micropore tape: ½-inch.

Notes

1. It goes without saying that all resuscitation equipment must be frequently checked and be in a state of instant readiness. There must be a system for restocking as items are used; the equipment itemized above has been deliberately restricted to be easily accommodated in a resuscitaire drawer. The more equipment the more difficult to find the item you need in a hurry.
2. Resuscitation should be carried out in a warm draught-free room in a good light.

Appendix 22

Equipment for exchange transfusion (*See also* Chapter 87)

M. F. Whitfield

Equipment

1. Resuscitation equipment (*see* Appendix 21).
2. Suitable environment for infant: incubator/operating table/radiant-heated intensive care crib such as Draeger Babytherm; this is most desirable, providing easy access and a warm, relatively draught-free, environment.
3. Drip stand with space for 2 bottles.
4. Oscilloscope cardiac monitor leads, electrodes and electrode jelly.
5. Anglepoise light or overhead phototherapy unit.
6. Electronic temperature monitor with rectal and skin probes.
7. Clock or watch with second hand.
8. 37°C (98.6°F) thermostatic water bath (if available).
9. Urine collecting bag (adult type) for collecting blood waste.
10. Input/output/heart rate record chart.

Drugs/IV fluids/containers

1. Blood 1 or 2 units of semipacked cells of appropriate cross-matched group <48 hours old (on no account >5 days old).
2. N saline (0.9% NaCl) 500 ml + 1000 units per ml heparin.
3. Calcium gluconate 10%, 10 ml ampoules.
4. Sodium bicarbonate 8.4% 10 ml ampules.
5. 1% lignocaine (for umbilical cut-down, if required).
6. 2 sequestrene tubes.
7. 2 serum tubes.
8. 2 universal containers (sterile).
9. Antiseptic.
10. Nobecutane.

Sterile equipment

2 20 ml syringes
1 4 way stopcock

or 2 3 way stopcocks
2 adult blood-giving sets
1 extension tubing (for waste) – (e.g. tubing from a drip set)
2 umbilical catheters, 5 and 8 FG
2 sterile towels, one with central hole
gauze swabs
2 gallipots
2 gowns
gloves sizes 6½–8.

Sterile instruments

4 pairs mosquito forceps
1 pair dissecting forceps (fine, untoothed)
1 pair stitch-holding forceps
1 vascular probe
4 towel clips
1 scalpel and blade
1 pair scissors
curved needle and 2/0 catgut
1 metal rule (centimetre graduation), unless supplied with disposable set.

Notes

1. It is usually convenient to use a disposable exchange transfusion pack. The Pharmaseal set can be obtained from most medical suppliers.
2. Exchange transfusion is a potentially hazardous procedure particularly in the hands of inexperienced operators and if the donor blood is more than 48 hours old. It is necessary to have a skilled assistant (doctor or nurse) who monitors the condition of the infant as well as keeping a close check on input and output. It is important to be as comfortable as possible but if the procedure is not carried out in an incubator or intensive care crib the air temperature in the room needs to be around 30°C (86°F) or more if the infant is not to lose heat.

Appendix 23

Guide to sizes of tracheal tubes

Table A23.1 Guide to sizes of tracheal tubes*

ENDOTRACHEAL			*TRACHEOSTOMY*			
Magill No.		*B.S. Diameter* (mm)	*Bronchoscope*	*Polyvinyl chloride*		
$\frac{Age}{2} + 1$	*Age*	$\frac{Age}{4} + 4.5$ *Int. Dia.* (mm)	*Negus*	*Great Ormond Street Int. Dia.* (mm)	*Ext. Dia* (mm)	*PORTEX FG*
000		2.5				
00		3.0				
0A	0–3 months	3.5	Suckling	3.5		
0	3–6 months	4.0		4.0		
1	6 months–2 years	4.5	Infant	4.5	6.0	0
2	2–4 years	5.0		5.0	7.0	0
3	4–5 years	5.5	Child			
4	5–7 years	6.0		6.0	8.0	24
5	7–8 years	6.5	Adolescent			
6	8–10 years	7.0		7.0	9.0	27
7	10–12 years		Small adult		10.0	30
8	12–14 years	8.0	Large adult		11.0	33
9	Adult	9.0			12.0	36
10	Adult					
11	Adult	10.0			13.0	39
12	Adult	11.0			14.0	42

* Modified from Browne, D. R. G. (1969). *Anaesthesia* **24**: 620.

Appendix 24

Useful general data

J. A. Black

Data on electrolytes from *Clinical and Resuscitative Data* (1977) by R. P. H. Dunnill and B. E. Crawley, Oxford; Blackwell Scientific Publications, by kind permission of the authors and publishers.

Central Venous pressure measurements: mm Hg (Torr) × 1.36 = cm H_2O

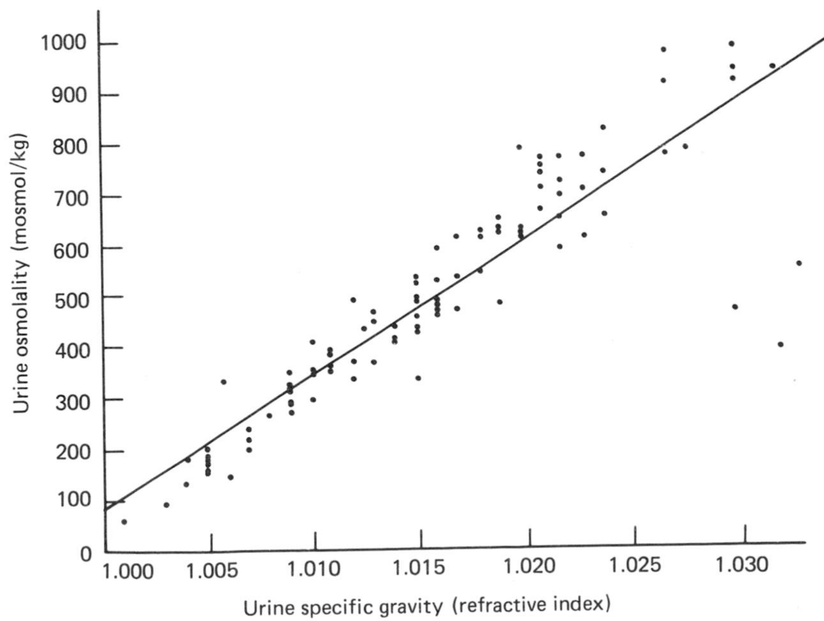

Figure A24.1 Relationship between urine specific gravity (refractive index) and urine osmolality. (Reproduced from Low and Tay (1978), with kind permission of authors and publishers.)

Electrolytes

Milligram to millimole to milliequivalent conversion equations

$$\text{Milliequivalents}/\ell = \frac{(\text{mg}/100\,\text{ml}) \times 10 \times \text{valency}}{\text{mol.wt}} = \text{mmol}/\ell \times \text{valency}$$

$$\text{Milligrams}/100\,\text{ml} = \frac{\text{mEq}/\ell \times \text{mol.wt}}{10 \times \text{valency}} = \frac{\text{mmol}/\ell \times \text{mol.wt}}{10}$$

$$\text{Millimol}/\ell = \frac{10 \times \text{mg}/100\,\text{ml}}{\text{mol.wt}} = \frac{\text{mEq}/\ell}{\text{valency}}$$

Molar values

1 g Na^+	contains 43.5 mmol Na^+
1 g Na chloride	contains 17.1 mmol Na^+
1 g Na bicarbonate	contains 12 mmol Na^+
1 g Na lactate	contains 8.9 mmol Na^+
1 g Na citrate	contains 10.2 mmol Na^+
1 g K^+	contains 25.6 mmol K^+
1 g K chloride	contains 13.5 mmol K^+
1 g K acetate	contains 10.2 mmol K^+
1 g K citrate	contains 9.3 mmol K^+
1 g K bicarbonate	contains 9.9 mmol K^+
1 g Ca^{2+}	contains 25 mmol Ca^{2+}
1 g Ca gluconate*	contains 2.3 mmol Ca^{2+}
1 g $CaCl_2$ + $2H_2O$	contains 6.8 mmol Ca^{2+} + 13.6 mmol Cl
1 g Mg^{2+}	contains 42 mmol Mg^{2+}
1 g Mg sulphate + $7H_20$	contains 4 mmol Mg^{2+}
1 g NH_4 chloride	contains 18.7 mmol NH_4

* 10 ml 10% calcium gluconate contains 1 g calcium gluconate

Calculation of plasma osmolality

$$1.89\,(\text{serum Na}^+ + \text{K}^+\ \text{mmol}/\ell) + \frac{\text{Blood glucose in mg}/100\,\text{ml}}{18} + \frac{\text{Blood urea in mg}/100\,\text{ml}}{4}$$

Infusion set volumes

Drop size depends upon:

1. The fluid being given.
2. The drip rate.
3. The type of drip set.
4. The nature of the added drugs.

Using the Baxter–Travenol C2071 giving set Bamber *et al.* (1983) found that for most IV solutions except for blood and haemaccel an average figure of 19 drops per ml was sufficiently accurate. Added drugs may also affect drop size; though, of a range of added drugs, Theakston, Brown and Allwood (1983) found that diazepam emulsion was the only drug which significantly affected drop size. Appleton *et al.* (1984) showed that drop size was only affected by high flow rates, such as 60–90 drops per minute. It is *in every case* important to calibrate the IV system when starting an infusion, otherwise large errors in fluid administration may occur. Particular care should be taken with lipid emulsions.

Example: (for simplicity) at 20 drops per ml:

20 drops per min = 1 ml/min = 60 ml/hour
∴ for this particular drop size:
Number of drops per min × 3 = number of ml per hour

Use of 5 or 10 ml syringes as measures of weight (Simmonds, Vaughan and Gunn, 1983)

3 ml = 3.5 g NaCl
3 ml = 2.5 g $NaHCO_3$
1.5 ml = 1.5 g KCl
30 ml = 20 g glucose
50 ml = 40 g sugar (sucrose)

Domestic measures

Volume: 1 teaspoon = 3.5–5 ml
(teaspoon length 4.5 cm and breadth 3.0 cm = 3.75 ml)
1 teacup = 150 ml
1 tumbler = 250–300 ml
1 mug = 200–300 ml
1 ounce = 28 ml (approx. 30 ml)
1 pint = 20 oz = 568 ml (average approx. 500 ml)
1 US pint = 16 oz = 454 ml

Weight: 1 level (5 ml) teaspoon = approx. 5 g water
Salt: 1 level (5 ml) teaspoon = approx. 5 g NaCl
Sugar: 1 level (5 ml) teaspoon = 4 g sucrose or glucose

Food additives that have been associated with urticaria

(Joint Reports of Royal College of Physicians and British Nutrition Foundation, 1984)
E numbers are manufacturers codes shown on label.

Antioxidants:
Butylated hydroxyanisole : E320
Butylated hydroxytoluene : E321

Colouring agents:

Amaranth	:	E123
Sunset yellow	:	E110
Tartrazine	:	E102

Preservatives:

Benzoic acid (and derivatives)	:	E210
Sodium metabisulphite	:	E223
Sodium nitrite	:	E250

Flavourings (no E numbers):

Menthol
Quinine

Others (no E numbers):

Papain (meat tenderizer)
Penicillin } as residues from the veterinary
Tetracycline } treatment of animals

References

APPLETON, G. A., BRADLEY, S. A., KIRBY, J. and LAWLER, P. G. (1984) Drop size of IV fluids. *British Journal of Parenteral Therapy,* **5,** 225

BAMBER, P. A., KIRBY, J., BRADLEY, S. A., KIRBY, J. and LAWLER, P. G. (1983) *British Journal of Parenteral Therapy,* **4,** 5–6

LOW, P. S. and TAY, J. S. H. (1978) Urine osmolality, refractive index and specific gravity. *Journal of the Singapore Paediatric Society,* **20,** 37–42

ROYAL COLLEGE OF PHYSICIANS AND BRITISH NUTRITION FOUNDATION (1984) Joint Report on Food Intolerance and Food Aversion. *Journal of Royal College of Physicians,* **18,** 83–123

SIMMONDS, S., VAUGHAN, P. and GUNN, S. W. (1983) *Refugee Community Health Care,* p. 156. Oxford University Press

THEAKSTON, F. J., BROWN, M. E. and ALLWOOD, M. C. (1983) Influences of added drugs on the drop size of intravenous fluids. *Journal of Parenteral Therapy,* **4,** 4–6

Index

The figures in **bold** refer to main sections.